ILLUSTRATED GUIDE TO MICROSURGICAL TECHNIQUES in the Rat

With Elements of Surgical Anatomy

ILLUSTRATED GUIDE TO MICROSURGICAL TECHNIQUES in the Rat

With Elements of Surgical Anatomy

(363 photos and 53 drawings)

PETROS MIRILAS

Pediatric Surgeon-Microsurgeon, 'Aghia Sophia' Children's Hospital, Athens, Greece

Diplomate in Micosurgical Techniques, University Paris XIII-Léonard de Vinci, France

Clinical Professor of Surgical Anatomy & Technique, Emory University, Atlanta, GA, USA

PREFACE

Marc Goldstein, MD, DSc (hon), FACS

Matthew P. Hardy Distinguished Professor of Reproductive Medicine, and Urology

Surgeon-in-Chief, Male Reproductive Medicine and Surgery

Weill Cornell Medicine, New York Presbyterian Hospital

New York, NY

TEXT EDITING

Maggie Hodges, MD • Clara Farley, MD

Lee Hugar, MD • Lindel Krige Dewberry, MD

Chun Li, MD • Vishes Mehta, MD

Thomas Hagopian, MD • Patrick Walker, MD

DRAWINGS

by the author and Edward M. Hagopian

P.M.P.

BROKEN HILL Publishers Ltd

Science is ever-changing

New research accomplishments and clinical experience has expanded the field of medical knowledge and represent an ongoing process. With this in mind,it is imperative that we make the appropriate changes as far as it concerns the course of action, in the treatment of our patients.
The content of this textbook reflects all the most recent knowledge and internationally accepted techniques as they are analyzed by experienced authors in the field, in each chapter.
Nevertheless, the authors and the editor acknowledge that every medical opinion is under the limitations of the time frame that this book was created, as well as possible mistakes that might have escaped their attention.
Readers of this textbook are encouraged to keep that in mind, while at the same time we hope that the information included will become a starting point for young colleagues or the more experienced ones, for new research projects, clinical trials or maybe an updated version of the book in the near future.

ISBN: 978-9925-563-84-5

9 789925 563845

16 Zenas Kanther Princess De Tyras Str.
1065 Nicosia, CYPRUS
e-mail: info@brokenhill.com.cy
website: http://www.brokenhill.com.cy

To my students

Preface

It is a pleasure to highly recommend this book on microsurgical techniques in the rat. Currently the trend in medical/surgical research is on molecular biology. Research on basic surgical/microsurgical techniques and pathophysiology have significantly declined over the past several decades. This guide to microsurgical techniques in the rat is beautifully presented and illustrated. It shows state of the art microsurgical techniques for experimentation in the rat. To my knowledge, this is the first book exclusively devoted to microsurgical experimental techniques in the rat.

Although current medical research focuses on molecular biology, the steady expansion of replant and transplant techniques, including digital replants, arm and hand replants, and now facial and penile transplants, make the attainment of good microsurgical technique essential.

Research and training in rats is mandatory prior to application in humans. Furthermore, the outcomes of microsurgical techniques in humans is very dependent on technical perfection, which is best attained by employing the techniques described in this outstanding book.

I strongly recommend that this book be in every microsurgical laboratory and every department that employs microsurgical techniques in humans and for research in animals.

Marc Goldstein, MD, DSc (hon), FACS
Matthew P. Hardy Distinguished Professor of Reproductive Medicine, and Urology
Surgeon-in-Chief, Male Reproductive Medicine and Surgery
Weill Cornell Medicine, New York Presbyterian Hospital
New York, NY

Instead of Prologue
by the author

I do not really like, not to say dislike, prologues. I always read them at the end, after I have absorbed the oeuvre. Often, I realize that the preface introduces ideas other than the ones I find in the book. Let it be, I surrender because the publisher asks for it and because, in Sophocles' Antigone, the prologue is not negligible as it takes 99 full lines (of course the parallelism is grotesque).

So, the *Illustrated Guide to Microsurgical Techniques in the Rat* (with elements of surgical anatomy) could serve as the manual of a microsurgery class. It is addressed to surgeons who want to learn microsurgery, while taking a class or working on their own in some laboratory, in order to use microsurgery in research or clinical practice. The elements of surgical anatomy present in the text are rather necessary because the microscope is going to magnify this lack of knowledge.

I had the chance to be a resident of Pediatric Surgery and doctoral student in Paris, France. During that time (more than 20 years ago), I completed the course of the University Diploma in Microsurgical Techniques in the University XIII-Leonard de Vinci of Paris, which was housed in the Laboratory of Microsurgery of the "Academy of Surgery of Paris Hospitals" (Ecole de Chirurgie des Hopitaux de Paris), located in the lovely quartier Fer à Moulin. I continued as a post-doc student for another year in the same laboratory. Of note, I was the only resident in Pediatric Surgery; all my colleagues were residents in Orthopedics or Plastic Surgery. My drive was to learn Microsurgery with the aim to use it in my research and perform experimental surgery in small animals. Practicing clinical microsurgery in neonatal and pediatric surgery came much later.

The Paris School of Surgery advanced microsurgery course is one of most well respected, classified together with the of London Northwick Park Institute and New York Columbia University.[1] The students of the University Diploma in Paris perform about 20 operations (exercises) in the rat. The curriculum of the Diploma includes 30 sessions, once a week for eight months, which makes a total of 120 hours. The exercises include end-to-end and end-to-side anastomoses of veins and arteries, with diameters 0.5 mm to 2 mm, arterio-venous anastomoses, bypasses, transplantations of flaps and organs. Procedures are not repeated; instead the trainee has to advance in more difficult operation each time. At the end of the course there are examinations (on some of the procedures); success was associated to hours of practice devoted by the student. The course had no manual book, only few notes with rough drawings.

In the suite of my career, I started to reproduce one by one all the procedures of the course and document them with photos and videos. In parallel, I was trained and then taught Surgical Anatomy at Emory University, USA. Thus, it become obvious to me that the surgical microscope requires and reveals much more details of the anatomy of the surgical field. The current work is the outcome of experience in microsurgical techniques and understanding of the surgical anatomy of the field, both gained during repeating, modifying and completing the procedures of the Ecole de Chirurgie.

For quite some time I was puzzled with the title of the book. The English "Manual" was fitting as a book of instruction, which it is, but the book is not small and comprises a thorough understanding of anatomy. Titles such as "Experimental Microsurgery" pointed to a textbook and did not correspond to the content. The solution was provided by some of my favorite reading, 'Guide to Cooking' by Nikolaos Tselementes (Athens, Greece, 1930). This guide describes the kitchen, cookware, preparations, and recipes, and each follows the other in order of increasing difficulty, without repetitions. Similar is the structure of the present book: the

1. Shurey S, Akelina Y, Legagneux J, Malzone G, Jiga L, Ghanem AM. The rat model in microsurgery education: classical exercises and new horizons. Arch Plast Surg 2014;41:201-208.

microscope, the instruments, the rat, the basic techniques, operations with increasing difficulty, and, lastly, the complicated transplantations, also without repetitions. Unexpectedly, Tselementes praises the ethical dimension of cooking (for that era), to bring the family together through satisfaction of one (or more) of the senses. The corresponding ethical value of microsurgery is the satisfaction of curiosity in the surgical field and satisfaction of the best possible result in terms of technique.

Dr Anastasia Mentessidou helped me in performing all the operations. I was also assisted by Dr Elissaios Kontis, who edited the photos and made some diagrams. The book was simultaneously written in Greek and English, to acquire the maximum audience. My students in Emory University, class 2014, undertook the editing of my (poor) English text—this process revealed errors and omissions in the Greek text: Dr Maggie Hodges edited Chapters 1-4; Dr Clara Farley, Chapters 7, 18-20; Dr Lee Hugar, Chapters 5, 6, 27-28; Dr Lindel Krige Dewberry, Preface, Chapters 9, 12-14; Dr Chun Li, Chapters 21, 31; Dr Vishes Mehta, Chapters 8, 10, 11, 15; Dr Thomas Hagopian did a lot of work with Chapters 17, 22-25, 29-30 (including editing of others); Dr Patrick Walker, Chapter 16. Our artist, Edward Hagopian, made some wonderful drawings and also corrected some of mine. These co-workers proved that my attitude to trust the mind of young people is correct. To all these young surgeons I am deeply grateful. My students corrected me as well as they interactively taught me through all these years.

I am also grateful to my friend, the publisher Christos Pashalides, who trusted me and took the risk of publishing this book in English and Greek. I want to express my gratitude to Ms Niki Panopoulou, who turned the manuscripts into books, for her professionalism and patience through all my endless corrections.

I wish to this book 'bon voyage' in the hands of new microsurgeons. It has departed from me, and does not belong to me any more. The feeling within me can be described as relief. The torch is yours, and if you teach, you will pass onto the next. This thought compensates the effort put in writing the book. Knowledge does not belong to us, as nothing belongs to us, according to my humble opinion.

Petros Mirilas

The Personality and Attitude of a Microsurgeon

Since the 1950s, studies have depicted surgeons (residents and specialists) as doctors capable of providing nearly instantaneous solutions to the problems presented to them; at the other end of the spectrum was the 'thoughtful' internist. However, in addition to their ability to think, process, and react rapidly and decisively, surgeons have also been described as being aggressive, ambitious, and lacking empathy.

The author's opinion is that such stereotypes–which have even become entrenched as prototypical descriptions of the surgical personality in academic literature–are only valuable as anecdotes, like the well-known tale regarding duck hunting: *Four doctors go duck hunting. A group of ducks suddenly flies over them. The psychiatrist wondered if the psychic trauma of losing a parent would be irreparable for the progeny; meanwhile the ducks flew away. The internist proposed the question as to whether they were ducks or geese, based on their differential characteristics; meanwhile the ducks flew away. Then the surgeon approached, replaced the rifle with a Kalashnikov, downed all of birds, and ordered the pathologist to posthumously determine which were ducks and which were geese.* The trainee microsurgeon with such a cavalier attitude cannot exist–it would be impossible to become a microsurgeon.

In contrast to the stereotypes above, the microsurgeon is a more thoughtful surgeon. He is required to have patience, persistence, and love for the world the surgical microscope will reveal: in the same way in which a scuba diver discovers a love for the world of the deep sea. An esteemed relationship with the teacher is very important because the mentor will both inspire the trainee microsurgeon and encourage him/her after inevitable failures. The trainee microsurgeon should possess a working knowledge of both the principles of microsurgery and the surgical anatomy of the field. However, despite proficiency in these principles, it is almost certain that the trainee will falter or fail during his/her first attempt suturing the very small vessels (e.g. femoral veins in the rat).

In the operating room or laboratory, an effective microsurgeon maintains an aura of calm. It is important for the microsurgeon to manage any nervousness or anxiety they may have, both to preserve their surgical finesse and to set the tone of the operating room. The motto 'gentle, yet firm' could well characterize both the practice and the persona of a successful microsurgeon. The nature of microsurgery favors surgeons possessing curiosity and ingenuity. Microsurgery provides the opportunity for identification and dissection of miniscule entities in the surgical field. It is also expected that the microsurgeon will come to recognize the defects of the microsurgical instruments they use; as such, it is not surprising that he/she may have the opportunity and cause to design new instruments during their career. Similarly, microsurgeons who have been exposed to other disciplines have the potential to become pioneers by integrating microsurgery into these other disciplines (e.g. recently, computer programs have been used for tremor abatement, and robotic surgery has been combined with microsurgery).

The microsurgeon, regardless of whichever specialty he/she comes from, has excellent future prospects; while it may not be perceived early in training, it may be discovered with time. The obvious benefit is that microsurgery, beyond its spectacular applications, will help the surgeon in detailed dissection resulting in avoidance of anatomical complications. The less apparent benefit is that microsurgery will constitute a connection to Science (for those who still believe that surgery is simply artisanal). Handling and operating upon laboratory animals, as required in the training to become a microsurgeon, forces the microsurgical trainee to become familiar with basic surgical science. In the laboratory, the microsurgeon will inevitably come in contact with experimental models, scientific protocols, doctoral and postdoctoral research. Thus, the microsurgeon is endowed with scientific capabilities, a very powerful weapon for an academic career.

How to Use this Book

This book can constitute the basic manual of an annual series of exercises in microsurgical techniques in the rat, in the setting of an organized class. Similarly, it can effectively be used by surgeons (residents–second year and above–and specialists) who want to learn microsurgery and have access to a laboratory of experimental surgery with the required specialized equipment, such as a surgical microscope, microsurgical instruments and sutures.

The *Illustrated Guide to Microsurgical Techniques in the Rat* is comprised of a series of lessons (course sessions), as shown in Table 1 at the end of this note.

Courses flow with increasing difficulty, from vessels of larger, 2 mm, diameter to smaller vessels of 0.5 mm diameter, from technically simple procedures to complicated ones, from larger to smaller suture (9/0, 10/0 11/0), while dissection of the surgical field becomes gradually more demanding. At the end of the series are the transplantations, which require a complex design. Therefore, the Guide is read following the order of the chapters, from the first to the last page as a whole and not in part. The knowledge of each chapter is prerequisite for following chapter(s), and is not repeated but briefly in the text with a referral to a previous chapter.

The trainee should begin from the basics, to get familiar with the surgical microscope, microsurgical instruments and sutures, and learn to handle the laboratory rat, prepare and anesthetize it, and follow it up postoperatively (Introductive part, Chapters 1-3). Then, he/she has to study the basic microsurgical techniques of suturing vessels and nerves (Chapters 4-7). The microsurgical procedures (Chapters 8-21) must be performed in order, and followed by the transplantations (Chapters 22-31), which are based on the earlier described microsurgical procedures.

Given the design of the book, the *list of contents* is not comprised of a mere listing of headings and pages as usually happens, but rather has a specific structure and significance: In every chapter, the complexity of the dissection is briefly described, followed by the design of the operation; at the end are listed in bold the diameter(s) of the vessel(s) anastomosed—which is not mentioned in the text—and the number and size of sutures used. Therefore, this catalogue of contents has the features of a tool and is recommended to be used together with the respective chapter of the text. It can also be used as an advisor for the technique to be followed given the diameter of the vessel, in case that the microsurgeon wishes to anastomose vessels of respective size during another operation, outside of the series of the exercises.

Each chapter is followed by a one or two-page *summary*. This is specifically designed to be used on the bench during the operation. It is advised to have the Guide open to the respective summary and placed on a stand while the procedure is being performed.

It is strictly recommended that the trainee advances onto the next procedure only if he/she has successfully completed the previous one. If working alone in a laboratory, this progression will depend on the trainee's personal schedule. If working in a training team (course), it will be necessary to return to the laboratory, outside of class hours, and repeat the operation until successfully completed. The writer followed this strategy during his training.

TABLE 1 - LIST OF COURSE SESSIONS IN MICROSURGICAL TECHNIQUES BASED ON THIS BOOK

Session number	Chapter number(s)	Exercise taught
1	1-2	Material and equipment (microsurgical instruments), surgical microscope
	3	Pre-operative preparation, anesthesia, and post-operative care of the laboratory rat
	4	Microsurgical technique for suturing vessels
2	5	Principles of end-to-end anastomosis of vessels
	6	Principles of end-to-side anastomosis of vessels
	7	Technique of microsurgical suturing of nerves
3	8	End-to-end anastomosis of the aorta
4	9	End-to-end anastomosis of the external jugular vein &
		End-to-end anastomosis of the common carotid artery
5	10	Interposition of external jugular vein graft in the abdominal aorta
6	11	Abdominal aorta bypass graft using the external jugular vein
7	12	Interposition of external jugular (deep tributary) vein into the common carotid artery
8	13	Common carotid artery bypass graft using the external jugular (deep tributary) vein
9	14	End-to-side anastomosis of the common carotid artery to the external jugular vein
10	15	End-to-end anastomosis between the aorta and right common iliac artery
11	16	End-to-side anastomosis of the portal vein to the inferior vena cava
12	17	Anastomosis of the sciatic nerve & Grafting of the sciatic nerve
13	18	End-to-end anastomoses of the femoral vessels
14	19	Interposition of superficial inferior epigastric vein graft in the femoral artery
15	20	Femoral artery bypass graft using the superficial inferior epigastric vein
16	21	End-to-end anastomoses of the superficial inferior epigastric vessels
17	22	Orthotopic autotransplantation of pedicled inguinal skin flap
18	23	Contralateral autotransplantation of pedicled inguinal skin flap
19	24	Autotransplantation of free inguinal skin flap to the neck
20	25	Autotransplantation of the posterior limb
21	26	Orthotopic autotransplantation of the left kidney
22	27	Orthotopic transplantation of the left kidney
23	28	Heterotopic (auto)transplantation of the left kidney
24	29	Autotransplantation of the uterine horn-fallopian tube-ovary
25	30	Transplantation of the ovary-fallopian tube
26	31	Heterotopic heart transplantation

Note: The number of 26 sessions was calculated on a basis of a 13 week academic semester. If it is desired to increase the 26 sessions to 30 (or more) to cover the program of a year, this can be done by splitting the 1st and 2nd sessions into additional sessions; the 23rd session (28th chapter, *Heterotopic transplantation of left kidney*) into two operations (anastomoses to the aorta-inferior vena cava, and in next session to the common iliac vessels); the 25th session (30th chapter, *Transplantation of the ovary-fallopian tube*) can be extended into three—or more—operations (e.g, anastomoses of common iliac vessels to aorta-inferior vena cava, anastomoses of common iliac vessels to common iliac vessels, and anastomoses of the graft's vessels of the uterine horn to common iliac vessels).

Little - Useful Advices

- Practice calmness and concentration (breathing exercises help), listen to the rhythm of your own body, and fully control your hands
- Stay away from coffee, caffeine containing drinks and smoking
- Alcohol can wait for Saturday evening (and with good company)
- Sleep well, sleep deprivation increases hand tremor
- A light breakfast, or a snack and sugar drink before surgery helps, low blood sugar causes tremor and decreases concentration
- Solve any problems with your colleagues before surgery; peace of mind is necessary
- Do not hesitate to tell your instructor that he/she is pressing you too hard
- Music in the room helps, gives peacefulness, but it is required that the kind of music is your favorite—if not, and irritates you, do not hesitate to ask to change the music (the writer prefers small ensembles of classical music, likes piano jazz, but imperatively asks to cease any techno, pop, rock, and rap)
- Forget all your problems with bills and your mother-in-law, the magic microscopic waits to calm you
- But if serious problems occur, ask to be replaced or postpone surgery
- Take breaks of 5-10 min every 1 hour, as the tension in microsurgery is high; human attention does not last for long—but your operation is going to last for a long time
- Do not hesitate to take a break to use the bathroom or drink an orange juice (the worst part is to wash your hands again)
- Do not struggle with time, the learning curve works by itself
- Failure is a challenge, cut the sutures and do it again—only here is it permitted to show your egoism, nowhere else
- Cease searching for 'bravo', your result speaks for itself

And one last piece of 'wisdom': cherish your child-like curiosity; this is going to nurture you as a scientist...

List of Contents

INTRODUCTIVE PART

1. Material and equipment 33

Laboratory equipment; surgical instruments; microsurgical instruments; sutures, laboratory animals; disposable surgical material

Usage and characteristics of microsurgical instruments

Microsurgical sutures and guidelines for choosing size in relation to the diameter of vessel or nerve

Maintenance and handling of microsurgical instruments

Microsurgeon positioning and posture in the laboratory and operating room

2. The surgical microscope 41

Principles of function of the surgical microscope

Basic components of the surgical microscope; types of surgical microscopes; accessories; basic functions (switches and knobs)

Personalized adjustment of the surgical microscope; adjustment of the distance between the head of the microscope and surgical field; adjustment of the optical path

3. Pre-operative preparation, anesthesia and post-operative care of the laboratory rat 51

Pre-operative alimentation

Induction and maintenance of anesthesia

Preparation of the operative field (hair cutting and shaving, antisepsis)

Post-operative care

Euthanasia

BASIC MICROSURGICAL TECHNIQUES

4. Microsurgical technique for suturing vessels 57

Handling of the microsurgical suture with the needle holder; suture needle's entry into and exit from the vessel with the aid of microsurgical forceps

Tying knots with the microsurgical forceps and the needle holder

5. Principles of end-to-end anastomosis of vessels 63

Placement of a yellow background beneath the vessel; application of the double vascular clamp; transection of the vessel; irrigation of the lumen with normal saline; removal of the adventitia; approximation of clamps

Placement of sutures (after the two corner sutures): depending on their number, use of the technique of 'dividing the gap' between previously placed sutures (for a total of 4 or 8 sutures); or the technique of placing the sutures at equal distances starting from the periphery–close to corner sutures–, by coming 'closer to closer,' toward the middle point (for a total of 6 or 10 sutures); or combination of the two techniques (for a total of 12 sutures)
Removal of the double clamp, gauze placement and wait
Patency test
Disproportion in diameter of vessels to be anastomosed: <50%: mechanical dilation of the smaller vessel; 50-100%: oblique section or 'fish-mouth' diametric insicions of the smaller vessel; >100%: conversion to end-to-side anastomosis
Problems (solutions): The double clamp cannot be rotated (suturing starts from the middle of posterior wall); gap after approximation of clamps (traction with suture on neighboring tissues or insertion of vein graft); very large blood leak after removal of the double clamp (additional suture); suspicion that a suture catches the opposite wall (suture cut and reposition) – if several sutures (removal of all sutures and redo)

6. Principles of end-to-side anastomosis of vessels 75
Placement of a yellow background beneath the vessels; application of the double vascular clamp and incision (transverse preferably, or longitudinal, or ellipsoid) on the side-anastomosed vessel; irrigation of the lumen with normal saline; preparation of the end-anastomosed vessel (placement of the single clamp, transection, irrigation, removal of the adventitia)
Placement of sutures: 1. (After the two corner sutures): If the end-anastomosed vessel (single clamp) can be rotated, the anterior surface is sutured first using the technique of 'dividing the gap' between previously placed sutures (for a total of 4 or 8 sutures); or the technique of placing the sutures at equal distances 'closer to closer' from the corner sutures toward the middle point (for a total of 6 or 10 sutures); or combination of the two techniques (for a total of 12 sutures). 2. If the end-anastomosed vessel cannot be rotated, but the posterior surface is accessible: placement of the 1st suture in the middle of the posterior surface and then of the rest sutures at equal distances, away from either side of the 1st suture and toward the median anterior suture from either side; posterior surface non accessible: continuous suturing of the posterior surface up to the corner sutures
Removal of the single and double clamp; gauze placement and wait
Patency test. 1. Blood flow toward the end-anastomosed vessel, 2. Blood flow toward the side-anastomosed vessel

7. Technique of microsurgical suturing of nerves 85
Neurolysis; transection of nerve, approximation of stumps
Principles of nerve suturing techniques: 1. suturing the epineurium, 2. suturing the perineuriums, 3. suturing the epineurium and the perineuriums

MICROSURGICAL PROCEDURES

8. End-to-end anastomosis of the aorta 93
Midline laparotomy; mobilization and arrangement of splanchna outside the abdomen (intestine), and inside the abdomen (liver, spleen)
Opening of the retroperitoneum; microsurgical dissection of the aorta; ligation and transection of the lumbar arteries

- **End-to-end anastomosis with 10 or 12 sutures 10/0**
- **Diameter of aorta: 1.2-1.5 mm**

Synopsis 107

9. **End-to-end anastomosis of the external jugular vein & end-to-end anastomosis of the common carotid artery** 109

External Jugular Vein

Transverse incision and superficial dissection of the neck; microsurgical dissection of the external jugular vein

- **End-to-end anastomosis with 8 or 10 sutures 10/0**
- **Diameter of external jugular vein: 1.9 mm (1.6-2.1 mm)**

Common Carotid Artery

Deep dissection of the neck; access of the common carotid artery: 1. by separation of sternohyoid muscles along the midline, 2. by transection of the sternal part of the sternocleidomastoid muscle and deep dissection from the lateral border of sternohyoid muscle; microsurgical dissection of the common carotid artery

- **End-to-end anastomosis with 8 sutures 10/0**
- **Diameter of common carotid artery: 0.7-1.2 mm**

Synopsis 125

10. **Interposition of external jugular vein graft in the abdominal aorta** 127

Transverse incision and superficial dissection of the neck; microsurgical dissection of the external jugular vein and of the tributary veins at its trifurcation

Midline laparotomy; placement of intestine outside the abdomen and arrangement of splanchna (liver, spleen). Opening of the retroperitoneum; microsurgical dissection of the aorta

Harvest and transfer of the graft (external jugular vein plus part of major tributary)

Transection of the aorta

- **Two simultaneous end-to-end anastomoses between vessels of different wall thickness, each with 10 sutures 10/0**
- **Diameter of external jugular vein: 1.9 mm (1.6-2.1 mm)**
- **Diameter of aorta: 1.2-1.5 mm**

Synopsis 133

11. **Abdominal aorta bypass graft using the external jugular vein** 135

Transverse incision and superficial dissection of the neck; microsurgical dissection of the external jugular vein and of the tributary veins at its trifurcation

Midline laparotomy; placement of intestine outside the abdomen and arrangement of splanchna (liver, spleen). Opening of the retroperitoneum; microsurgical dissection of the aorta

Harvest and transfer of the graft (external jugular vein plus part of major tributary)

Transverse incisions on the aorta

- **Two simultaneous end-to-side anastomoses between vessels of different wall thickness, each with 10 or 12 sutures 10/0; the end-anastomosed vessel can be rotated**
- **Diameter of external jugular vein: 1.9 mm (1.6-2.1 mm)**
- **Diameter of aorta: 1.2-1.5 mm**

Ligation of the aorta between the anastomoses

Synopsis 140

12. **Interposition of external jugular (deep tributary) vein into the common carotid artery** 143

Transverse incision and superficial dissection of the neck; microsurgical dissection of the external jugular vein and of the tributary veins at its trifurcation

Deep dissection of the neck; access of the common carotid artery by transection of the sternal part of the sternocleidomastoid muscle; microsurgical dissection of the common carotid artery

Harvest and transfer of the graft (major tributary of the external jugular vein)
Transection of the common carotid artery
- **Two simultaneous end-to-end anastomoses between vessels of different wall thickness, each with 8 sutures 10/0**
- **Diameter of common carotid artery: 0.7-1.2mm, almost equal to the deep tributary vein**

Synopsis 151

13. Common carotid artery bypass graft using the external jugular (deep tributary) vein 153
Transverse incision and superficial dissection of the neck; microsurgical dissection of the external jugular vein and of the tributary veins at its trifurcation
Deep dissection of the neck; access of the common carotid artery by transection of the sternal part of the sternocleidomastoid muscle; microsurgical dissection of the common carotid artery
Harvest and transfer of the graft (major tributary of the external jugular vein)
Transverse incisions on the common carotid artery
- **Two simultaneous end-to-side anastomoses between vessels of different wall thickness, each with 8 sutures 10/0; the end-anastomosed vessel can be rotated**
- **Diameter of common carotid artery: 0.7-1.2 mm, almost equal to the deep tributary vein**

Ligation of the common carotid artery between the anastomoses
Synopsis 157

14. End-to-side anastomosis of the common carotid artery to the external jugular vein 159
Transverse incision and superficial dissection of the neck; microsurgical dissection of the external jugular vein
Deep dissection of the neck; access of the common carotid artery by transection of the sternal part of the sternocleidomastoid muscle; microsurgical dissection, peripheral ligation and transection of the common carotid artery
Transverse incision on the external jugular vein
- **End-to-side anastomosis between vessels of different wall thickness with 8 sutures 10/0; the end-anastomosed common carotid artery can not be rotated**
- **Diameter of common carotid artery: 0.7-1.2 mm**
- **Diameter of external jugular vein: 1.9 mm (1.6-2.1 mm)**
- **Model of arterio-venous fistula**

Synopsis 164

15. End-to-end anastomosis between the aorta and right common iliac artery 165
Midline laparotomy; placement of intestine outside the abdomen and arrangement of splanchna (liver, spleen); opening of the retroperitoneum; microsurgical dissection of the aorta, which is continued until the first branch of the right common iliac artery
Transection of the aorta; transection, rotation and mechanical dilatation of the right common iliac artery
- **End-to-end anastomosis with 10 sutures 10/0**
- **Diameter of aorta: 1.2-1.5 mm**
- **Diameter of common iliac artery: 0.7-0.9 mm**
- **Model of anastomosis between vessels of different size**

Synopsis 173

16. End-to-side anastomosis of the portal vein to the inferior vena cava 175

Midline laparotomy; placement of intestine outside the abdomen; rotation of middle and right lobes of the liver cephalad

Opening of the retroperitoneum; microsurgical dissection of the inferior vena cava between left and right renal veins; ligation and transection of lumbar veins

Microsurgical dissection of the portal vein; ligation and transection of tributary veins; ligation and transection of portal vein close to the hilum of the liver

Transverse incision on the inferior vena cava

- **End-to-side venous anastomosis with 10 or 12 sutures 10/0; the end-anastomosed portal vein can not be rotated**
- **Diameter of portal vein: 1.5 mm**
- **Diameter of inferior vena cava: 1.5-3 mm**
- **Anastomosis to be completed within 30 min since portal vein occluded**

Synopsis 186

17. Anastomosis of the sciatic nerve & grafting of the sciatic nerve 189

Mid-thigh transverse incision; separation of the tensor fasciae latae muscle from the biceps femoris muscle; exposure and dissection of the sciatic nerve (neurolysis)

Transection of the nerve and microsurgical dissection of the epineurium

- **Anastomosis of the nerve with 4 sutures 9/0**
- **Grafting of the nerve: two simultaneous anastomoses, each with 4 sutures 9/0, without placement of vascular clamp**
- **Diameter of sciatic nerve: 2 mm**

Synopsis 196

18. End-to-end anastomoses of the femoral vessels 197

Subinguinal incision; opening of the deep fascia; microsurgical dissection of the femoral vessels and transection of their branches/tributaries from the origin/confluence of the superficial inferior epigastric vessels up to the inguinal ligament; transection of the femoral vessels

- **Two simultaneous end-to-end anastomoses: artery with 6 sutures 11/0, vein with 6 or 8 sutures 11/0**
- **Diameter of femoral artery: almost 1 mm (0.7-0.9 mm cephalad to the origin of the superficial inferior epigastric vessels)**
- **Diameter of femoral vein: approximately 2 mm**

Synopsis 209

19. Interposition of superficial inferior epigastric vein graft in the femoral artery 211

Subinguinal incision; opening of the deep fascia; microsurgical dissection of the femoral artery—and transection of branches—from the origin of the superficial inferior epigastric artery for at least 1 cm cranially

Microsurgical dissection of the superficial inferior epigastric vein for at least 1 cm from its confluence with the femoral vein

Harvest and transfer of the graft (superficial inferior epigastric vein)

Transection of the femoral artery
- **Two simultaneous end-to-end anastomoses between vessels of different wall thickness, each with 6 sutures 11/0**
- **Diameter of superficial inferior epigastric vein: approximately 1 mm**
- **Diameter of femoral artery: approximately 1 mm**

Synopsis 219

20. Femoral artery bypass graft using the superficial inferior epigastric vein 221

Subinguinal incision; opening of the deep fascia; microsurgical dissection of the femoral artery from the origin of the superficial inferior epigastric artery for at least 1 cm cranially
Microsurgical dissection of the superficial inferior epigastric vein for at least 1 cm from its confluence with the femoral vein
Harvest and transfer of the graft (superficial inferior epigastric vein)
Transverse incisions on the femoral artery
- **Two simultaneous end-to-side anastomoses between vessels of different wall thickness, each with 6 sutures 11/0; the end-anastomosed vessel can be rotated**
- **Diameter of superficial inferior epigastric vein: approximately 1 mm**
- **Diameter of femoral artery: approximately 1 mm**

Synopsis 225

21. End-to-end anastomoses of the superficial inferior epigastric vessels 227

Subinguinal incision; opening of the fatty layer of superficial fascia; microsurgical dissection and separation of the superficial inferior epigastric artery and vein
- **End-to-end arterial anastomosis with 4 sutures 11/0**
- **Diameter of superficial inferior epigastric artery: approximately 0.5 mm**
- **End-to-end venous anastomosis with 6 sutures 11/0**
- **Diameter of superficial inferior epigastric vein: approximately 1 mm**

Synopsis 232

TRANSPLANTATIONS

22. Orthotopic autotransplantation of pedicled inguinal skin flap 235

Subinguinal incision; dissection of a skin flap 4x2 cm supplied by the superficial inferior epigastric vessels
Microsurgical dissection of femoral vessels from the inguinal ligament up to and including the final part of the saphenous vein; transection of all their branches/tributaries except for the superficial inferior epigastric vessels. Ligation and transection of the femoral vessels distal to the junction of the superficial inferior epigastric vessels, so that the vascular pedicle of the flap is composed by the superficial inferior epigastric–femoral vessels. Transection of the femoral vessels midway between inguinal ligament and junction of the superficial inferior epigastric vessels
- **Two simultaneous end-to-end anastomoses: femoral artery with 6 sutures 11/0, femoral vein with 8 sutures 11/0**
- **Diameter of femoral artery: approximately 1 mm**
- **Diameter of femoral vein: approximately 2 mm**

Synopsis 245

23. Contralateral autotransplantation of pedicled inguinal skin flap 247

Subinguinal incision; dissection of a skin flap 4x2 cm supplied by the superficial inferior epigastric vessels. Microsurgical dissection of femoral vessels from the inguinal ligament to the saphenous vein; transection of all branches/tributaries except for the superficial inferior epigastric vessels. Ligation and transection of the femoral vessels distal to the junction of the superficial inferior epigastric vessels, so that the vascular pedicle of the flap is composed by the superficial inferior epigastric – femoral vessels

Contralateral subinguinal incision; microsurgical dissection of femoral vessels from the inguinal ligament to the junction of the superficial inferior epigastric vessels; transverse arteriotomy and venotomy

Flap harvest (ligation and transection of femoral vessels close to the inguinal ligament); transfer to the other side

- **Two simultaneous end-to-side anastomoses: femoral arteries with 6 sutures 11/0, femoral veins with 8 sutures 11/0; the end-anastomosed vessels can be rotated**
- **Diameter of femoral artery: approximately 1 mm**
- **Diameter of femoral vein: approximately 2 mm**

Synopsis 255

24. Autotransplantation of free inguinal skin flap to the neck 257

Subinguinal incision; dissection of a skin flap 4x2 cm supplied by the superficial inferior epigastric vessels. Microsurgical dissection of femoral vessels from the inguinal ligament to the saphenous vein; transection of all branches/tributaries except for the superficial inferior epigastric vessels. Ligation and transection of the femoral vessels distal to the junction of the superficial inferior epigastric vessels, so that the vascular pedicle of the flap is composed by the superficial inferior epigastric – femoral vessels

Opening and superficial dissection of the neck; microsurgical dissection of the external jugular vein. Access to the common carotid artery by separation of sternohyoid muscles along the midline; microsurgical dissection; transverse arteriotomy

Flap harvest (ligation and transection of femoral vessels close to the inguinal ligament); transfer to the surgical field of the neck

- **End-to-side anastomosis between femoral artery and common carotid artery with 6 sutures 11/0; the end-anastomosed vessel can be rotated**
  Diameter of femoral artery: approximately 1 mm
  Diameter of common carotid artery: 0.7-1.2 mm

Rearrangement of the surgical field; transverse incision on the external jugular vein

- **End-to-side anastomosis between femoral vein and external jugular vein with 6 or 8 sutures 11/0; the end-anastomosed vessel cannot be rotated, the anastomosis starts from the middle of the posterior surface**
- **Diameter of femoral vein: approximately 2 mm**
- **Diameter of external jugular vein: 1.9 mm (1.6-2.1 mm)**

Synopsis 270

25. Autotransplantation of the posterior limb 273

Subinguinal incision; microsurgical dissection of femoral vessels; transection of anterior muscles; microsurgical dissection and transection of the sciatic nerve; transection of posterior muscles and skin; occlusion and transection of femoral vessels; transection of the femur

Rejoining of the femur with internal fixation; suturing of posterior muscles

- **Suturing of sciatic nerve with 4 sutures 9/0**
- **Diameter of sciatic nerve: approximately 2 mm**

- **Two simultaneous end-to-end anastomoses: femoral artery with 6 sutures 11/0, femoral vein with 6 or 8 sutures 11/0**
- **Diameter of femoral artery: approximately 1 mm**
- **Diameter of femoral vein: approximately 2 mm**

Suturing of anterior muscles and skin

Synopsis 281

26. Orthotopic autotransplantation of the left kidney 283

Midline laparotomy; placement of the intestine to the right of the rat. Opening of the retroperitoneum and renal fascia. Microsurgical dissection and removal of the perirenal fat. Microsurgical dissection–removal of perivascular fat and separation–of renal vessels and their branches/tributaries (diameter of the latter: 0.5-1 mm), from their origin from/confluence with the aorta/inferior vena cava up to and including the renal hilum. Ligation and transection of extrarenal branches/tributaries of renal vessels: inferior adrenal vein and artery, gonadal vein, deep tributary veins. Opening of a 'window' between ureter and periureteral fat in the site of planned transection

Transection of renal vessels and ureter

- **Two simultaneous end-to-end anastomoses: renal artery with 8 sutures 11/0, renal vein with 10 or 12 sutures 10/0; the graft can be rotated**
- **The anastomoses must be completed within 30 minutes since occlusion of renal vessels**
- **Diameter of renal artery: 0.7-0.8 mm**
- **Diameter of renal vein: 1.5-2 mm**
- **Anastomosis of the ureter without clamp, with 4 sutures 11/0**

Synopsis 297

27. Orthotopic transplantation of the left kidney 299

In donor and recipient: Midline laparotomy; placement of the intestine to the right of the rat. Opening of the retroperitoneum and renal fascia. Microsurgical dissection and removal of the perirenal fat. Microsurgical dissection–removal of perivascular fat and separation–of renal vessels and their branches/ tributaries (diameter of the latter: 0.5-1 mm), from their origin from/confluence with the aorta/inferior vena cava up to and including the renal hilum. Ligation and transection of extrarenal branches/tributaries of renal vessels: inferior adrenal vein and artery, gonadal vein, deep tributary veins. Dissection of the ureter off the periureteral fat at the site of planned transection

In donor: Dissection of the aorta, ligation above and below the origin of renal artery; transection of the renal vein. Flushing of the kidney with injection of cold heparin solution in the aorta

Graft harvest (transection of renal artery and ureter); transfer to the recipient. Removal of recipient's kidney

- **Two simultaneous end-to-end anastomoses: renal artery with 8 sutures 11/0, renal vein with 10 or 12 sutures 10/0; the graft can be rotated**
- **The anastomoses must be completed within 30 minutes since occlusion of renal vessels**
- **Diameter of renal artery: 0.7-0.8 mm**
- **Diameter of renal vein: 1.5-2 mm**
- **Anastomosis of the ureter without clamp, with 4 sutures 11/0**

Synopsis 307

28. Heterotopic (auto)transplantation of the left kidney 311

Midline laparotomy; placement of the intestine to the right of the rat. Opening of the retroperitoneum and renal fascia. Microsurgical dissection and removal of the perirenal fat. Microsurgical dissection–removal of perivascular fat and separation–of renal vessels and their branches/tributaries (diameter of the latter: 0.5-1 mm), from their origin from/confluence with the aorta/inferior vena cava up to and including the renal hilum. Ligation and transection of extrarenal branches/tributaries of renal vessels: inferior adrenal vein and artery, gonadal vein, deep tributary veins. *Ureter not dissected if only vessels anastomoses are practiced

I. TRANSPLANTATION WITH ANASTOMOSES IN THE AORTA - INFERIOR VENA CAVA 311

Microsurgical dissection of the aorta and inferior vena cava from the renal vessels to the bifurcation. Transverse arteriotomy and venotomy

Harvest of the graft (transection of renal vessels)

- **Two simultaneous end-to-side anastomoses: renal artery-aorta with 8 sutures 11/0, renal vein-inferior vena cava with 10 or 12 sutures 10/0; the graft can be rotated**
- **The anastomoses must be completed within 30 minutes since occlusion of renal vessels**
- **Diameter of renal artery: 0.7-0.8 mm**
- **Diameter of renal vein: 1.5-2 mm**
- **Diameter of aorta: 1.2-1.5 mm**
- **Diameter of inferior vena cava: 1.5-3 mm**

II. TRANSPLANTATION WITH ANASTOMOSES IN THE THE COMMON ILIAC VESSELS 320

Microsurgical dissection of the caudal part of the aorta and inferior vena cava and bifurcation (with transection of middle sacral vessels), which is continued in the common iliac vessels until the origin of the internal iliac artery. Alternatively, dissection of the common iliac vessels only (with preservation of middle sacral vessels)

Harvest of the graft (transection of renal vessels)

- **Two simultaneous end-to-side anastomoses: renal artery-common iliac artery with 8 sutures 11/0, renal vein-common iliac vein with 10 or 12 sutures 10/0; the graft can be rotated**
- **The anastomoses must be completed within 30 minutes since occlusion of renal vessels**
- **Diameter of renal artery: 0.7-0.8 mm**
- **Diameter of renal vein: 1.5-2 mm**
- **Diameter of common iliac artery: 0.7-0.9 mm**
- **Diameter of common iliac vein: approximately 2 mm**

III. REMARKS ON ALL KIDNEY TRANSPLANTATIONS 325

1. Transplantation of kidney with vessel variation
   A. Anomalies (variations) of renal arteries: accessory artery, double artery, long branch of renal artery
   B. Anomalies of renal veins
2. Flushing of the graft in autotransplantation

Synopsis 331

29. Autotransplantation of the uterine horn-fallopian tube-ovary 333

Midline laparotomy; placement of the intestine outside the abdomen, on the left side. Opening of the retroperitoneum. Microsurgical dissection of the right common iliac vessels (starting from aorta-inferior vena cava at the bifurcation) and of all their branches and tributaries

Ligation and transection of all branches and tributaries of the right common iliac vessels–except for the vessels of the uterine horn–and of right gonadal vessels, so that the only vascular supply to the complex

'uterine horn-fallopian tube-ovary' become the vessels of the horn (the only branches of right common iliac vessels retained)
Transection of the upper part of the uterine horn. Mobilization of the graft with ablation of mesometrium-mesovarium attachments. Transection of the right common iliac vessels

- **Two simultaneous end-to-end anastomoses: common iliac artery with 8 sutures 10/0, common iliac vein with 8 or 10 sutures 10/0; the graft can be rotated**
- **Diameter of common iliac artery: 0.7-0.9 mm**
- **Diameter of common iliac vein: approximately 2 mm**
- **Anastomosis of the uterine horn: 8 or 10 sutures 9/0**

Synopsis 356

30. Transplantation of the ovary-fallopian tube 357
Note: the graft includes the cranial part of the uterine horn
Donor's preparation
Median incision; placement of intestine outside the abdomen, on the left side; opening of retroperitoneum. Microsurgical dissection of the aorta, left common iliac artery, and right common iliac vessels and their branches/tributaries
Ligation and transection of all branches and tributaries of right common iliac vessels–except for the vessels of the uterine horn–and of ipsilateral gonadal vessels, so that the only vascular supply to the complex 'uterine horn-fallopian tube-ovary' become the vessels of the horn (the only branches of common iliac vessels retained)
Recipient's preparation
Median incision; placement of intestine outside the abdomen; opening of retroperitoneum. Microsurgical dissection of the aorta and inferior vena cava, from the renal vessels to the bifurcation; transverse arteriotomy and venotomy
Graft harvest (donor)
Flushing of the graft with injection of cold normal saline in the aorta, after ligation of the aorta and left common iliac artery and transection of the right common iliac vein.
Harvest of the graft by transecting the horn at the upper part, after cutting the vertical branches of the horn vessels up to the upper part of it; ablation of mesometrium-mesovarium attachments; transection of the right common iliac artery.
Graft implantation (recipient)

- **Two simultaneous end-to-side anastomoses: common iliac artery of the graft to aorta of recipient, and common iliac vein of the graft to inferior vena cava of recipient, each with 10 sutures 10/0; the graft can be rotated**
- **Diameter of common iliac artery: 0.7-0.9 mm**
- **Diameter of common iliac vein: approximately 2 mm**
- **Diameter of aorta: 1.2-1.5 mm**
- **Diameter of inferior vena cava: 1.5-3 mm**

Removal or the right 'upper part of the horn-fallopian tube-ovary' after transection of the gonadal vessels and vessels of the horn

- **Anastomosis of the uterine horn: 8-10 sutures 9/0**

Synopsis 372

31. Heterotopic heart transplantation 375
Recipient's preparation
Midline laparotomy; placement of intestine outside the abdomen; opening of retroperitoneum. Microsurgical dissection of the aorta and inferior vena cava, from the renal vessels to the bifurcation

Graft harvest (donor)
Bilateral, U-type thoracotomy; removal of the heart en block with vessels, lungs, trachea, esophagus
Flushing of the graft with cold normal saline via the inferior vena cava
Separation of the heart from lungs, trachea, esophagus
Microsurgical dissection, ligation and transection of superior and inferior vena cava, of all pulmonary vessels–except for left pulmonary artery–, and of the three branches of the aortic arch
Graft implantation (recipient)
Transverse incision on the aorta and inferior vena cava
- **Two simultaneous end-to-side anastomoses: graft aorta-recipients's aorta with 10 or 12 sutures 10/0, graft left pulmonary artery-recipient's inferior vena cava with 10 sutures 10/0; suggested technique as if the graft cannot be rotated**
- **Diameter of aorta: 1.2-1.5 mm**
- **Diameter of inferior vena cava: 1.5-3 mm**
- **Diameter of pulmonary artery: 1 mm**
- The heart beats but does not work as a pump (left ventricle not used)

Synopsis....400

PART I

INTRODUCTION

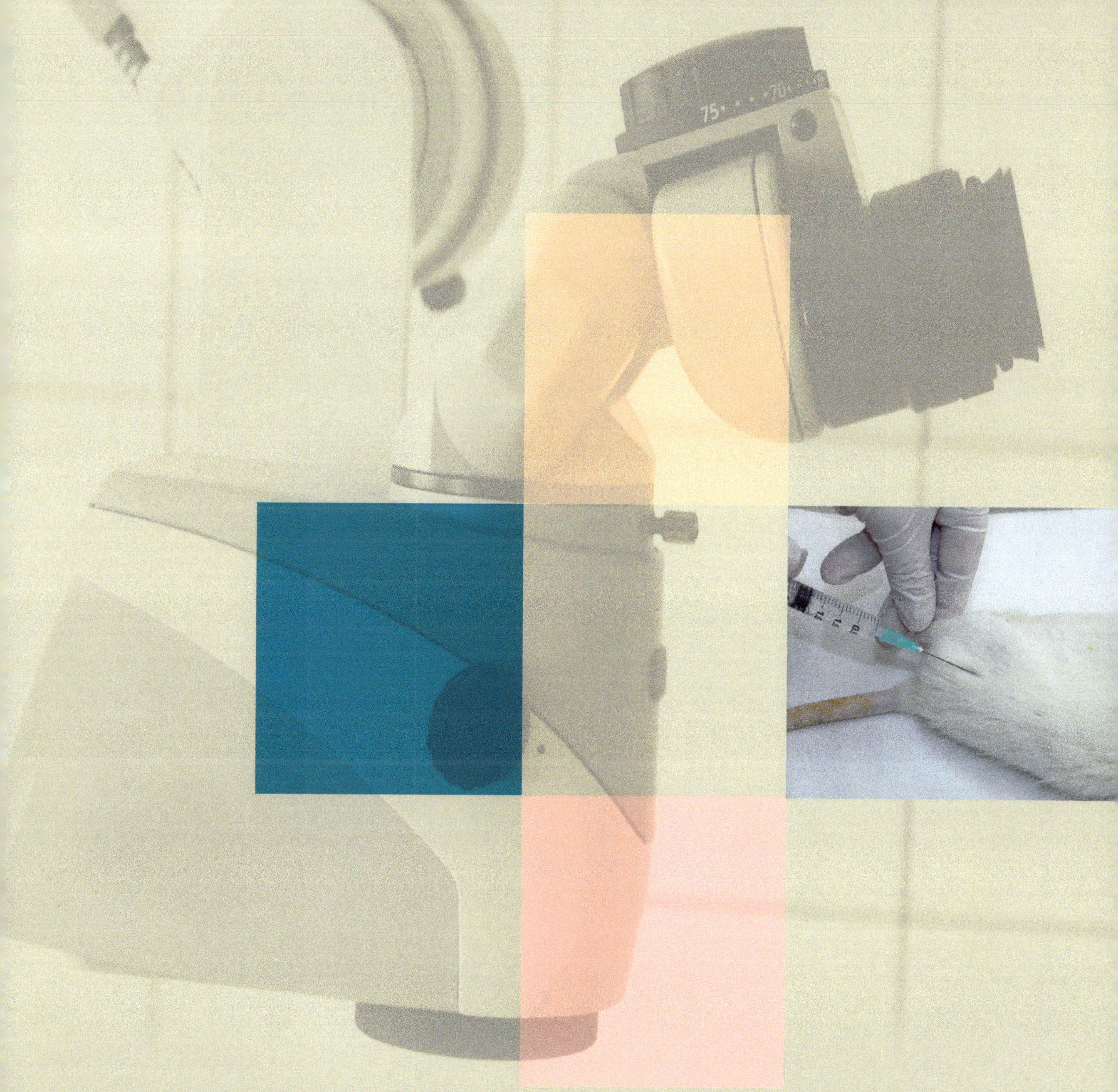

1

Material and equipment

A. Equipment

Laboratory equipment (Fig. 1-1)

1. Surgical microscope with a magnification range of 4× to 40×. The microscope should be equipped with a co-observation system for assisted surgery as well as a digital recording camera and a photo camera.
2. Computer (preferably, with a large monitor), equipped with appropriate software (compatible with the camera) for the recording and editing of video and photos.
3. Chair of adjustable height, with arms (for resting the elbows upon to improve the stability of the surgeon's hands).
4. Table of 90 cm (35.4 inches) height.
5. Waterproof working surface, dimensions 30 cm × 20 cm.
6. External cold light source, with ability to control light.
7. Closed glass chamber (with a maximum diameter of 8 cm) within which to induce anesthesia for the rat.
8. Electric razor.
9. Monopolar diathermy, single use, battery operated (used in Ophthalmology).

Surgical instruments (Fig. 1-2)

I. Non-microsurgical instruments

1. Surgical scalpel (with additional removable blades)
2. One surgical forceps
3. Two anatomical forceps
4. Needle holders for sutures from 2/0 to 7/0
5. One pair of Metzenbaum dissecting scissors
6. One pair of sharp scissors (curved or straight)

II. Microsurgical instruments

1. Two jewelers forceps, Dumont No. 3 and No. 5
2. A Barraquer needle holder, curved, without lock
3. A pair of dissecting scissors, 11-15 cm long, ring handled, with blunt tips and slightly curved blades

4. A pair of cutting scissors (also known as adventitia scissors), 11-15 cm long, flat handled, with pointed tips and straight blades
5. Single and Double vascular clamps
6. Very fine surgical forceps (Adson or Bunny type)

Sutures

Required sutures include:

- 2/0 non-absorbable sutures
- 3/0 non-absorbable sutures
- 7/0 & 8/0 prolene sutures, round needle in cross-section
- 9/0 nylon: suture diameter 35 μm (in cross-section), round needle of diameter 100 μm
- 10/0 nylon: suture diameter 25 μm, round needle of diameter 50 or 75 μm
- 11/0 nylon: suture diameter 25 μm, round needle of diameter 50 μm

Laboratory animals

Sprague Dawley rats of mean age 90 days and mean weight 200 g.

Disposable surgical material

1. Normal saline, 10 ml vials, warmed (to body temperature)
2. Gauze pads, 5 × 5 cm and 10 × 10 cm
3. Surgical sponges (peanut-like, or other)
4. Antiseptic solution (iodine based or chlorexidine, not alcohol based)
5. Adhesive elastic bands (small size, to fix the rat's legs to the working surface)
6. Syringes: 20 ml, 5 ml, 2.5 ml and 1 ml
7. Sterilized, absorptive paper for covering the working surface
8. Examination gloves (nitrile or latex)
9. Sterile surgical gloves
10. Surgical gowns

Additional disposable material may be required for specific microsurgical procedures and will be mentioned in the respective Chapters.

B. Usage and characteristics of microsurgical instruments and sutures

Ergonomic characteristics of microsurgical instruments

- Instruments should be 11-15 cm in length, to facilitate ease of use and to minimize fatigue.
- Most instrument handles should be round, in order to roll the instrument easily with the fingers, as opposed

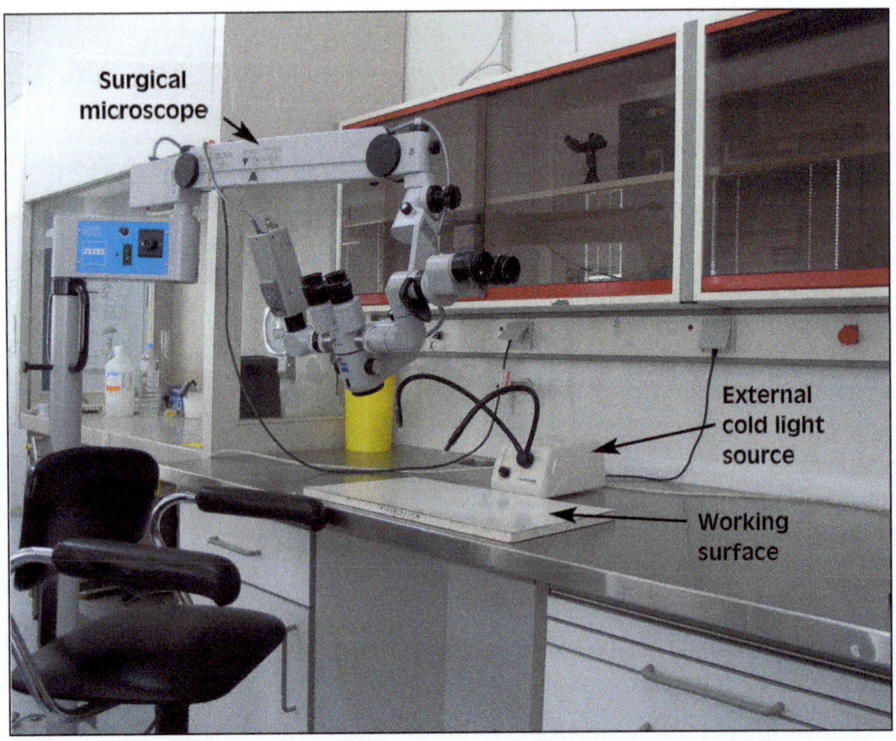

Figure 1-1

Proposed arrangement of the basic laboratory equipment. (From author's photo library)

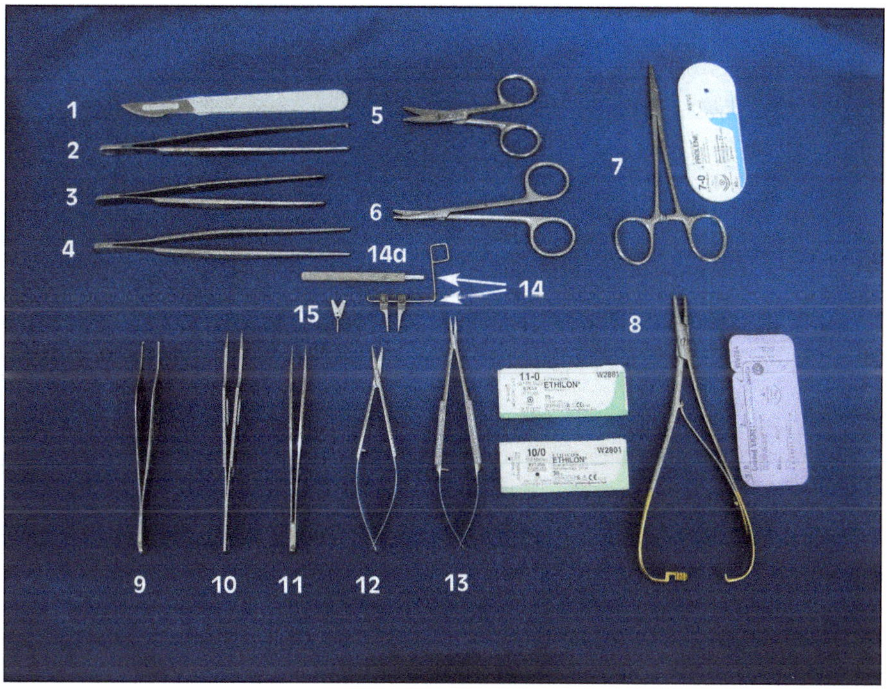

Figure 1-2

The surgical and microsurgical instruments required for a microsurgical procedure: **1.** scalpel, **2.** surgical forceps, **3 & 4.** anatomical forceps, **5.** sharp scissors, **6.** blunt scissors (baby-Metzenbaum), **7.** short needle holder for sutures 2/0 to 7/0, **8.** needle holder for sutures 2/0 to 4/0, **9.** fine surgical forceps (Adson or Bunny type), **10 & 11.** microsurgical forceps, Dumont No. 3 and No. 5, **12.** microsurgical scissors, **13.** Barraquer needle holder, 14 cm long, curved, without lock, for sutures 8/0 to 11/0, **14.** Gilbert's double vascular clamp, **14a.** driver for opening/closing the jaws of the Gilbert's double vascular clamps. **15.** single microsurgical vascular clamp. (From author's photo library)

to relying upon movement of the wrist to provide rotational range of motion.
Cutting microscissors can be flat-handled to allow for improved precision.

- Instruments must have the proper weight for comfortable use. Heavy instruments will contribute to increased fatigue. At the same time, if instruments are too light (e.g. wolframium-made), they are also better avoided.
- Instruments with a matte finish are preferable, in order to avoid reflections and glare.

Forceps

The Dumont forceps used in microsurgery originate from jeweler's forceps and are used for grasping and handling of both sutures and needles, dissection of tissues, dilation of vessels, and testing of post-anastomosis vessel patency. Microsurgical forceps may have either straight tips or curved tips. There are also forceps with grasping tips; however, instead recommend using fine surgical forceps.

Dumont No. 3 forceps are mostly used for tissue dissection, while also being used to test the patency of vessels after microsurgical anastomosis.

Dumont No. 5 forceps are mostly used for detailed dissection, and for dilation of the lumen of very small vessels.

Needle holders

Microsurgical needle holders are used for placement of sutures, as well as for dissection of small vessels due to their fine and rounded tip. These needle holders are equipped with a system of pressure calibration designed to protect the suture needle from deformation.

The two basic types of microsurgical needle holders are the Barraquer and Castroviejo. The latter has flat handle, whereas the Barraquer is round-handled and thus preferred because it can be rotated more easily between the finger tips.

Microsurgical needle holders are available with the following characteristics:

- Locking or non-locking: When using a locking microsurgical needle holder, locking the jaws of the needle holder immobilizes the needle while a second, closing, movement of the handles releases the needle. Note that the locking mechanism of the needle holder must not be used to help pass the needle through a vessel wall. On the contrary, during passage of the needle through a vessel wall, the needle holder should be unlocked and the needle should be controlled only by pressure applied to the handles of the needle holder. Close attention should also be paid to the motion of unlocking the needle holder, as it could cause unwanted movement during a critical moment. In general, locking needle holders are not recommended for use in microsurgery, both for the reasons described above and for their functional limitations: for example, the needle cannot be loaded on to the holder when pressed in the middle of its arch while on a flexible surgical field (as described below). Furthermore, a locking needle holder can become dangerous when in the hands of a beginner, particularly if he/she forgets to unlock it (e.g., drawing the suture through the vessel wall, while keeping the suture locked into the needle holder, may tear the vessel at the location where the suture is already attached).

- Straight or curved tips: Both are very useful. Needle holders with curved tips facilitate the ability to load the needle when it lies in the surgical field at an angle to the main axis of the needle holder. Needle holders with curved tips are also useful for suturing smaller vessels and find frequent application in terminolateral anastomoses.
- Smooth or serrated jaws: As a rule, all microsurgical instruments used to grasp or hold should have smooth surfaces; otherwise, the serrated jaws risk destroying the needle or the suture.
- Jaws (tips) of various sizes: It is advisable that an additional needle holder with fine jaws be available for 11/0 sutures (and 12/0 sutures, if used).
- Variable length: Needle holders utilized in microsurgery can be found with lengths ranging from 14.6 to 18 cm (5.75 inches to 7 inches). Short needle holders are generally preferred.

Scissors

Blunt tipped scissors are used for dissection of tissues, but can also be used closed, as a dissection probe. These scissors are also especially useful during dissection of vessels, as they help to avoid trauma to the vascular wall. The blunt tipped scissors are equipped with rounded handles, allowing for easy rolling; additionally, the surfaces of the scissor handles are serrated for better, non-slip handling, while the blunt, rounded tips help to avoid traumatizing the surrounding tissues. The blades of the blunt tipped scissors are curved in order to provide better access to the posterior surfaces of tissues or organs, and are especially useful when dissecting layered components from one another, e.g. adventitia from the vessel wall.

Sharp cutting scissors are used to cut vessels, to obtain clean edges. These scissors are used for detailed dissection, trimming, and reshaping of structures that have been already been dissected free using blunt scissors; we usually recommend sharp scissors with flat handles to afford improved stability and precision. The sharp scissors are preferred when working under higher magnifications, where the straight blades and the sharp tip provide the surgeon with a better view of the entities being cut; this view can be obscured by the blunt tips and curved blades of dissecting scissors. However, close attention must be paid to using sharp scissors in order to avoid trauma to surrounding structures and tissues.

We recommend using blunt tipped microsurgical scissors to cut sutures from 10/0 to 12/0. Non-microsurgical scissors should be used to cut sutures 9/0 and lower. Other authors suggest having a third pair of scissors available and designated for cutting all suture, irrespective of suture size, while still others recommend that all microsurgical sutures above 8/0 should be cut using sharp microsurgical scissors.

Vascular clamps

In general, the duration of use of vascular clamps is suggested not to surpass 1 hour in order to avoid trauma to the vessel. Even when vascular clamps are said to be atraumatic (flat jaw surfaces), they produce histological lesions to the vascular walls.

There are clamps specific for arteries and others specific for veins. However, this distinction does not apply for clamps used in rats because of the small size of their vessels.

There are single and double clamps. All of the microsurgical techniques described in this book use Gilbert's double clamp (**Fig. 1-3**). Gilbert's double clamp is essentially composed of two microvascular clamps mounted on a double bar. The clamps can be moved along the bars, thus the distance between the clamps is adjustable; this delineates the length of the vessel between the clamps. The jaws of each clamp open and close by turning the head of a screw (right for tightening, left for loosening) with the use of a specific driver, thereby adjusting the pressure applied to the vessel wall.

Gilbert's double clamp is robust enough for use by the beginner in microsurgery. As expected, there is a learning curve in its application, especially in relation to pressure applied by the clamp jaws on the vessel. This double clamp is very useful for anastomoses performed on uneven surfaces, deep in the surgical field. After use, the double clamp requires meticulous cleaning to remove tissue debris and blood clots, with particular attention paid to cleaning debris not only from the jaws of the clamp, but also from the bars along which the clamps move, and from the screws which tighten the clamps.

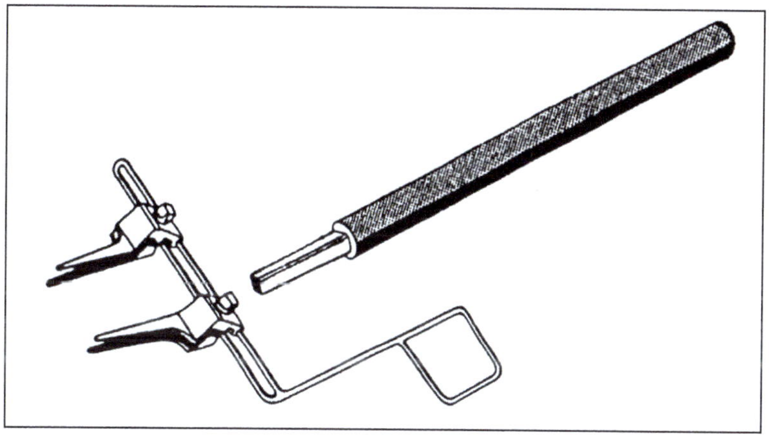

Figure 1-3

Gilbert's double vascular clamp (drawing), depicted with the driver for opening/closing the jaws of the clamps. (From Teot T, Dupoirieux L, Tassin X. Techniques d' Entrainement à la Microchirurgie. Montpellier: Sauramps Medical, 1991)

Diathermy

In the above catalog of laboratory equipment, the 'Monopolar diathermy, single use, battery operated (used in Opthalmology)' is listed, because of its relatively low cost. However, the diathermy of choice in microsurgery is the bipolar coagulator, as the monopolar diathermy produces a wider area of coagulation due to the spread of heat to surrounding tissues. Bipolar diathermy can more precisely be applied to vessels less than 1 mm in caliber, with appropriate adjustments in power. For vessels with a diameter greater than 1 mm, ligation with 6/0 or 7/0 suture is preferred. However, the trainee should keep in mind that veins are better ligated, irrespective of size.

The fine tips of the diathermy must be intact in order to coagulate small vessels with accuracy. Given that the tips are quite vulnerable, they must be inspected before beginning the operation. Finally, a replacement diathermy must be available in case of diathermy damage or malfunction.

Irrigation

In microsurgery, frequent irrigation of the surgical field with warm normal saline is necessary (although some microsurgeons prefer Ringer's Lactate). For irrigation, a 10 ml syringe is used, to which a 21 gauge (21G) angiocatheter, or smaller, is attached. We usually use a 27G venocatheter (abbocath). It is wise to have two such syringes on the table, so that at least one is available at any given moment.

A common joke in microsurgery is that we work 'underwater.' Periodical irrigation is important in order to keep tissues from desiccating during long microsurgical procedures; this is especially true for the edges of vessels to be anastomosed. Irrigation also eases the handling of sutures, which readily attach to tissues when the surgical field is dry (both because the suture is so thin and because of static electricity in the field). The adhesion of suture to the surrounding tissues can lead to breaking of the suture or tearing of the vessel edges during an anastomosis.

Aspiration

Absorption of fluid from the surgical field is performed using small handmade swabs of rolled gauze, prepared before the operation. These same swabs are also used for removing small clots.

The classic suction device utilized in macrosurgery is not used in microsurgery (not even with the smallest possible tip). With such powerful suction, there is a catastrophic risk of aspirating very thin vessels (at any stage of the procedure: whether they are dissected, undergoing anastomosis, or whether they have already been anastomosed).

Background material

Background material is placed under the vessels to be anastomosed, after they have been dissected free of the surrounding tissues. We use a piece of a surgical glove, with approximate dimensions 2 cm × 3 cm (varying according to the size of the surgical field). The light yellow color of the surgical glove offers a nice contrast with the vessels. Another solution is to use a similar piece of soft, plastic, yellow sheeting (preferably with a matte finish to avoid glare). Before placement behind the vessels, the background material must be moistened with warm normal saline.

Retractors

For use in the laboratory rat, we use retractors handmade from simple paper clips of various sizes. The paper clip is opened in the middle, and then one edge is bent twice with pliers at any angle (if we bend the paper clip using two, 90° angles, the edge of the retractor will be U-shaped). This U-shaped configuration is appropriate for keeping open the abdominal wall following a median incision (No. 1, **Fig 1-4**). However, the second angle of the paperclip may also be acute, or both angles can be acute, to create a retractor used in a median incision (No. 2, **Fig. 1-4**). To create a retractor aimed at retracting the edge of the liver or the spleen, the paper clip can be bent using an obtuse angle and a 90°angle (No. 3, **Fig. 1-4**). The bent edge of the retractor may be enveloped with gauze to be less traumatic. The other edge of these retractors is bound to an elastic band (No. 4, **Fig. 1-4**), which is adhered to the working surface with adhesive tape; the elastic band, with various degrees of stretchiness, allows for varying tensions to be applied to the opening of the abdominal wall or to retracting abdominal splanchna in the surgical field.

Microsurgical Sutures

The following guidelines can be used for choosing the

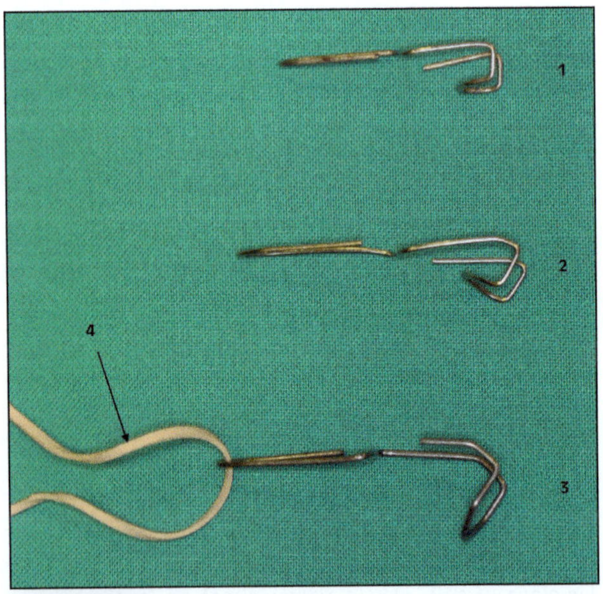

Figure 1-4

Hand made retractors from paper clips. **1.** U-shaped, two 90° bends, **2.** clip with two acute bends (alternatively, the 1st bend may be 90°, and the 2nd bend may be at an acute angle). Retractors No. 1 and No. 2 are usually applied to the edges of the insicion. **3.** clip with 1st bend of 90° and 2nd bend at an obtuse angle (e.g. for retracting a liver lobe or the spleen), **4.** elastic band bound to the clip, to be adhered to the working surface, allowing adjustable tension to be applied to the retractor. (From author's photo library).

appropriate size of suture in relation to the size of the vessel or nerve to be anastomosed:

Vessels
- **diameter <1 mm: 11/0**
- **diameter> 1 mm: 10/0**

Nerves
- **epineurium: 9/0 (or 10/0 if the diameter of the nerve is <1mm)**
- **perineurium: 10/0**

The needles of microsurgical sutures are round (in cross-section), atraumatic, 3-5 mm in length, and their arch length is 3/8 of a circle.

The sutures most often used in microsurgery are non-absorbable Nylon monofilaments (Ethilon, Ethicon). Table 1 shows the characteristics of sutures, ranging from 12/0 (smallest) to 9/0 (larger). This numbering of sutures is performed according to the American U.S.P. (United States Pharmocopeia) classification, while the metric system classifies the sutures according their diameter (measured in micrometers, μm or μ).

As can be seen in Table 1, the needle diameter is disproportionately larger than the suture diameter, which has been the main criticism of Nylon microsurgical sutures. The inequity of the two diameters is due to the construction of these sutures (i.e. how the end of the suture enters the base of the needle). As a result of this size mismatch, the hole in the vascular wall created by the needle is larger than the suture that is passed through it, leading to micro-leakages (happily, these do not appear to be surgically significant due to their rapid healing time. Additionally, the base of the needle is the area experiencing the greatest strain; therefore, surgical maneuvers often lead to deformation of the needle and/or rupture of the suture where it enters the needle's base.

Some microsurgeons use absorbable sutures such as:
- VICRYL: Its use reduces the inflammatory reaction (and necrosis) of vascular walls. For this reason, the risk of postoperative aneurysm is lessened.
- DEXON: This suture is more durable than Nylon; however, its blue-green color makes it difficult to use.
- PDS: The blue-purple color of this suture offers a nice contrast with entities within the surgical field. However, PDS has the disadvantage of high deformation memory, meaning that the suture does not easily straighten after manipulation, but can remain curled. Furthermore, surgical knots can be voluminous when using this suture.

Table 1. Characteristics of microsurgical sutures

No of suture	Needle diameter	Suture diameter	Needle length	Suture length
12/0	50 µ	14 µ	4,1 mm	13 cm
11/0	50 µ	18 µ	4,1 mm	13 cm
11/0	70 µ	18 µ	5,1 mm	13 cm
10/0	50 µ	22 µ	4,1 mm	13 cm
10/0	70 µ	22 µ	5,1 mm	13 cm
10/0	100 µ	22 µ	5,1 mm	13 cm
10/0	140 µ	22 µ	6,4 mm	45 cm
9/0	100 µ	35 µ	5,1 mm	13 cm
9/0	140 µ	35 µ	6,4 mm	45 cm

From: Teot T, Dupoirieux L, Tassin X. Techniques d' Entrainement à la Microchirurgie. Montpellier: Sauramps Medical, 1991.

Maintenance of microsurgical instruments

Immediately after every use, microsurgical instruments must be placed in a cup full of heparinized normal saline, to remove any adherent blood clots. Careful attention must be paid to prevent instruments from touching one another, especially at their delicate tips. To this end, a piece of soft elastic material should cover the bottom of the cup, which assists with suspension of the instruments in the heparinized solution, while minimizing the chance of accidental impacts that will deform the tips of the instruments.

At the end of the operation, all microsurgical instruments must be cleaned thoroughly, and a small soft brush and warm normal saline are useful to wash them of debris. Cleaning must be done very meticulously, removing any tissue debris and blood clots from the fine tips. Particular attention should be paid to brushing not only the delicate tips, but also to other specialized parts, such as articulations, screws, the bars of the double clamps, etc. Obviously, during this procedure all tips and jaws of scissors, needle holders, and forceps—i.e., any kind of grasping or holding instrument—must be wide open, in order to be cleaned appropriately. Following cleaning, these instruments are then left to dry, open, on a smooth surface covered with absorptive paper. Finally, the instruments are polished by a soft cotton cloth to remove any marks that may remain from washing.

It is very important to cover the tips of the instruments with a small plastic cylinder (which can be handmade from an intravenous line tubing) before re-stocking them in their case. Instruments should be stored in a stainless steel case lined with silicone rubber, with finger mats which keep the instruments immobile and separated from both each other and from the walls of the case.

The case containing the instruments is sterilized with the cover left open. A flash sterilization of 20 minutes duration is adequate for use in a human; however, this step is not necessary for use with laboratory rats.

From time to time, the instruments should be lubricated with an oil designed for maintenance of surgical instruments. Requests for sharpening and further repairs need to be addressed to the manufacturer.

Handling of microsurgical instruments

- Microsurgical instruments should be held using a pencil grasp. This handling offers stability while performing microsurgical dissection and anastomoses.
- Instruments with rounded handles (e.g., Barraquer needle holders) are rolled between the tips of the thumb and the index finger.
- Short microsurgical instruments (11-14 cm) are best handled with the thumb, index and middle finger; if the instruments are longer (greater than 14 cm) they are supported within the thenar space.

  Please note, the handling of microsurgical instruments is quite different from the handling of macrosurgical instruments, which are controlled more by motion at the wrist.
- Grasping the needle of microsurgical sutures with the needle holder requires specific attention: the needle must be grasped in the middle of its arch. If the ne-

edle is held near the tip, rotation is difficult; if the needle is held more towards the end of the arch, the user risks deforming the needle with the effort required to pass the needle through the tissue.

- If the needle lies upon a flexible surface in the surgical field (i.e., upon tissue), a useful trick is to first grasp the needle in the middle its arch before pressing it gently against the underlying surface, without completely closing the jaws of the needle holder, thereby allowing the needle to rotate. This maneuver should rotate the direction of the needle, allowing it to then, easily, be grasped correctly.
- If the needle lies on a surface that is incompressible, the maneuver described above cannot be applied; the user is then required to grasp the needle with forceps in order to appropriately load it on the needle holder.
- If the suture is new, and still in its pack, the needle holder should always be used to grasp the needle in the middle of its arch.

In all of the circumstances described above, the jaws of the needle holder should be perpendicular to the long axis of the needle. The needle should be grasped and immobilized in the jaws, with the needle set approximately 1 mm from the edge of the tips of the needle holder.

C. Microsurgeon positioning & posture

1. In the laboratory

For the duration of all microsurgical procedures, the elbows and the arms of the microsurgeon should rest comfortably on the armrests of their chair and/or upon the bench on which their working surface is found (the armrests of the chair are brought at the height of the working surface). The continuous contact of the surgeon's arms with either the bench and/or the working surface is necessary for eliminating (or at least minimizing) hand tremors.

The microsurgeon should sit with a straight back (comfortably supported by the back of the chair) and with relaxed shoulders. Both feet should be placed flat on the floor and their posture must be relaxed, facilitating the proper positioning of the arms on the working surface (as described above). To this end, the height of the seat of the chair should be adjusted according to each surgeon's physical requirements. The goal of the surgeon's positioning is to place the elbows at the height of the working surface, with the upper arms found at right angles to the forearms. The personalized positioning of the microscope will follow (described in Chapter 2).

While satisfying the above requirements, the assistant's positioning should also be comfortable. The best placement of the two surgeons (either co-surgeons or surgeon and trainee) is opposite from one another, facing each other across the surgical field.

The microsurgical instruments are always arranged in the same order, and at an ergonomic position found adjacent to the working surface, prior to starting the operation. Classical surgical instruments are placed separately, but also in a specific order and in an ergonomic, easily accessible position.

2. In the operating room

As in the laboratory, the microsurgeon operates while seated in an armchair (preferably an armchair, but at least a chair with a back), and the same applies for the assistant or co-surgeon. The surgeons' arms should be steady while resting on the patient's body, with the forearms always held at a right angle to the body. In the operating room, a firm surface for the surgeons' arms to rest upon is not as readily available as it is in the laboratory, and attention must also be paid to prevent the arms of the surgeons from placing undue pressure on the patient, and from interfering with intravenous lines, catheters, ECG cables, ground cords, etc.

Adjusting the height of the surgeons' chairs and of the table must be done prior to starting any operation. In making these adjustments, table and chair height should be based upon the needs of the primary surgeon, while also attempting to accommodate the comfort of the co-surgeon or assistant. The adjustment of the height of the head of the surgical microscope will be discussed in Chapter 2.

For most microsurgical procedures, the surgical procedure begins as a classical surgery (macrosurgery), transitions to the microsurgical portion of the case, and is then continued and completed as a macrosurgical case. The microsurgical instruments are therefore prepared and arranged on a separate table, in ergonomic position in relation to the primary surgeon. It is useful to remember that the personnel within the operating room usually have no microsurgical training, and might therefore need continuous guidance regarding the handling of microsurgical instruments. For the sake of the integrity of the microsurgical instruments which are often the surgeon's personal belongings, the assistant or the surgeon himself (despite his/her fatigue) will frequently undertake the task of cleaning and storing the microsurgical instruments following completion of the operation.

2 The surgical microscope

This Chapter describes the basic steps for adjusting a surgical microscope; for details on the fine adjustments of your surgical microscope, please study the microscope's specific instruction manual.

The surgical microscope is a very intricate, large, and expensive device. Etymologically, the term 'microscope' comes from the Greek 'mikros', meaning 'small', and 'skopion', which is derived from the verb 'skopein', meaning 'to look, see'. The surgical microscope is therefore the instrument used for 'viewing and operating upon that which is small'; thus, it is an indispensable tool for microsurgery.

The surgeon's familiarity with the surgical microscope is of extreme importance for the sucess of an operation. It is imperative that the surgeon understands the microscope's basic functions, is adept in the use of the individual controls (focus, zoom, etc.), and takes the necessary precautions during use of the microscope. For these reasons, it is suggested that the surgeon read not only this introductive Chapter, but also the instruction manual that accompanies the microscope, while also spending the appropriate time to familiarize himself/herself with the microscope's use. If the microsurgeon lacks mastery of his/her microscope, the microsurgical operation can be exhausting, and handling minuscule anatomic entities can become cumbersome, posing catastrophic risks.

A. Principles of function

The surgical microscope is a complex instrument which consists of a combination of optical elements, providing the surgeon with a stereoscopic, high quality, magnified image of the small structures of the surgical field. The optical elements found in the head of the microscope and their arrangements are shown in **Figure 2-1.**

The following description follows the path of light from the object of interest to the eyes of the surgeon. Light from the object first passes through the lenses of the *focus system* (objective lens) (No. 1, **Fig. 2-1**). The distance between the focus system (objective lens) and the magnification system (No. 3, **Fig. 2-1**), which is found next in the light's path (see below), is adjusted by turning the *focus control knob* (No. 2, **Fig. 2-1**). The *focal distance,* or *working distance,* (i.e. the distance between the object and the objective lens within which the microscope can focus) is restricted, and in most surgical microscopes ranges from 20 cm to 40 cm. If the working distance is less than 20 cm or greater than 40 cm the microscope cannot focus on this object, and the head of the microscpe must be adjusted in order to place the object within the microscope's working distance. When this is achieved, it is possible to adjust the focus upon the object using the focus control knob.

As can be seen in **Figure 2-1**, the focus system (objective lens) is composed of one unit, and is the common starting place for light entering the surgical microscope. However, after passing through the objective lens, the beam of light is subsequently split. All of the optical components following the objective lens are therefore twinned, with duplicate components guiding each beam of light toward each of the surgeon's eyes.

Following the focus system, the *magnification system* (No. 3, **Fig. 2-1**) is comprised of a series of lenses, both converging and diverging, arranged in a specific order. The magnification system is adjusted by using the *magnification control knob* (No. 4, **Fig. 2-1**) (please bear in mind that there are actually two magnification control knobs on most stereotactic surgical microscopes, one on either side of the head). The knobs controlling the magnification turn together, both clockwise and counterclockwise, and stop at positions that bear the designations 0.4, 0.6, 1.6, and 2.5. The magnification control knob is used to adjust, in a stepwise fashion, the distance between the lenses of the magnification system. In this way, the image of the object appears larger or smaller to the eyes of the surgeon.

A common fallacy is that the designation found on the magnification control knob represents the actual magnification of the objects on the surgical field. While the author of this text once wondered why the 2.5 designation of the surgical microscope provided significantly greater magnification than his, albeit cheap, 2.5× loupes, he later learned that the true magnification afforded by the surgical microscope is a composite effect of *all* of the lenses of the magnification system. For this reason, the true magnification of the objects on the surgical field can be calculated only by using an equation specific to each surgical microscope-the inputs of which include numerous parameters, only one of which is the designation found on the control knob.

Instead of the mechanical magnification control knob (with the preset positions described above), many modern surgical microscopes use an electronic system of magnification adjustement (i.e., a motorized 'zoom'). The motorized 'zoom' feature is controlled by pressing one of two buttons that act to seamlessly increase or decrease the effective magnification. While a surgical microscope equipped with a motorized zoom system has the disadvantage of taking up more space and increasing the height of the microscope (which thereby narrows the operable working distance) the 'zoom' fea-

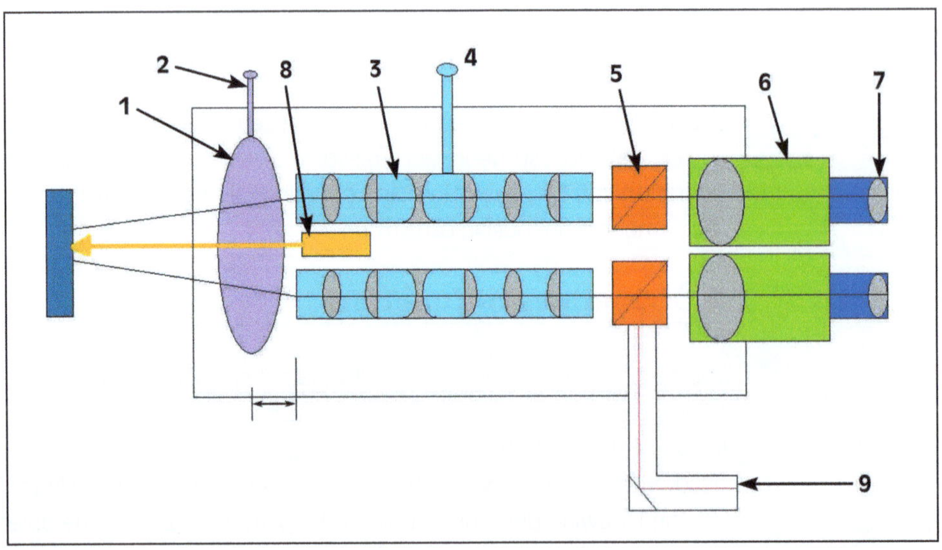

Figure 2-1

Diagrammatic representation of the arrangement of the optical components within the head of the surgical microscope. The yellow arrow shows the course of light from the light source to the surgical field. The two continuous lines passing through all of the lenses and prisms depict the optical path of light from the surgical field to each eye. The two-way arrow indicates the adjustable distance between focus system and magnification system (i.e., the focus control). **1.** focus system (objective lens), **2.** focus control knob, **3.** magnification system, **4.** magnification control knob, **5.** prisms, for bending of the optical path, **6.** binocular tube system, **7.** eyepiece, **8.** light source, **9.** outlet allowing for co-observation, videography, or photography (Diagram: E. Kontis) ture allows for swift, seamless magnification changes whithout the 'blackouts' experienced when shifting between settings on a manual surgical microscope. In our opinion, the advantages of a motorized 'zoom' feature far outweigh the minor impact of the increased height of the surgical microscope.

After leaving the aforementioned magnification system, the path of light through most surgical microscopes then travels through *prisms* (No. 5, **Fig. 2-1**). These prisms permit an image to pass through them, while bending the image at a specific angle, allowing for the addition of a *co-observation system* (No. 9, **Fig. 2-1**), a video camera, or a photography camera (these prisms have an angle of deviation of 90°).

Next in the path of light through the surgical microscope is the *tube system* (No. 6, **Fig. 2-1**) (often mentioned as *binocular tubes*), followed by the *eyepiece* (ocular lens) (No. 7, **Fig. 2-1**). The binocular tubes also contain multiple lenses that act to orient the image as it travels from the objective lens (focus system) to the ocular lens (eyepiece).

The total course of the light from the objects on the surgical field to the eye–through the focus system, the magnification system, the binocular tubes, and through the eyepieces of the surgical microscope–is known as the *optical path* of the object.

The surgical microscope offers a *stereoscopic view*, meaning the surgeon is afforded a three-dimensional view of the surgical field. This three-dimensional view is provided when the surgical microscope directs one of the two optical paths from the surgical field into each eyepiece, respectively. This binocular viewing system creates two slightly offset images of the object, due to the different positioning of the observer's eyes in their head; this provides a perception of depth (stereopsis). General speaking, there are two types of stereoscopic microscopes: the one most commonly used in surgical microscopes has a single objective lens, followed by two parallel paths of light from the magnification sysetm to the eyepieces; this system is referred to as telescope system (**Fig. 2-1**). The other type of microscope has two objective lens (i.e. two, independent optical paths) and is mostly used in examination microscopes, and is referred to as a Greenough's system.

When passing through the prisms, the light from the surgical field is deviated from its original path. If the light from only one optical path is deviated toward the co-observation tube (as in **Figure 2-1**), the co-observation tube is only able to provide a two-dimensional image of the surgical field; in this case, either a monocular tube or binocular tubes can be attached to the accessory outlet of the microscope, but without stereopsis. If both optical paths are deviated, then the image is viewed through binocular tubes and is three-dimensional, allowing for the assistance of a co-surgeon. The existence of a second system of binocular tubes does not mean that they are stereoscopic; this can only be understood if ones looks through these binoculars.

Surgical microscopes are illuminated by a *cold light source* (No. 8, **Fig. 2-1**). Cold light sources utilize fiberoptic cables to deliver light to the operative field; the light source is most commonly located elsewhere (as in the base of the microscope). The light path is coaxial to the optical path, in order to avoid casting shadows onto the surgical field. Cold light sources provide a brighter source of illumination when compared to the alternative light sources (direct light sources). The heat emitted by direct light sources can interfere with the image produced by the microscope.

However, the 'cold light' is not truly cold: it is only slightly cooler than directly transmitted light. Therefore, attention should be paid toward minimizing extended, direct exposure of unprotected tissues to the 'cold light' in order to avoid the heating and desiccation of tissue. To this end, frequent irrigation of the surgical field is necessary (irrigation is also necessary in order to avoid adhesion of microsurgical sutures to tissues, as discussed in Chapter 1).

Given that the light reflected by the objects of the surgical field composes the image presented by the surgical microscope, the microscope can 'function' using only normal room lighting, without the aid of additional illumination. However, surgical microscopes require a focused, intense light source, and this need is further increased as the magnification is increased. Often, a surgeon will experience the sensation that the lights have dimmed as he/she has increased the magnification of the surgical field. This subjective 'dimming' is the result of increased loss of light due to refraction, which occurs when the distance between the lenses of the magnification system is increased. Therefore, when using greater degrees of magnification, the surgeon may want to concomitantly increase the intensity of the light provided by the light source.

B. Basic components of the surgical microscope - Types of surgical microscopes

The surgical microscope is comprised of three basic

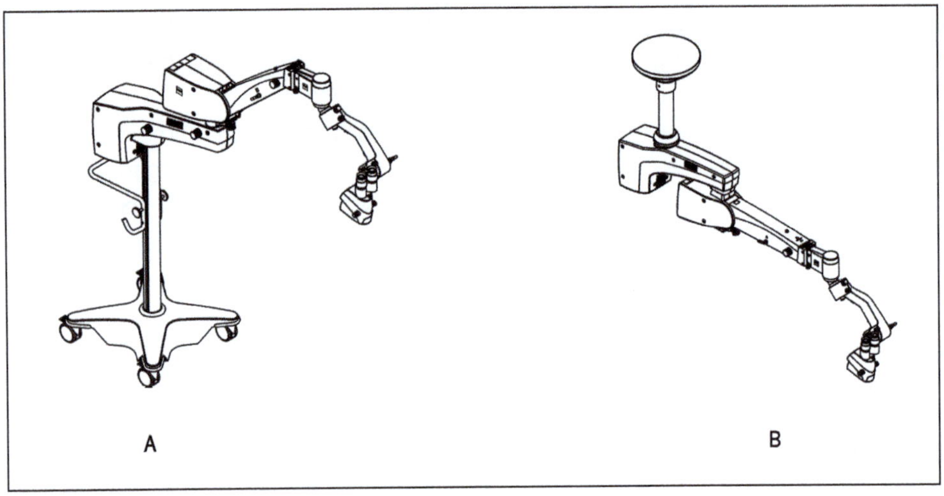

Figure 2-2

Types of surgical microscopes according to the mounting of the base. **A.** Mobile, mounted on a floor stand. **B.** Ceiling-mounted. (From: OPMI Movena Surgical Microscope on S7 Suspension Systems, Instructions for use, Carl Zeiss Surgical GmbH, 73446 Oberkochen, Germany, 2007)

components: the head, the articulated arm which suspends the head, and the base to which the arm is attached. Depending on the mounting of the base, microscopes can either be on a mobile floor stand or immobile (ceiling-mounted or wall-mounted) (**Fig. 2-2**).

Of the two designs, surgical microscopes mounted on mobile floor stands are the most frequently found. These surgical microscopes are set upon a stand with a rolling base, equipped with brakes to enable immobilization of the microscope (**Fig. 2-2A**).

Ceiling-mounted surgical microscopes have an immobile base suspended from the ceiling of the operating room or laboratory (**Fig. 2-2B**). Thus, the base of the microscope is fixed and only the arm and the head of the microscope are mobile. Ceiling-mounted surgical microscopes occupy less space in the operating room, but afford the surgeon less freedom than the mobile surgical microscopes on floor stands. Ceiling-mounted surgical microscopes are designed for procedures requiring a specific position of the surgeon, such as eye surgery or neurosurgery, whereas wall-mounted microscopes (where the base of the microscope is suspended on a wall) are often of the simplest design, and used for training in schools of microsurgery.

The mobile surgical microscope, mounted on a floor stand, is (as mentioned above) is the type most commonly used by microsurgeons in the laboratory and operating room. The mobile surgical microscope is comprised of the following parts (**Fig. 2-3**):

- By necessity, the base is the heaviest part of the microscope. Its weight serves to stabilize the microscope and minimize vibration. The base also houses the light source and is usually where the power switch is located.
- The articulated arm is usually made up of two, smaller arms. The articulated arm serves to both suspend and move the head of the microscope in all directions over the surgical field; the range of motion can be greater than 1.5 m in the horizontal plane (depending on the microscope), more than 60 cm in the vertical plane, and allows a 360° rotation around the vertical axis of the base. The articulated arm also includes a system to minimize vibration, offering improved stability to the head of the microscope. Furthermore, the articulations of the arm automatically re-stabilize when the head of the microscope is adjusted to another position.
- The head is the most important and delicate part of the surgical microscope, as it includes the optical apparatus requisite for the basic functions of the microscope (focus, magnification, stereoscopic vision). The buttons and knobs that control the basic functions of the surgical microscope are also found on the head, and the surgeon should be familiar with their position in order to effortlessly reach them during the operation, preferably without taking his/her eyes away from the eyepieces.

C. Accessories

Although mentioned as accessories, the items described below are necessary components of a surgical microscope. Found on the head of the microscope are two accessory outlets (**Fig. 2-4**) that can be used to add:

- a system for co-observation or assisted surgery (as described above)
- a photo camera or video camera, ideally connected to a computer capable of recording and/or projecting the operation onto a larger screen.

The surgeon can connect these accessories to the available outlets. If needed, the system for co-observa-

Figure 2-3

A typical mobile surgical microscope, mounted on a floor stand. **1.** floor stand, **2.** base of the microscope, **3.** articulated arm for suspension of the head, **4.** head, **5.** binoculars for co-observation/co-surgery, **6.** power switch. (Modified from: http://www.optos.com/Products/Medical-surgical-devices/Surgical-Microscopes)

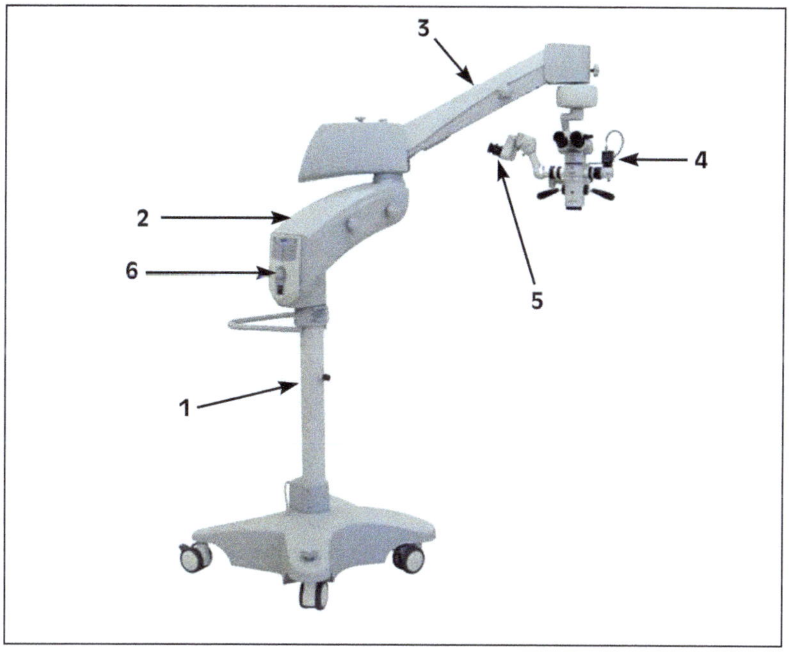

tion or assisted surgery can be removed from an outlet and replaced by an additional system for recording images or movies.

D. Basic functions

- Power switch (No. 6, **Fig. 2-3**): This switch is usually found on either the base or the articulated arm. In some models the same switch has a potentiometer function, allowing the surgeon to adjust the light source's intensity.
- Setting the tilt angle of the microscope to achieve the best viewing position: This is done by turning a knob that is typically found on the front end of the arm (or on the articulation between the arm and the head of the microscope). This is a gross adjustment that might need to be further fine-tuned after obtaining a clear vision of the surgical field. In the laboratory, the tilt angle of the microscope is usually fixed for each species of animal that is operated on. In the operating room, the tilt angle is one of the very first settings the surgeon should seek to adjust at the start of each case (with the exception being if he/she operates consistently on the same part of the body).
- Setting the interpupillary distance: In modern surgical microscopes, this can be accomplished by turning a knob (No. 1, **Fig. 2-5A**). When using simple training microscopes, the surgeon or trainee has to manually adjust the distance between the binocular tubes. The correct interpupillary distance has been set when the separate images delivered by the eyepieces merge into a single, clear image.
- Eyecups and diopter settings (No. 2, **Fig. 2-5A**): The eyecups should be adjusted in such a way that the surgeon is able to obtain a full, focused view of the surgical field. If a surgeon requires eyeglasses or contact lenses, but does not wish to use them when operating with the surgical microscope, he/she should begin adjusting the ring controlling the diopter setting by screwing in the eyecups (toward the microscope, to their fullest extent). While looking through the eyepieces, the surgeon should then slowly unscrew

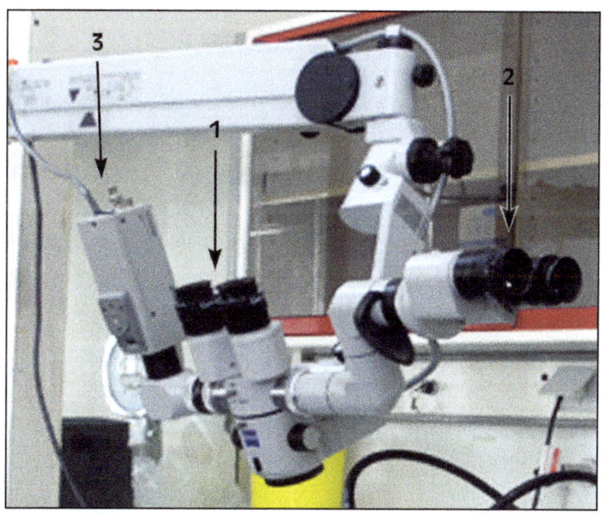

Figure 2-4

The head of the surgical microscope. **1.** surgeon's binocular eyepieces, **2.** binocular eyepieces allowing for co-observation or co-surgery, **3.** video camera. (From author's photo library)

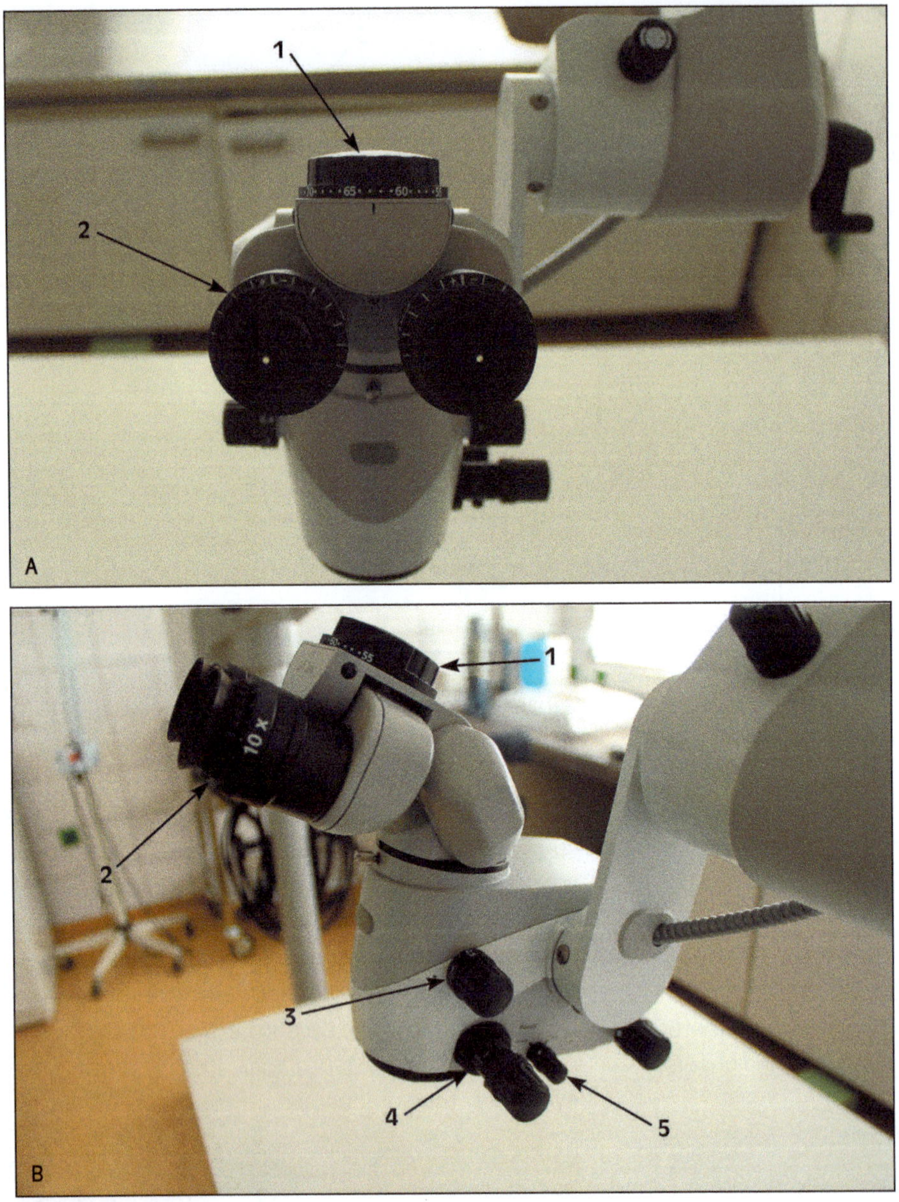

Figure 2-5

Photo of the head of the surgical microscope showing the controls of basic functions of the surgical microscope. **A.** Frontal view. **B.** Lateral view. **1.** knob for adjusting the interpupillary distance, **2.** ring controlling the diopter setting, **3.** magnification control knob, **4.** focus control knob, **5.** focus lock knob. (From author's photo library)

the eyecups (away from the microscope) until he/she is able to clearly see the full field of view. If the surgeon prefers wearing his/her eyeglasses or contact lenses, the diopter ring should be set to 0. The eyepieces of surgical microscopes are typically able to correct for refractive errors that range from -8 D (Diopters) to +5 D, depending upon the microscope.

- Magnification control knob (No. 3, Fig. **2-5B**).
- Focus control knob (No. 4, **Fig. 2-5B**).
- Control of light intensity: This is a potentiometer, whose position may vary based on the brand or type of microscope. As previously mentioned, the control of the light source intensity is usually found on the base of the microscope, often near or combined with the power switch; however, it can also be located on the arm of the surgical microscope.

Some surgical microscopes are equipped with additional controls. The surgeon must be aware of where they are, what they do, and how to safely and effectively utilize them. A few examples include (but are not limited to):

- Power switch for the accessory lamp, in the event of primary lamp failure.
- Focus lock knob (No. 5, **Fig. 2-5B**), which isolates the focus control knob (preventing the focus from changing despite possibly incidental turning of the focus control knob).
- Knob for adjusting the width of the illuminated field. Changing the width of the illuminated field is achieved by adjusting the width of the diaphragm located in front of the light source.

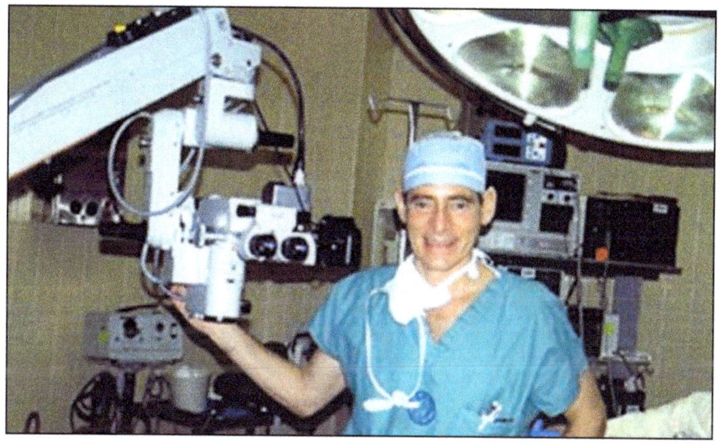

Figure 2-6

Marc Goldstein with his surgical microscope at New York Hospital- Cornell Medical Center (From: www.maleinfertility.org/new-varicocelectomy.html)

E. Personalized adjustment of the surgical microscope

Microsurgical procedures can be both long and exhausting. The microsurgeon, more than any other surgeon, must have a comfortable, ergonomic working environment. Therefore, it is necessary to optimize and individualize the microscope settings for the principle surgeon. This process includes many adjustments, from gross positioning of the microscope to fine tuning of the focus. The author has frequently found himself bemoaning when younger co-workers or students have changed something on 'his' microscope. Most likely, the readers will also develop a similar affectionate relationship with their surgical microscope. Photos can often be found of famous microsurgeons, seen smiling and hugging their trusty microscope (**Fig. 2-6**).

Positioning of the surgical microscope in the laboratory or operating room

The surgical microscope is usually positioned on the non-dominant side of the surgeon (i.e., for right-handed surgeons, the microscope is positioned on the surgeon's left side). The microsurgical instruments are then typically positioned on the surgeon's dominant side, so that the arm and the head of the surgical microscope do not obstruct the surgeon's view of his/her instruments.

The microscope should be far enough from the surgical field to allow for comfortable, unhindered working. If microsurgery is performed under aseptic conditions (as in the operating room), the arm of the microscope should be directed away from the sterile field. A simple, empirical rule to follow is that the distance between the head and the base of the microscope should be equal to the length of the surgeon's upper limb (as demonstrated in **Figure 2-7**), allowing the surgeon to

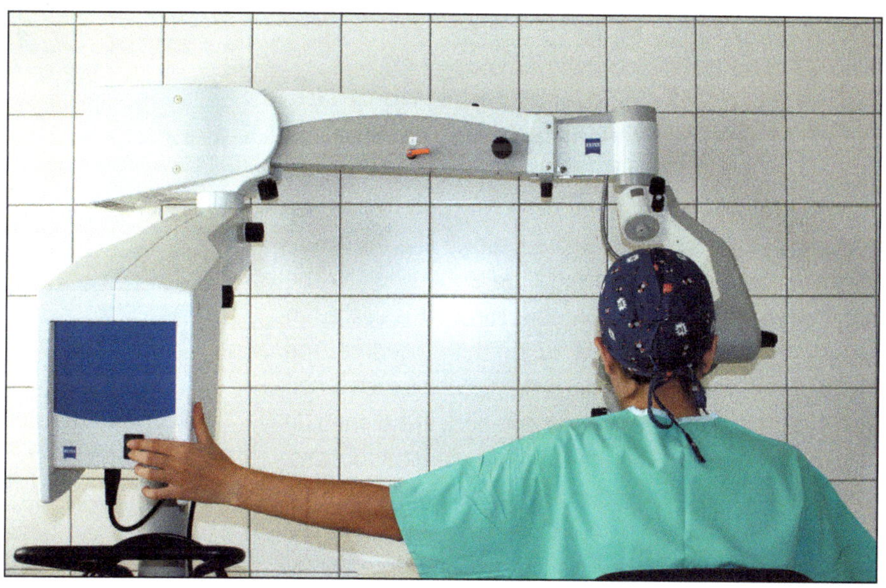

Figure 2-7

The distance between the head and the base of the microscope should be set equal to the length of the surgeon's upper limb. (From author's photo library)

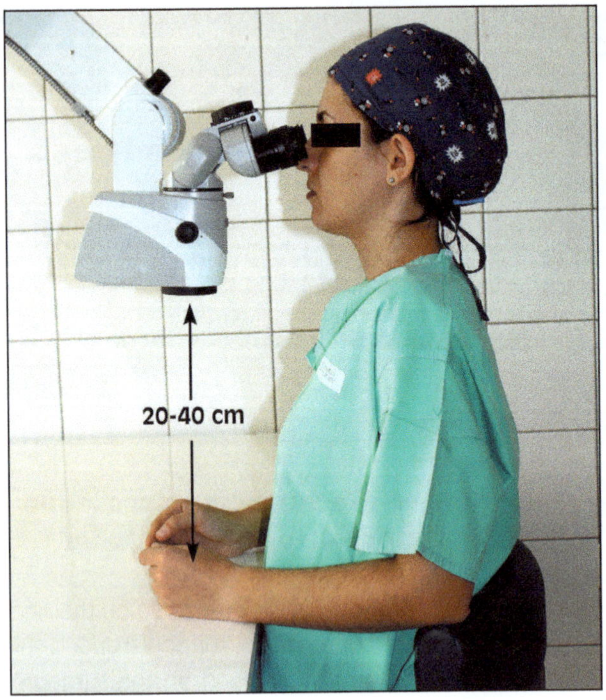

Figure 2-8

The surgeon, while in appropriate working postion. The head and the spine should be aligned. The arms should be horizontal. The elbows rest on the arms of the chair, which should be adjusted to the same height as the working surface. (From author's photo library)

easily reach the switches found on the base of the surgical microscope.

When moving the surgical microscope, it is safest to push or pull the base of the surgical microscope (at the level of the floor stand), engaging the wheel brakes after each move will further stabilize the microscope. Specific attention should be paid to avoid striking or bumping the head of the surgical microscope while either adjusting it or moving it.

Adjustment of the distance between the head of the microscope and surgical field

Adjusting the positioning of the head of the microscope over the surgical field must be done prior to the start of the operation, while the surgeon is seated in the position he will maintain during the procedure. The head of the microscope should be placed at such a height so that the surgeon's head and back are aligned, in order to avoid fatiguing the surgeon's cervical muscles. The distance of the head of the microscope from the surgical field is usually 20-40 cm, because this is the usual range of the focal distance (working distance) of most surgical microscopes (**Fig. 2-8**). If this distance needs to be maximized, the head of the microscope should be set 40 cm above the surgical field, and the seat of the surgeon's armchair may need to be elevated, with the arms lowered to the level of the surgical field (as seen in **Fig. 2-9**). Alternatively, if the working distance needs to be minimized, the surgeon's chair will need to be lowered, while the arms of the chair may need to be elevated. Regardless, when working within the focal distance of the surgical microscope, the microsurgeon should not hesitate to change the height of either the seat or the arms of his/her chair to suit his/her needs.

When working in the laboratory with rats, the adjustment of the head of the microscope is done in reference to the height of the working surface. Because the rat's body is narrow, the distance from the surgical field to the working surface is minimal (only a few centimeters). In contrast, in the operation room, the width of a

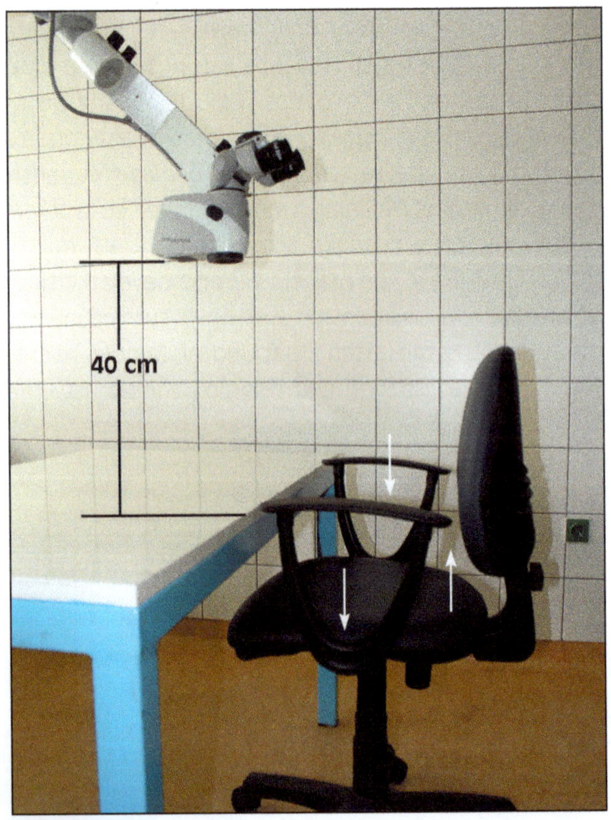

Figure 2-9

Adjustment of working position at the maximum focal (working) distance. With the head of the microscope set at 40cm from the working surface (or from the surgical field with the rat appropriately positioned), the seat of the chair may need to be elevated (as indicated by the upward arrow), and the arms of the chair may need to be lowered to the level of the working surface (as indicated by the downward arrows). (From author's photo library) human body is far from negligible; the adjustment of the head of the microscope must be performed with the patient on the table, allowing for consideration of the depth of the surgical field during the planned operation.

Adjustment of the optical path

In order to obtain the optimal view of the detailed, miniscule structures of the surgical field, it is necessary to correctly adjust the parameters of the optical path. The optical path is appropriately adjusted when it is possible to obtain a crisp, clear image of all components of the surgical field, at any magnification. Before proceeding with adjusting the optical path, please ensure that you have identified the position of the following: 1) the knob that controls the distance between the eyepieces (interpupillary distance), 2) the diopter setting, 3) the magnification control knob, and 4) the focus control knob.

The adjustment of the parameters of the optical path is performed before the operation, in the following order:

1. Set the magnification control knob to the lowest designation.
2. Adjust the distance of the eyepieces in order to view a single, complete image of the surgical field (No. 1, **Fig. 2-5A**).
3. In microscopes with a ring controlling the diopter setting (No. 2, **Fig. 2-5A**):
   - Surgeons not wearing eyeglasses or contact lenses should set the ring to 0.
   - Surgeons operating with their eyeglasses or contact lenses should also set the ring to 0.
   - Surgeons requiring the use of corrective lenses, who will be operating without their eyeglasses or contact lenses, should set each diopter according the degree of correction needed for the corresponding eye. For example, if a surgeon requires 3 degrees of correction for myopia of the left eye and 2.5 degrees of correction for myopia of the right eye, the surgeon should set the left diopter setting to +3 and the right diopter setting to +2.5.

   If the microscope does not have rings controlling the diopter settings, surgeons requiring corrective lenses should wear their glasses or contact lenses in order to operate.
4. Next, set the magnification control knob (No. 3, **Fig. 2-5B**) to the highest designation and then adjust the focus control (No. 4, **Fig. 2-5B**) until you are able to see the details of objects on the surgical field (e.g. letters and numbers on a key).

   Bear in mind, when the magnification is changed, the focus must be re-adjusted using the focus control knob (No. 4, **Fig. 2-5B**).

3

Pre-operative preparation, anesthesia and post-operative care of the laboratory rat

A. Pre-operative alimentation

Pre-operative fasting is not necessary when using rats as the operative subjects, as vomiting does not occur in rats. In contrast, pre-operative fasting is required when using several other species as operative subjects (dog, cat, pig, etc.), in order to reduce associated vomiting.

However, fasting is recommended for the 12-24 hours prior to surgery when surgery on the digestive system is planned for the rats, so that the gastrointestinal tract is as empty as possible prior to instrumentation. In these cases, it is wise to give the rats a glucose solution in order to avoid hypoglycemia. If surgery is planned on the liver, specific attention should be paid to the metabolic state of the animal.

B. Anesthesia

Anesthesia of the laboratory rat includes two phases:

1. Induction in anesthesia

Induction of anesthesia is performed using either ether (as described here) or other volatile anesthetics, e.g., halothane or isoflurane. To begin, the ether is poured into a cylindrical, wide-mouthed container made of glass, with a cap (e.g. jar). Before introducing the rat in to the container, a compact and absorptive piece of cotton wool is placed over the ether to prevent the rat from coming into direct contact with the ether. The effects of direct contact with the ether can be detrimental to the rat, to the point of producing fatal shock. Care must be taken to ensure that the rat stays on top of the cotton pad and does not 'tunnel' under it, thereby coming into contact with the ether.

The rat will need to stay in the jar for several minutes; after approximately 3-4 minutes it will be seen to slump down. At this stage, if the rat makes no attempt to raise or move its head when the jar is tilted, the rat is considered adequately anesthetized and can be removed from the jar. There is a risk for respiratory arrest when using ether for induction because the ether suppresses the respiratory center of the medulla oblongata; therefore, the surgeon must closely observe the rat the entire time that it is kept in the jar. Close attention should also be paid in order to avoid keeping the rat in the jar for longer than is necessary-the aim of induction anesthesia is only to achieve a level of anesthesia that will permit the administration (by injection) of the medications used to maintain anesthesia for the duration of the operation.

The best way to understand whether the rat is adequately anesthetized is to observe the rat's vibrissae, which are the longer and thicker hairs near the nose and the upper lip of the rat (mystacial vibrissae, also called whiskers). In the rat, the vibrissae are sensory organs for orientation, and have a rich innervation. When the rat is alert, vibrissae can move in either a random or coordinated manner. However, when anesthesia is achieved, the vibrissae stop moving. This cessation of movement of the vibrissae is the sign that the rat should be removed from the jar containing the ether.

Two points must be emphasized: 1) The anesthetic effect of ether is attained quickly, but also subsides rapidly. Therefore, the syringe with the maintenance anesthetic medications, which will be the next medications administered, must be ready before the rat is placed in the jar. 2) When the rat demonstrates that it is anesthetized (by cessation of all vibrissae movement), it has already inhaled a substantial quantity of ether and is near the point of respiratory arrest; therefore, the rat should be immediately removed from the jar when vibrissae movement halts.

2. Maintenance of anesthesia

Anesthesia is maintained by intramuscular injection of a combination of ketamine hydrochloride and chlorpromazine hydrochloride; this particular anesthetic combination ensures a depth of anesthesia suitable for proceeding with surgery.

Ketamine belongs to the group of general anesthesia drugs and is a lipophilic drug metabolized in the liver, which produces a 'dissociative state' whereby the rats are observed to appear awake, but are without consciousness and feel no pain. Ketamine causes deep analgesia and amnesia, without affecting the laryngeal reflexes and respiratory cycle; therefore, no endotracheal intubation is required. However, ketamine can increase arterial pressure and muscle tone due to associated central nervous system sympathetic stimulation.

Chlorpromazine is a phenothiazine, belonging to the family of typical antipsychotic drugs that act as antagonists of dopamine receptors, but which also has anticholinergic, antihistaminic and antiadrenergic actions. It is also lipophilic and metabolized in the liver. Chlorpromazine acts as a sedative, with this activity exacerbated by the concomitant administration of anesthetics.

The recommended dosages for preparation of the maintenance anesthetic mixture, for application in the rat, are:

- 44-100 mg ketamine/kg of weight (intramuscular administration, i.m.)
- 3-35 mg chlorpromazine/kg of weight (i.m.)

More precisely, after much experience, the dosages that we use are:

- **50 mg ketamine/kg of weight (i.m.)**
- **15 mg chlorpromazine/kg of weight (i.m.)**

➢ Always have a syringe, filled with at least one repeat dose, available in the event the initial sedation wears off.

Preparation of this anesthetic solution is very simple: using the labels on the vials of ketamine and chlorpromazine, identify the concentration of each drug (the number of milligrams present in each mL of solution). Taking into consideration the recommended dosages for the anesthesia, as described above, calculate how many mL of each of the two solutions are required given the weight of the rat. Then, using one syringe, aspirate the calculated volume of each drug to produce the desired mixture of the drugs. It is advisable to change needles before aspirating from a vial containing a different drug, in order to avoid mixing of the drugs in the other vials.

Other recommended drug combinations are:

- ketamine (i.m.) – midazolam (4 mg/kg, intraperitoneal or subcutaneous)
- ketamine – xylazine (2.5 mg/kg); both intraperitoneal

The best site for intramuscular administration is the external surface of the thigh, because of the muscular architecture of the rear limb (**Fig. 3-1**). After the needle is inserted into the muscles, aspiration must preceed injection in order to verify that the anesthetic solution will not be administered into a vessel.

Surgical anesthesia is achieved in only a few minutes and lasts for approximately three hours. If longer anesthesia is required, one-third (1/3) of the initial anesthetic dose can be repeated. The repeat dose should be prepared at the same time as the initial dose, and the syringe containing it should be available on the table next to the instruments. Thus, if the rat awakes during the operation, the surgeon will be prepared to immediately inject additional anesthetic. Until this injection again takes effect, a mask containing ether can be used. The easiest way to create such a mask is to place a piece of

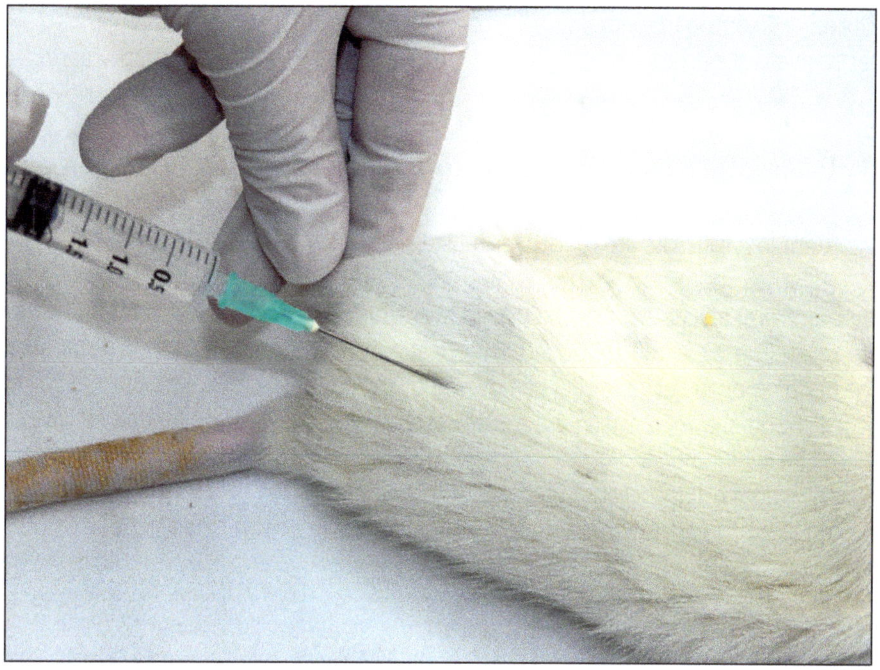

Figure 3-1

In the rat, the ideal site for intramuscular injection of anesthetic medications is the lateral surface of the thigh. (From author's photo library)

gauze saturated with ether at the bottom of a 20 ml or 50 ml syringe (**Fig. 3-2**), into which the rat's nose can be inserted in order to again induce anesthesia.

It should be noted that injection (intramuscular) anesthesia is utilized in all microsurgical operations described in this book; mask (ether) anesthesia has only the accessory role desribed above. However, in portocaval anastomosis mask anesthesia with ether is indicated, because in this operation the blood flow to the liver is impaired. Due to the compromised blood flow associated with procedures involving portocaval anastomosis, the usual drugs (ketamine-chlorpromazine) are not able to reach the liver in order to be metabolized.

C. Preparation of the operative filed

Preparation of the opertaive field entails cutting and shaving the overlying hair, and cleaning the skin with an antiseptic solution. This preparation is performed after the injection of maintenance anesthetic drugs. Close attention should be paid to avoiding incidental lacerations incurred while using the electric razor, because the skin of the rat is very thin and thus prone to injury.

Then the skin is cleaned with a piece of gauze saturated with an alcoholic solution; in general betadine use is not advised. However, if betadine is used it should be

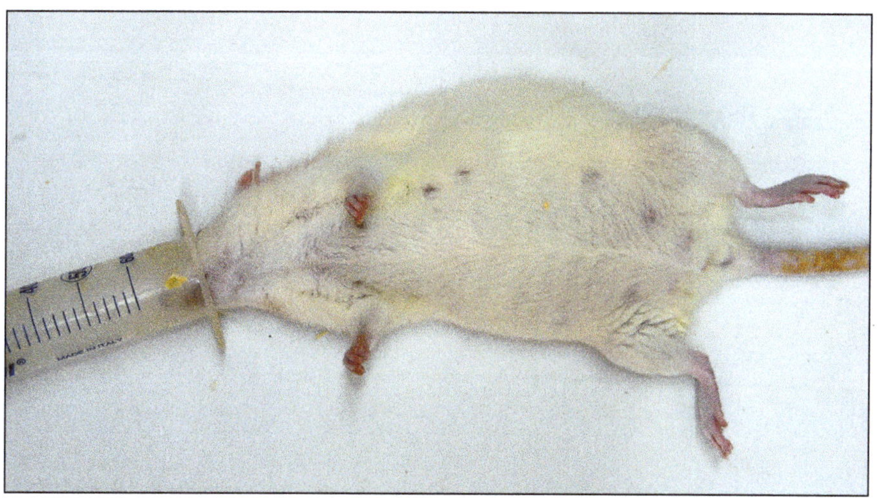

Figure 3-2

Anesthesia of the rat using a mask (made of a syringe) containing ether; for use during repeat induction anesthesia, or for portocaval anastomosis. (From author's photo library)

diluted 1:5 (one part betadine to 5 parts water), in order to avoid skin irritation.

D. Post-operative care (2 hours)

The room in which rats are to recover must be warm (27-30°C). Typical room temperature is often not high enough; therefore, a heat lamp can be placed over the cage of the rat or the cage can be placed on a heating surface. The bedding of the cage should be covered by absorptive paper; wood-shavings, which are otherwise widely used, should be avoided during post-operative care because they are irritant and dangerous for airway obstruction.

The signs to be monitored during recovery are:

- Respiratory rate (normally 85/min)
- Color of mucosae
- Mydriasis
- Reflex of rear limbs flexion on stimulus

The primary sign of post-operative pain in a rat is stillness (immobility). After major operations it is necessary to administer analgesic medications to the rat for 24-72 hours. Evidence of complete recovery can be recognized by the onset of eating or drinking.

Rats that have been operated upon must be kept in a separate cage for a few days, until they have recovered from the operative trauma, in order to avoid the phenomena of cannibalism. In our own laboratory, maternal cannibalism has been observed quite a few times when baby-rats have been returned to their mother to be fed after being operated upon.

E. Euthanasia

Euthanasia is the act of killing an animal with minimal physical and mental suffering, and is both ethically and legally mandated as the laboratory animal is protected by law. In organized laboratories, the surgeon will not be responsible for this unfortunate duty; technicians in the animal facilities department will take care of it.

In the event the surgeon has to euthanize the rats at either the end of the operation or during the course of an experiment, specific attention must be paid as to how euthanasia will be performed. One recommended method of euthanasia is the use of a 65% CO_2/35% O_2 gas for 45 sec followed by 100% CO_2 for 20 min. Another recommended method of euthanasia is the intravenous administration of pentovarvital (or pentovarvitone) (100 mg/kg). Others suggest intracardial administration of KCl after induction of anesthesia by ether. If euthanasia is required at the completion of the operation, while the rat is still under surgical anesthesia the inferior vena cava and the aorta are cut and the rat dies from massive hemorrhage. We should emphasize that the surgeon must know, and obey fully, the details of legislation regarding the euthanasia of laboratory animals; this legislation may vary between countries.

Part II

Basic Microsurgical Techniques

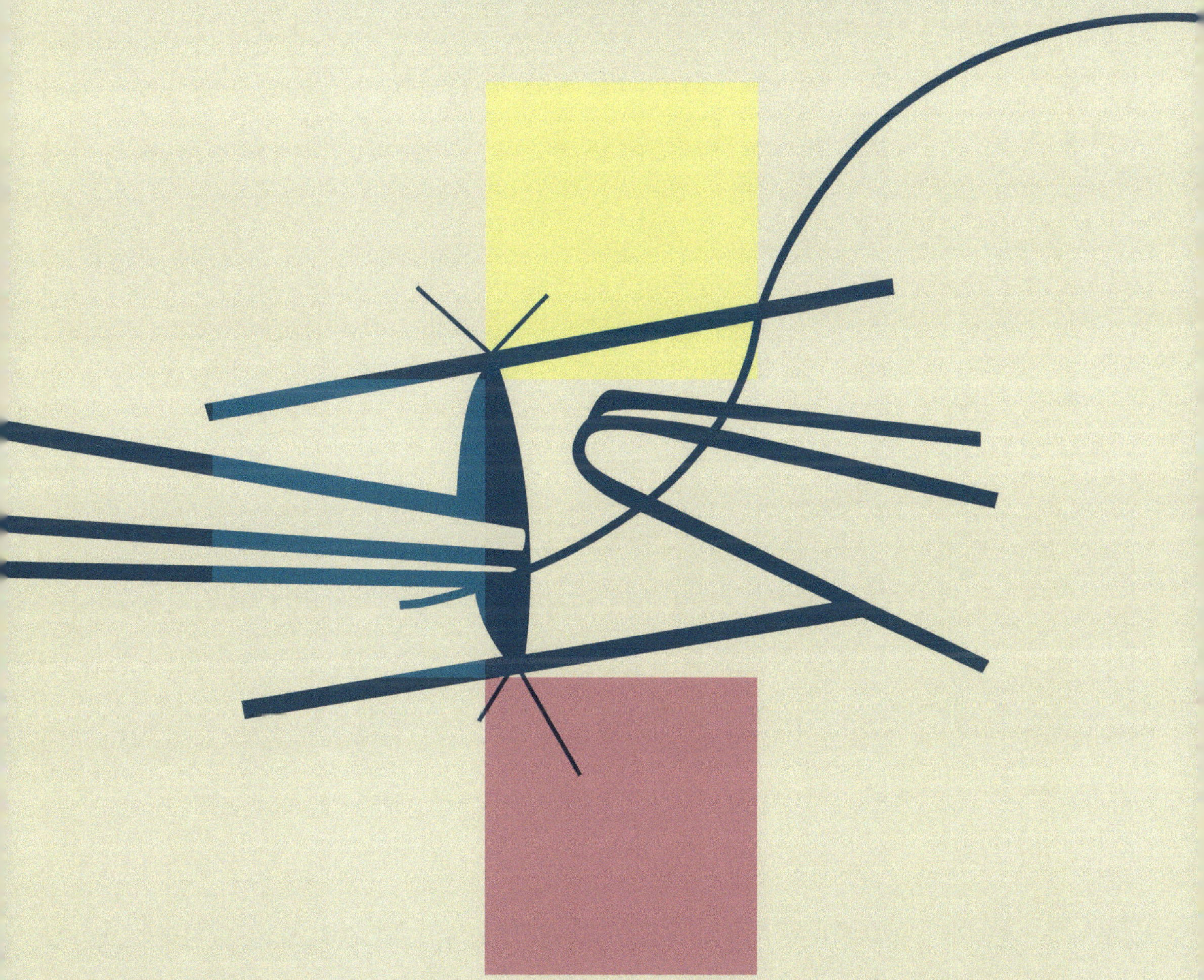

4 Microsurgical technique for suturing vessels

Warning: *When watching an expert microsurgeon, the technique for suturing vessels appears deceivingly simple. However, as beginners, it is likely that you will initially struggle. Do not become disappointed with this initial failure. Repeat your attempt with continued self-confidence, and remember to adhere to the rules described below.*

The first question voiced by the trainee in microsurgery is often whether or not the microsurgical technique for suturing differs from the suturing techniques of classical surgery. The answer is dual: microsurgical techniques for suturing are both similar to classic surgical suturing techniques–using both interrupted and continuous sutures–but are also significantly different with regard to knot tying, as well as other fine details.

When beginning to use the surgical microscope, the trainee will notice he/she seems to have entered an entirely different world; movements are tremendously magnified and working to overcome hand tremors can seem an insurmountable task. Furthermore, trainees often initially notice significant difficulty adjusting for the effects of magnification on hand-eye coordination. Despite these difficulties, trainees should remain encouraged; the guidelines detailed below will provide insight into mastering microsurgical techniques.

Microsurgical technique for suturing vessels

To begin, the needle holder is held in the surgeon's dominant hand. Most surgeons operate right-handed, therefore the descriptions of techniques which follow are framed for right-handed operating. Among the surgeons who are left-handed, there are a few who are able to operate ambidextrously. However, surgeons who are purely left-handed should use the instructions below as a guide, but should instead invert (symmetrically) the positions of the instruments in each hand.

Before beginning to suture, it is preferable that the suture be taken completely out of its paper or plastic envelope (removed from the envelope by grasping the needle with the needle holder) and irrigated or bathed in normal saline before entering the surgical field to minimize adherence to the surrounding tissues. A long thread might be unwieldy; however, one should take into account the not-insignificant cost of microsurgical sutures before cutting suture to a shorter length. Our practice is to avoid sacrificing any length of suture, even if this becomes troublesome for the surgeon. We also save remnants of sutures for use when an unexpected gap is noted in an anastomosis. For this reason, all suture packs and remnants are kept available until the completion of the operation.

When beginning training, it is often difficult to grasp the needle of the microsurgical suture with the needle holder when in the surgical field; when attempting this, the trainee will note that the needle often twists, escapes, or jumps out of his/her grasp. Instead of attempting to directly grasp the needle, let it lie on a pliable surface in the surgical field (for example, muscle), gently push into the middle of the arch of the needle, and the concavity of the needle will rotate upward. Then, grasp the needle with a needle holder or angulated forceps approximately 2/3 of the distance along the needle's arch, toward the base.

Before beginning to suture the vessel, the tips of the Dumont No. 3 forceps are inserted into the vessel lumen 1-2 mm beyond the edge of the cut vessel, with the jaws slightly open, thereby gently elevating the vessel wall. The needle is then passed through the vessel wall between the jaws of the forceps (**Fig. 4-1**). Close attention should be paid to avoid overstretching the vessel during this maneuver.

- ➢ Alternatively, the Dumont No. 3 forceps may be used to lift the vessel by the adventitia in order to facilitate the passage of the needle and suture.
- ➢ Holding the full thickness of the vessel wall between the jaws of the forceps should be avoided at all costs; this will cause great damage to the vessel wall and can result in failure of the anastomosis.

The needle should penetrate the vessel wall obliquely–indeed, almost horizontally (**Fig. 4-1**)–in order to avoid catching the posterior wall of the vessel in the suture, which is risked when the needle is passed through the vessel wall perpendicularly. This motion is accomplished primarily by rotation of the wrist, and may be completed by simultaneous rotation of the needle holder between the tips of the fingers. If the posterior wall of the vessel is captured in the suture, and this error is not immediately recognized and corrected, then failure of the anastomosis is guaranteed.

- ➢ The distance between the edge of the vessel stump and the point of entrance of the needle through the vessel wall (often referred to as the 'bite') should be equal to the thickness of the wall of the vessel (**Fig. 4-2**).

In the beginning, it is best for the trainee to pass the needle completely through the wall of one vessel stump, regrasp the needle after it has passed into the

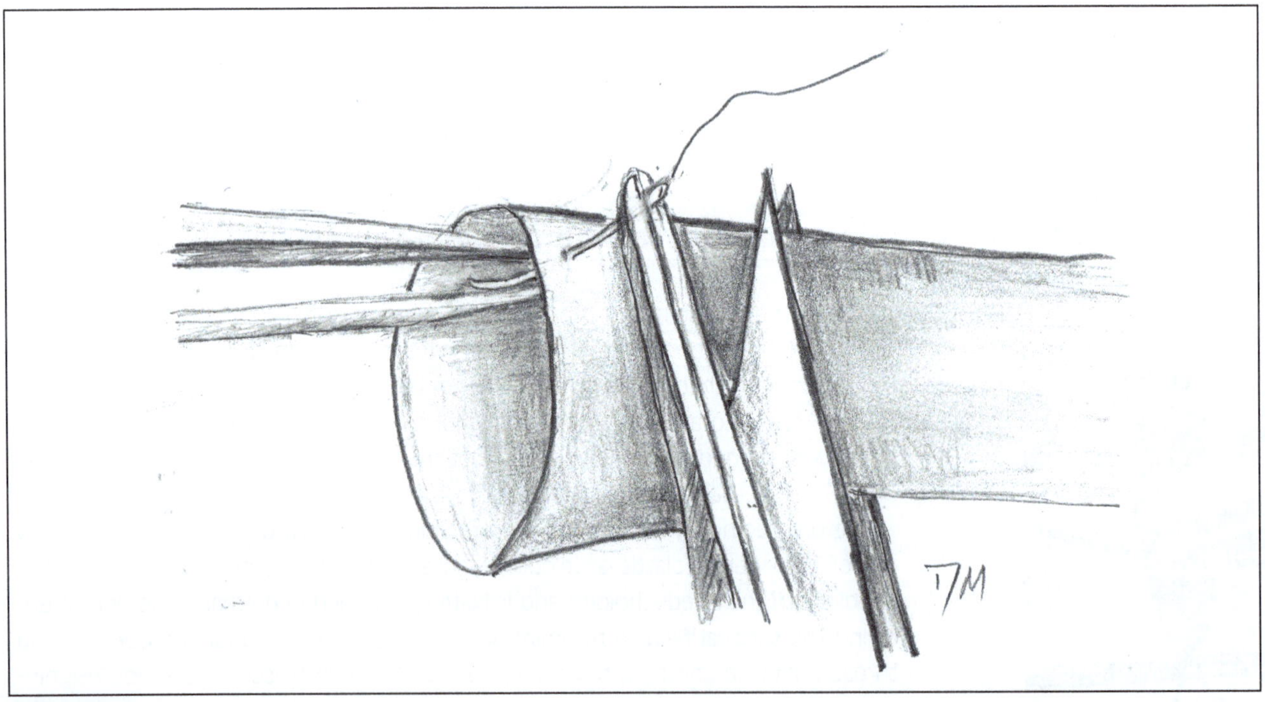

Figure 4-1

Demonstration of the entrance of the suture needle into the lumen of one of the two vessel stumps to be anastomosed. The needle holder drives the needle obliquely through the vessel wall. Dumont No. 3 forceps is inserted, open, into the lumen of the vessel and used to place gentle upward pressure against the wall of the vessel, allowing the needle to pass between the tips of the forceps. (Drawing by the author) lumen, and then pass the needle through the wall of the second vessel stump; this is the two-step technique. With practice, it will become easier to complete this motion using only one smooth passage of the needle through the walls of the vessel stumps, as opposed to the two-step technique described above. However, even with experience, the two-step technique is recommended when placing the corner- or stay-sutures (at 12 o'clock and 6 o'clock on the vascular anastomosis), as well as whenever there is fear that the posterior wall of the vessel may be inadvertently caught by the needle (as may happen in veins anastomosis).

When using the two-step technique, the Dumont No. 3 forceps is used to grasp the needle after it has entered the lumen of the vessel stump (having been driven from the outside of the vessel into the vessel lumen). The forceps is then used to pull the needle through the vessel wall (being sure to follow the curvature of the needle) and then to stabilize the needle, allowing it to be grasped again by the needle holder. The forceps can then be used to correct the position of the needle in the jaws of the needle holder; ideally, the needle should be grasped along the arch, 2/3 of the distance from the needle tip to the end of the needle, and the angle between the axes of the needle and needle holder should be 90°. Then, the needle is driven through the wall of the opposite vessel stump, from inside to outside (again obliquely), to complete the stitch.

- The distance between the point of exit of the needle from the vessel and the edge of the vessel stump –the 'exit bite'–should be equal to the bite at the entrance of the needle; both bites should be equal to the thickness of the vessel wall. If the bites are unequal, the edges of the vessel stumps will become everted, jeopardizing the anastomosis.

When passing the needle through the vessel wall of the opposing vessel stump, from inside of the lumen outwards, the Dumont No. 3 forceps can be used to gently lift the adventitia of the vessel, thereby keeping the lumen of the vessel open and assisting passage of the needle (this maneuver is rather necessary for veins, whose lumen is usually collapsed). Alternatively, the forceps can be used to apply gentle external pressure on the vessel wall, allowing the needle to be driven through the vessel wall, with the needle exiting between the tips of the forceps (**Fig. 4-3**).

Then, the needle holder is first used to push the needle through the vessel wall, from the lumen outwards. When 2/3 of the needle's length has been driven through the vessel wall, the needle holder is shifted toward the tip of the needle and used to pull the needle all of the way through the wall of the vessel. At this point, the surgeon can lower the magnification of the surgical microscope in order to obtain a wider view of the surgi-

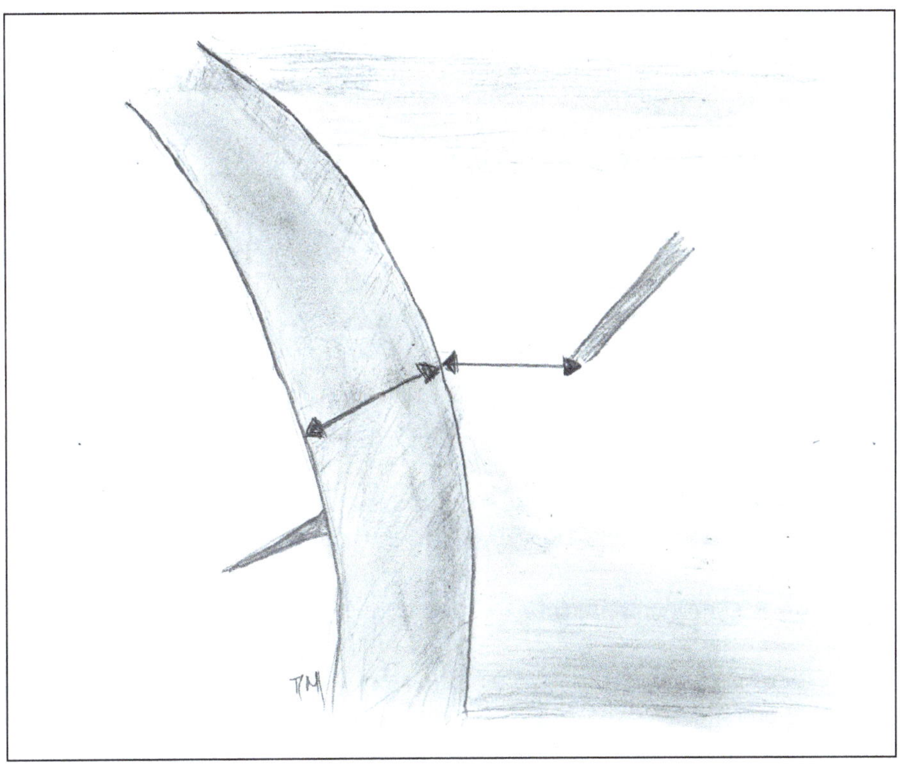

Figure 4-2

The distance between the point of entrance of the needle and the edge of the vessel stump–the 'bite'–should be equal to the thickness of the wall of the vessel (as shown by the bidirectional arrows). (Drawing by the author)

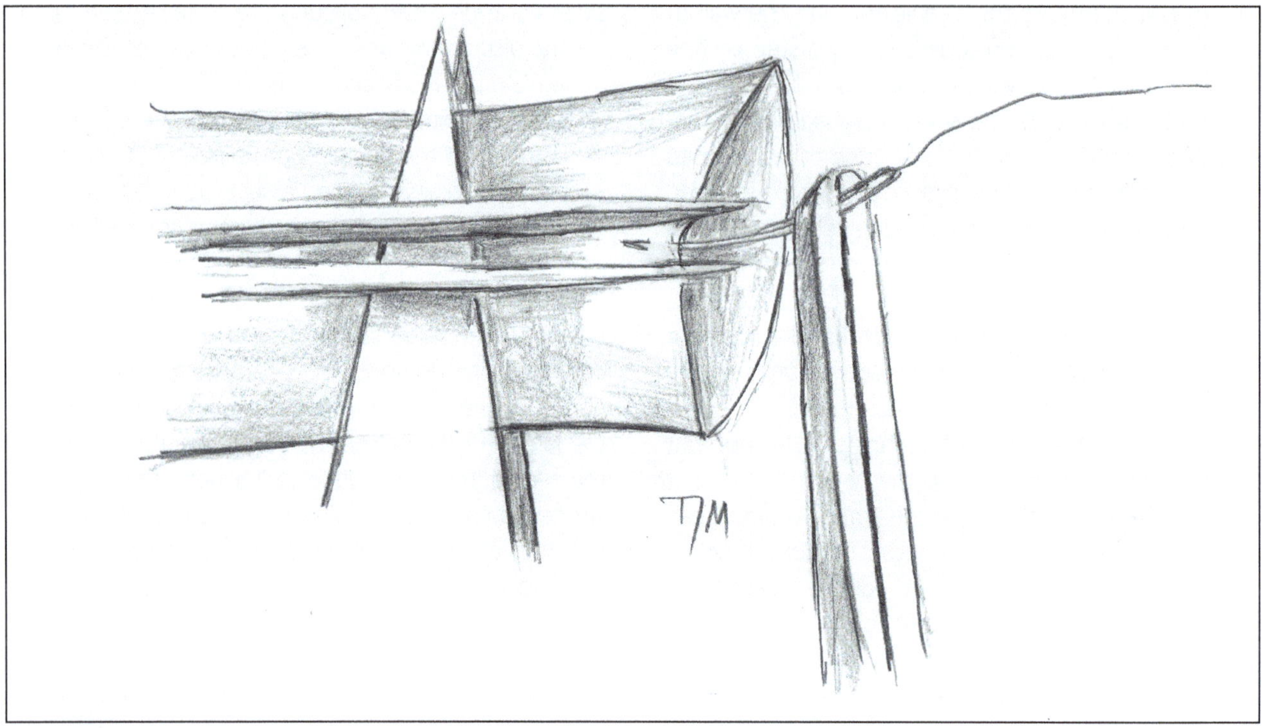

Figure 4-3

Demonstration of the suture needle's exit from the lumen of the opposing vessel stump. The needle holder drives the needle obliquely through the wall of the vessel, ideally at a distance from the edge of the vessel equal to the bite distance of the suture needle entering the opposing vessel (see Figure 4-1). The open Dumont No. 3 forceps is used to externally support the wall of the vessel, allowing the needle to pass between the tips of the forceps. (Drawing by the author)

cal field. The needle is grasped with the forceps and pulled through the vessel wall until the end of the suture is seen in the surgical field of the microscope; at this point the suture is pulled more slowly. The needle holder is then used to grasp the end of the suture; if this end is inadvertently drawn through the vessel, the stitch should be restarted. When drawing the suture through the vessel wall, the needle holder can be positioned where the suture enters the first vessel stump, with the jaws open (one jaw touching the external surface of the vessel), so that the thread passes between them as it is drawn through the vessel wall. When the end of the suture is seen, the jaws are then closed to prevent drawing the suture completely through the vessel wall. With experience, this use of the needle holder to secure the end of the suture can be omitted, as the trainee will be better able to judge the distance to the end of the thread.

Meanwhile, by using the forceps to draw the suture through the vessel wall the needle has likely passed out of sight (beyond the visual field). When the end of the suture is appropriately placed, the needle can be secured in place within the surgical field, preferably near the anastomosis. We propose anchoring the needle in an adjacent muscle, so that it can be readily re-grasped without requiring lowering of the magnification or repositioning of the microscope.

If the suture's thread is long, forceps can be used at the point of entrance into the vessel wall, to slow its passage; otherwise, pulling a long suture quickly through the vessel wall risks tearing the vessel. It is important to regularly irrigate the suture and the surgical field with warm normal saline, remove all debris from the area of tissue dissection, and arrange the instruments back into position for further use.

Knots: 3 simple, flat

The first knot is made as follows: The No. 3 forceps is used to lift the thread of the suture approximately 2 cm from the vessel wall (on the end attached to the needle), while the tips of the needle holder are placed over the thread (with the jaws closed and the tips pointed towards the exit of the suture) (**Fig. 4-4**). The needle holder is moved in order to create a loop of thread resting around the needle holder, while the left hand holds the

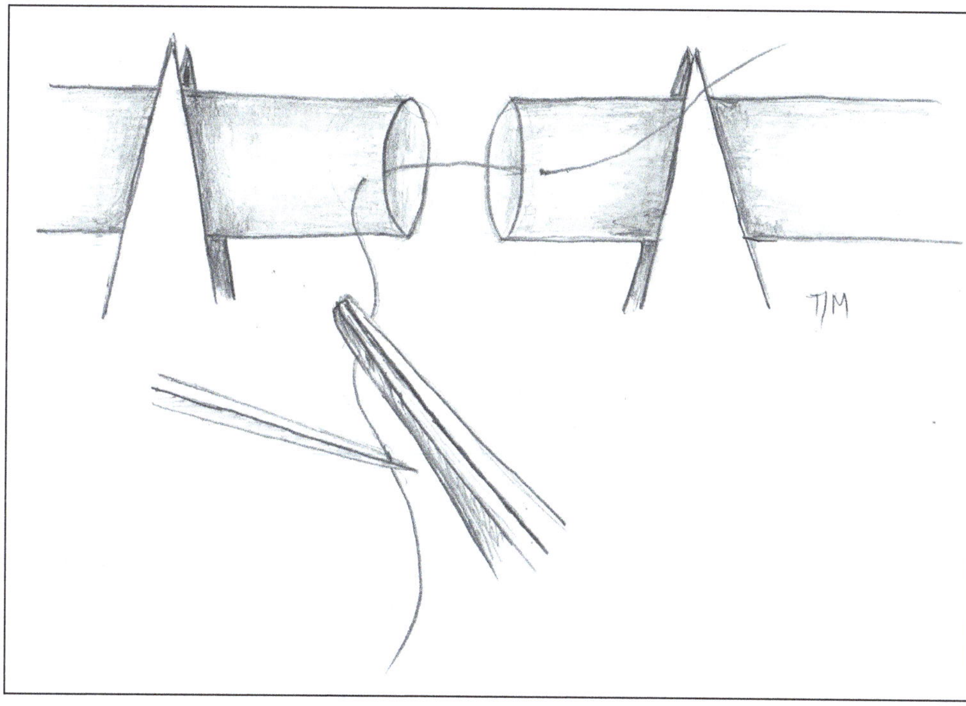

Figure 4-4

Preparation for beginning the first simple, flat knot. The proximal length of suture thread (closest to the needle) is held by the forceps. An adequate length of the proximal suture thread (usually 2 cm) is left between the forceps and the vessel wall in order to form a loop around the needle holder. The tips of the needle holder are placed over the suture thread, pointing upwards. (Drawing by the author)

forceps (with the thread) still. Others suggest, conversely, that the forceps (holding the thread) should be used to create a loop of suture around the still needle holder.

While making this loop of suture, the tips of the needle holder should point upwards; for the beginner, this positioning will help prevent the loop of suture from sliding off of the tips of the needle holder. Furthermore, the loop of suture should not be too tight or too close to the tips of the needle holder. Care should be taken to place the loop of suture in such a way that the needle holder can grasp the distal, short end of the suture.

Then, while the loop on the needle holder, by turning their wrist, the surgeon uses the needle holder to grasp the distal end of the thread—the jaws of the needle holder are opened before or during this movement. The distal end of the suture should be short enough to stand up, allowing it to easily be picked up from the surrounding tissues without difficulty. This process is more challenging if the distal suture is not long enough, is not visible, is difficult to be picked up due to resting at a peculiar angle, or is adhered to surrounding tissues; this difficulty can either be prevented when placing the suture, or corrected when encountered. When struggling with a short distal suture, release the needle holder from the loop and lengthen the distal suture. While then attempting to form the first throw of the knot, take care to again leave enough length for the loop of suture, otherwise the distal suture may once again be too short. If the distal suture lies at an angle that makes it difficult to grasp, again release the needle holder and correct the position of the distal suture by using the needle holder or the forceps. Similarly, if the distal suture is adherent to neighboring tissues, the needle may need to be released in order to use the needle holder to adequately mobilize the distal suture.

In order to tie a simple, flat knot, the hands are crossed with the needle holder and the forceps simultaneously pulling the distal and the proximal ends of the suture in opposite directions, along the long axis of the vessels (**Fig. 4-5**). The knot should be placed along the long axis of the vessel, and care should be taken to avoid making the knot too tight; otherwise, the edges of the vessels will overlap each other, thereby compromising the anastomosis.

It may surprise the beginner that the completion of the final knot is accomplished with the addition of only two further simple, flat knots–exactly the same as the first knot–for a total of three knots. There is no first double knot, no reversed second knot, and no fourth or fifth knot. Amazingly, these three knots serve their purpose well. The only case where we suggest utilizing a reversed second knot is when the anastomosis is performed under tension.

After completing the knot, the tails of the suture should be cut short (maximum length of 1 mm) to avoid becoming entangled in subsequent sutures. In or-

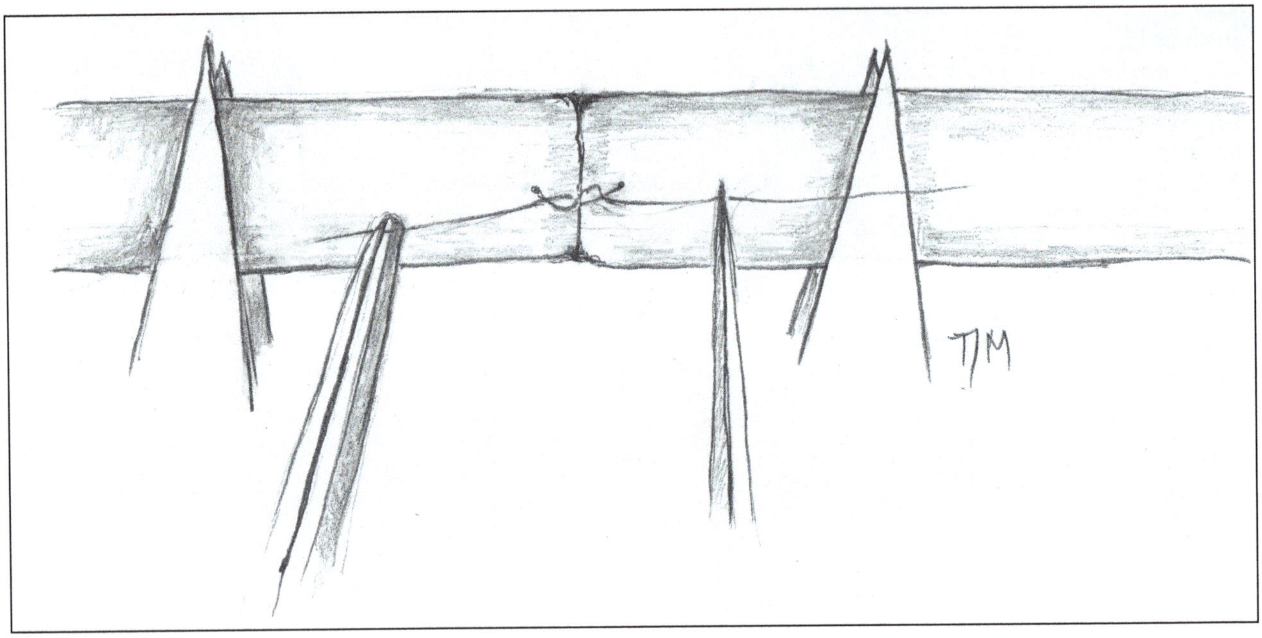

Figure 4-5

Demonstration of completing the first simple, flat knot. The needle holder grasps the distal end of the suture and a simple, flat knot is created by drawing the instruments in opposite directions (the forceps and needle holder will cross each other). Compare the current position of the needle holder with the position seen in Figure 4-3; it is found on the other side of the forceps. To tighten the knot, the instruments are gently pulled away from each other with the same force. (Drawing by the author)

der to safely and methodically retrieve the needle, the ends of suture are cut in the following order: first, the distal tail is cut and the suture debris is removed from the surgical field. Next, the forceps grasps the proximal, long tail of the suture, and the suture is cut close to the knot, while the forceps is used to maintain a hold of the remaining suture (and needle). By moving the forceps, the needle is brought back into the visible surgical field. Of note, if the needle was previously anchored on an adjacent muscle, it should be freed before attempting to move this proximal end of the suture into the surgical field.

5

Principles of end-to-end anastomosis of vessels

Before any vessel dissection, the surgical field may be irrigated with xylocaine solution 2%. Xylocaine is a powerful vasodilatative drug in the rat. Irrigation with xylocaine solution 2% has been reported to cause a 30-35% increase in artery diameter within 3-4 min of administration. We use xylocaine solution only electively in vessels of small diameter. Xylocaine has little effect on veins.

Another solution for microscopic vascular surgery, to be used during the anastomosis (after vessel transection but before suturing) is heparin solution in Ringer's Lactate at a concentration of 25,000 IU/L. This solution is not toxic to endothelium.

1. Placement of a yellow background beneath the vessel

After dissecting and mobilizing, the vessel is gently lifted with Dumont forceps. A piece of yellow, flexible plastic (or a piece of surgeon's glove) is placed beneath the vessel as a background. A yellow backgroung offers a strong color contrast with the vessel wall and provides better resolution of fine details at vessel's end. It is much easier to place a background if both the background and surgical field have first been irrigated with warmed normal saline.

2. Application of the double vascular clamp

Gilbert's double clamp, used here, constists of two microvascular clamps that can move along a double bar, and the jaws of each clamp open and close by turning the head of a screw by a specific diriver (see **Figure 1-3**). When applying the Gilbert clamp, the two clamps are placed in the surgical field perpenticular to the vessel and with their jaws opened wide enough to comfortably accept the vessel. Make sure that the vessel is adequately dissected from surrounding tissues so that the douple clamp can be easily applied. If the clamp cannot be applied without causing undue stress or increased tension on the vessel, it is necessary to withdraw the clamp and further dissect around the vessel. The clamp should be applied without difficulty.

Once placed in the desired position, the vessel is placed as close as possible to the tips of the jaws so that the vessel can rotate. Vessel rotation is important during the anastomosis so that the surgeon has a better view of the posterior surface. The upstream clamp is applied first in order to interrupt blood flow in the direction of the downstream clamp. The downstream clamp is then applied. This sequence avoids entrapment of blood in the length of vessel between the two clamps.

An adequate distance, usually of 1 cm, must be left between the two clamps of the double clamp, because the vessel will shrink after transection. Most often it is required to approximate the clamps.

Additionally, it is crucial that the minimum pressure is applied on the vessel by the clamp jaws (their open-close is controlled with the specific driver, see **Figure 1-3**). Excessive pressure will crush the tissue and destroy the endothelium. This injury will lead to thrombosis and failure of the operation.

3. Transection of the vessel

Once the vessel is clamped, it can be transected. The vessel should be trancescted with straight scissors brought down vertically and perpendicular to the vessel. The transection of the vessel must always be done midway between the two clamps. The cut must be 'clean,' meaning that the scissors blades close once and the vessel is swiftly cut across to create neat edges. If the edges of the vessel are rough, there is a great possibility that parts of the adventitia or vessel wall will be entraped in the lumen resulting in thrombosis after the anastomosis.

It is almost always observed that the vessel shrinks after transcection, causing the two edges to separate by a distance. This gap will be relatively small during experimental microsurgery in rats. In human microsurgery, however, a long gap will form when a portion of the vessel often has to be removed due to trauma. The solution to this problem is discussed at the end of the Chapter.

4. Irrigation of the vessel lumen with normal saline

Immediately after transection, the lumen of the vessel is irrigated with normal saline in order to wash away the remaining blood and to avoid clot formation. It is important that the normal saline be body temperature, as vessels constrict when subjected to cold temperatures. The smaller the lumen of the vessel, the more difficult suturing becomes.

Irrigation is performed by drawing up a full 5 ml syringe with body temperature normal saline. If the needle of the syringe is kept for the irrigation (bent at a right or obtuse angle), it should not enter the lumen, not to traumatize the endothelium, which would result in thrombosis when the blood flow will be reestablished. But usually the needle is replaced by a 27G pediatric angiocatheter, which is connected to the syringe (the needle of the catheter is removed, and the catheter is bent). The angiocatheter is cut obliquely so that its tip be sharpened and can enter the lumen. Care must be taken to avoid trauma to the endothelium. Try to wash the lumen using only pressure from the angiocatheter, very gently place the catheter in and out of the vessel, and achieve a high enough washing pressure to assure that all old blood is cleaned from the lumen.

5. Removal of the adventitia

The outer vessel wall is referred to as the adventitia. Its removal is necessary, because adventitial debris can become entraped in the lumen during anastomosis. This will cause clot formation and certain failure of the anastomosis.

If dissection and transection of the vessel are correctly performed, i.e the vessel has been fully cleaned from adjacent tissue and cut perpendicularly, the edge of the adventitia should be aligned with the edge of the transected vessel. To distinguish the adventitia from the rest of the layers, irrigate the edge of the vessel with normal saline under light pressure. This will cause the adventitia to 'float' away from the inner layers of vessel wall.

Once identified, the adventitia is folded (reflected back) onto the wall of the vessel (**Fig. 5-1**). This is similar to rolling up one's shirt sleeve, with the sleeve analogous to the adventitia and one's arm being the remaining layers of the vessel wall. As will be described in future Chapters, two Dumont forceps are used; one to hold the vessel and the other to 'roll up' the adventitia. Compared to working on arteries, folding the adventitia of a vein much more difficult; most of the times, ad-

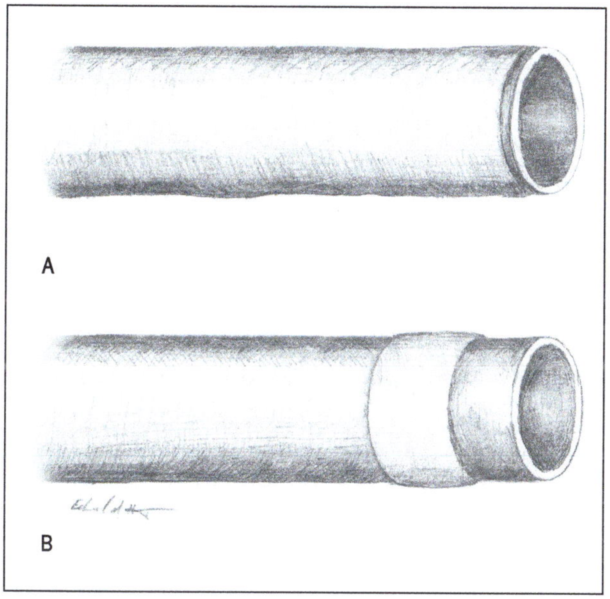

Figure 5-1

Folding the adventitia. **A.** Adventitia, lying on the rest layers of the wall of the artery (after it has been detached from them). **B.** Adventitia has been reflected away from the cut edge of the vessel. (Drawing by Edward M. Hagopian)

ventitia removal in veins will be done by pulling and cutting parts of the adventitia.

If you face difficulties in folding the adventitia of an artery, the 'sleeve amputation' technique may be applied. In this technique, the adventitia of all around the vessel (anterior and posterior surface) is pulled with forceps past the edge of the vessel stump. While keeping the adventitia under tension, cut it perpendicular to the vessel axis with straight, sharp scissors. This will allow removal of a ring of adventitia. The remaining adventitia will retract, exposing a ring of the rest layers of the vessel wall. This technique is not suggested for veins, because it is difficult to pull a whole ring of adventitia from the rest of the wall. Most likely, as said above, removal will be done in piecemeal by pulling and cutting off parts of the adventitia.

Avoid exaggerated removal the adventitia. Only a ring near the edge of the vascular stump needs to be removed in order to place the sutures. Overstripping risks trauma to the vessel and may impaire blood supply to the vessel wall.

6. Approximation of clamps

Before suturing the anastomosis, the two clamps of the double clamp carrying the vessel edges should be approximated. Placing sutures under tension may cause the vessel edges to rotate and become improperly oriented (loss of symmetry at the approximated edges). There is also the risk or tearing the vessel wall. Finally, if there is tension, knots will probably be loose or not bring the edges into contact, resulting in a leaky anastomosis when blood flow is reestablished.

7. Suturing technique in end-to-end anastomosis

The level of magnification used by the surgeon is constantly changed to fit his/her needs during microscopic vascular anastomosis:

- Sutures are placed under 25x magnification. Magnification can be increased to 40x to help the surgeon make sure that an anterior wall suture did not catch the internal layer of the posterior wall of the vessel. High magnification may also be necessary for difficult sutures.
- Knot tying is done under 16x magnification. Magnification can decrease in order to find the end of a long thread in the surgical field.

First the two sutures at 12 o'clock and 6 o'clock are placed (Nos. 1 and 2, **Fig. 5-2 A-E**) [the open lumen of a vessel is imagined as a clock, with the top of the clock, i.e. 12 o'clock lying upwards and 6 o'clock clock downwards]. These sutures are referred to as the 'corner sutures' and are of great imprortance because they help properly orientate the vessel edges. When the suture line is vertical (with the vessel horizontal), the 12 o'clock suture is placed first, followed by the 6 o'clock suture.

The anastomosis continues by placing the sutures of the anterior surface.

➲ **Be careful** not to catch the posterior surface with any stitch of the anterior surface!

After the anterior wall is finished, rotate the double clamp with the enclosed vessel is flipped over and the posterior surface of the sutured anterior wall is visible (**Fig. 5-3**). Before suturing the posterior surface, verify that there is no cacth of the posterior surface. Then, in the same way as in the anterior surface but in mirror image–since the vessel has been reversed–, are placed sutures of the posterior surface.

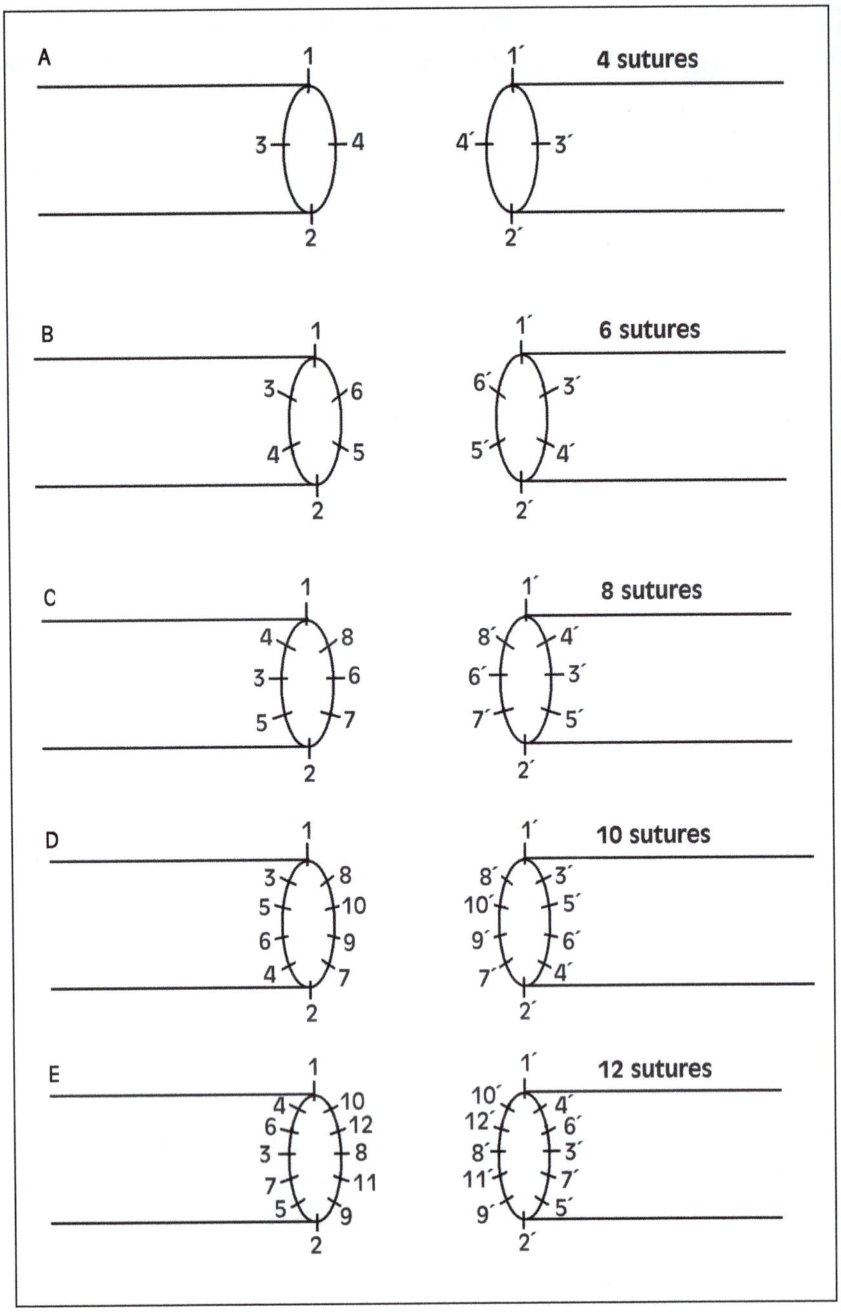

Figure 5-2

Order of suture placement during end-to-end anastomosis based on total count of sutures. Numbers show the position and order of suture placement; accented numbers show the symmetric position of these sutures on the other stump. According to the text, corner sutures (12 o'clock and 6 o'clock) are placed first, the anterior half of the vessel is sutured, the double clamp is rotated, and then posterior half of the vessel is sutured. The numbers on the posterior surface are in mirror order because of the rotation of the clamp.

A. 4 sutures, 2 corner sutures, 1 in the middle of each semicircle.

B. 6 sutures, 2 corner sutures, 2 equally spaced in each semicircle (first is placed the upper suture).

C. 8 sutures, 2 corner sutures, 3 in each semicircle of which the first is placed in the middle of each semicircle followed by one suture in the middle of each quadrant; the suture in the upper quadrant is placed first.

D. 10 sutures, 2 corner sutures, 4 equally spaced in each semicircle; of the latter, the two peripheral sutures closest to the corner are placed first (the upper first), followed by the two central sutures (the upper first). The same apply for the posterior surface.

E. 12 sutures, 2 corner sutures, and 5 in each semicircle; the median suture (No. 3) is placed in the middle of the semicircle, with the remaining placed at equal distances (from the corner sutures and between themselves) in a closer to closer fashion: first the peripheral sutures Nos. 4 and 5 (upper first), and then the medial Nos. 6 and 7 (upper first) are placed. The same apply for the posterior surface. (Diagram: E. Kontis)

Two different techniques can be used to place the remaining sutures (beyond the corner sutures) and completing the anastomosis:

1. ***Dividing the gap:*** The distance between two sutures is divided in half, and the next suture is placed in the middle of the distance. Thus, by subsequent dividings of the gaps, the anterior and then the posterior surface of the vessel are sutured.
   Once the corner sutures are secured, the median suture in the middle of the semicircle of the anterior surface is placed. The same applies for each quadrant, the median suture is placed in the middle, and so forth, until completing suturing of the anterior surface. The vessel is rotated and the posterior surface is sutured in the same way.
   The advantage of this technique is that the sutures are spontaneously placed at equal distances from each other. Therefore, tension on the vessel wall is also divided equaly, resulting in a tight anastomosis.

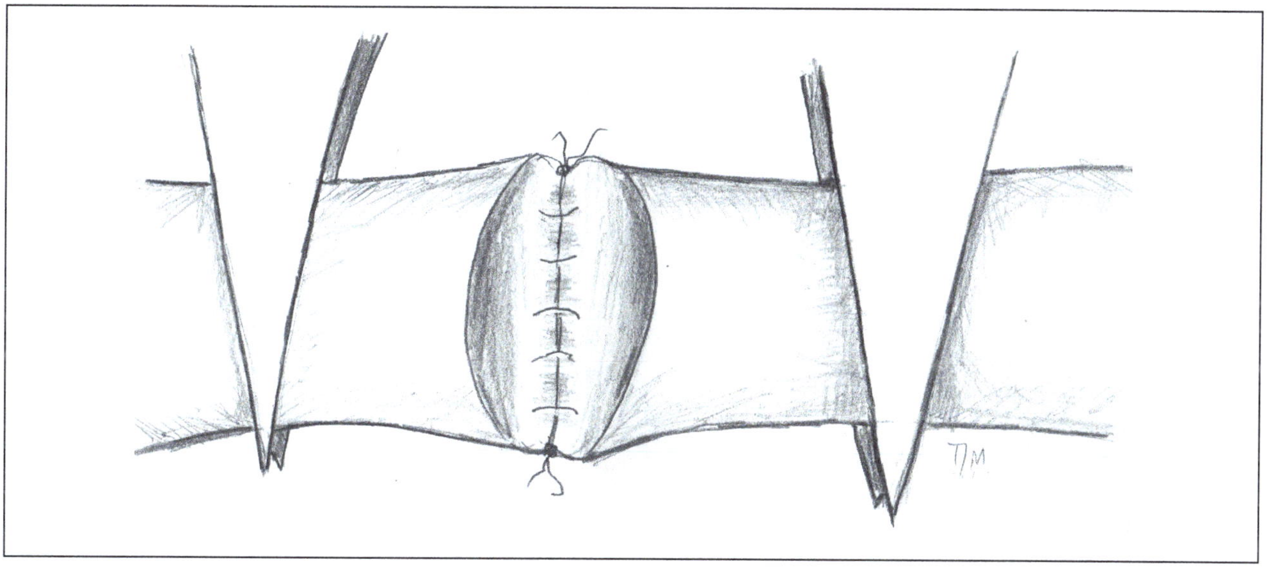

Figure 5-3

Posterior view of the sutured anterior wall of the end-to-end anastomosis. After the anterior surface has been completed, the double clamp is rotated and the correct placement of sutures is examined. (Drawing by the author)

2. **Technique 'de proche en proche'** ('closer to closer'): In this technique, the sutures are placed at estimated equal distances from the previous sutures and between themselves. The lateral sutures (those closest to the corner sutures) are placed first, followed by the more central sutures (those toward the middle of the semicircle). In French this technique is called 'de proche en proche' ('closer to closer'). This name reveals the strategy of narrowing the gap by coming closer and closer to the midway point of the corner sutures.

This technique is applied when the previous technique of 'dividing the gap' is not applicable because an even number of sutures are required to cover the distance between corner sutures sutures (or between corner and median suture if the technique of 'dividing the gap' was applied for the semicircle, see below). The technique 'de proche en proche' requires more planning in advance because it is important to assure that the distance between sutures is equal.

Depending on the number of sutures required after the placement of the corner sutures, the proper technique will be chosen:

- For a odd number of sutures per semicircle, each time 'divide the gap'
- For an even number, go 'closer to closer', from the periphery to the center of the semicircle, in equal distances
- For 5 sutures per semicircle, the two techiques need to be combined (see below, 'Total number of 12 sutures,' which is the maximum number of sutures in the techniques presented in this book)

Hereafter, we descibe in detail the technique of suture placement in relation to their total count (according to the operations that will be described in the following chapters).

Total number of 4 sutures

After placement of the 2 corner sutures (12 o'clock and 6 o'clock), 2 more sutures follow, each put in middle of each semicircle (semicircles refer to the anterior and posterior surfaces) (**Fig. 5-2A**).

Total number of 6 sutures

After placement of the 2 corner sutures (12 o'clock and 6 o'clock), there are 4 remaining, i.e. 2 for each semicircle of the anterior and posterior surface. The two sutures of the anterior surface are placed in equal distances from the corner sutures, which are equal to the distance between themeselves. In both surfaces, the upper sutures are put first and the the lower follow (**Fig. 5-2B**).

Total number of 8 sutures

After placement of the 2 corner sutures (12 o'clock and 6 o'clock), there are 6 remaining, i.e. 3 for each semicircle of the anterior and posterior surface. The median suture is placed first in the middle of the semicircle, and each of the 2 remaining is put in the middle of each quadrant (**Fig. 5-2C**).

Total number of 10 sutures

After placement of the 2 corner sutures (12 o'clock and 6 o'clock), there are 8 remaining, i.e. 4 for each semicircle of the anterior and posterior surface. Here the strategy 'de proche en proche' ('closer to closer') is indicated: first are placed the 2 lateral (toward the corner sutures) and then the 2 more central, all in equal distance (between themselves and from the corner sutures). In both the anterior and posterior surfaces, in each of the 2 pairs, first are placed the upper and then the lower sutures [for a vertical suture line] (**Fig. 5-2D**).

Total number of 12 sutures

After placement of the 2 corner sutures (12 o'clock and 6 o'clock), there are 10 remaining, i.e. 5 for each semicircle of the anterior and posterior surface. From these, the median is placed in the middle of the semicircle, and 2 in each quantrant in in equal distances (between themselves and from the median and corner sutures). Lateral sutures (toward the corner suture) are placed first, and then the more central ones. In both the anterior and posterior surfaces, first are placed the upper and then the lower sutures [for a vertical suture line] (**Fig. 5-2E**). Some surgeons, however, prefer to finish suturing each of the quadrants after placement of the median suture in the middle of the semicircle. This techique is acceptable but not preferable.

Note: *all the above directions depicted in* ***Figure 5-2*** *refer to a vertical suture line, and the upper sutures are placed first. If the vessels stumps are vertical and the suture line is placed horizontal, a right-handed surgeon will most likely follow suturing from left to right.*

After the anastomosis is finished, rotate back the clamp back and forth to examine the anastomosis. It should look completely sealed on both the posterior and anterior surfaces. If a gap is present, do not hesitate to place an extra suture, even if this surpasses the number of sutures given in the guidelines of this book for each operation. The integrity of the anastomosis is more important than the number of sutures that must be used.

8. Removal of the double clamp

When removing the Gilbert clamp, it is important that the distal (downstream) clamp be released first. Release of the distal clamp will allow blood to flow backwards, backfilling to the proximal (upstream) clamp. This normal backflow of blood will have a hemostatic effect on the suture line and is the first indication of a patent anastomosis.

9. Gauze placement

Small leaks from the gaps between sutures are expected after clamp release. In fact, the anastomosis may immediately become submerged in blood. After the double clamp is completely released, a piece of gauze is placed on the anastomosis. The gauze is left in contact with the anastomosis for three to four minutes without applying any pressure. During this time, clots are formed between sutures and sealing of the anastomosis results.

10. Patency test

The operation is succeful only if the anastomosis is patent. The patency test is performed using two forceps placed one next to the other distal to the anastomosis (**Fig. 5-4A**). Then, the upstream forcesps, closest to the anastomosis, stops the blood flow, while the downstream forceps is slid distally for a few millimeters. using a 'milking' action, thus emptying the lumen between the two forceps and closes at final position (**Fig. 5-4B**). Finally, the upstream forceps is released while the downstream forceps stays in place. Rapid filling of the emptied portion of vessel to the downstream forceps is proof that the anastomosis is patent (**Fig. 5-4C**). A delay in filling of the vessel shows that the anastomosis is not fully patent and may be due to a suture that caught the anterior and posterior surfaces. In such a case, complete obstruction of the lumen will follow shortly. Only the rapid filling is a valid prood of patency of the anastomosis.

At the end of the operation, irrigate the surgical field and remove any blood or clots. Also, look for remnants of sutures or other foreign bodies, because these will have an undesired vasoconstrictive effect.

Veins

The technique of end-to-end anastomosis of veins is not different from that of arteries. However, some important differences do exist due to the thinner wall and the larger size of veins. In general, the risk of thrombosis is greater in veins.

- Due to a thinner medial wall layer, it is much more diffuclt to detach and reverse the adventitia of veins without injuring the rest of the wall. That's why, as said above, adventitia removal in veins will be done in piecemeal by pulling and cutting parts of the adventitia.
- The thin vein walls collapse very easily after transection of the vessel, making suturing more difficult and increasing the chance that both anterior and posterior walls are caught in a suture, leading to throbosis after anastomosis. As a result, it is advised to irrigate the surgical field with normal saline frequently during anastomosis.
- The larger size of the vein requires an increased number of sutures compared with arteries. In the techniques described in the following Chapters, the reader will observe that very often two more sutures are necessary for the vein. In addition, the vein size also varies, and the surgeon will have the option to use two more sutures (e.g., 8 or 10 sutures for the external jugular vein in Chapter 9). The wider lumen of the veins in some cases will require suture of larger caliber compared with the artery (e.g. renal vessels in Chapter 26).

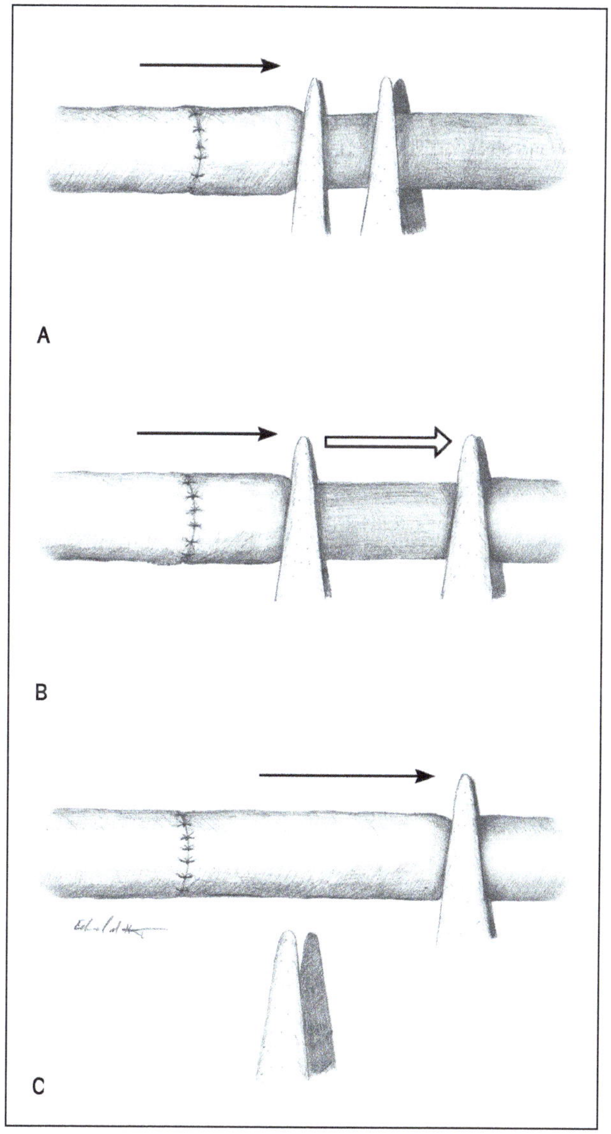

Figure 5-4

Patency test of an end-to-end anastomosis. The black-filled arrow shows the blood flow, and the arrowhead shows where the flow ends. The empty arrow shows the movement of the downstream forceps. **A.** The upstream forceps occludes the vessel distal to the anastomosis and a second forceps is placed further distally (downstream). **B.** The second forceps gently slides downstream for a short distance, 'milking' the intervening segment of vessel of its contents, and stays closed at final position. **C.** The first forceps is removed, allowing blood to flow in to the emptied length of vessel. If the emptied portion rapidly fills up to the second forceps, the anastomosis is patent. (Drawing by Edward M. Hagopian)

Disproportion of Lumen Size

A fairly common problem in vascular microsurgery is a disproportion in diameter of the vessels to be anastomosed. However, since experimental micrsurgery is performed under ideal, prescheduled conditions, this problem may be easily addressed. In clinical microsurgery conditions are more demanding. Regardeless of the setting (experimental or clinical), it is important that the microsurgeon know how to solve this problem. There are various proposals depending on how much the vessel diameters differ.

Difference of vessel diameters <50%

Mechanical dilation of the lumen

If the vessels to be anastomosed differ in diameter by <50%, performing mechanical dilation of the lumen on the smaller of the two vessels can rectify this problem. After the vessels have been thoroughly dissected and placed in the double clamp, and the adventitia has been removed, the closed tips of a forceps are inserted in to the lumen of the smaller vessel and gradually opened (**Fig. 5-5**). For large vessels in the rat, Dumont No. 3 is the proper forceps; for smaller ones use Dumont No. 5 forceps.

The tips of the forceps are inserted in the lumen of the vessel for a few mm; this distance varies with the size of the vessel. A few repetitions of inserting and gradually opening the instrument are required. Gradual, controlled opening of the forceps is important; if the forceps is allowed to spring open, the abrupt force may traumatize the vessel wall. Moreover, proper forceps size is crucial, as fine forceps may puncture the wall of larger vessels.

The lumen should not be dilated at maximum to totally match the diameter of the larger vessel. A small difference in vessel diameters can be tolerated and we want to avoid traumatizing the smaller vessel. Small mismatches in diameter can be corrected by placing sutures farther apart on the larger vessel (longer 'steps') and closer together (smaller 'steps') on the smaller vessel.

Difference of vessel diameters 50-100%

1. Oblique section of the smaller vessel

Mechanical dilatation of the smaller vessel is not an option to correct the size disparity when it reaches >50% of the larger vessel diameter. For disparities of 50 to 100%—up to the point where the smaller vessel is half the size of the larger vessel—the technique of choice is the oblique section of the smaller vessel (**Fig. 5-6**). The angle at which the oblique section is made is of great importance. This angle is formed by the cut edge of the vessel (oblique section line) and a line which is perpendicular to the longitudinal axis of the vessel (**Fig. 5-6A**). This angle will be the angle at which the smaller vessel deviates after the anastomosis (angle between the longitudinal axes of the vessels) (**Fig. 5-6B**).

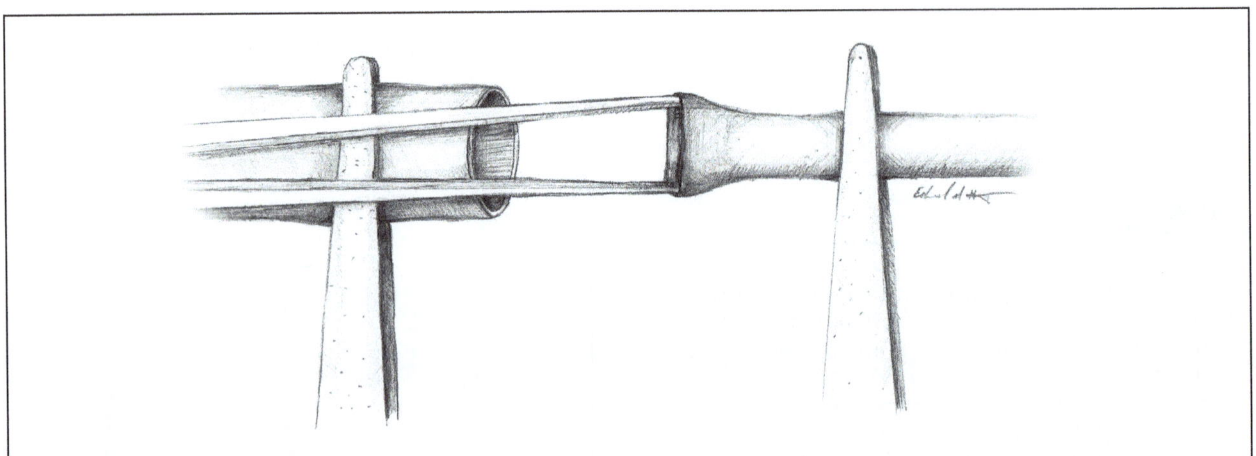

Figure 5-5

Dilation of the smaller vessel to rectify a disproportion of vessels diameters <50%. A relatively blunt forceps, Dumont No. 3 or No. 5 depending on vessel size, is inserted into the lumen with tips closed, and gently allowed to open gradually. The process can be repeated a few times. (Drawing by Edward M. Hagopian)

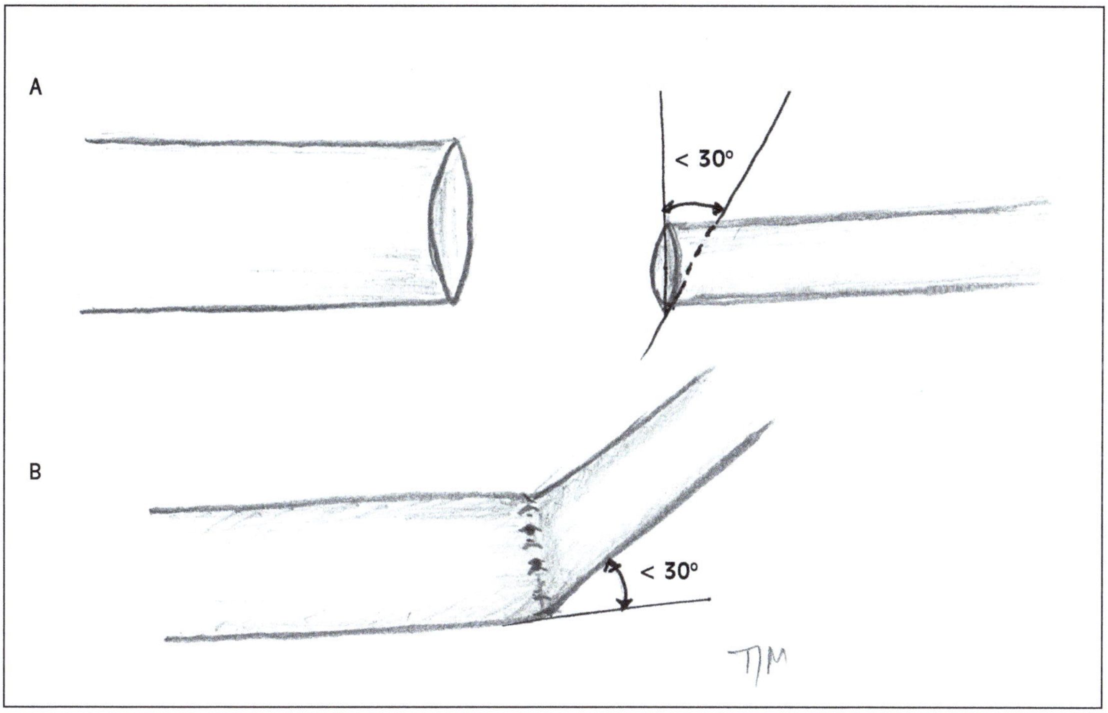

Figure 5-6

Oblique section of the smaller vessel to correct a 50-100% difference in vessels diameters **A.** The angle of the oblique section should be <30°, otherwise blood supply to the remaining stump of the smaller vessel will be impaired. **B.** The angle of oblique section is equal to the angle of deviation of the longitudinal axis of the smaller vessel from the longitudinal axis of the larger vessel at the site of the anastomosis. (Drawing by the author)

➤ The angle of oblique section of the smaller vessal should not surpass 30°

If the angle is >30°, blood supply to the remaining triangular stump of the smaller vessel may be impaired, resulting in post-operative aneurism at that site.

2. 'Fish-mouth' diametric insicions on the smaller vessel

Another technique available to rectify a 50-100% diameter disproportion is to make two small, 'fish-mouth' longitudinal incisions on the smaller vessel at the 3' and 9 o'clock positions (**Fig. 5-7**). This rcsluts in a spcctacu lar increase in vessel width. No other correction, e.g. cutting 'ears' (corners), is required. Attention is required when suturing on the smaller vessel due to the crooked shape of this modified opening.

Difference of vessel diameters >100%

End-to-side anastomosis

When the diameter of the smaller vessel is less than half the size of the larger vessel—a >100% disparity in diameter—an end-to-end anastomosis is not technically possible. Therefore, the planned procedure must be aborted and an end-to-side anastomosis should be performed.

Trouble Shooting

Below are solutions to a few usual problem that may be encountered during end-to-end anastomoses. These little 'secrets' in microsurgey are conquered with experience, and there are many others that you will discover yourselves.

The double clamp cannot be rotated (verify before start suturing)

Once the vessel stumps has been placed in the double clamp, verify that the clamp can be rotated before placing corner sutures. In some instances, the arrangent of the surgical field lessens or prevents rotation of the clamp. In such cases, the posterior wall is sutured first. To start, place the first suture on the posterior wall, in the middle of the semicircle. The knot is

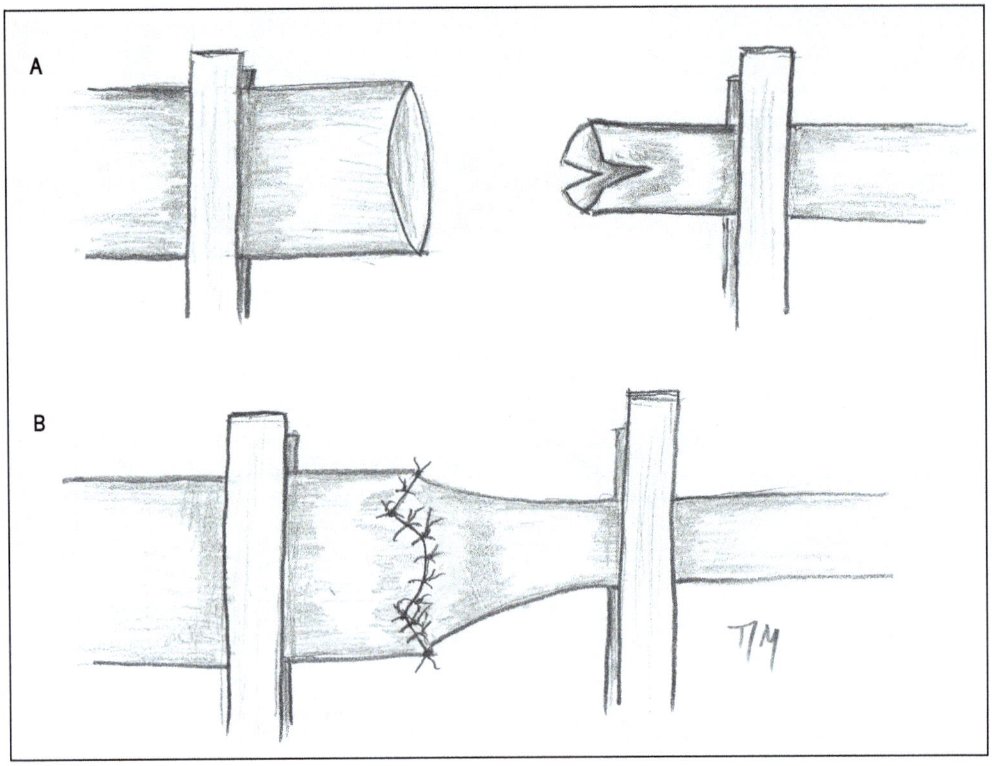

Figure 5-7

'Fish-mouth' longitudinal incisions of the smaller vessel to correct a 50-100% difference in vessels diameters. **A.** After cutting diametric longitudinal incisions, before anastomosis. **B.** After making the anastomosis. Observe the crooked line of sutures that requires specific attention. (Drawing by the author)

placed external to the lumen by first passing the needle from outside to inside the lumen, and then inside to outside the lumen (**Fig 5-8**). The median suture may be tied and left long, or may not be tied, in order to be used as a stay suture to facilitate the placement of the other sutures. Then, the two corner sutures may be placed, and left untied. Placement of the remaining posterior wall sutures follow, always placing the knots outside the lumen. Use the appropriate technique—*dividing the gap, closer to closer, or combination*—depending on the number of sutures required. After suturing the posterior wall including the corner sutures, the surgeon proceeds with the anterior wall sutures.

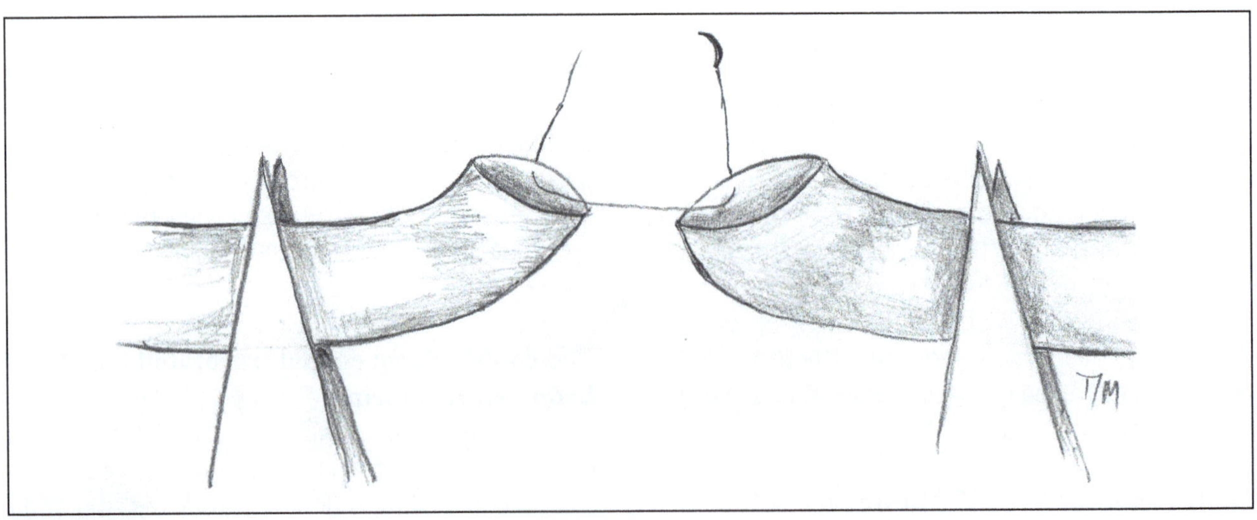

Figure 5-8

Posterior to anterior approach to suturing if the double clamp cannot be rotated. The first suture is placed in the middle of the posterior semicircle. The suture passes from outside to inside the upstream lumen, and from inside to outside the downstream vessel lumen. This places the knot on the external surface of the vessel. (Drawing by the author)

A portion of the vessel has to be excised, resulting in a gap that cannot be rectified by approximation of the clamps

There are two solutions to consider in this situation. The first is to try reducing tension on the anastomosis by applying traction on the upstream stump. The upstream stump is pulled towards the downstream stump and secured to its surroundings by placing a few sutures between its wall (not in the lumen) and the neighboring tissues. This technique may have serious consequenses via inadvertent vessel puncture or narrowing of the lumen. Both of these problems impair blood flow and increase the risk of thrombosis. If the gap is too large, a second solution—insertion of a vein graft—may be used to bridge the gap.

Very large blood leak after removal of the double clamp

In this scenario, there is most likely a gap in the suture line. Place the double clamp back onto the vessel and close it. Irrigate with normal saline to remove all blood and clots. When the surgical field is clean and the anastomosis can be clearly visualized, open slightly the upstream clamp to allow blood flow to the anastomosis, and close it again. This will help to find exactly where the leak is. Irrigate the surgical field and place an additional suture at the site of the gap. Pay attention not to catch the opposite wall of the vessel.

Suspicion that a suture catches the opposite wall

Correct this immediately. With the double clamp in place, cut the offending suture and place another in the same position; careful not to catch the opposite wall again. If you suspect that another suture has also caught the opposite wall, there is no other solution than to remove all sutures and start the anastomosis from the beginning. Good luck!

6 Principles of end-to-side anastomosis

End-to-End anastomosis is a prerequisite for End-to Side anastomosis. Therefore the reader is invited to read the previous Chapter. Important details are not repeated here.

1. Placement of a yellow background beneath the vessels

After the vessels have been dissected and mobilized, they are lifted up by Dumont forceps and a flexible yellow plastic background is placed underneath, centered at the site where the anastomosis is going to be performed. The yellow background serves to increase color contrast, thereby improving visualization of the vessels. The background and surgical field should be irrigated with warm normal saline. The field for an end-to-side is usually larger than that for an end-to-end anastomosis, because both the single clamp placed on the vessel that is going to be anastomosed terminally, and the double clamp placed on the vessel that is going to be anastomosed laterally, are better viewed and handled when both lie on the background.

2. Application of the double vascular clamp

The double clamp is applied on the vessel that is going to be anastomosed laterally. The principles of this application are the same as in the previous Chapter on end-to-end anastomosis.

3. Incision of the side-anastomosed vessel

An important rule for end-to-side anastomoses is that the size of the incision made on the side-anastomosed vessel must be equal to the diamenter of the vessel anastomosed at its end. This rule must be strictly followed by the beginner. Otherwise, trying to make the vessels fit will result in tearing or making suture holes that result in hemorrhage or will lead to stenosis of the anastomosis.

➢ The best way to judge the size of the the incision of the side-anastomosed vessel is to bring the lumen of the end-anastomosed vessel adjacent to the site of incision. This allows one to directly measure the incision size.

This means that the end-anastomosed vessel has to be prepared first (in this Chapter, however, it is described to be prepared second to the the side-anastomosed vessel, see below, section No. 5). In relatively simple operations with end-to-side anastomoses, the end-anastomosed vessel can be prepared first (Chapters 14, 23). In complicated operations such as the portocaval anastomosis (Chapter 16), the side-anastomosed vessel is prepared first. In heterotopic transplantation of the kidney (Chapter 28) or ovary (Chapter 30), receiver vessels that will be side-anastomosed are prepared first and end-anastomosed graft vessels follow. The opposite happens in the heterotopic transplantation of the heart, where graft vessels are prepared first (Chapter 31). On other occasions, preparation of the two side-anastomosed vessels of the receiver may not be performed simulteously, as in transplantation of inguinal dermal graft in the neck (Chapter 24), where the artery is prepared first, the arterial anastomosis is performed, and follows the vein-receiver incision and the veins anasrtomosis.

The incision of the side-anastomosed vessel can be made in one of three ways—transverse, longitudinal, or ellipsoid—with the transverse incision being recommended for most cases.

A. Transverse incision

This incision is performed transversally using sharp and straight microsurgcal scissors. Start by bringing scissors perperdicular to the longitudinal axis of the vessel (**Fig. 6-1**). The vessel is lifted with microsurgical forceps (**Fig. 6-2**). The ensuing incision includes all vessel layers—starting with adventitia, then media, and finally intima—until the vessel lumen is exposed (**Fig. 6-1**).

The beginner must must also be careful not to transect the side-anastomosed vessel when performing the incision. However, this serious accident does happen from time to time. The solution is to perform an end-to-end anastomosis to repair the cut vessel and chose a new site on which to perform the end-to-side anastomosis.

B. Longitudinal incision

On rare occasions, a longitudinal incision (along the length of the vessel) is chosen for the side-anastomosed vessel. To make it, microsurgical straight, sharp scissors or a pointed scalpel are used (**Fig. 6-3**). The vessel is slightly lifted up by microsurgical forceps.

The longitudinal incision is not recommended for the trainnee as it has many disadvantages. For one, the incision itself is difficult to make. In a transverse incision, the

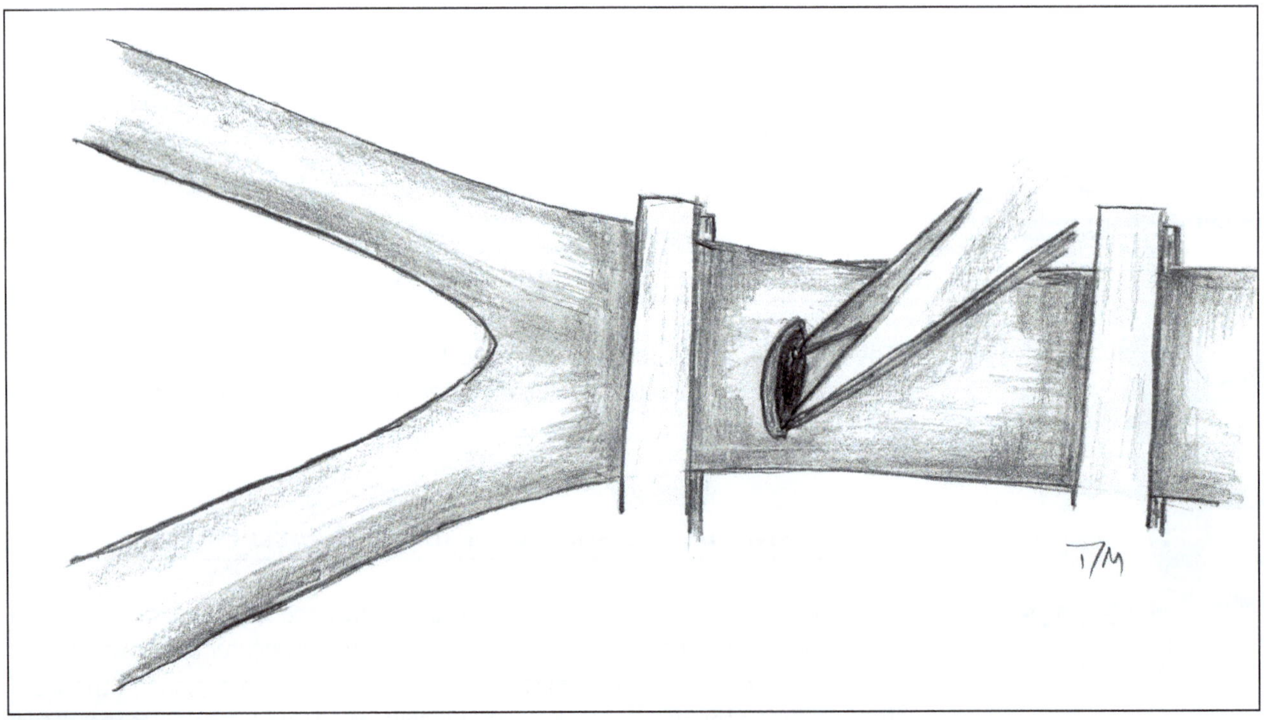

Figure 6-1

Transverse incision of the side-anastomosed vessel. (Drawing by the author)

Figure 6-2

Transverse incision of the side-anastomosed vessel. The vessel has been dissected and a background (a piece of surgeon's glove) has been put underneath it. The double clamp can be seen obstructing the vessel. The vessel is lifted up by curved microsurgical forceps and microsurgical scissors are brought perpendicular to the long axis of the vessel to make a transverse incision. (From author's photo library)

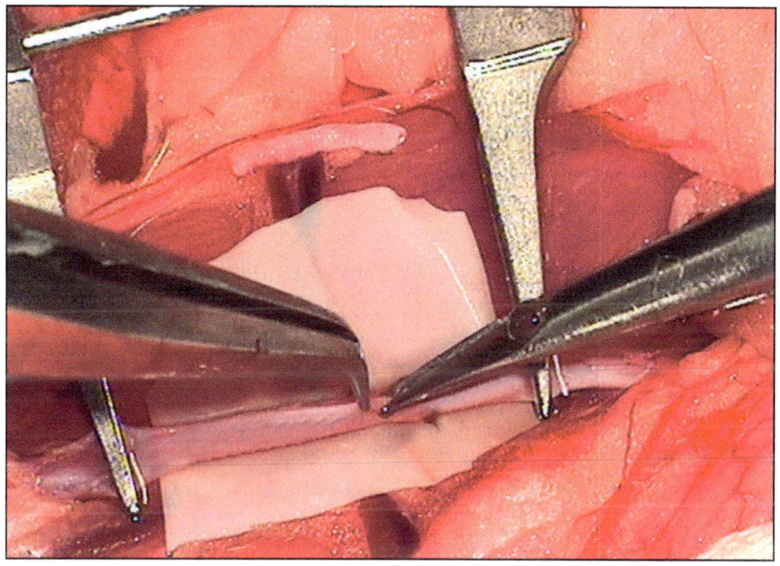

forceps lifts the vessel wall perpendicular to the planned incision and creates a tension line across which we can cut. In a longitudinal incision, however, the act of holding the vessel with forceps does not create this same helpful line of tension and thus does not offer support to the scissors as they cut in the same direction (the incision line is parallel to the tension line). After a longitudinal incision is made, the apperture is not held open by the natural tension lines of the vessel (as happens in tranverse incisions). This prevents direct vision of the lumen of the vessel and makes suturing difficult. Finally, dissecting adventitia around a longitudinal incision is much more difficult and there is increased risk that debris remains inside the lumen, resulting in thrombosis after the anastomosis.

In general, the longitudinal incision is not recommended for the trainnee. As its only possible application, we consider only the case of a vein of small caliber as the end-anastomosed vessel.

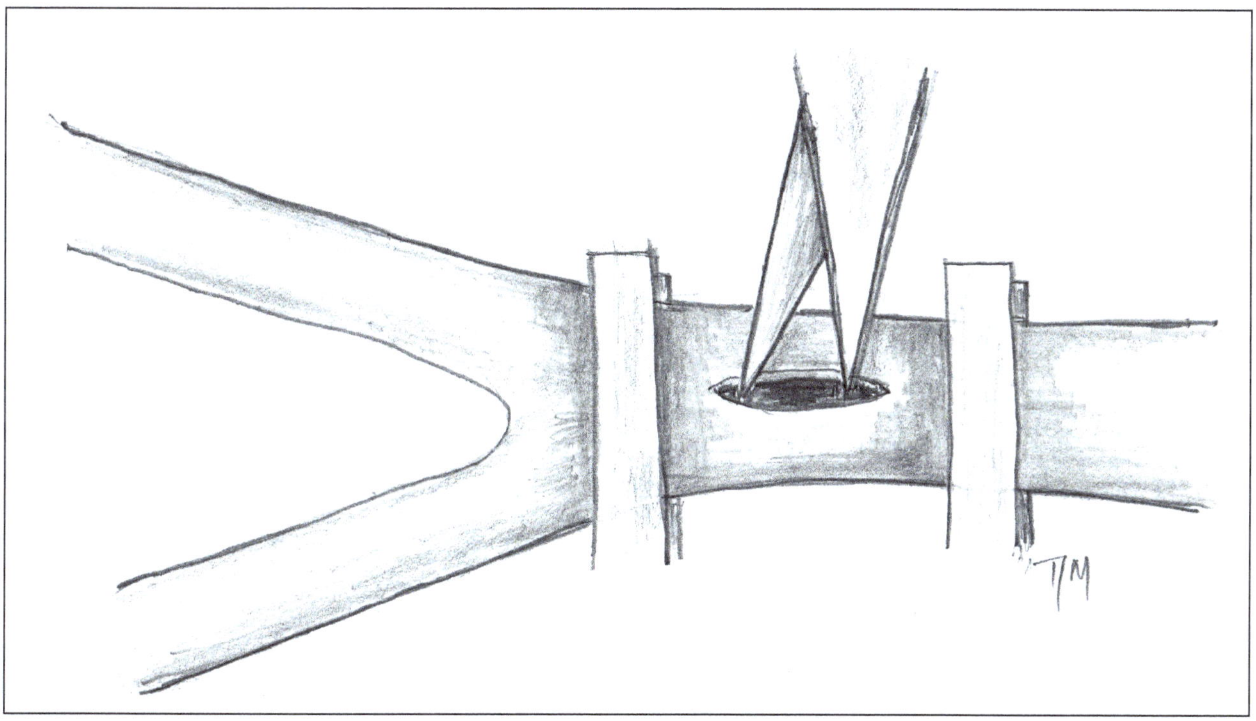

Figure 6-3

Longitudinal incision of the side-anastomosed vessel. (Drawing by the author)

C. Ellipsoid incision

To begin this technique, a stay suture is placed in the middle of the part of the vessel to be excised–usually in the midline of the anterior wall of the side-anastomosed vessel–and is lifted up for support. The apperture is created with two incisions–one on either side of the stay suture–using straight sharp scissors brought in at a 45° to 60° angle with respect to the longitudinal axis of the vessel. The cut starts lateral to the stay suture, extends transversely through the anterolateral wall of the vessel, and ends at an equal distance from the stay suture on the opposite side (**Fig. 6-4**). Other surgeons choose to pull up on the stay suture and perform both cuts simultaneously, with one closure of the scissors' legs. This is the 'tranverse' ellipsoid incision. Another alternative is the 'longitudinal' ellipsoid incision, which is performed with the scissors longitudinal axis placed parallel to the vessels longitudinal axis (**Fig. 6-4 Inlet**).

The maximum length of this ellipsoid aperture is allowed to be up to 30% larger than the diameter of the end-anastomosed vessel (this widening of the anastmostis facilitates blood flow through it).

As can be perceived from the details of this technique, the ellipsoid incision is addressed to the expert microsurgeon. It is usually applied when widening of the anastomosis is required. The beginner risks opening a hole in the side-anastomosed vessel that will be much too large to be anastomosed.

4. Irrigation of the lumen - Removal of the adventitia of the side-anastomosed vessel

As described in the prior Chapter, the vessel lumen must be irrigated under pressure with warm normal saline to wash away remaining blood clots. Remember that the 27G angiocatheter must not be inserted into the lumen.

Next, a small amount of adventitia (outer wall layer) is cut away all along the perimeter of the incision. This provides clean edges along the oval opening, where the anastomosis will be performed. Removal of the adventitia is not just a detail; it is crucial. Adventitial debris, if left behind, may get entrapped in the vessel lumen and result in thrombosis is. Adventitia removal is easier in arteries than in veins, because in artteries the adventitia is more prominent and can be detached. In larger veins, adventitia must also be removed in the perimeter of the incision; often to achive this, pieces of the adventitia are cut off the outer wall of the vein in the perime-

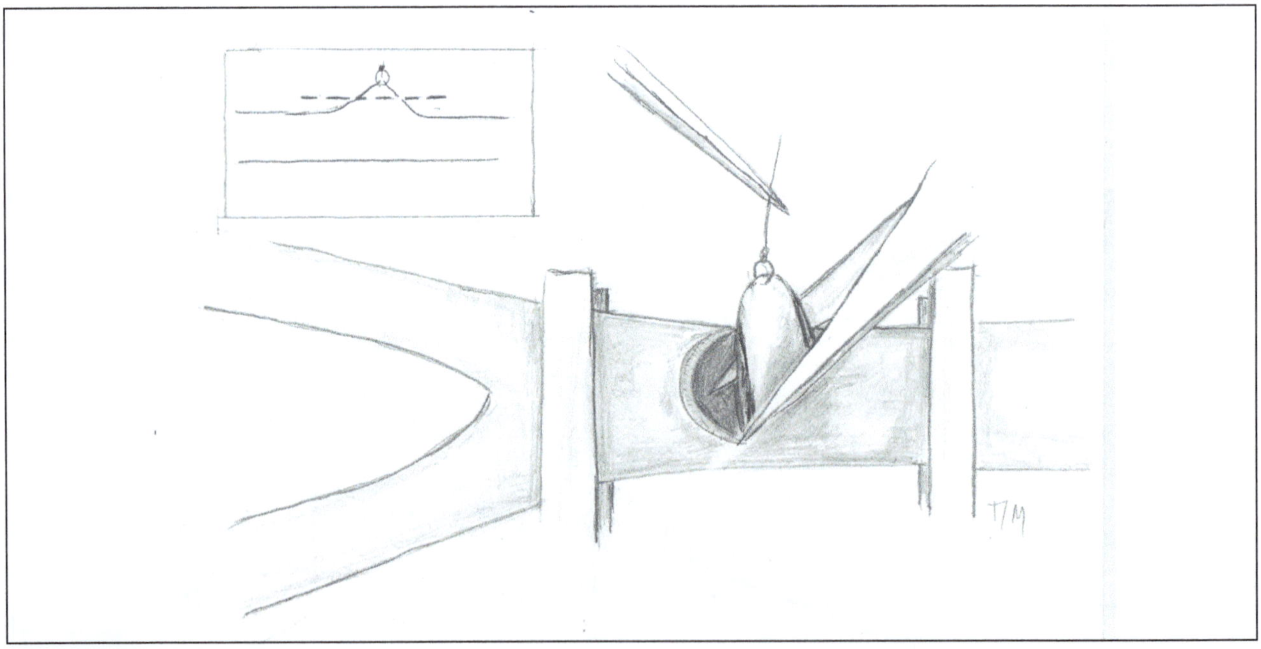

Figure 6-4

Transverse ellipsoid incision of the side-anastomosed vessel (aorta, above the bifurcation). A stay suture is placed midline in the part of the vessel to be excised and is lifted with Dumont forceps. A transverse cut has been performed with scissors caudal to the stay suture, starting from one side and ending at an equal distance on the opposite side. The ellipsoid incision will be completed by transecting the lifted flap of vessel wall on the cranial side of the stay suture (shown here). **Inlet:** Longitudinal ellipsoid incision. The suture pulls up the vessel wall and the incision (dashed line) is made parallel to the longitudinal axis of the vessel. (Drawing by the author) ter of the incision. In small veins. this step is extremlly difficult and can be omitted; the edges of the incision, however, must be clear.

5. Preparation of the end-anastomosed vessel

One end of the vessel is suture ligated, and the other occluded with the single vascular clamp. Whether clamp on the upstream or downstream side of the vessel, with suture ligation on the opposite side, depends on the design of the operation and the desired direction of blood flow through the anastomosis: artery to artery, artery to vein, vein to vein, and vein to artery. When a design includes veins, take into consideration that the presence of valves prevent retrograde blood flow, i.e. the blood flow though the vein cannot be reversed.

Once the correct approach and orientation of the end-anastomosed vessel is chosen, the end-anastomosed vessel is transected close to the ligation site with adequate lenght left towards the clamp. Leaving enough vessel length toward the clamp helps arrange for an easy anastomosis. The lumen of the vessel is irrigated with warm normal saline and the adventitia of the vessel is then folded (in the case of arteries) or removed (in the case of veins) as described in Chapter 5.

6. Suturing technique in end-to-side anastomosis

6.1. If the end-anastomosed vessel can be rotated, the anterior surface is sutured first

- Place the two corner sutures at 3 o'clock and 9 o'clock

These are the two basic sutures that will correctly orient the vessels. At 3 o'clock (toward the right hand of the surgeon), the suture first passes through the wall of the side-anastomosed vessel (from outside to inside the lumen) and then through the wall of the end-anastomosed vessel (from inside to outside the lumen). This allows the surgeon to keep the knot tied on the outside of the lumen. At 9 o'clock (toward the left hand of the surgeon), the suture first passes through the end-anastomosed vessel (from outside to inside the lumen), and then exits from the lumen passing through the side-anastomosed vessel. As with the 3'clock suture, the knot is tied external to the vessels wall. A knot inside the vessel lumen will cause the anastomosis to fail.

On the anterior wall, the sutures usually pass through the wall of the end-anastomosed vessel into the lumen (outside-inside) and exit through the side-anastomed vessel (inside-outside). Again, all knots are tied outside the lumen. The anterior surface is sutured by following either the principle of dividing the gap or estimated equal distances (closer to closer) (see Chapter 5.7 for suturing techniques). Depending on the total count of sutures required, either technique or a combination of the two is followed.

Once the anterior wall sutures are placed, the vessel is rotated and the suture line is inspected. The surgeon should look for any sutures that entrapped the posterior wall. Next, the posterior surface of the anastomosis is sutured in the same way as the anterior wall.

What follows is a detailed description of suture placement technique in relation to the total count of sutures requiered.

Total number of 4 sutures

After placement of the two corner sutures (3 o'clock and 9 o'clock), the 3rd suture is placed in the middle of the anterior surface semicircle.The end-anastomosed vessel is rotated and the 4th suture is placed in the middle of the posterior surface (**Fig. 6-5A**).

Total number of 6 sutures

After placement of the two corner sutures (3 o'clock and 9 o'clock), there are four left (two for each semicircle of the anterior and posterior surfaces). The two sutures of the anterior surface are placed at equal distances from the corner sutures, which are equal to the distance between themeselves.The end-anastomosed vessel is rotated and the two sutures of the posterior surface are placed in the same way (**Fig. 6-5B**).

Total number of 8 sutures

After placement of the two corner sutures (3 o'clock and 9 o'clock), there are six left (three for each semicircle). First, the median suture is placed in the middle of the anterior semicircle. The remaining two sutures for the anterior semicircle are placed in the middle of each quadrant. The end-anastomosed vessel is rotated and the three sutures of the posterior surface are placed in the same way (**Fig. 6-5C**).

Total number of 10 sutures

After placement of the two corner sutures (3 o'clock and

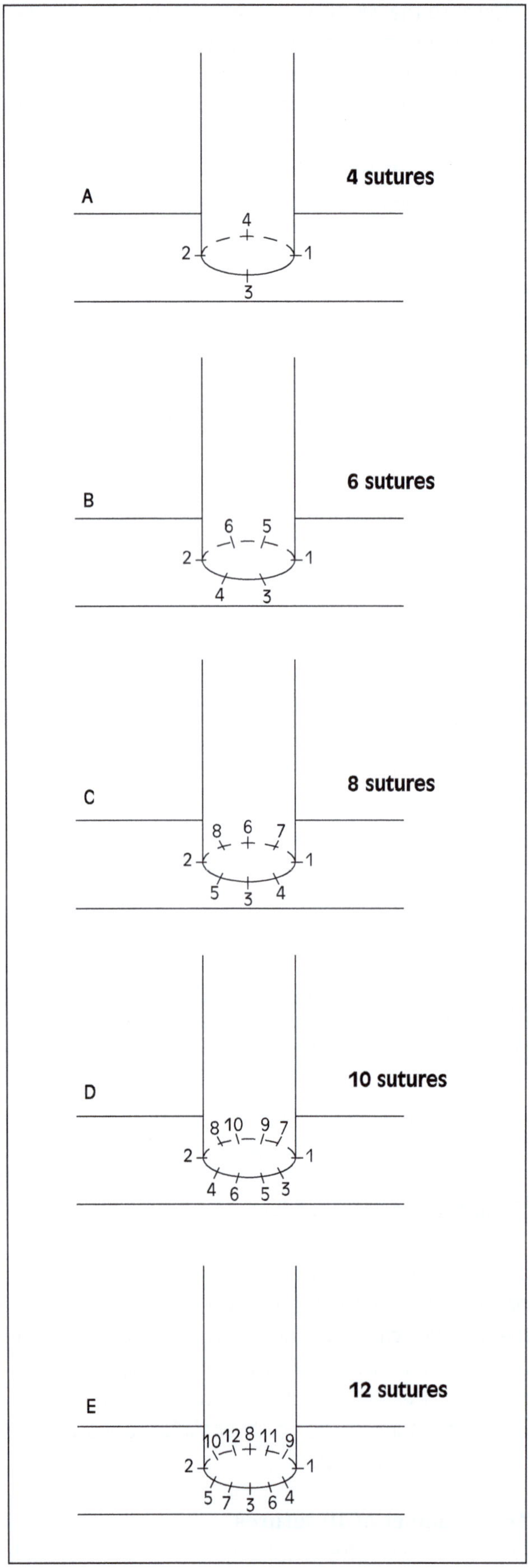

Figure 6-5

Order of suture placement depending on total count in end-to-side vascular anastomosis if the end-anastomosed vessel can be rotated. The anterior surface is sutured first, the vessel is rotated and suturing of the posterior surface follows. Numbers show the position and order of suture placement. The posterior surface of the end-anastomosed vessel is shown with a dash line. The corner sutures are those at 3 o'clock and 9 o'clock (numbered 1 and 2, respectively). All knots are placed external to the vessels wall.
A. Total of **4 sutures:** 2 corner sutures, and 1 in the middle of each semicircle.
B. 6 sutures: 2 corner sutures, and 2 placed at equal distances in each semicircle.
C. 8 sutures: 2 corner sutures, and 3 in each semicircle; the first of which is placed in the middle of the semicircle followed by one in the middle of each quadrant.
D. 10 sutures: 2 corner sutures, and 4 in each semicircle, all at equal distances. The first two are placed peripherally (close to the corner sutures) and the remaining two are placed medially.
E. 12 sutures: 2 corner sutures, and 5 in each semicircle. The first is placed in the middle of the semicircle followed by two more in each quadrant, at equal distances (between themselves and from the middle and corner sutures). First are placed the peripheral sutures (close to the corner sutures), and then the more medial sutures. (Diagram: E. Kontis)

9 o'clock), there are four left for each semicircle. The four sutrures of the anterior surface are placed at estimated equal distances, between themselves and the corner sutures. Here, the strategy to be used is closer to closer (de proche en proche, see Chapter 5). First, the two lateral sutures are placed (those closest to the corner sutures), followed by the two medial sutures. The end-anastomosed vessel is rotated and the four sutures of the posterior surface are placed in the same way (**Fig. 6-5D**).

Total number of 12 sutures

After placement of the two corner sutures (3 o'clock and 9 o'clock), there are 10 left (five for each semicircle). On the anterior surface, the first of these five is placed in the middle of the semicircle, followed by two more in each quantrant, placed at equal distances (between themselves, the corner suture, and the middle suture). Lateral sutures, those closest to the corner suture, are placed first. Then the more medial sutures are placed. The end-anastomosed vessel is rotated and the five sutures of the posterior surface are placed in the same way (**Fig. 6-5E**).

6.2. If the end-anastomosed vessel cannot be rotated, the posterior surface is sutured first

I. Posterior surface accessible

By 'accessible' we mean that sutures can be placed on the posterior surface and the knots can be tied outside of the lumen.

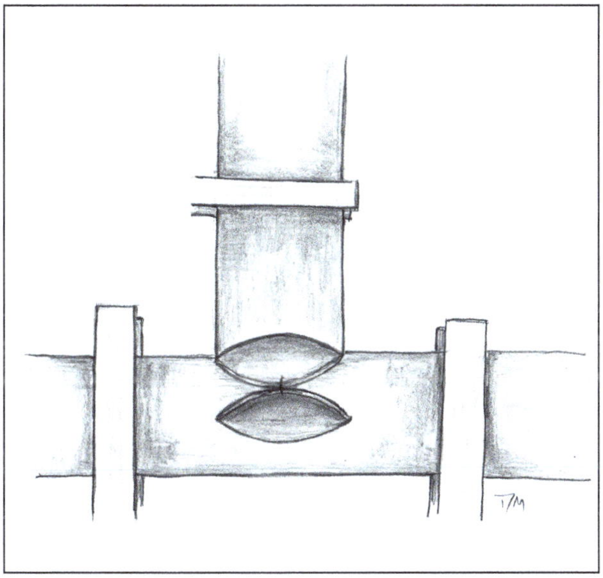

Figure 6-6

Placement of the 1st suture when the vessel cannot be rotated but the posterior surface is accessible in an end-to-side anastomosis. This suture is placed in the middle of the posterior surface. The suture passes from outside the lumen to inside the lumen of the side-anastomosed vessel, and then is passed from inside to outside the lumen end-anastomosed vessel. The knot is tied outside the lumen. (Drawing by the author)

➢ The anastomosis starts with placement of the 1st suture in the middle of the posterior surface (**Fig. 6-6**)

This suture passes from the outside the lumen of the side-anastomosed vessel into the lumen, and then exits by passing from inside to outside the lumen of the end-anastomosed vessel. The suture can also be placed in the reverse way, passing first though the end-anastomosed vessel, if needed. Either way is acceptable and the decision depends on how the vessels are oriented in the surgical field. Regardless of how the first suture is placed, the remaining sutures of the posterior surface are best placed by passing through the side-anastomosed vessel first. Proceeding in this manner is easier because the side-anastomosed vessel is held steady in the double clamp. As always, knots are to be tied on the outside surface of the vessel.

The second and third sutures are placed on either side and at equal distances from the first. The fourth and fifth sutures are then placed on either side and at equal distances from second and third sutures. The total suture count will determine whether corner sutures are placed or not. This strategy follows the principle of *away from either side of the median posterior suture and toward the median anterior suture from either side.*

What follows is a description of suture placement depending on their total count (**Fig. 6-7**). Placement of a total of **4 sutures** is not shown because it is rarely used in this case and is evident: the first suture is placed in the middle of the posterior surface, the second and third sutures are the corner sutures, the fourth suture is put in the middle of the anterior surface of the anastomosis.

Total number of 6 sutures

After placement of the 1st suture in the middle of the posterior semicircle, the 2nd and 3rd sutures are placed on either side at equal distances. At the same distances from those, the 4th and 5th sutures are placed in the anterior surface. The 6th suture is placed in the middle of the anterior semicircle, midway between the 4th and 5th sutures (**Fig. 6-7A**). There are no corner sutures placed in this scenario. Attention is needed to assure that all distances between any pair of sutures are the same.

Total number of 8 sutures

After placement of the 1st suture, the 2nd and 3rd sutures are placed on either side, at equal distances from the 1st. Given that the 4th and 5th sutures are placed as corner sutures, it is evident that the 2nd and 3rd suture are placed in the middle of each quadrant of the posterior surface. Similarly, on the anterior surface, the 6th and 7th sutures are placed equal distances from the corner sutuers (in the middle of each quadrant), and the 8th suture is placed in between the 6th and 7th sutures (in the middle of the anterior semicircle) (**Fig. 6-7B**).

Total number of 10 sutures

Making an anastomosis that requires 10 sutures, when the vessel cannot be rotated, is the most difficult case. After placement of the 1st suture, the 2nd and 3rd sutures are placed on either side at equal distances. The 4th and 5th sutures are similarly placed at the same distances. There are no corner sutures in this case.

On the anterior surface of the anastomosis, the 6th and 7th sutures are placed on either side at same distances. Similarily the 8th and 9th sutures are placed toward the middle of the semicircle. In the middle of the distance between the 8th and 9th suture is where the 10th suture is placed (in the middle of the anterior semicircle) (**Fig. 6-7C**). Attention is needed that all distances between any pair of sutures are the same.

When placing the last three sutures in this scenario, the median suture can be placed first and each of the last two at equal distances from the middle. However, the view of posterior luminal wall is restricted when the middle anterior suture is placed before sutures 8 and 9.

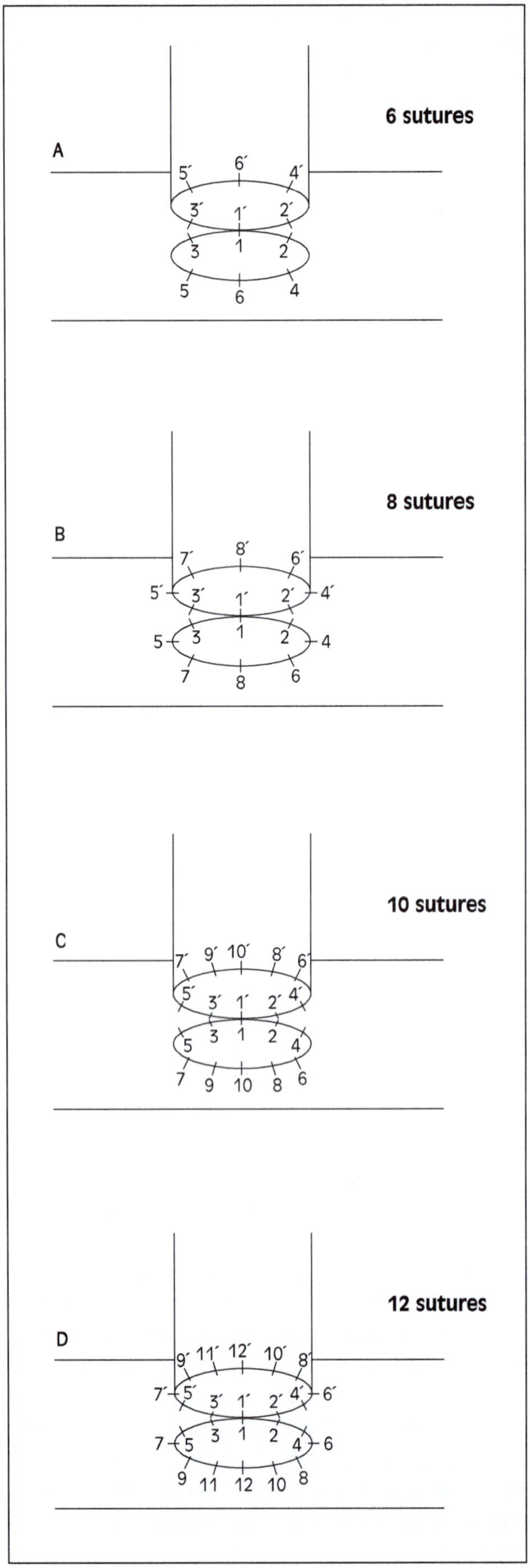

Figure 6-7

Order of suture placement depending on their total count in end-to-side vascular anastomosis, if the end-anastomosed vessel cannot be rotated. Numbers show the position and order of suture placement on the side-anastomosed vessel. Accented numbers show the symmetric position and order of sutures (points of exit) on the end-anastomosed vessel. All sutures first pass through the wall of the side-anastomosed vessel. Knots are tied outside the lumen. All sutures are equidistant from adjacent sutures.
A. 6 sutures: The 1st is placed in the middle of the posterior surface. The 2nd and 3rd sutures are placed on either side of the 1st. Similarly, the 4th and 5th sutures are placed on the anterior surface, with the 6th placed in between them.
B. 8 sutures: The 1st is placed in the middle of the posterior surface. The 2nd and 3rd sutures are placed on either side of the 1st The 4th and 5th are corner sutures. The 6th and 7th are placed on the anterior surface, with the 8th in the middle of the anterior semicircle. The sutures 2, 3, 6, 7 are placed in the middle of each quadrant.
C. 10 sutures: The 1st is placed in the middle of the posterior surface. The 2nd and 3rd are placed on either side of the 1st, and similarly the 4th and 5th sutures. The 6th and 7th follow on either side on the anterior surface. The 8th and 9th follow, more medially, and the 10th is placed last in between them.
D. 12 sutures: The 1st is placed in the middle of the posterior surface, the 2nd and 3rd on either side, and similarly the 4th and 5th sutures. The 6th and 7th are the corner sutures. The 8th and 9th are put on either side in the anterior surface and similarly the 10th and 11th more medially, with the 12th in between the previous two. (Diagram: E. E. Kontis)

Total number of 12 sutures

After placement of the 1st suture, the 2nd and 3rd sutures are placed on either side of the 1st suture, and similarly the 4th and 5th suture, all at equal distances. The 6th and 7th sutures are placed as corner sutures.

On the anterior surface of the anastomosis, the 8th and 9th sutures are placed on either side, at a distance from the corner sutures that equals the distances between previous adjacent sutures. Similarly, the 10th and 11th sutures are placed toward the middle of the semicircle. In the middle of their distance is placed the 12th suture (in the middle of the anterior semicircle) (**Fig. 6-7D**).

Alternatively, the median suture of the anterior surface can be placed first, thus leaving two remaining sutures for each quadrant. This strategy has the benefit of allowing the surgeon to better estimate distances between adjacent sutures. However, as previously noted it restricts the view of the posterior surface and makes it difficult for the surgeon to correct a mistake should the posterior wall be cought by an anterior suture.

II. Posterior surface not accessible

If it is not possible to place and tie interrupted sutures in the posterior surface of the anastomosis, then the posterior semicircle of the anastomosis must be created using a continuous (running) suture from inside the lumen. This technique begins with the placement of two corner sutures at 3 o'clock and 9 o'clock. The needle end of the 3 o'clock suture is kept long and then tied. This suture is used to close the posterior wall with a running stitch. The 9 o'clock suture is placed as an interrupted stitch, but the needle end is cut long enough so that the surgeon can easily tie it to the end of the continuous suture.

The continuous, 'running' suture is performed as follows. After the knot has been tied external to the lumen at 3 o'clock, the needle passes in situ from outside to inside the lumen of the side-anastomosed vessel. Then it passes from inside to outside, through the wall of the end-anastomosed vessel, and then from the exterior of the end-anastomosed vessel to internal of the side-anastomosed vessel, and so forth (**Fig. 6-8**). When the final suture passes adjacent to where the 9 o'clock corner suture is placed, the needle will be found on the inside of the lumen. At this point, it must pass in situ from inside the lumen to outside the lumen of the side-anastomosed vessel so that it can be tied to the longer tail of the 9 o'clock corner suture.

The anterior wall is sutured with interrupted sutures as previously described, depending on the necessary total count of sutures.

7. Release of the clamps

In principle, the downstream clamp is released before the upstream clamp, so blood does not accumulate within and put undue pressure on the anastomosis. In situations where the direction of blood flow is toward the side-anastomosed vessel, the double clamp is released first. This is followed by releasing the single clamp on the end-anastomosed vessel (the upstream clamp). If the direction of blood flow is in the direction of the end-anastomosed vessel, the single clamp is released before the double clamp.

8. Gauze placement

After the clamps have been released, a gauze is placed on the anastomosis. The gauze is left in place for 3 minutes, without applying any pressure, to allow for hemostasis of any leaks within the anastomosis.

9. Patency test

The patency test is performed in one of two ways, depending on the direction of blood through the anastomosis.

1. Flow is toward the end-anastomosed vessel. When the direction of blood flow is toward the end-anastomosed vessel, two forceps are used to test patency similar to an end-to-end anastomosis (see Chapter 5.10). The first forceps (closer to the anastomosis) stops blood flow. Next, a second forceps slides half-closed along the vessel a few millimeters di-

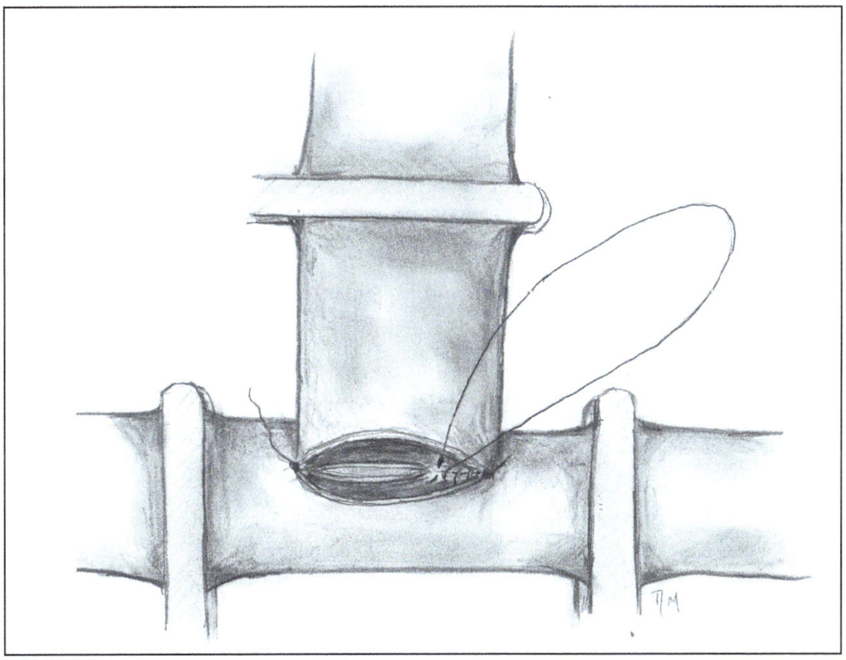

Figure 6-8

Continuous suturing of the posterior semicircle if the posterior wall is not accessible in an end-to-side anastomosis. Two corner sutures are placed, with the 9 o'clock suture cut long and the needle of the 3 o'clock suture left on. The needle of the latter suture enters in situ the lumen of the side-anastomosed vessel and a continuous suture follows (from inside-outside the end-anastomosed vessel, then from outside-inside the side-anastomosed vessel). At the end the suture exits in situ the lumen and is tied with the 9 o'clock suture. (Drawing by the author)

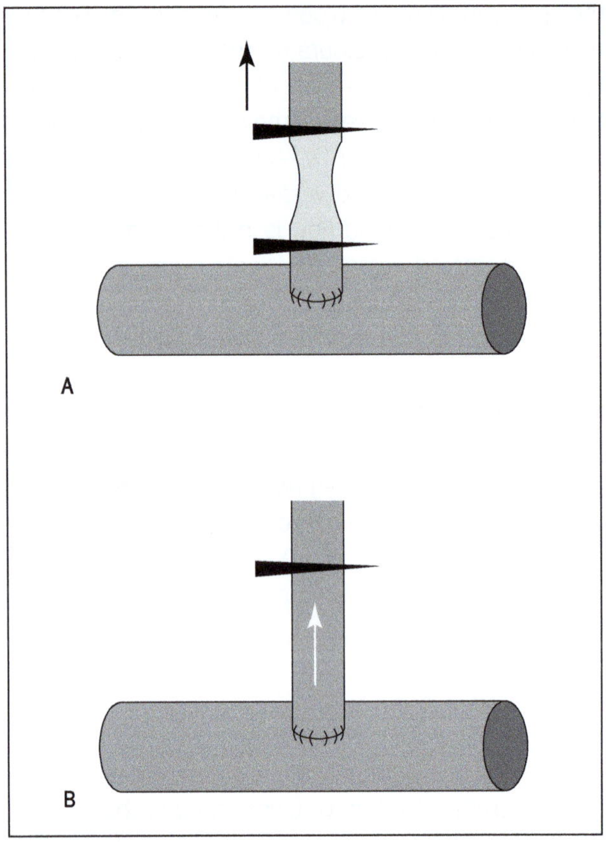

Figure 6-9

Patency test of an end-to-side anastomosis when direction of blood flow is toward the end-anastomosed vessel. The black arrow shows the movement of the downstream forceps and the white arrow the direction of blood flow. **A.** The central forceps occludes the vessel; a second forceps is placed peripherally and slides distally thus emptying the vessel, and occlude it after a short distance. **B.** The central forceps is removed. If the anastomosis is patent, the lumen is rapidly filled up to the second forceps. (Diagram: E. Kontis)

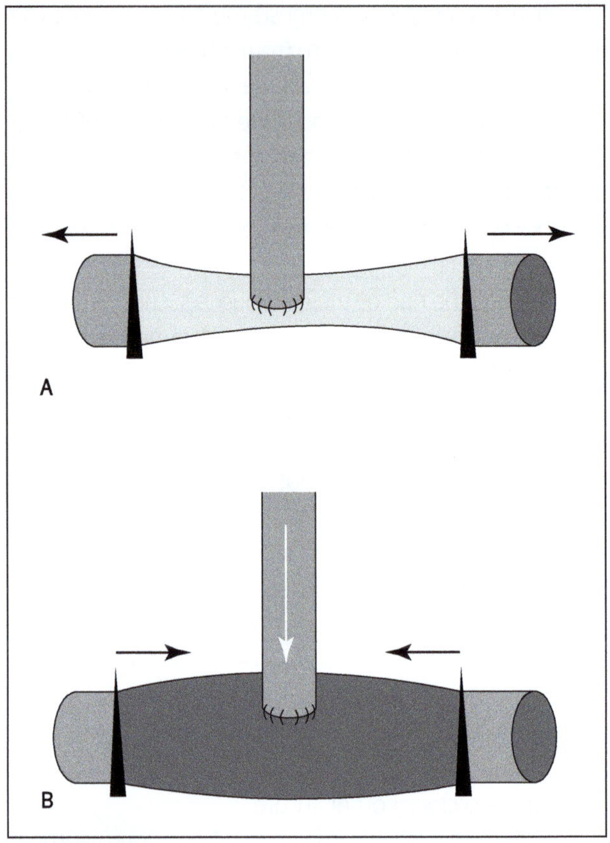

Figure 6-10

Patency test of an end-to-side anastomosis if the direction of blood flow is toward the side-anastomosed vessel. The black arrows show the movement of the forceps and the white arrow the direction of blood flow. **A.** The two forceps slide half-closed in opposite directions on the side-anastomosed vessel and empty the lumen; they close after a short distance. **B.** The closed forceps approach each other. If the anastomosis is patent, the lumen is rapidly filled between the forceps. (Diagram: E. Kontis)

stal to the first, in order to empty the lumen of blood in a 'milking' action. After a few millimeters of 'milking', the second forceps occludes the vessel (**Fig. 6-9A**). The first forceps is removed, keeping the second in place. If the anastomosis is patent, the end-anastomosed vessel will immediately fill with blood up to the second forceps (**Fig. 6-9B**).

2. Flow is toward the side-anastomosed vessel. If the direction of blood flow is toward the side-anastomosed vessel, two forceps are used to simultaneously empty this vessel. The forceps slide in opposite directions, not totally closed but still applying enough pressure to empty the vessel ('milking' motion). The forceps close at their final position (**Fig. 6-10A**). Then, the two closed forceps are brought closer to each other with a quick movement. If the anastomosis is patent, the side-anastomosed vessel will rapidly fill between the forceps (**Fig. 6-10B**).

7

Technique of microsurgical suturing of nerves

Basics of nerve microanatomy

Peripheral nerves are ensheathed by an outer covering of connective tissue called the epineurium. The epineurium carries small blood vessels (vasa nervorum) that serve as the blood supply to the nerve. In addition to covering the nerve, the epineurium continues as several dividing walls (septa) between the bundles of nerve fibers within each axon. The nerve bundles are surrounded by a complete sleeve (a layer of flat cells), called the perineurium (**Fig. 7-1**).

The trainee in microsurgery should be able to recognize the epineurium and the perineurium. It is advisable to gain this experience in the laboratory before attempting a nerve suturing.

Nerve preparation

During preparation of nerves, the surgical field is regularly irrigated with 2% xylocaine solution. Normal saline is not used because it causes edema of nerve membranes.

Neurolysis, i.e. mobilization and dissection of the nerve, can be easily executed in the ideal conditions of the experimental laboratory. However, neurolysis in the clinical setting may prove difficult, particularly in a surgical field with scar or fibrosis. The epineurium can be recognized by its white, pearly color and the presence of the small vessels of the vasa nervorum on the surface (**Fig. 7-1**). If mobilization of the nerve and the epineurium proves to be impossible, then the epineurium can be opened. This technique is called internal neurolysis. Because the epineurium lies between the bundles of nerve fibers within each axon, it is conceivable that a surgical plane can be created in this space. Said plane will provide adequate exposure to each perineurium, likely with a small amount of surrounding epineurium. The technique used to approximate and suture each perineurium will be discussed in detail below.

Nerve transection should be performed perpendicular to the nerve using sharp scissors. Transection should be done with a clear cut to obtain clean edges of the stumps. Otherwise, the bundles of nerve fibers will extend beyond the border of the cut and 'overflow' (like toothpaste out of a tube), due to their jelly-like consi-

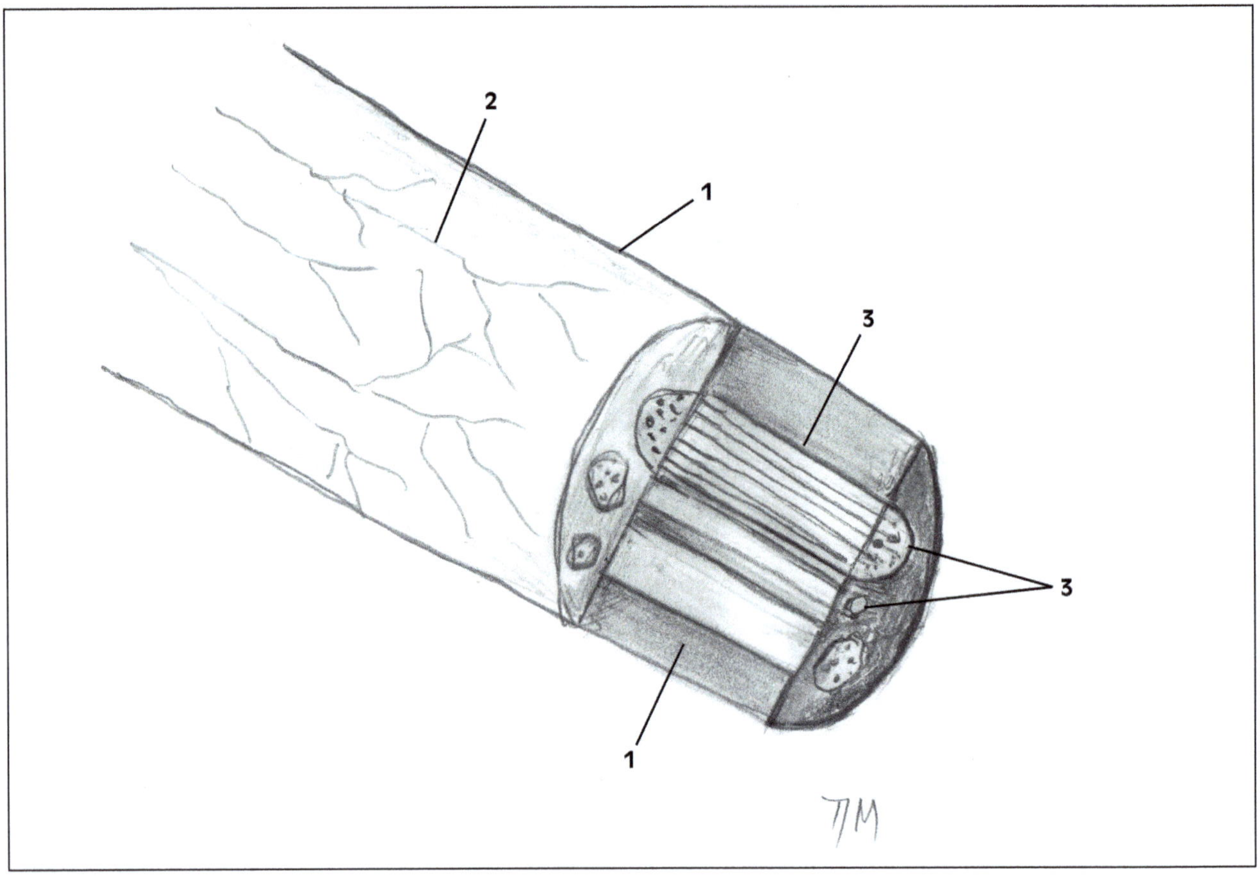

Figure 7-1

Microanatomy of a peripheral nerve. The nerve has been cut perpendicular to the long axis and stepwise along the axis to show its internal structure. **1.** epineurium, covers the external surface of the nerve and fills in the space between each perineurium (grey area), **2.** vessels (vasa nervorum) on the epineurium, **3.** perineurium, around each bundle of neural fibers; one bundle is shown as opened and nerve fibers are seen as thin lines. (Drawing by the author)

stency. If this happens, the borders of the perineuriums will be lost, requiring an additional transection to obtain clean edges.

Approximation of the stumps of the nerve

Once the nerve is transected, the two ends of the nerves retract and move away from each other. The edges need to be re-approximated as soon as possible, otherwise the nerve fibers will 'overflow' out of the perineuriums.

- A double vascular clamp should never be used for the approximation of the nerve stumps. The pressure applied by this clamp would cause significant damage to the small vessels of the epineurium.

Some microsurgeons use fine needles (e.g. 28G) to approximate the stumps of the nerve. This technique, however, is traumatic and, in the hands of a trainee, may result in longitudinal tear of one or both stumps.

Another acceptable, non-traumatic technique is to approximate the stumps of the nerve using a 10/0 Nylon stay-suture (**Fig. 7-2**). The suture needle enters the epineurium at a distance of 1-1.5 cm from the right edge (for right-handed surgeons) and a knot is made at the distal end of the thread. The needle is pushed along the axis of the nerve and a Dumont forceps is then used to grasp the needle. The needle is then passed to the needle driver and pushed into the lumen of the

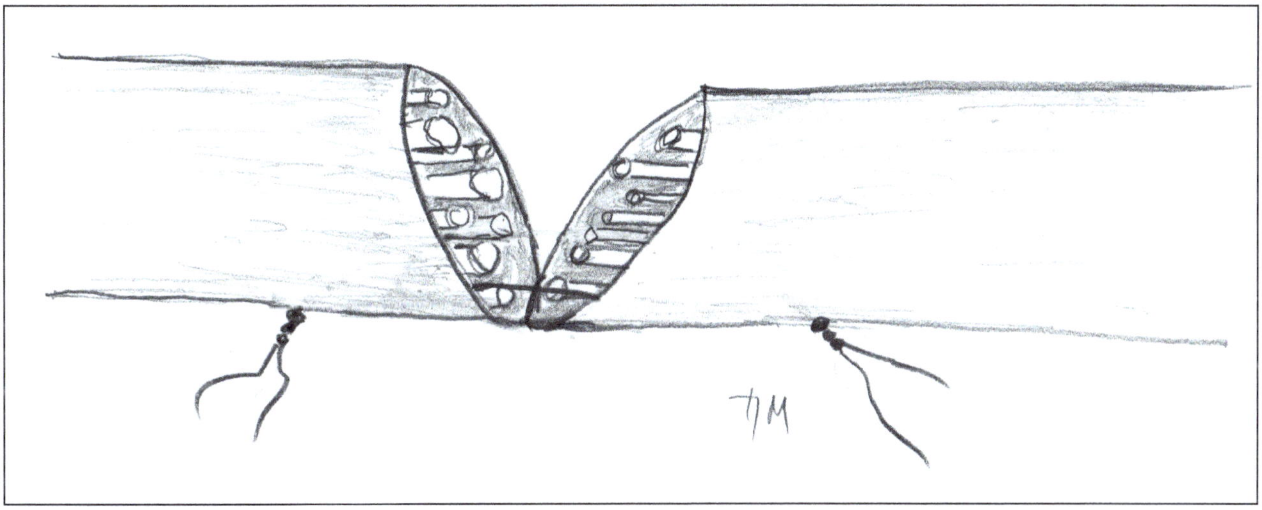

Figure 7-2

Placement of a stay suture for approximation of the nerve stumps. A Nylon 10/0 suture enters the epineurium at 1-1.5 cm from the edge and a knot is made at the distal end. The suture exits at an equidistant location on the opposite stump and is tied once the edges of the nerves are approximated. The suture will be removed once the nerve is sutured to completion. (Drawing by the author)

other nerve stump. The needle then exits the epineurium at a distance of 1-1.5 cm from the left edge. By pulling the needle, or the suture, the two stumps of the nerve approximate. Once the stumps come into contact, a knot is made at the exit of the epineurium on the left edge of the nerve. The ends of suture at both knots are left long as this is a stay suture and only of temporary use. The stay suture is removed once the nerve has been sutured to completion. Suturing of the nerve is discussed below.

Principles of nerve suturing techniques

Proper suturing of the nerve must align the nerve stumps, correctly orient each bundle to its counterpart and ensure an airtight closure. Use of a monofilament Nylon suture is recommended as it does not cause sclerosis or fibrosis of the neural tissue.

1. Suturing the epineurium

The technique used to suture the epineurium is the same as the technique used for vascular microsuturing, but as mentioned before, the double clamp cannot be used due to its damaging effect on the vasa nervorum. Therefore, the following needs are born asking for solutions:

- The stumps of the nerve must be approximated to each other. To this end, the previously described stay suture can be used (**Fig. 7-2**).
- The stumps of the nerve must be approximated without rotation about the longitudinal axis, otherwise the course of the nerve fibers will not be aligned. Alignment can be obtained by following the course of the vasa nervorum on the epineurium (**Fig. 7-1**).
- Once aligned, the stumps of the nerve must then be able to rotate in order to suture the posterior surface. To facilitate rotation, two sutures are placed on the epineurium and tied in the middle of the anterior surface and in the middle of the posterior surface (9 o'clock and 3 o'clock) (**Fig. 7-3**). These suture ends will initially be left long to assist with handling the nerve and placing the rest of the sutures. The suture ends will be cut short once the epineurium has been sutured to completion.

Suturing of the epineurium is performed under high magnification in the rat. If the diameter of the nerve is less than 1 mm, Nylon 9/0 or 10/0 suture should be used.

The disadvantage of suturing the nerve by suturing

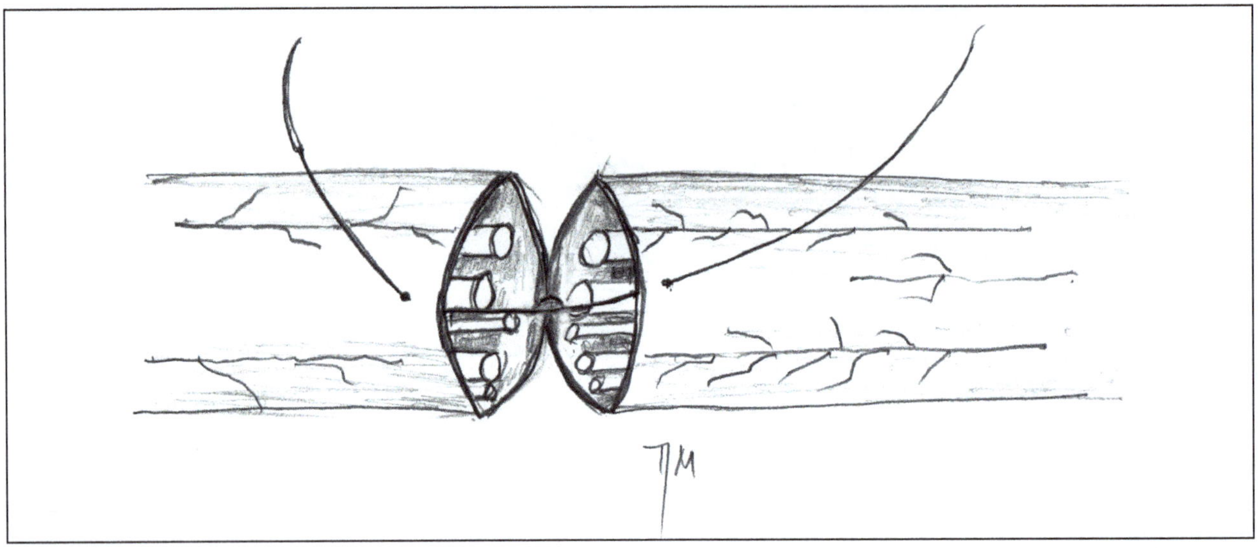

Figure 7-3

Suturing of the epineurium. The vessels on the epineurium are used to identify the correct positioning of the two nerve stumps and avoid rotation around the longitudinal axis. One suture has been placed in the middle of the posterior surface, with the knot external to the epineurium. The second suture passes in the middle of the anterior surface of the epineurium. (Drawing by the author)

the epineurium is that, beyond following the rough course of the vessels on the epineurium as a means to align the bundles of nerve fibers, there is no other certainty that the nerve fibers will be aligned correctly. Therefore, it is possible that the corresponding nerve fibers do not come into contact, or that only a portion of fibers find their counterparts. Additionally, the nerve fibers may erroneously come in contact with fibers of a different bundle which would have detrimental effects in the setting of a mixed nerve (i.e., a motor fiber aligned to a sensory fiber).

2. Suturing the perineuriums

The perineuriums within the nerve are recognized by a white, pearly color and elastic consistency, while their content, the bundles of nerve fibers, are jelly-like in consistency. The surgeon's main concern is to identify, based on size, the perineurium of one stump that corresponds to the correct perineurium of the other stump. This task requires great care to avoid mistakes.

Suturing of the perineurium is performed under maximum magnification. Nylon 10/0 or 11/0 sutures are used. One or two sutures are placed on each perineurium, depending on its size (**Fig. 7-4**).

While some surgeons do not suture the epineurium upon closure of the perineuriums we recommend performing this additional step. To perform this step correctly, it is important to avoid placing the suture line of the epineurium directly atop the suture 'line' of the perineuriums. Of note, this 'line' is rarely straight in nature, as the sutures tend to move following approximation, as shown in **Figure 7-4**. To avoid overlapping the two suture lines, the epineurium can be sutured at a small distance from the suture line of the perineuriums. This step may require a Z-plasty incision along the epineurium.

3. Suturing the epineurium and the perineuriums

After each perineurium bundle has been matched by size, and the two nerve stumps have been aligned by the course of vessels on their surfaces, sutures are placed passing through the epineurium and each perineurium. Each suture enters the epineurium on one stump, enters the lumen of the nerve and passes through an individual perineurium. In the other stump, the suture passes through the corresponding perineurium and then externally through the epineurium at a symmetrical

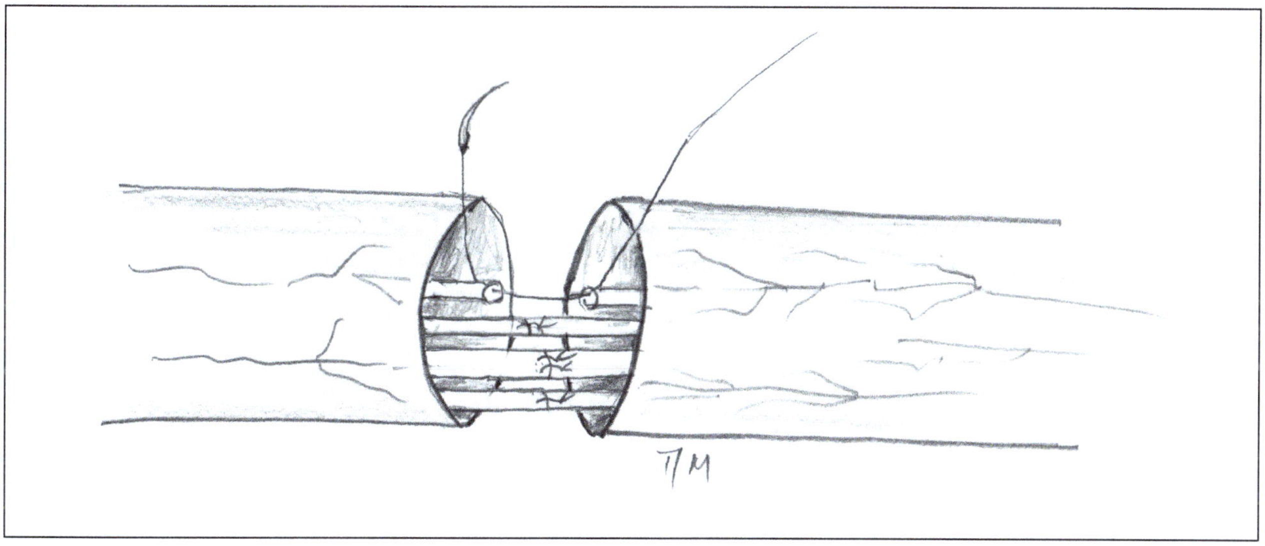

Figure 7-4

Suturing of the perineurium. The perineriums of each stump are matched by size. One or two Nylon 10/0 or 11/0 sutures are placed on each perineurium. (Drawing by the author)

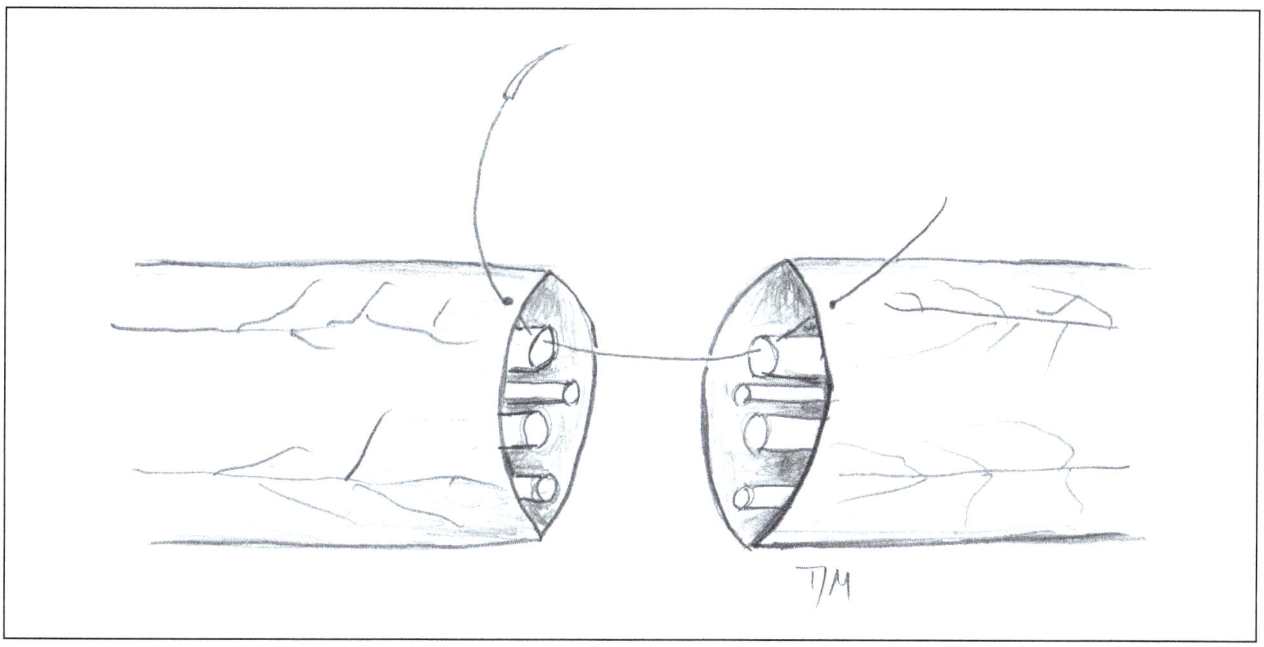

Figure 7-5

Suturing of the epineurium and the perineurium. For proper orientation of the nerve, the vessels on the epineurium are aligned and the perineuriums are matched by size of the bundles of nerve fibers. Each suture passes through both the epineurium and perieurium. All knots are placed on the external surface of the epineurium. (Drawing by the author)

distance to the previous stump (**Fig. 7-5**). The suture is then tied with the distal end of the thread, placing the knot external to the epineurium. In similar fashion, additional sutures are placed.

Supporters of this technique argue that it has the advantage of correctly orienting all bundles of nerve fibers and avoids placing knots in contact with the perineurim of each bundle of nerve fibers.

Part III

Microsurgical Procedures

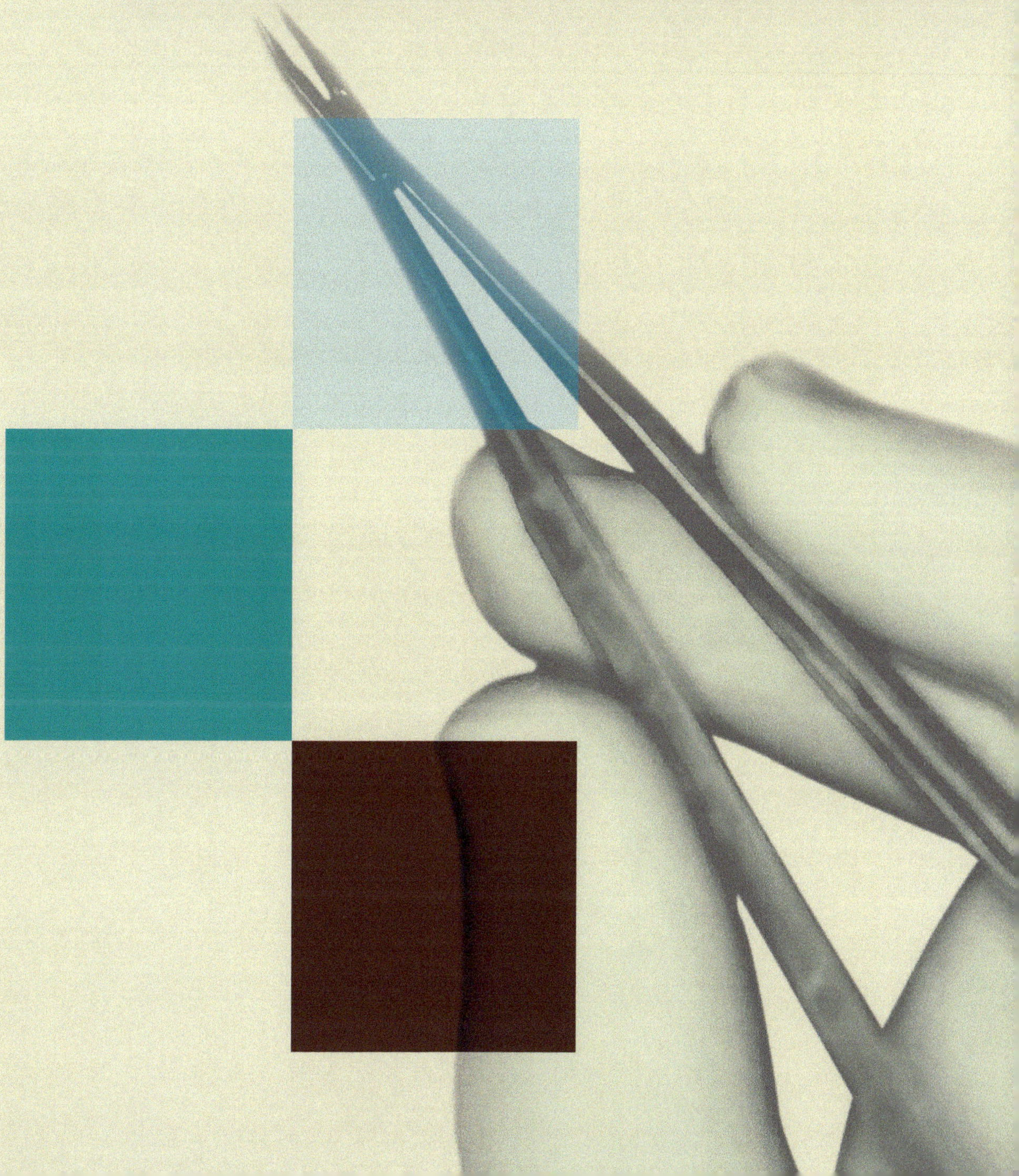

8

End-to-End anastomosis of the aorta

(below the renal arteries)

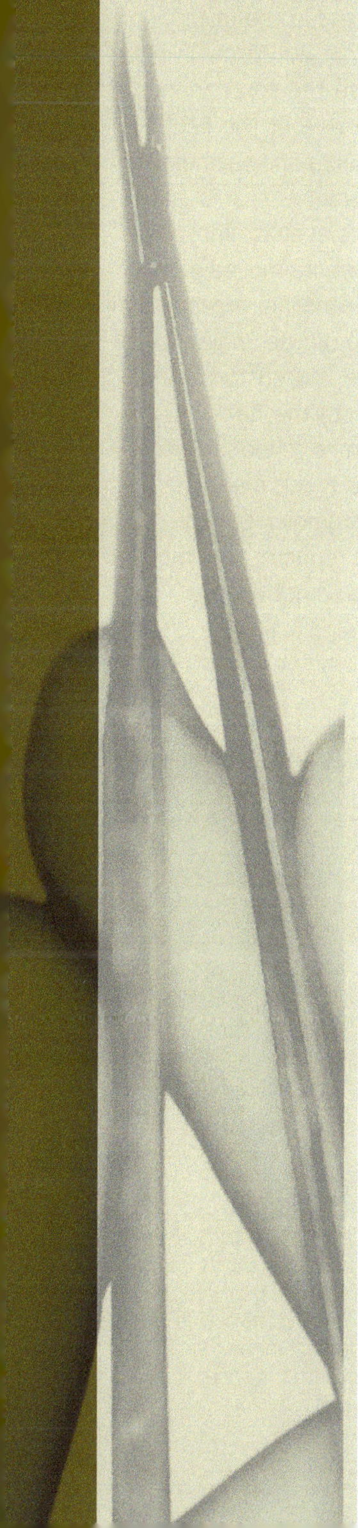

A. Positioning of the rat

The rat is placed in dorsal decubitus (supine) position on the working surface. The long axis of the body of the rat is parallel to the frontal (coronal) plane of the surgeon's body and the rat's head is placed on the surgeon's left. The limbs of the rat are immobilized on the working surface with adhesive tape.

B. Preparation of the surgical field

1. Opening of the abdominal wall

A midline incision is performed in the skin. The incision starts from 5 mm below the xiphoid cartilage (the caudal part of the xiphoid process is cartilaginous in the rat) and ends 5 mm above the pubic symphisis. The skin and superficial fascia are detached from the investing fascia of the muscles using blunt scissors (baby-Metzenbaum). If a small vessel of the superficial fascia bleeds, diathermy may be used.

Abdominal rectus muscles must be separated exactly on the linea alba. For the incision of the linea alba, a scalpel or scissors (baby-Metzenbaum) can be used. The two can be combined, i.e. opening may start with the scalpel and continue with scissors. For the trainee we recommend exclusive use of the scissors. The abdominal wall is pulled up at the midline with fine teeth surgical forceps, and a small transverse incision is made in the midline with the scissors. Air immediately enters the abdominal cavity and the abdominal wall separates from the splanchna. Then, while lifting the incision edge with the forcpes, one blade of the scissors enters the abdominal cavity and incision of the linea alba is completed.

➢ Access through the linea alba, if done correctly, is bloodless.

If you come across hemorrhage, this means you did not follow the linea alba and have entered the rectus muscles. If this occurs, cauterize to stop the bleeding—or place a hemostatic suture if needed. Then, come back in the midline to continue the incision of the linea alba correctly.

➤ Cephalad, during the incision of the linea alba, you are going to come across the border of the liver. Take care not to traumatize it.

Normally, the scissors will slide over the lobes of the liver. Do not try to remove the liver lobes now, this will be done after the paper clip retractors will be in place (see below).

Paper clip retractors are placed on either edge of the incision. They should be placed symmetrically and under the same traction force, otherwise the surgical field will be asymmetric and pose difficulties in maneuvers. Alternatively, four retractors (two on each edge) can be placed. More retractors do not necessarily produce a better surgical field and may hinder the surgeon's maneuvers. The optimal surgical field results from correct positioning and symmetry of the retractors.

2. Mobilization and arrangement of splanchna

After opening the abdomen and placement of the retractors, the surgeon obtains full view of the abdominal viscera (**Fig. 8-1**). Before any manipulation, a few drops of warm normal saline are sprinkled in the abdomen. Using two atraumatic (anatomical) forceps, the organs are moved and identified.

Handling of the liver

The rat liver occupies a great part of the abdominal space and has more lobes than the human: right, middle, left and quadrate (see **Figure 16-2**). In contrast to the human, these lobes are separated by true, deep fissures, and are therefore mobile. The falciform ligament courses between the left and the middle lobes, but is not encountered during the median incision.

The lobes of the liver that protrude in the surgical field must be moved. For dissection of the aorta below the left renal artery (see below) [and in the majority of the operations in the abdomen that will follow in next Chapters], it is adequate to move the spontaneously protruding lobes that disturb the view of the field, without specific recognition of the lobes and segments of the rat liver (as is necessary in operations near/or at the porta hepatis, such as the portocaval anastomosis, see Chapter 16.C). The protruding lobes are moved away or rotated upward with very gentle handling; a paper clip retractor that has been bent at an obtuse angle (No. 3, **Fig. 1-4**) and enveloped by gauze is used to this end. The goal is just to move them from the field, not the complete cephalad inversion. In some schools of microsurgery rotation of the liver lobes is not mentioned at all in the dissection for aorta anastomosis, but the protruding lobes are moved with the retractor that mobilizes the intestine (see below), which is not wrong.

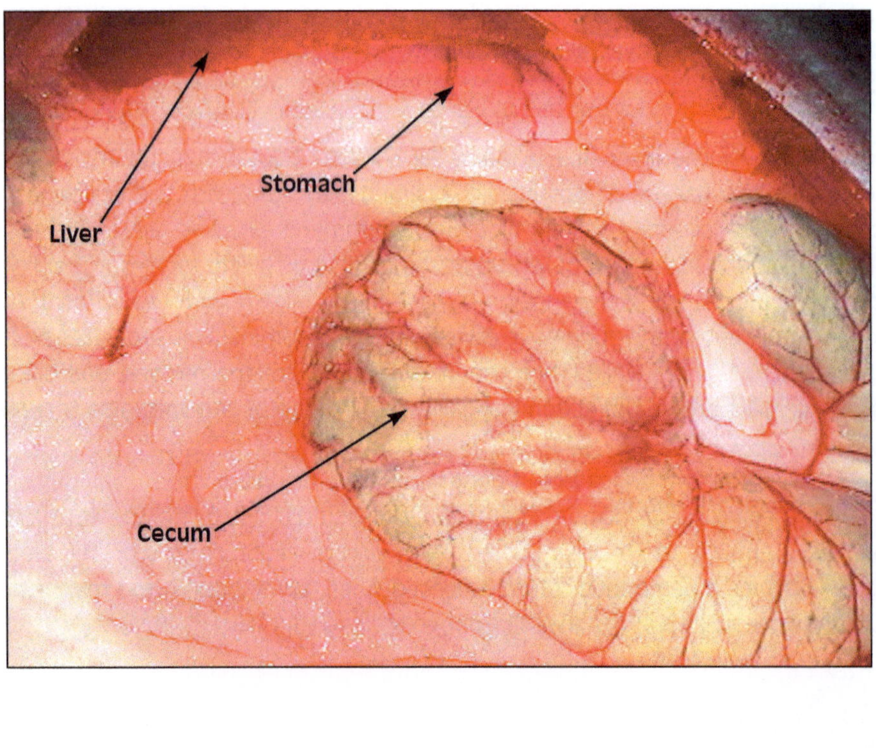

Figure 8-1

View of the visceral organs of the abdomen after opening of the abdominal wall in the rat. Note the medial position of the cecum and the abundant fat in the mesentery. (From author's photo library)

➢ Pay specific attention not to traumatize the liver during these maneuvers: use an obtusely bent retractor (dressed with gauze), broader atraumatic forceps, and do not grasp the lobes of the liver with forceps, they are fragile.

Mobilization of the intestine

The cecum is the largest and the most distended part of the colon in the rat. Endowed with a long mesentery, the cecum is totally mobile and found medially in the abdominal cavity. In order to move the intestine out of the abdomen, the cecum is grasped and pulled out. As it is being moved, the exit of the cecum from the abdomen is followed by exit of the ascending colon and small intestine, because of the continuous mesentery. The relations of the mesenteries of the small and large intestines in the rat are shown in **Figure 8-2.**

- The cecum and the ascending colon are not attached to the posterior peritoneum. They are mobile due to their long mesentery that is attached at the root of the superior mesenteric artery from which they are fed, and does not adhere to the parietal peritoneum of the posterior abdominal wall.

  In the human, during development, these organs get attached to the posterior peritoneum, the visce-

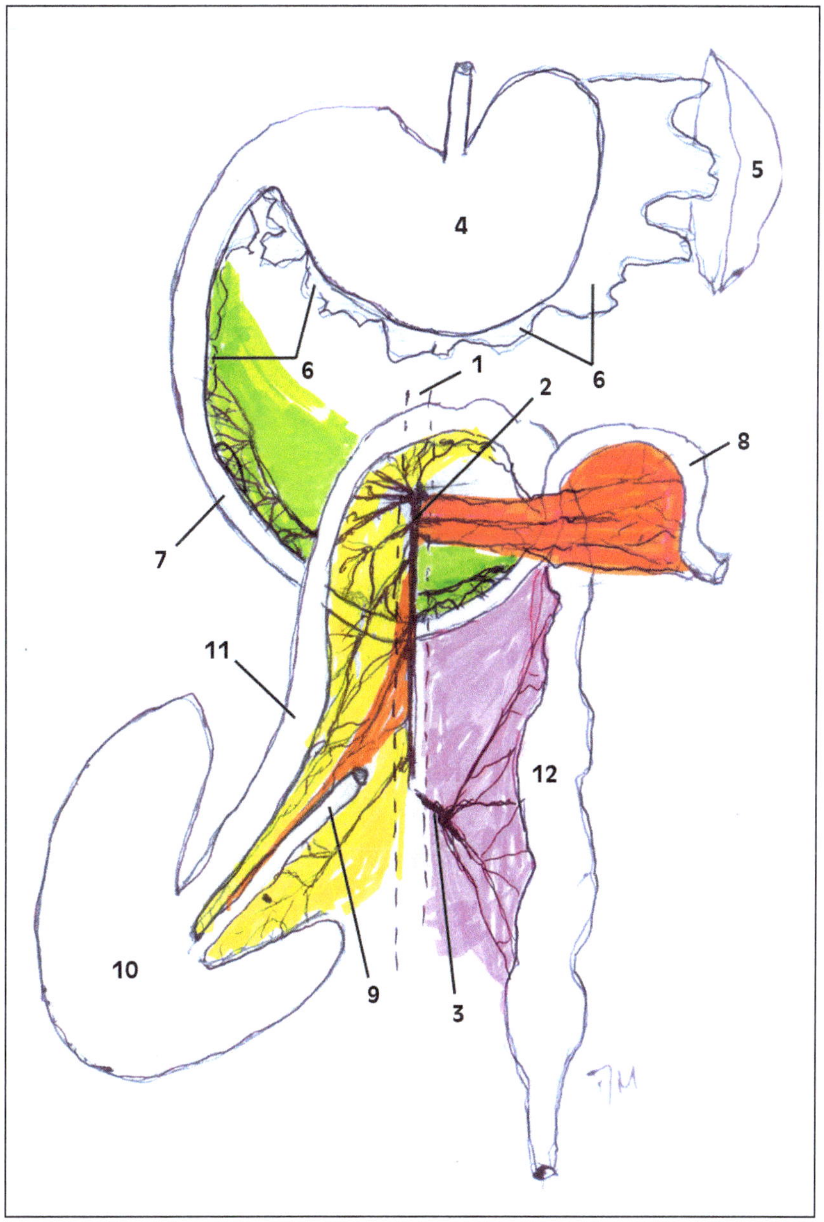

Figure 8-2

Mesenteries of the small and large intestine in the rat. The cecum and the ascending colon are not fixed to the posterior peritoneum as in the human, but are mobile because of their free long mesentery (painted **yellow**), which is continuous with the mesentery of the mobile ileum (painted **light orange**). The jejunum, due to its free mesentery (painted **dark orange**), is fully mobile as far as the 3rd part of the duodenum. The mesentery of the 2nd and 3rd part of the duodenum (painted **green**) is attached to the posterior peritoneum, therefore they are fixed. Note that in this image the duodenal loop is presented enlarged and the 2nd and 3rd parts longer than in reality. The mesentery of the descending colon (painted **pink**)–which is fixed to the posterior peritoneum in the human – is presented here as extending to the left. However, in the rat this mesentery is actually short, connecting the descending colon to the aorta anteroposteriorly. **1.** aorta, **2.** superior mesenteric artery, **3.** inferior mesenteric artery, **4.** stomach, **5.** spleen, 6. pancreas, **7.** duodenum, **8.** jejunum, **9.** ileum, **10.** cecum, **11.** ascending colon, **12.** descending colon. (Drawing by the author) ral and parietal peritonea fuse, and these organs become secondarily retroperitoneal. In order to mobilize the ascending colon and the cecum in the mature human, an incision is performed in the right paracolic fossa, and the visceral peritoneum is detached from the parietal; essentially, the embryonic mesentery is thus reconstructed. The surgical plane between the two leaves of the peritoneum—visceral and parietal—is evidently avascular, because the vessels of the intestine are contained in the mesentery, and those of the retroperitoneum are behind the parietal peritoneum.

This dissection is not needed in the rat. Due to the fact that they are not attached to the posterior peritoneum, the cecum and ascending colon of the rat have a long free mesentery (see yellow-painted in **Figure 8-2**), and therefore are easily moved out of the abdominal cavity.

- The ileum follows the exit of the cecum and ascending colon because it has a free mesentery, which is continuous with the mesentery of the right colon (see light orange-painted in **Figure 8-2**). These parts of the intestine, up to the middle-left transverse colon, are fed by the superior mesenteric artery whose branches are contents of these mesenteries.
- The jejunum follows the exit of the ileum. Evidently, the long mesentery of the jejunum (see dark orange-painted in **Figure 8-2**) is continuous with the mesentery of the ileum. The jejunum is free to move out of the abdomen up to the 3rd part of the duodenum.

The 3rd and 2nd part of the duodenum will not follow the exit of the small intestine because they are attached to the posterior peritoneum. During development, the C-shaped duodenum originates at the midline plane and has a distinct mesentery in the concavity. Then, the duodenum bends to the right. This move brings the mesentery of the 2nd and 3rd part of the duodenum to attach and fuse with the posterior peritoneum (see green-painted in **Figure 8-2**). Thus these duodenal parts become secondarily retroperitoneal.

In order to mobilize the initial part of the jejunum from the retroperitoneum, an incision is made along its attachment with the posterior peritoneum, at the antimesenteric border, towards the adjacent descending colon (**Fig. 8-3**). Since there are no clear borders between start of jejunum and terminal 3rd part of the duodenum, it is very possible that the incision of the posterior peritoneum is extended to the terminal 3rd part. This maneuver is secure because all vascular supply of the jejunum and 3rd part comes from the diametric mesenteric border. Attention, however, is needed with the adjacent rat pancreas. In contrast to the human, the rat pancreas is a 'semi-liquid' organ of irregular shape. It extends behind the stomach into the hilum of the spleen, and at the 2nd and 3rd part of the duodenum (**Fig. 8-2**). These irregular pancreatic parts, which may also be found at the posterior surface of the

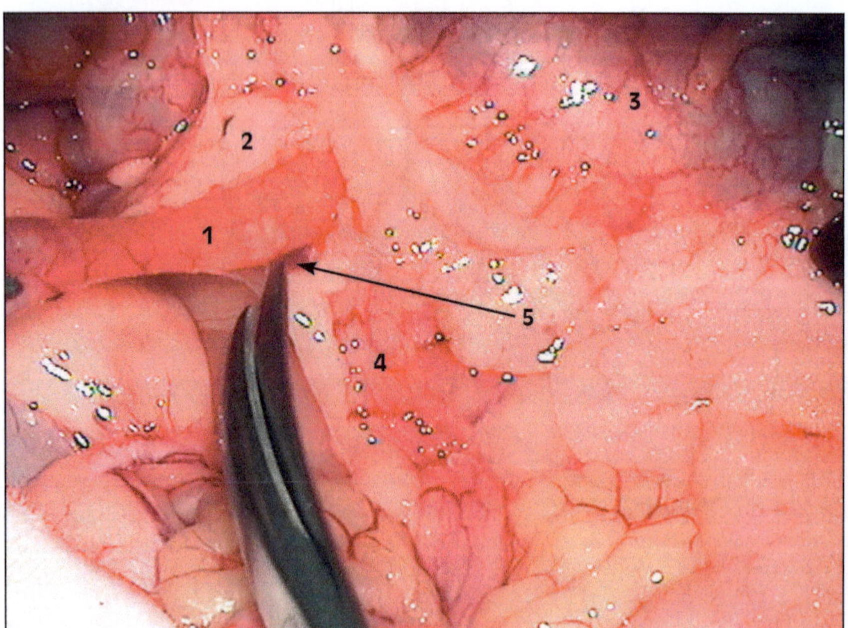

Figure 8-3

Mobilization of the initial part of the jejunum with incision of the posterior peritoneum at the antimesenteric border of the jejunum. The initial jejunum (and most likely also the final 3rd part of the duodenum, as suggested by the position of the pancreas) is pulled to the right side and straightened with forceps Dumont No. 3. The baby-Metzenbaum scissors cut the transparent posterior peritoneum, which continues towards the adjacent descending colon, so here the incision of the posterior peritoneum looks like 'between initial jejunum and descending colon'. **1.** initial part of the jejunum, **2.** pancreas, **3.** stomach, **4.** descending colon **5.** posterior peritoneum leaf. (From author's photo library)

3rd part of the duodenum, should not be traumatized during the incision of the posterior peritoneum for mobilization of the initial part of the jejunum.

- The descending colon remains in the abdomen. In the human, the mesentery of the descending colon attaches to the posterior peritoneum during development, and is detached similarly to the right colon as mentioned above; the sigmoid retains its mesentery and remains mobile.
  In the rat, the descending colon and sigmoid have a median position, over the aorta (No 4, **Fig. 8-3**, and No 1, **Fig 8-4**) and the sigmoid does not have a long mesentery. The mesentery of the left colon is short, although for didactic reasons, this mesentery is presented long, from midline to the left, in **Figure 2** (pink-painted). No specific technique is required to mobilize the left colon out of the field of the aorta in the rat. This is done grossly while opening the retroperitoneum with two gauzes (see below, **Fig 8-5**). For the aorta dissection, the descending colon and the inferior epigastric branches contained in its mesentery are moved to the right side (No 5, **Fig. 8-5B**). For other operations the left colon can be moved to the left.

After the intestines have been mobilized, they are placed on a gauze pad saturated with warm normal saline, on the right side of the rat. Be careful not to traumatize the intestines with the liver retractor found underneath. To mobilize the intestines, two broad atraumatic forceps are used. Avoid grasping the same part of the intestine repeatedly to minimize trauma to the intestinal wall. Microsurgical forceps should be avoided when handling the intestine, because they exert high pressure over a small surface area and can easily damage the intestinal wall.

Once the intestines have been moved out of the abdomen, they are covered with a gauze and irrigated with warm normal saline. Throughout the operation, it is very important to irrigate the packed intestines and the peritoneal cavity with warm normal saline to prevent heat loss and avoid dehydration and electrolyte disturbances. The peritoneum is known for its great absorption ability. If left without saline irrigation, the rat intestines will obtain a characteristic look as the serosa becomes matte and hardens.

Mobilization of the intestines permits a thorough view of the retroperitoneum, which contains abundant fat (**Fig. 8-4**). The descending colon and rectum are in the midline, the right kidney is clearly visible, and the spleen is on the left at the lower part of the stomach.

Handling of the spleen

The spleen is proportionally larger in the rat than in the human. In the rat, the spleen is not attached to the diaphragm (there is no spleno-phrenic ligament) or to the colon (there is no spleno-colic ligament). The spleen is mobile and occupies a large part of the abdominal cavity on the left. It is clearly seen when the intestines have been removed from the abdominal

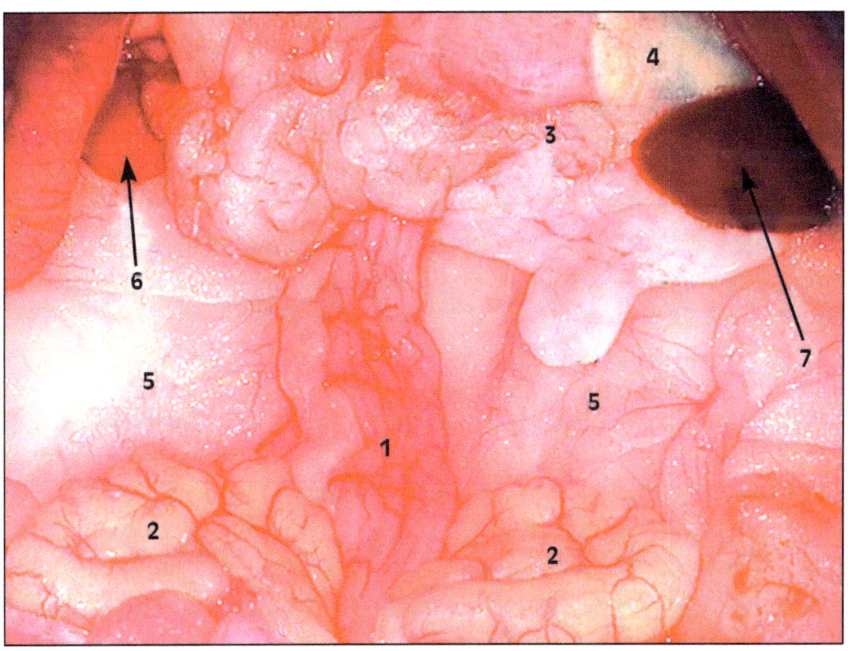

Figure 8-4

The peritoneal cavity after moving the intestines out of the abdomen. Note the rectum in the midline, the right kidney, and the abundant fat in the retroperitoneum. **1.** rectum, **2.** seminal vesicles, **3.** pancreas, **4.** stomach, **5.** retroperitoneal fat (covered by the posterior parietal peritoneum), **6.** right kidney, **7.** spleen. (From author's photo library)

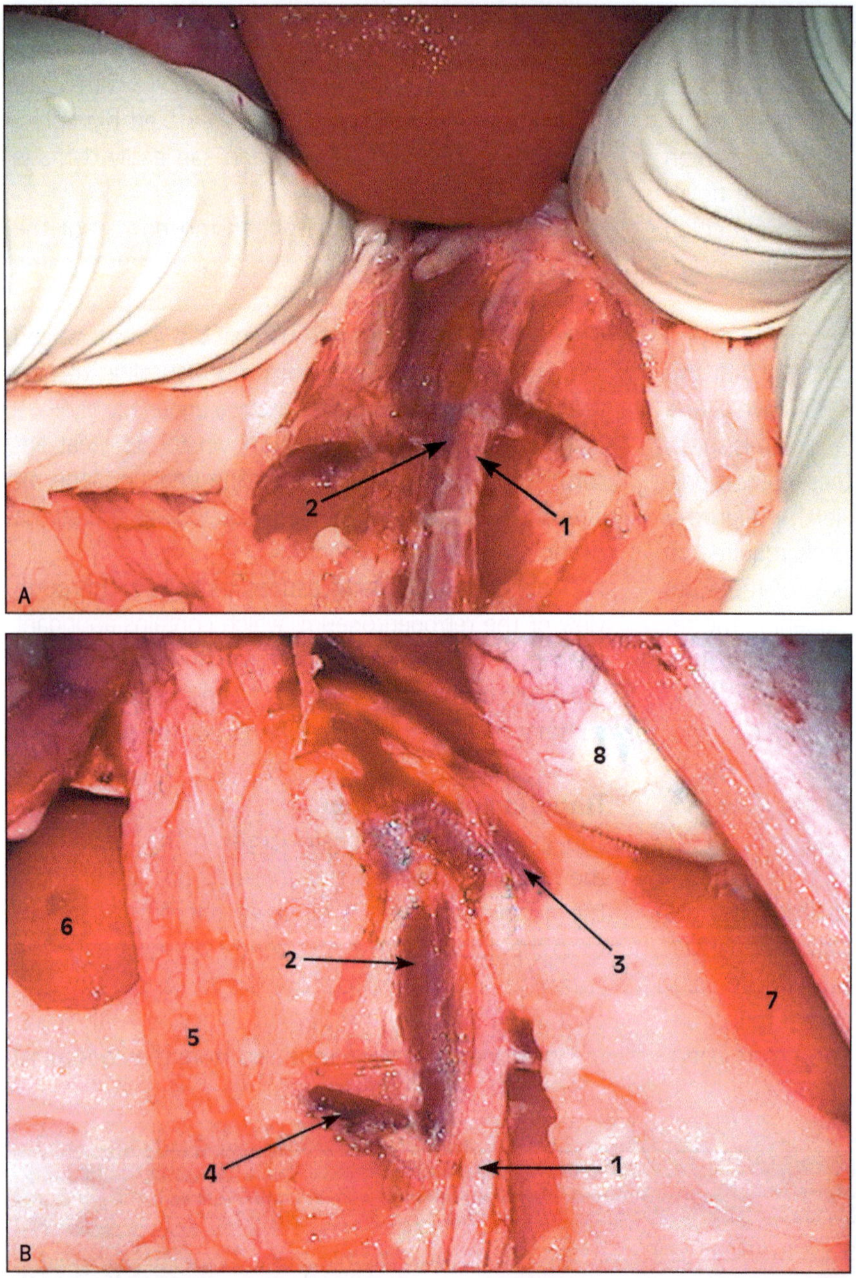

Figure 8-5

Opening of the retroperitoneum in the rat. **A.** Two gauzes saturated with warm normal saline are used. By application of light pressure the two gauzes are drawn laterally with two fingers. The retroperitoneum is opened and the aorta **(1)** and the inferior vena cava **(2)** can be seen. **B.** View of the microsurgical field of the aorta and the inferior vena cava after opening of the retroperitoneum with the gauzes, prior to any further dissection. **1.** aorta, **2.** inferior vena cava, **3.** left renal vein, **4.** right lumbar vein, **5.** rectum, **6.** right kidney, **7.** left kidney, **8.** stomach. (From author's photo library)

cavity (No. 7, **Fig. 8-4**). Using another paper clip retractor bent at an obtuse angle (No. 3, **Fig. 1-4**) and enveloped by a gauze pad, the spleen is pushed to the left, away from the surgical field of the aorta. The existing paper clip retractor(s) put on the left edge of the abdominal wall can also be used for moving the spleen. In this case the spleen is packed under the wall retractor and moved to the left and cranially, out of the surgical field of the aorta. Specific attention is paid to the pancreas that reaches the hilum of the spleen. In the rat, as said, the pancreas is proportionally larger, and a much more mobile and diffuse organ than in the human (No. 3, **Fig. 8-4**).

C. Preparation of the microsurgical field and microsurgical dissection of the aorta

1. Opening of the retroperitoneum

The retroperitoneum is opened manually using two gauzes saturated with warm normal saline that are drawn laterally, on either side, moving away from the midline, thus tearing the posterior peritoneum (**Fig. 8-5A**). This technique permits the blunt dissection of the retroperitoneum. If applied correctly, it exposes the microsurgical field of the inferior vena cava (IVC) and aorta (**Fig. 8-**

5B). For this technique, the surgeon should not apply a vertical force to the retroperitoneum (as if to open a hole in it). In contrast, apply the force horizontally, trying to draw the gauzes across the posterior parietal peritoneum.

Alternatively, the retroperitoneum can be opened and dissected using blunt microsurgical scissors and microsurgical forceps. This dissection method, however, requires expertise because the great vessels are covered by a layer of fibro-fatty connective tissue, which is difficult to remove. Careless application of microsurgical scissors may result in trauma to the IVC, aorta, or lumbar tributaries/branches of these two vessels. Other microsurgeons may also use two microsurgical forceps and a combination of blunt dissection and a tearing action. These alternative techniques are not suggested for the trainee.

2. Microsurgical dissection of the aorta

The aim of the microsurgical dissection is to separate the aorta and its branches from the IVC and its tributaries. The outer layers of the IVC and aorta are attached at all places the two great vessels come into contact; it is hard to separate them. The same applies for their branches and tributaries. For this reason the dissection must be done meticulously, taking care not to harm the veins, whose wall is more vulnerable and easily ruptured.

The dissection of the aorta starts just proximal to the bifurcation of the aorta into common iliac arteries, and extends cephalad up to the left renal vein. Dissection begins by opening a 'window' in the connective tissue between the aorta and IVC, as follows (**Fig. 8-6**): The adventitia of the aorta is grasped with Dumont forceps No. 3 and pulled up under enough tension to stretch the connective tissue between aorta and IVC. With their tip closed, the blunt microsurgical scissors can detect the weakest area of the connective tissue, which is also more transparent. With the tip of the scissors make one or several lateral movements (always closed) and open a window. This window is extended with a combination of mainly blunt and occasionally sharp dissection, until a clear plane of complete separation between the aorta and IVC is achieved. It is advised not to cut tissue that is not transparent, and not to remove 'connective tissue'. This fibrofatty tissue contains all the preaortic autonomic plexuses and lymphatics; therefore, it should be preserved and moved away from the plane of dissection.

Developing the plane of dissection between the aorta and IVC, the surgeon has to confront the lumbar vessels. Though the actual number may vary, in the rat there are usually 3 lumbar arteries and 2 lumbar veins. As

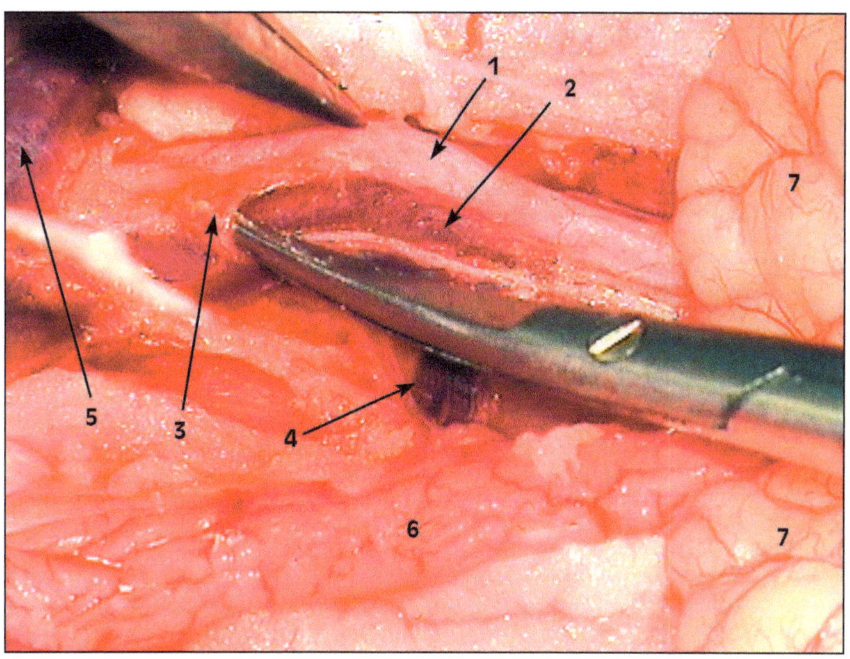

Figure 8-6

Opening of the surgical plane between the aorta and inferior vena cava. Blunt microsurgical scissors create a 'window' between the fused outer layers of the aorta and inferior vena cava. **1.** aorta, **2.** inferior vena cava, **3.** common outer layer of 'connective' tissue (see text), **4.** lumbar vein, **5.** left renal vein, **6.** rectum, **7.** seminal vesicles. (From author's photo library)

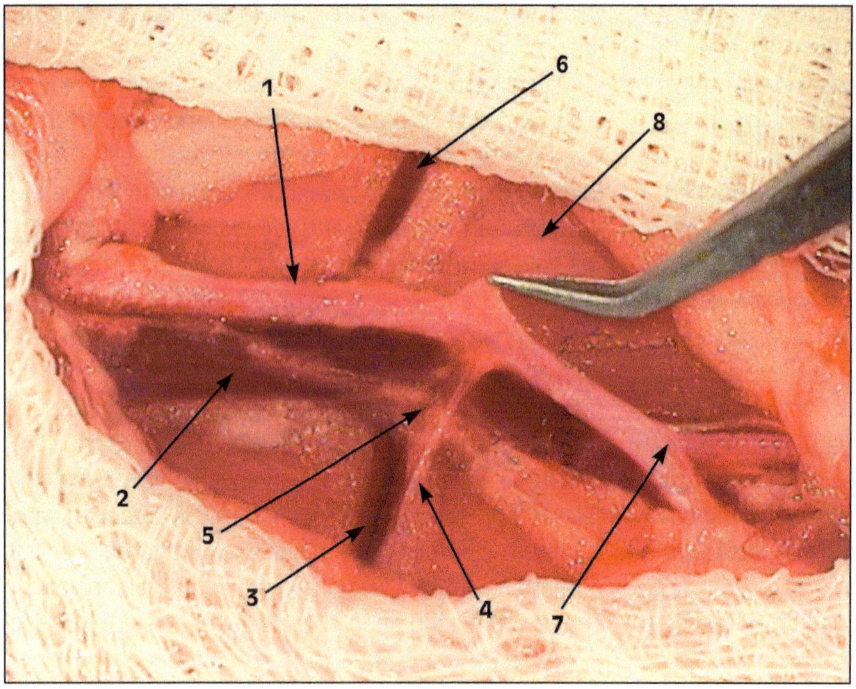

Figure 8-7

Expansion of the surgical plane between aorta and inferior vena cava and pulling up the aorta with microsurgical forceps, reveals the fibrofatty attachment of the outer layers between a lumbar artery and the respective vein (similar to the attachment between aorta and inferior vena cava). **1.** aorta, **2.** inferior vena cava, **3.** right lumbar vein, **4.** right lumbar artery, **5.** fibrofatty attachment of outer layers of lumbar artery and vein, **6.** left lumbar vein, **7.** aorta bifurcation, **8.** left psoas muscle. (From author's photo library)

with the aorta and IVC, the outer coatings of arteries and veins attach to each other in areas of contact between the two vessels (when paired) (**Fig. 8-7**). In order to separate the two vessels, the usual technique is to expand between them the plane of separation developed between aorta and ICV. After separation from the corresponding vein, each lumbar artery has to be fully dissected (**Fig. 8-8**). Sometimes, dissection reveals that lumbar veins are double and converge to a short vein that empties in the IVC (**Fig. 8-9**), or, more rarely, that the two closely adjacent lumbar veins will stay separate and empty independently.

After dissection, every lumbar artery should be double-ligated with suture and transected between ligations. Lumbar arteries can also be cut directly with the cautery without ligations (**Fig. 8-10**). Attention must be paid not to cause tissue trauma due to heat transmission to adjacent structures. Cauterization can

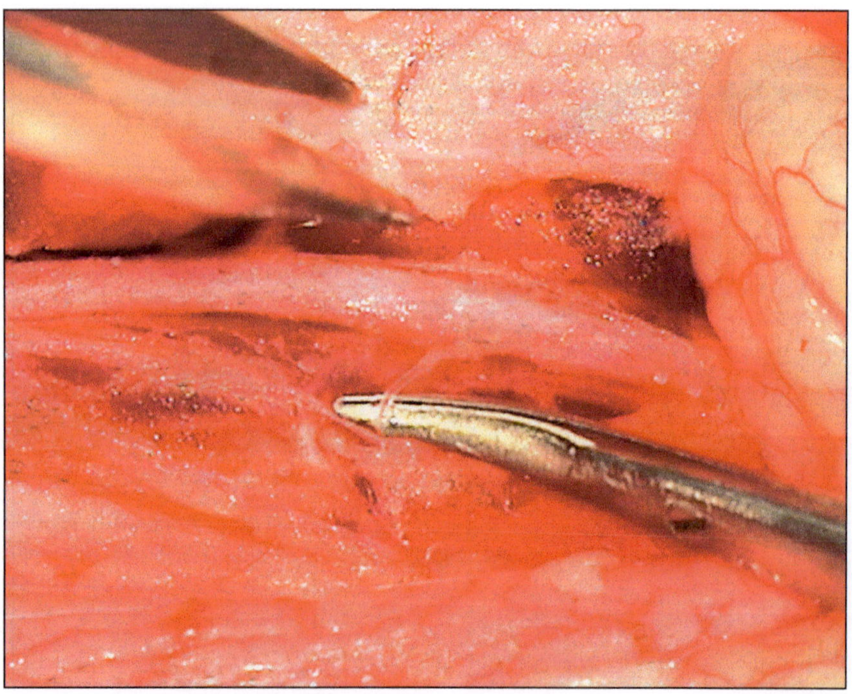

Figure 8-8

Dissection of a lumbar artery and separation from the respective lumbar vein. Blunt microsurgical scissors have entered the plane between the two vessels and lift up the lumbar artery. (From author's photo library)

Figure 8-9

Bilateral double lumbar veins. The two veins converge into one vein, which empties in the inferior vena cava. Dumont forceps No. 3 grasps the adventitia and lifts up the aorta. **1.** aorta, **2.** inferior vena cava, **3.** right double lumbar vein, **4.** right lumbar artery, **5.** fibroareolar attachment between aorta inferior vena cava that extends between lumbar arteries and corresponding lumbar veins, **6.** left double lumbar vein. (From author's photo library)

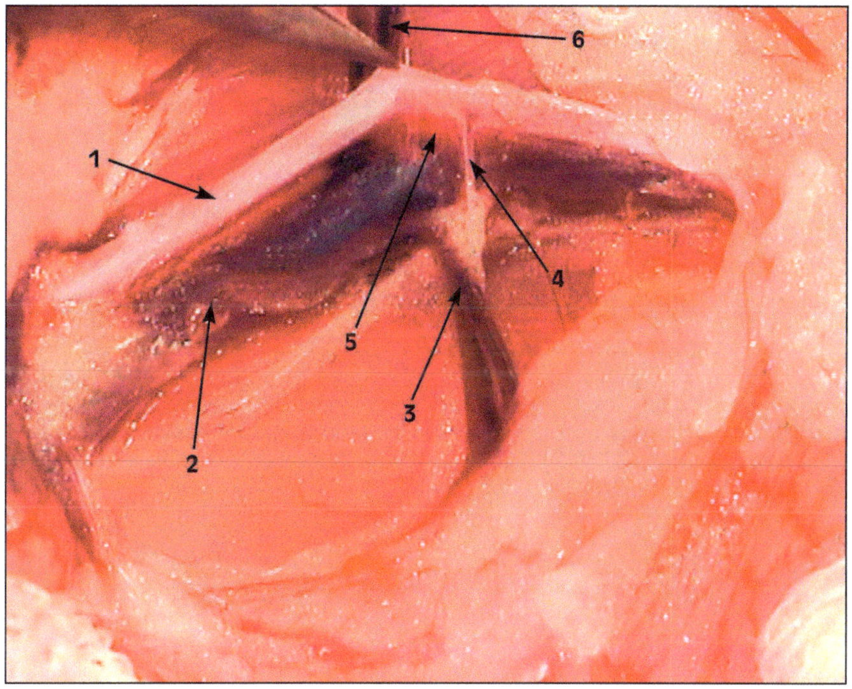

also result in catastrophic hemorrhage from rupture of the IVC or a lumbar vein. Cauterization for division of lumbar veins without ligations is forbidden [this is not necessary for aorta anastomosis, but may be performed in other operations that require IVC mobilization. It is mentioned here for completeness]. Lumbar veins, and for the trainee, lumbar arteries should also be double-ligated with 9/0 suture and then cut between ligations using microsurgical scissors. As trainees admit, ligation of lumbar vessels is an important exercise for familiarization with microsurgical manipulations.

After the aorta has been fully dissected, all lumbar arteries have been cut, and the aorta has been completely separated from the IVC (from the bifurcation to the left renal vein), the surgical field is irrigated with warm normal saline and a plastic yellow background is placed under the aorta (**Fig. 8-11**).

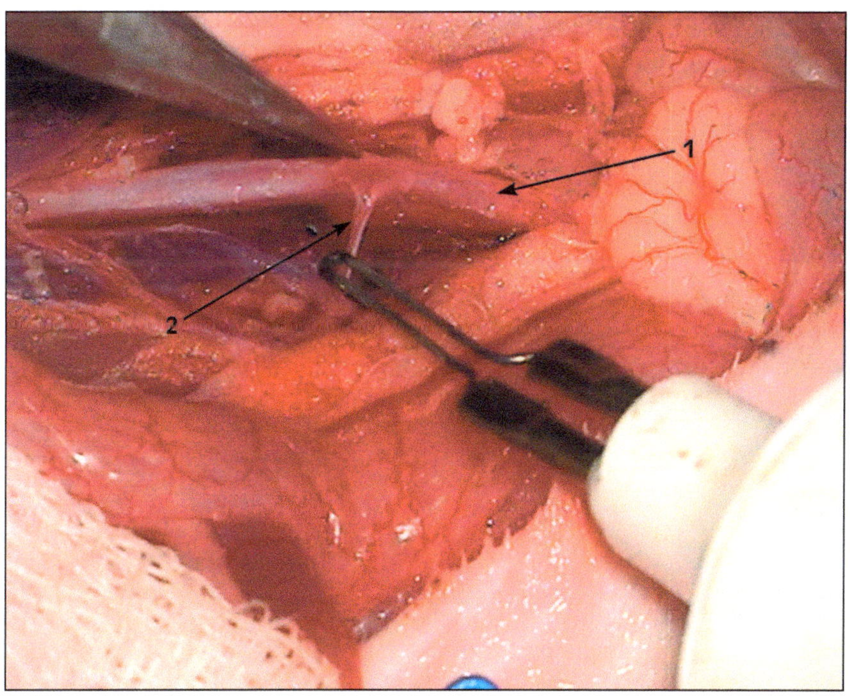

Figure 8-10

Cauterization of a lumbar artery using the diathermy of single use. Dumont forceps No. 3 lifts the aorta (by grasping the adventitia) and with it the dissected lumbar artery. **1.** aorta, **2.** lumbar artery. (From author's photo library)

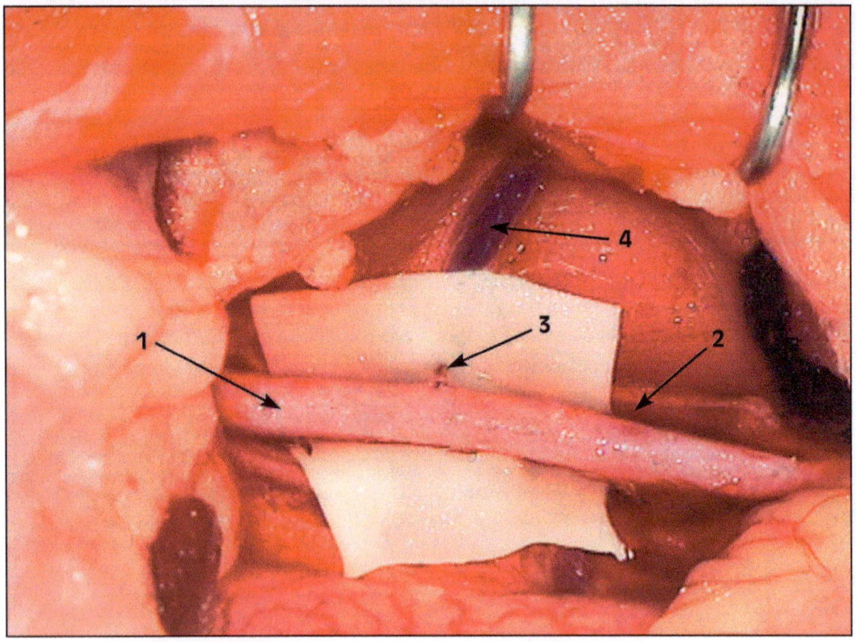

Figure 8-11

Placement of a yellow plastic background under the aorta, after the aorta has been separated from the inferior vena cava and fully dissected from its bifurcation to the level of the left renal artery; the lumbar arteries have been divided. The anatomic relation of aorta and inferior vena cava has been altered with placement of the aorta on the background. **1.** aorta, **2.** inferior vena cava, **3.** stump of a left lumbar artery (has been divided with cautery, no ligation sutures placed), **4.** corresponding left lumbar vein. (From author's photo library)

D. End-to-End anastomosis

The reader is asked to read Chapter 5 for a complete description of the end-to-end anastomosis technique.

- The anastomosis will be performed by placing **10 or 12 sutures 10/0**

Alternatively, the anastomosis can be done with 8 or 10 sutures 9/0. We suggest the use of sutures 10/0.

The steps of the process of the end-to-end anastomosis are as follows:

1. Placement of the double vascular clamp (**Fig. 8-12**).
2. Transection of the vessel (**Fig. 8-13**).
3. Irrigation of the lumen with normal saline (**Fig. 8-14**). For the aorta, the irrigation is done using a 5 ml syringe, the needle of which is replaced with an angiocatheter (Abbocath, orange, 27G). The length of the angiocatheter can be trimmed and the tip can be cut diagonally; this helps with injecting saline into the lumen.
4. Removal (folding) of the adventitia. Dumont No. 3 forceps immobilizes the vessel and Dumont No. 5 forceps folds the adventitia (**Fig. 8-15**).
5. Reapproximation of the two clamps of the double clamp.

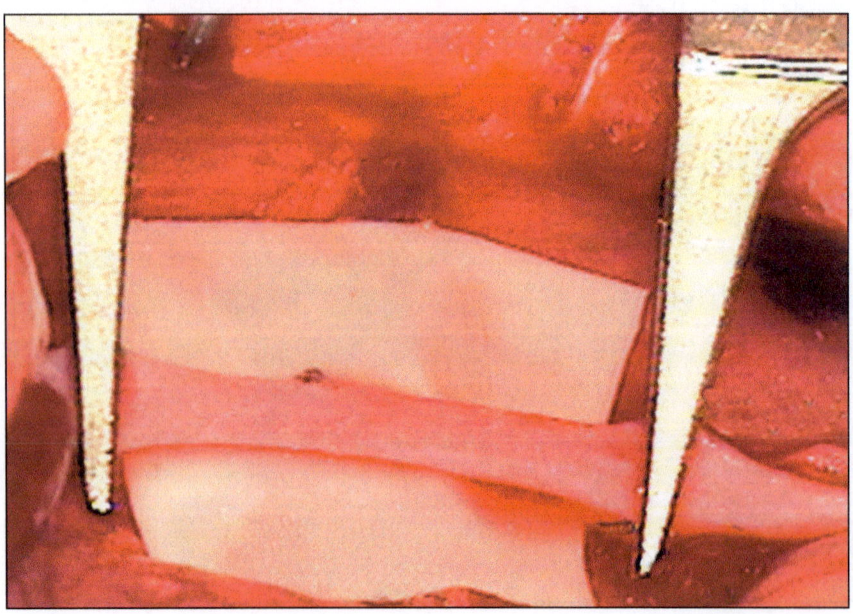

Figure 8-12

Placement of the double vascular clamp on the aorta. The vessel should be placed toward the tips of the jaws, so that the clamp can be rotated. (From author's photo library)

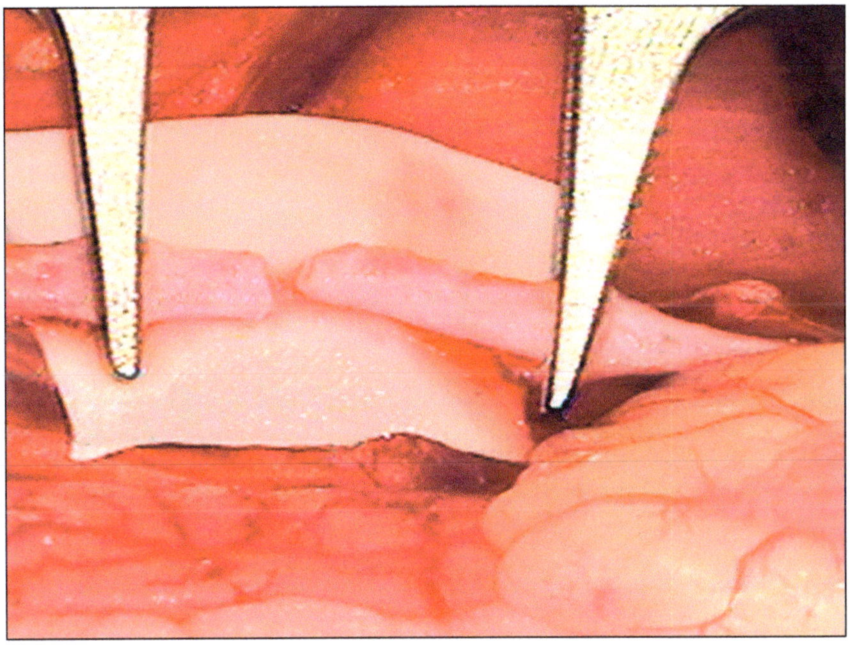

Figure 8-13

Transection of the aorta must be performed with a clean cut to obtain neat edges at the stumps. Note that the stumps shrink and the edges move away from each other. Approximation of the two clamps will bring the vessel stumps in contact. (From author's photo library)

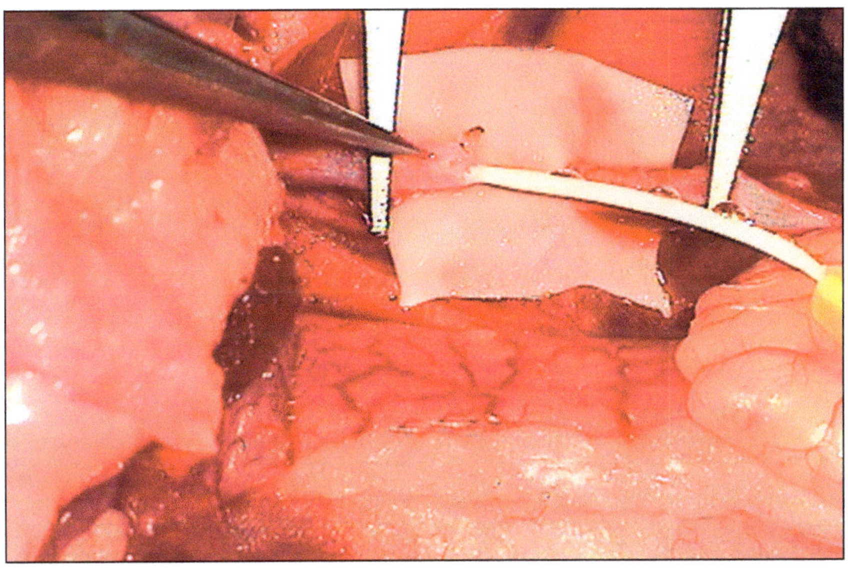

Figure 8-14

The lumen of the cranial stump of the aorta is irrigated with warm normal saline to wash out blood and clots. Dumont No. 5 forceps holds the vessel from the adventitia, and the catheter, without entering the lumen, injects saline under pressure. (From author's photo library)

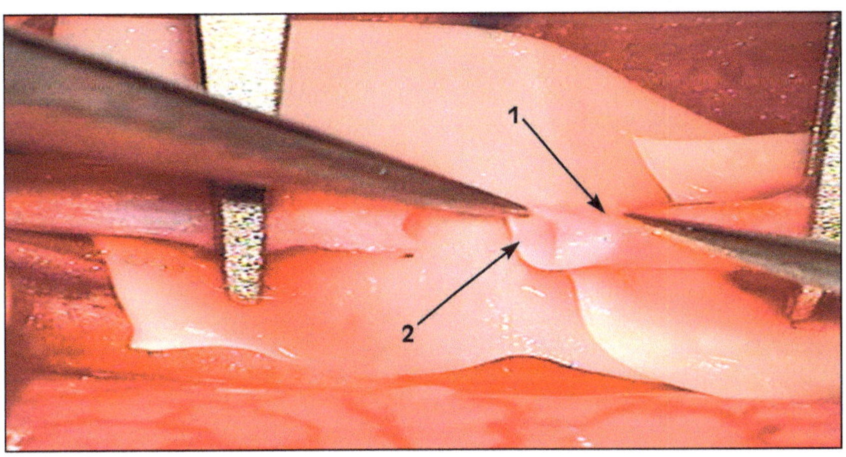

Figure 8-15

Folding of the adventitia of the aorta. Dumont forceps No. 5 folds the adventitia (**1**), while Dumont forceps No. 3 immobilizes the vessel by grasping the external surface of the vessel (**2**) to avoid traumatizing the edge or the lumen. Note the whitish and glistening wall of the vessel deprived of adventitia near the edge. (From author's photo library)

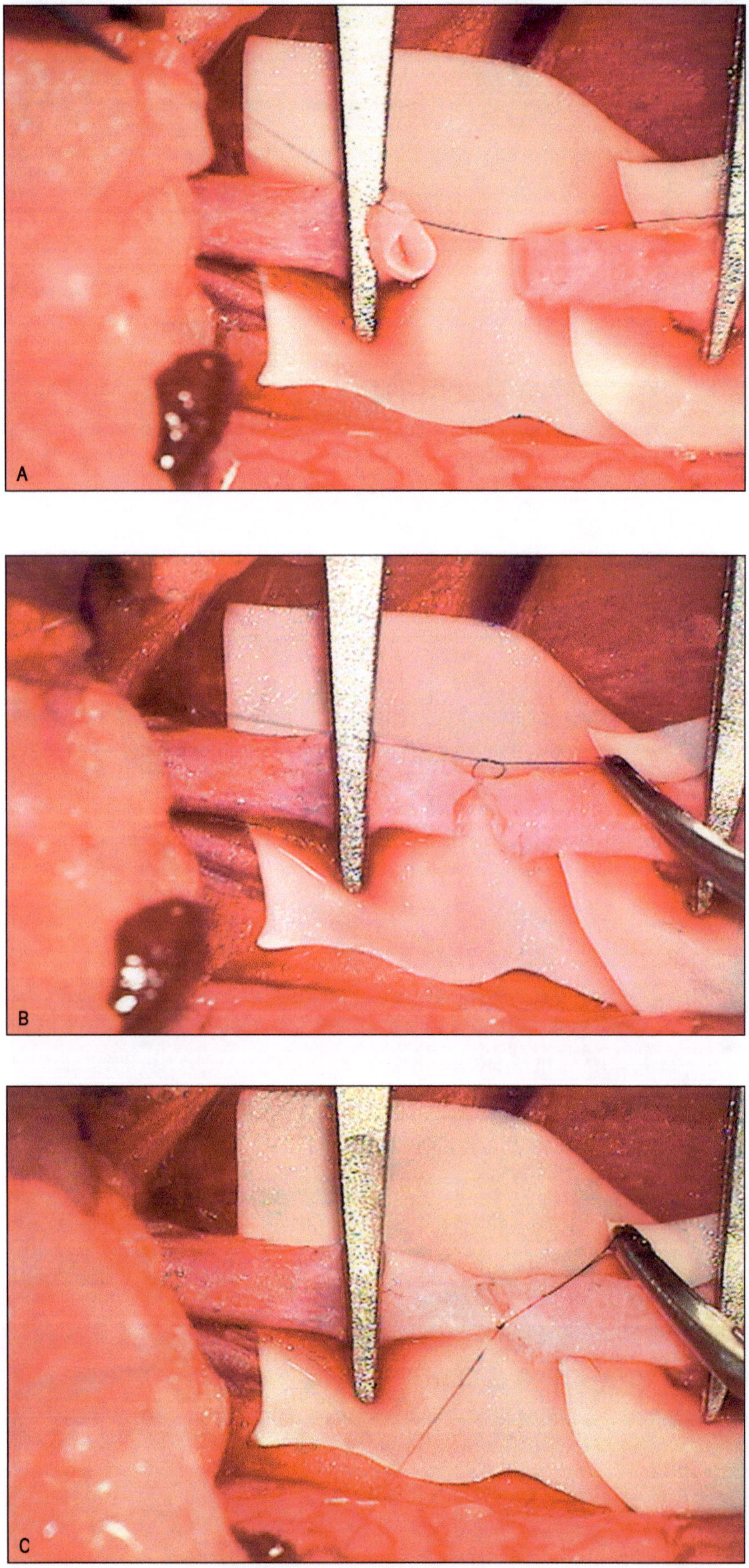

Figure 8-16

Placement of the corner sutures. **A.** The first 12 o'clock suture is placed (up). **B.** First simple knot at 12 o'clock. **C.** Tying the knot at 6 o'clock (down). (From author's photo library)

Figure 8-17

Completed suturing of the anterior surface. (From author's photo library)

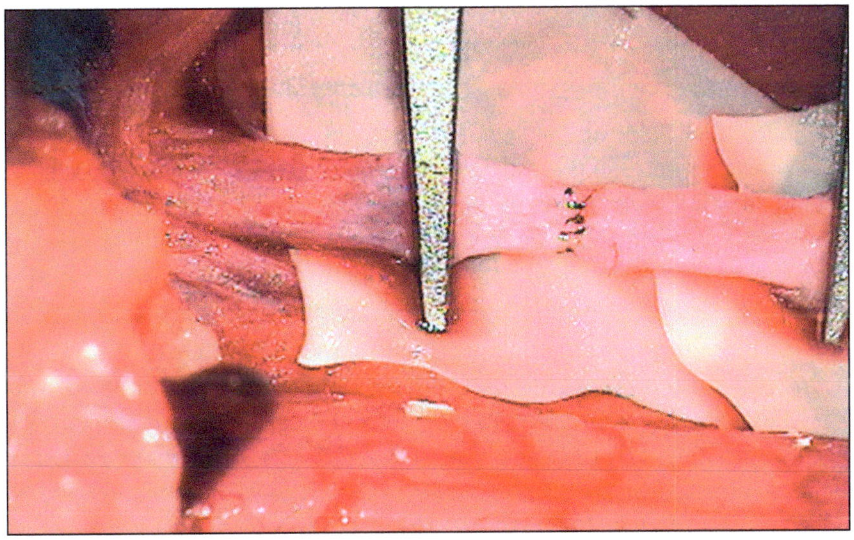

6. Placement of the two corner sutures (12 o'clock and 6 o'clock) that will orient the vessel stumps (**Fig. 8-16**).
7. Suturing of the anterior surface is completed (**Fig. 8-17**). If 10 sutures will be placed, there are 4 remaining per surface, from which the first 2 are placed lateral (toward the corner sutures), the 2 next more central, all at equal distances (from the corner sutures and between themselves). If 12 sutures will be placed, there are 5 remaining per surface, from which the median is put in the middle of the semicircle, and 2 in each quadrant in equal distances (from the corner sutures and between themselves).
8. Rotation of the double clamp and checking that the sutures of the anterior surface have been placed correctly.
9. Suturing of the posterior surface is completed, using the same technique as in the anterior surface (**Fig. 8-18**).
10. Release of the vessel from the double clamp.
11. Gauze (wet) placement on the anastomosis for 3 minutes.
12. Patency test.

    The patency test is performed as described in Chapter 5.10 (see **Figure 5-4**). In short, distal to the anastomosis toward the aorta bifurcation, a first, upstream forceps occludes the aorta and a second, downstream forceps is placed initially next to the first forceps and then moves distally while half-closed, thereby 'milking' the vessel, and finally remains closed. The upstream forceps is removed, and if there is patency, the vessel is immediately filled up to the downstream forceps.
13. Withdrawal of the yellow background.

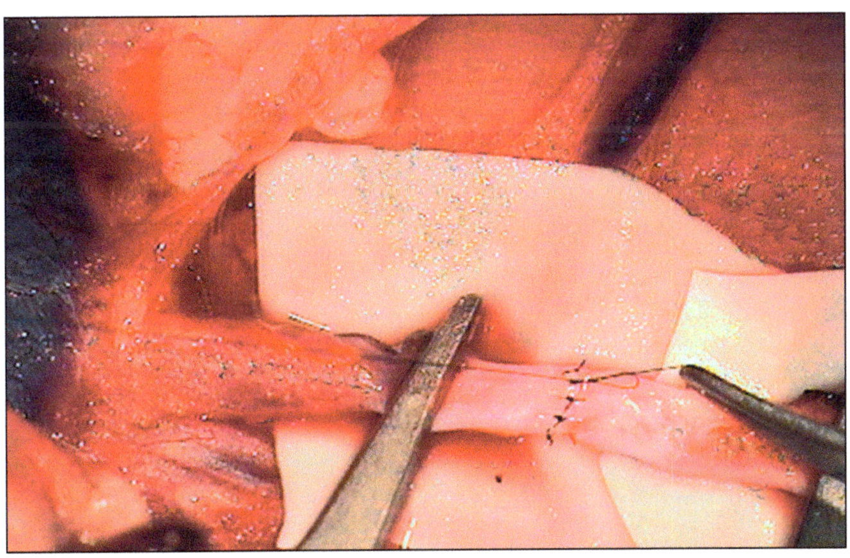

Figure 8-18

Rotation of the clamp and suturing of the posterior surface of the anastomosis. Here, the last suture is placed. The suture above it is the peripheral suture towards 12 o'clock (first are placed the peripheral sutures and then the more central ones). The corner suture of 12 o'clock is not seen here because of the rotation of the clamp and the angle under which the photo was taken. (From author's photo library)

E. Return of splanchna - Closure of surgical trauma

The gauze enveloping the intestines is removed. The small intestine returns in the abdomen first and the colon and cecum follows. This order of repositioning aims to restore the anatomical position of intestines seen when the abdomen was opened: the small intestine deep, and the cecum superficial and medially in the abdominal cavity.

The paper clip retractor holding the lobes of the liver is removed. The liver lobes return in the abdomen pushed smoothly with broad anatomical forceps. If a separate retractor was used to hold the spleen, it is removed followed by the abdominal wall retractors.

The abdominal cavity is irrigated once more with warm normal saline. The viscera and the abdominal walls are inspected for hemorrhage. Check that no gauze has been left in the abdomen.

Closure of the abdominal wall follows, in two layers (muscles – superficial fascia and skin) with non-absorbable 2/0 sutures. Creation of a continuous muscle layer can also be done. If you prefer to place absorbable sutures, use those with slow absorption in order to minimize the risk of abdominal wall dehiscence.

It is important that the animal be totally cleansed of blood on its body. The smell of blood is very irritating for animals. Rats will very often be 'occupied' with their trauma or the trauma of some other rat returned the same cage. For this reason, it is strongly suggested that animals be isolated after the operation.

Synopsis...

... of end-to-end anastomosis of the aorta

A. Position of the rat: Laid on its back, head on the surgeon's left. The limbs are immobilized on the working surface with adhesive tape.

B. Preparation of the surgical field: A median incision is performed, from the xiphoid to the pubic symphysis and the linea alba is opened. Paper clip retractors are placed at the edges of the incision. The lobes of the liver protruding in the field are packed with another retractor. The intestines (cecum, ascending, transverse colon, small intestine) are moved out of the abdomen and packed in a gauze, placed to the right of the rat. The peritoneal cavity and the removed splanchna are regularly irrigated with warm normal saline.

C. Preparation of the microsurgical field and microsurgical dissection of the aorta: The retroperitoneum is opened with two wet gauzes. A plane of separation between the aorta and inferior vena cava is created and the aorta is completely mobilized, from the bifurcation to the left renal vein. All lumbar arteries are dissected, cleaned and divided either between two ligations (9/0 suture) or using cautery. A yellow plastic background is put under the aorta.

D. End-to-end anastomosis: 10 or 12 sutures of 10/0

1. Placement of double vascular clamp.
2. Transection of the aorta.
3. Irrigation of the lumen with normal saline
4. Folding of the adventitia.
5. Reapproximation of the two clamps of the double clamp.
6. Placement of the two corner sutures (12 o'clock and 6 o'clock).
7. Suturing of the anterior surface: 4 sutures at equal distances, first the 2 peripheral. Or 5 sutures, the median first and 2 in each quadrant, at equal distances.
8. Rotation of the clamp and checking sutures of the anterior surface.
9. Suturing of the posterior surface, similar to anterior.
10. Release of the double clamp.
11. Placement of a wet gauze on the anastomosis for 3 minutes.
12. Patency test.
13. Withdrawal of the yellow plastic background.

E. Return of the splanchna and closure of the abdominal wall in two layers with non-absorbable sutures 2/0: continuous or interrupted in the muscles, interrupted in the subcutaneous-skin.

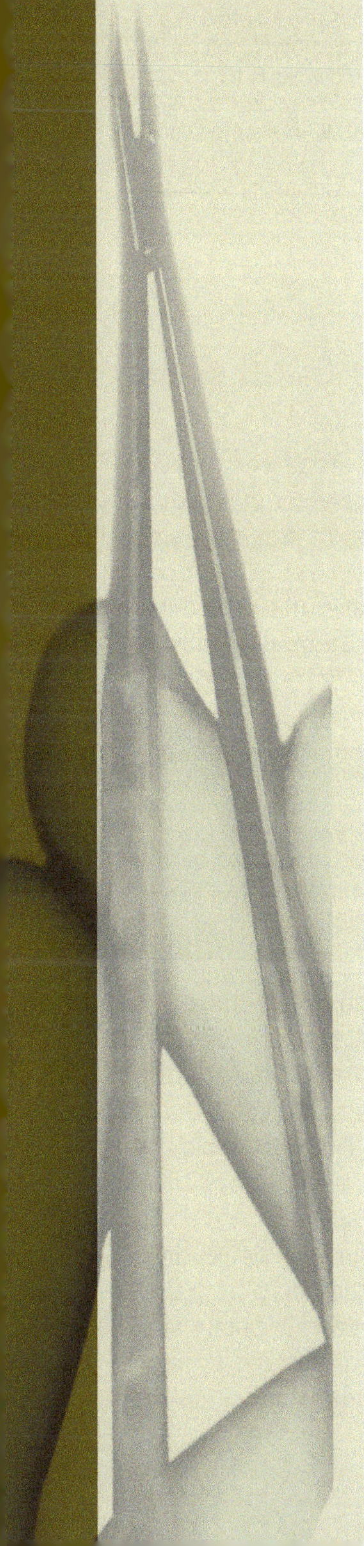

9

End-to-end anastomosis of the external jugular vein & End-to-end anastomosis of the common carotid artery

The procedures are described here for the vessels of the right side of the neck. They can identically be applied to vessels of the left side.
The two procedures can be performed separately, as described in this chapter. Usually, however, they are done in sequence, starting with the vein.

I. EXTERNAL JUGULAR VEIN

A. Positioning of the rat

The rat is placed in supine position (dorsal decubitus) on the working surface. The long axis of the body of the rat is parallel to the frontal (coronal) level of the surgeon's body, and the rat's head is placed on the surgeon's left. The limbs of the rat are immobilized on the working surface with adhesive tape.

B. Preparation of the surgical field

A transverse incision is performed at the base of the neck, extending from shoulder to shoulder. The incision includes the skin, platysma and a large part of the fat of the superficial fascia. As a reminder, the superficial fascia of the neck extends in depth from the subcutaneous tissue to the investing fascia of the muscles (deep fascia). The superficial fascia includes fat, the platysma, the submandibular salivary glands and the system of superficial veins that includes the external jugular veins with their tributaries and anastomoses with other veins.

On either side of the incision, the fatty layer of the superficial fascia of the neck is detached and removed with two gauzes saturated in warm normal saline. The surgeon exerts light pressure and draws the gauzes in opposite directions craniocaudally, in order to remove the fat of the superficial fascia. Thus, the superficial external jugular veins and their tributaries, as well as the submandibular salivary glands, are revealed (**Fig. 9-1**). Attention must be paid not to traumatize the external jugular vein or one of the tributaries. It is advised to include the contralateral external jugular vein in this dissection, so that the surgeon does not have to come

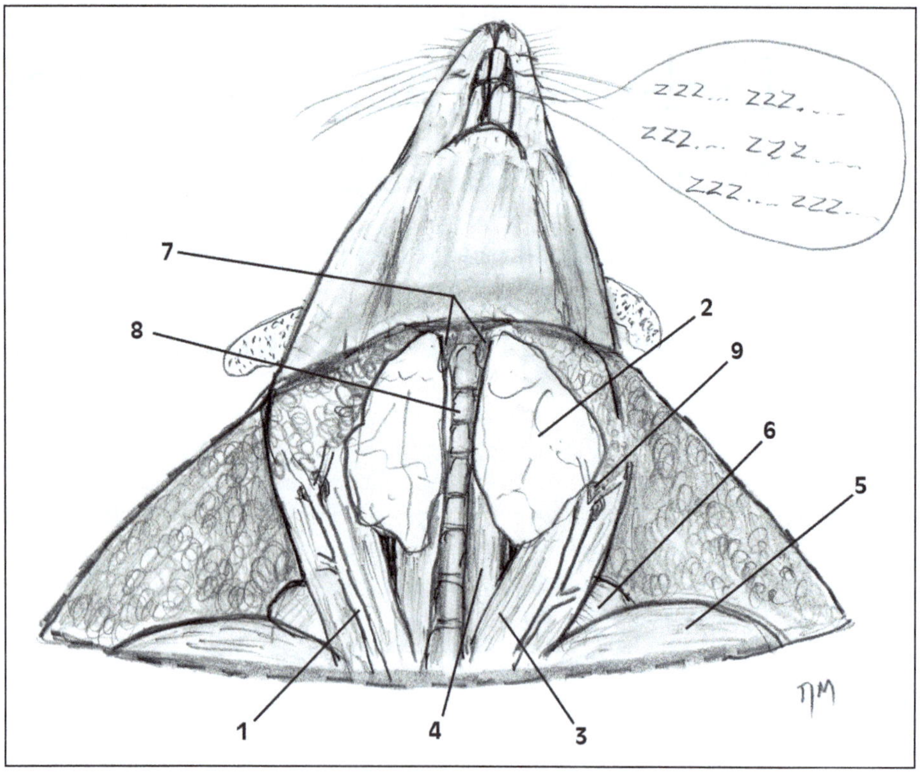

Figure 9-1

The surgical field of the neck in the rat, after incision of the skin and and initial removal of the fatty layer of superficial fascia (including the platysma) with the use of gauze pads. After further dissection and retraction of the superficial fascia, the submandibular g-lands will be removed cranial-ly.**1.** external jugular vein, **2.** submandibular salivary gland, **3.** sternocleidomastoid muscle, **4.** sternohyoid muscle, **5.** deltoid muscle, **6.** trapezius muscle, **7.** thyroid gland, **8.** trachea, **9.** small lymph node at the trifurcation of the external jugular vein. (Drawing by the author)

back if he/she needs to repeat the anastomosis in the contralateral vein. Further dissection and cranial removal of the superficial fascia with the gauzes will also remove submandibular salivary glands, found in this surgical layer.

Then, a paper clip retractor is placed in the middle of the incision, along the midline, pulling cranially the upper edge of the incision. At the other end of the retractor a piece of rubber is attached, which is adhered on the working surface, beyond the nose of the rat. The retractor pulls up the skin, the platysma, the fat of the superficial fascia, and the submandibular salivary glands.

The above dissection reveals in the surgical field the external jugular vein (No. 1, **Fig. 9-1**), which, as in humans, courses along the ipsilateral sternocleidomastoid muscle. Cranially, at the trifurcation of the external jugular vein, a lymph node is usually found (No. 9, **Fig. 9-1**), distinguished from the fat by its darker purple color. A nice view of the underlying neck muscles can be seen in **Figure 12-1B.**

C. Microsurgical dissection of the external jugular vein

Dissection of the external jugular vein is performed with Dumont No. 3 forceps and blunt microsurgical scissors (**Fig. 9-2**). The forceps grasps and extends the fibro-fatty tissue surrounding the vein, and the scissors enter the weakest area on top of the vein wall, initially closed and then open to develop the plane. This blunt dissection will be enough for the most part of the cleaning of the vein. In some areas, however, sharp dissection will be required, i.e. cutting a piece of fat, pulled up by forceps, with scissors. The dissection aims to provide a completely clean vein.

- Meticulous dissection of the vein is not a waste of time. The cleaner the vein wall, the easier the anastomosis.

Dissection of the external jugular vein starts from the upper border of the pectoralis major muscle and reaches the mandible, including the tributary veins of the 'trifurcation' of the external jugular vein, i.e. the lingual, mandibular, and facial veins (**Fig. 9-3**). As said above, the location of the trifurcation is marked by a lymph node (No. 9, **Fig. 9-1**, and No. 4, **Fig 9-4**).

In the course of the microsurgical dissection of the external jugular vein from the pectoralis muscle to the trifurcation, 2-3 other smaller tributary veins are met (**Fig. 9-4**). These will be cauterized or (more securely) ligated with two 9/0 sutures and cut in bet-

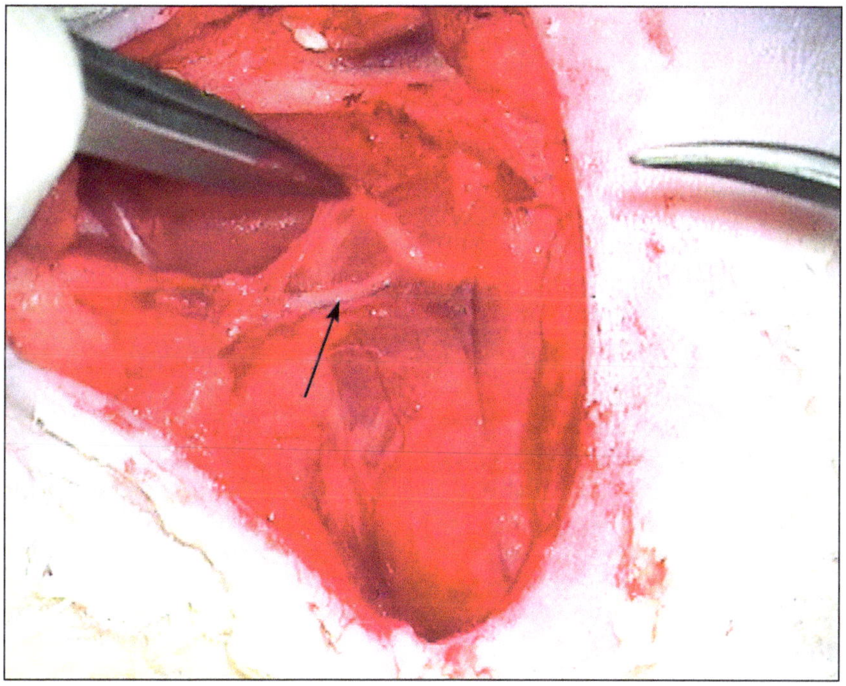

Figure 9-2

Microsurgical dissection of the right external jugular vein. The arrow shows the external jugular vein in the fatty layer of the superficial fascia of the neck. The skin, platysma, and submandibular salivary glands have been moved cranially with a paper clip retractor. Dumont No. 3 forceps holds a sheet of fat, just dissected off the external jugular vein with the microsurgical scissors (its tip can be seen on the right). (From author's photo library)

ween. Attention must be paid to the tributary found at the lower part of the external jugular vein, above the edge of the pectoralis muscle. This vein is quite large and often divides in two smaller veins emptying into the posterior surface of the external jugular vein (**Fig. 9-4**). It is advised to double-ligate and then divide the vein or each or the two smaller veins (separately) and not to cauterize and divide them. For ligation, smoothly lift up the external jugular vein, holding it from the adventitia with forceps Dumont No. 5; do not lift the tributary vein. Also, do not lift up the external jugular vein by grasping the stump of some other cauterized tributary found cranially, because it can bleed. If this happens —the author has done

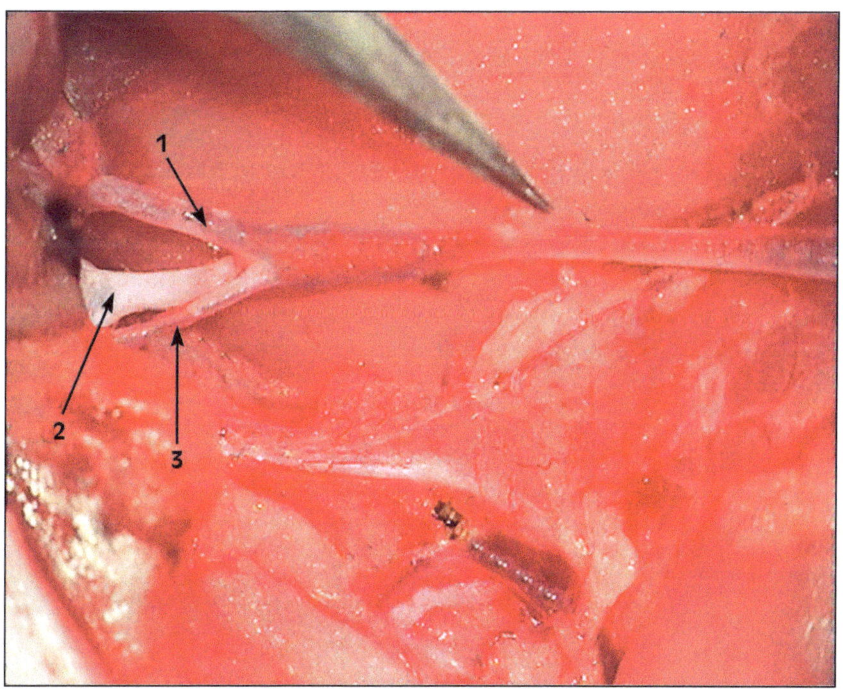

Figure 9-3

Right external jugular vein fully dissected, from the base of the neck to the mandible. Dumont forceps No. 5 lifts the external jugular vein. In the 'trifurcation' of the external jugular vein converge a right, a left and a deep vein: **1.** lingual vein, **2.** mandibular vein, **3.** facial vein. (From author's photo library)

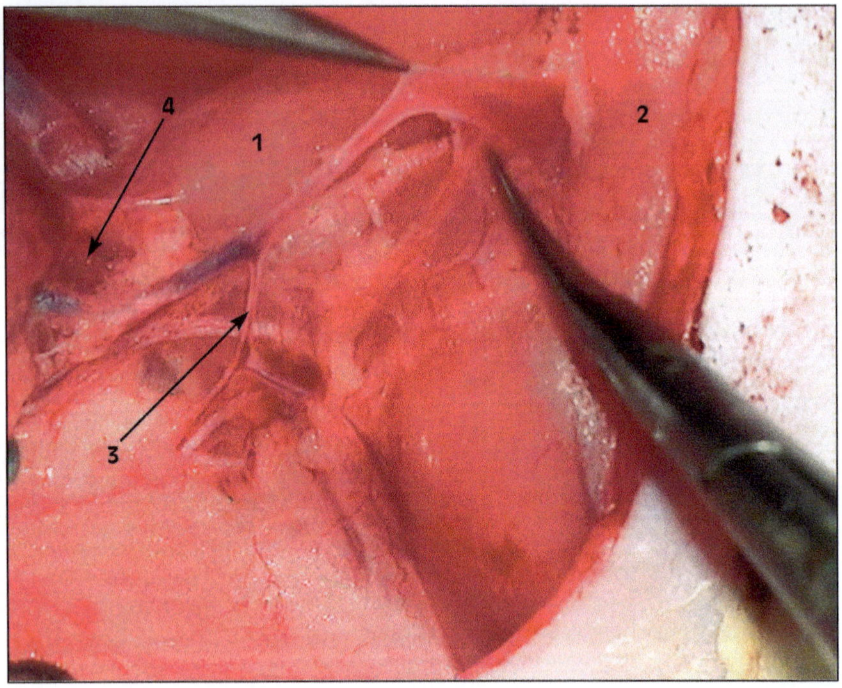

Figure 9-4

Dissection of the tributaries of the right external jugular vein between its trifurcation and the upper edge of pectoralis major muscle. The forceps lifts the external jugular vein and the scissors point to a tributary vein dividing in two small veins emptying in the posterior surface of the exterior jugular vein. Cranially to this dissection, another dissected lateral tributary vein (3) can be seen below the trifurcation. **1.** sternocleidomastoid muscle, **2.** pectoralis major muscle, **3.** tributary vein, observe the two smaller veins emptying in it and coursing in the remaining superficial fascia, **4.** characteristic lymph node at the trifurcation of the external jugular vein. (From author's photo library)

this mistake more that once—do not try to cauterize it, you risk a more serious hemorrhage (this has also happened to the author!). Ligate again the stump of the tributary vein as usual with a free 9/0 or 10/0 suture (use a free piece of suture or the end opposite to the needle), or place a passing-through suture (suture ligate) if it is large enough. Although the detailed microsurgical dissection easily reveals the small lateral tributaries, the subsequent cutting after double ligation or cauterization (**Fig. 9-5**) require specific attention because the vein wall is deprived of a muscle layer, therefore much more fragile than that of arteries.

The adventitia, i.e. the outer layer, of the external jugular vein should also be removed from the wall of the vessel. The dissection can be done either with the

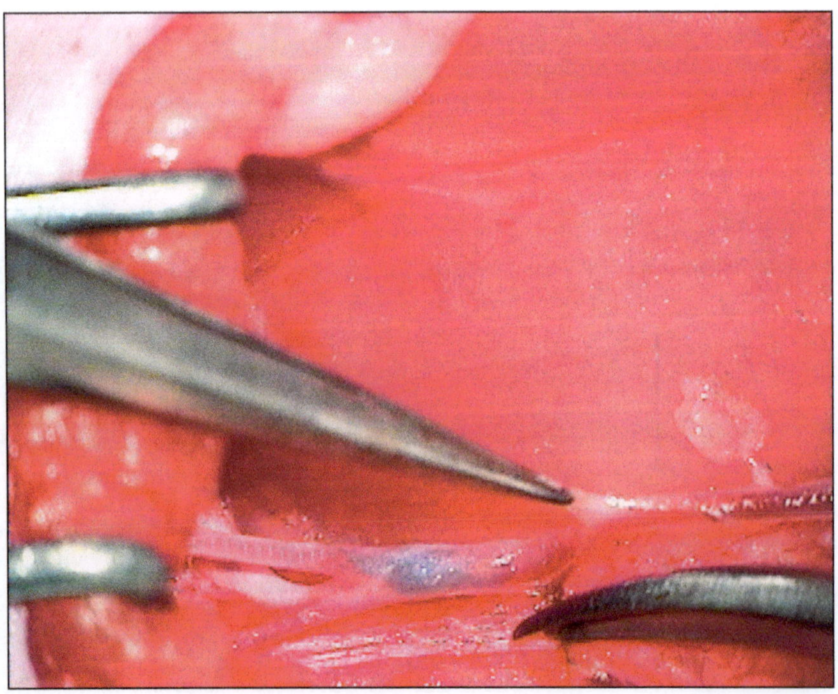

Figure 9-5

Transection of a small lateral tributary vein after electrocoagulation. The right external jugular vein is lifted from the adventitia with forceps Dumont No. 5 and the coagulated tributary is transected with scissors. (From author's photo library)

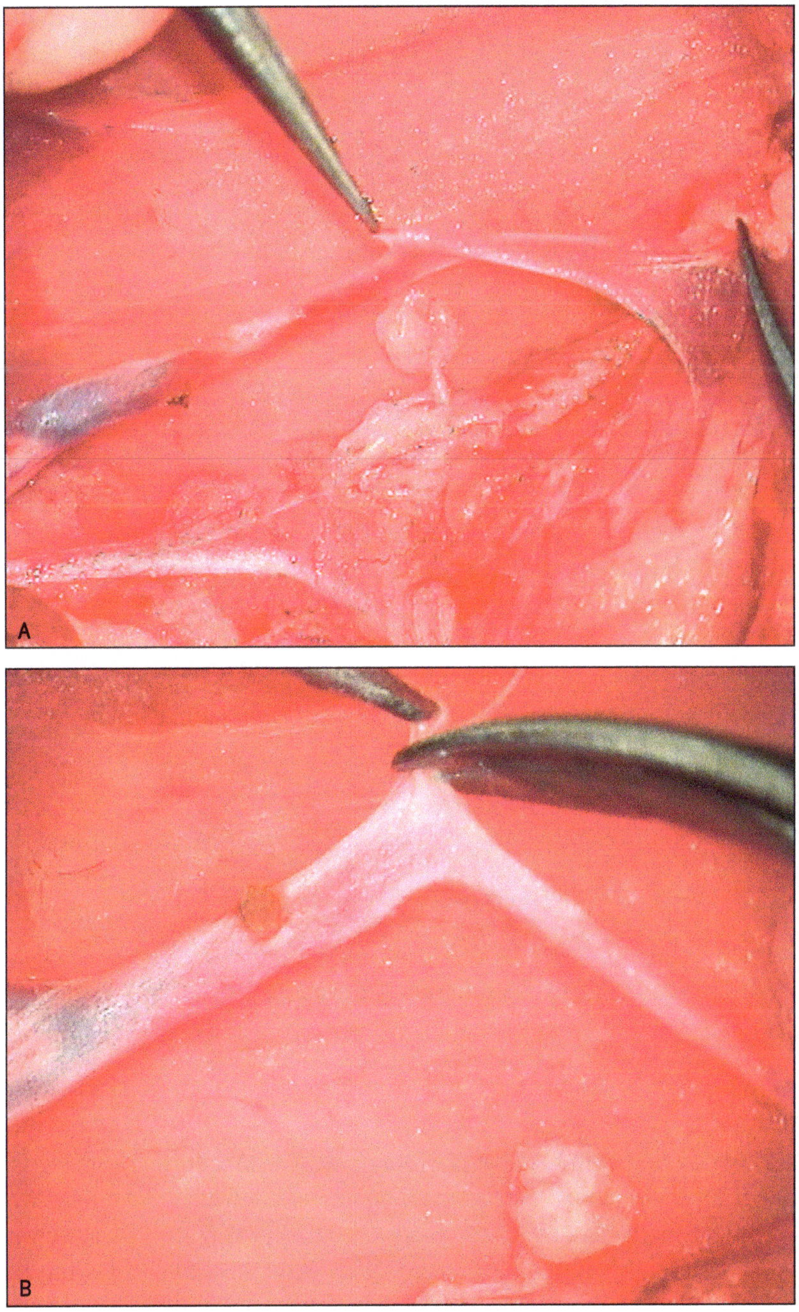

Figure 9-6

Dissection of the adventitia (outer layer) of the right external jugular vein. **A.** Forceps Dumont No. 5 detaches the adventitia, while microsurgical blunt scissors press the vein against the upper edge of the pectoralis muscle. **B.** Forceps Dumont No. 5 holds and scissor cut the adventitia of the external jugular vein. (From author's photo library)

two microsurgical forceps No. 3 and No. 5, or with the forceps No. 5 and the microsurgical scissors (**Fig. 9-6**). Dissection with scissors must be performed with great attention because it is very easy to traumatize and rupture the vein. Also, the vein should not be pulled strongly, because this may lead to thrombosis. The goal of this step of the dissection is to obtain 1 cm of length of vein free of adventitia. Then, a small sheet of yellow plastic background is put underneath the external jugular vein (**Fig. 9-7**).

Note: The dissection of the external jugular vein presented above comprises its full length, including dissection of the three tributaries cephalad to the trifurcation. For the end-to-end anastomosis of the external jugular vein, which requires a minimum of 1 cm clean vessel, dissection of the three tributaries may not be necessary. It is presented for completeness and because it is necessary for other operations in the rest of this book.

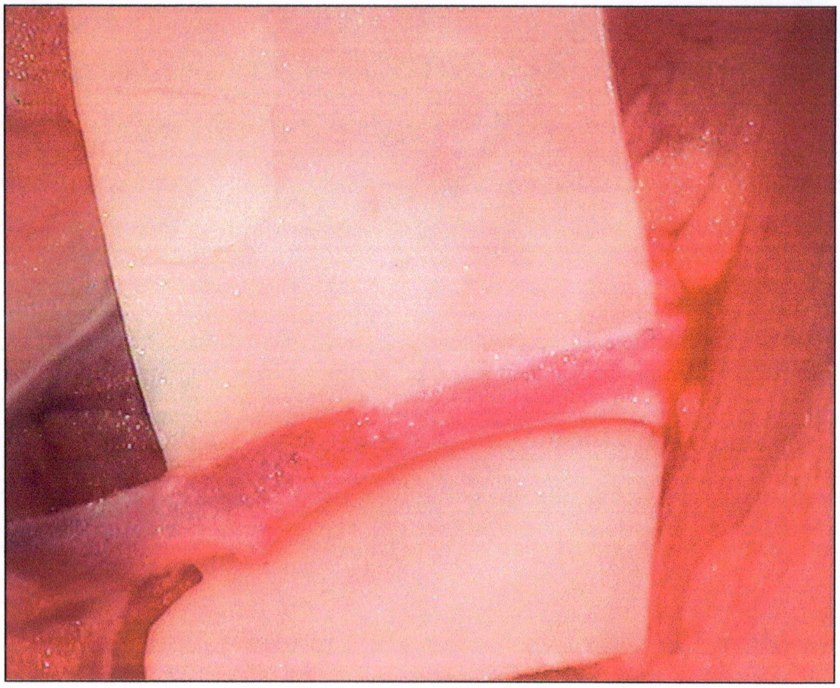

Figure 9-7

The right external jugular vein after dissection of the adventitia, isolated on a plastic background. (From author's photo library)

D. End-to-end anastomosis

The full-length technique of the end-to-end anastomosis of vessels is described in Chapter 5.

- The anastomosis will be performed by placing **8 or 10 sutures 10/0 (usually 8 sutures are placed).**

The steps of the process of the end-to-end anastomosis are as follows:

1. Placement of the double vascular clamp.
2. Transection of the vessel, performed at a distance from the edge of the pectoralis major muscle that gives enough space for the patency test (see 11.b, below).
3. Irrigation of the lumen with normal saline. Warm normal saline is injected into the lumen of the vein using a syringe attached to an angiocatheter 27G.
4. Reapproximation of the clamps of the double clamp.
5. Placement of the two corner sutures (12 o'clock and 6 o'clock) that will orient the vein stumps (**Fig. 9-8**).
6. Suturing of the anterior surface is completed. If 8 sutures are placed, there are 3 remaining per surface, from which the median is placed in the middle of the semicircle, and each of the next two in the middle of each quadrant. If 10 sutures will be placed, there are 4 remaining per surface, which will be placed with the first 2 laterally (toward the corner sutures), then 2 more centrally, all at equal distances (from the corner sutures and between themselves).
7. Rotation of the double clamp and checking that all sutures on the anterior surface have been placed correctly.
8. Suturing of the posterior surface is completed, using the same technique as in the anterior surface.
9. Release of the vessel from the double clamp.
10. Gauze (wet) placement on the anastomosis for 3 minutes.
11. Patency test.
    a. Normally, as described in Chapter 5.10 (**Fig. 5-4**), the patency test will be performed with two microsurgical forceps, initially placed on the vessel one next to the other after the suture line, following the blood flow. The upstream forceps (closest to the sutures) occludes the vessel, while the downstream moves half-closed, milking the vessel and closes again at final position. The upstream forceps is withdrawn while the downstream forceps stays in place. If there is patency across the suture line, the vessel will be immediately filled up to the downstream forceps.
    b. If the anastomosis of the external jugular vein is performed close to the edge of the pectoralis muscle (very low), then there may be not enough space to put the two forceps there and per-

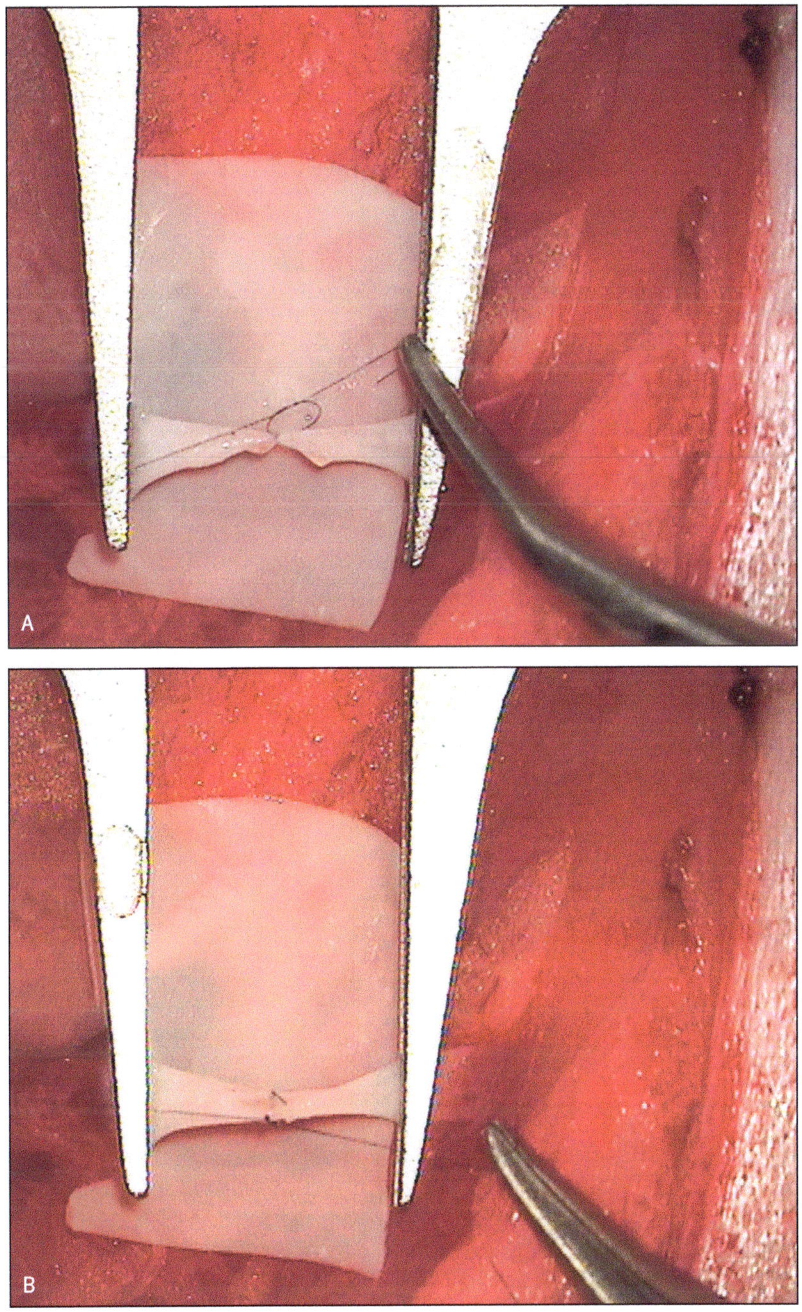

Figure 9-8

Placement of the two corner sutures of the anastomosis of the two stumps of the right external jugular vein. **A.** Descending of the first simple knot on 12 o'clock (up). **B.** Tightening the tie of the third knot on 6 o'clock (down). (From author's photo library)

form the classic patency test. For such cases we present here an alternative technique of the test: A first forceps is placed upstream, cranial to the suture line and closes the vein. Next to it and toward the suture line, is placed a second forceps, which is drawn downstream 'half-closed' over the anastomosis, to stop and remain closed near the pectoralis muscle. The movement of this forceps empties the lumen of the vein (**Fig. 9-9 A**). The upstream forceps is removed and the blood flow is freed. If there is patency in the anastomosis, the vein will be immediately filled up to the downstream forceps (**Fig. 9-9 B**). It is evident that the forceps moving 'half-closed' over the suture line can cause trauma of the suture line or take out a suture if the movement is violent. This is the disadvantage of this technique, and therefore care must be taken in applying it.

12. Withdrawal of the yellow background.

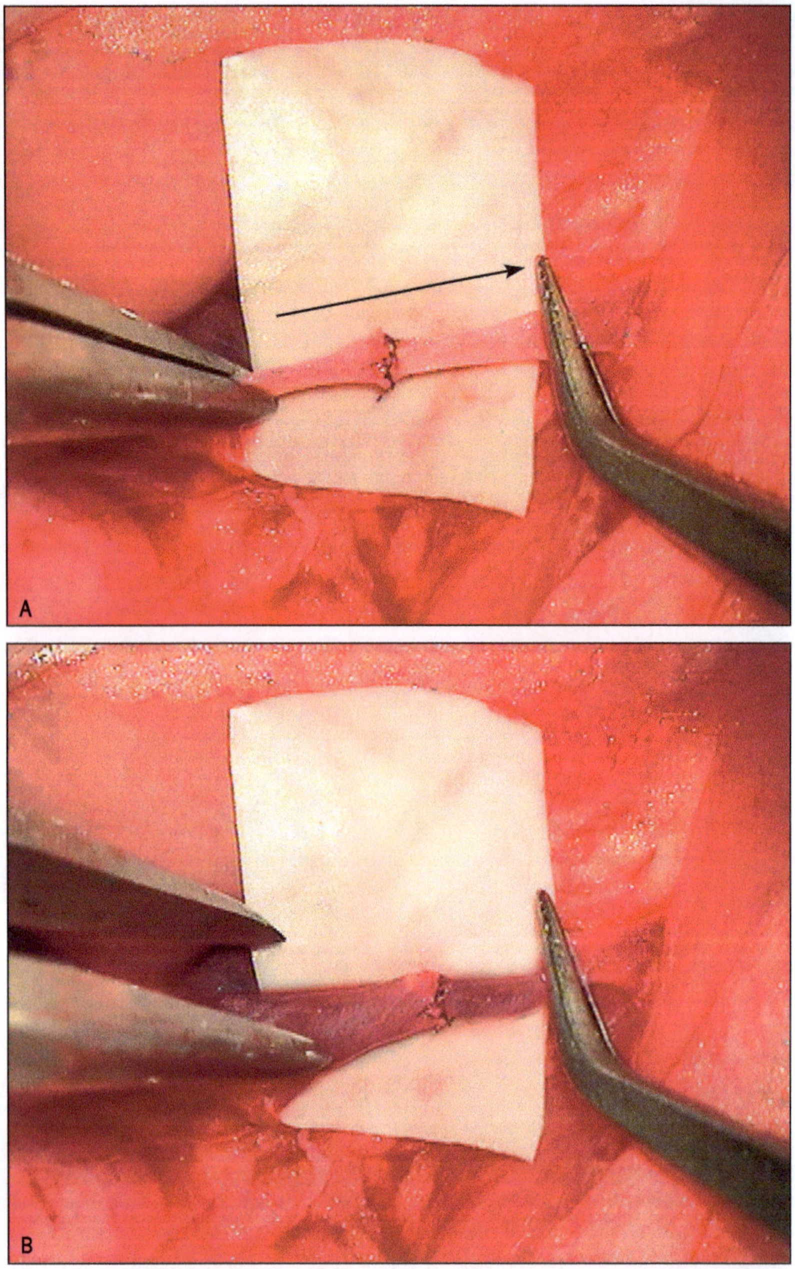

Figure 9-9

Alternative patency test of the end-to-end anastomosis of the right external jugular vein, if there is no space cranial to the border of the perctoralis major to perform the classic test of Figure 5-4. **A.** Dumont No. 5 forceps is placed upstream, cranial to the suture line and interrupts the flow in the vein. The curved microsurgical forceps is initially placed next to Dumont f'half-closed' downstream (toward the heart), thus emptying the lumen of the vein. The arrow shows the movement of the curved forceps. **B.** When Dumont forceps is removed and the blood flow is freed, the lumen of the vein is immediately filled up to the curved forceps, showing the patency of the anastomosis. (From author's photo library)

E. Closure of surgical trauma

Closure of the surgical incision is done in one layer, suturing the skin and superficial fascia (platysma included) with interrupted, non-absorbable 2/0 sutures.

II. COMMON CAROTID ARTERY

A. Positioning of the rat

As in I.A.

B. Preparation of the surgical field and microsurgical dissection of the common carotid artery

Incision at the base of the neck, dissection of the superficial fascia, and placement of the paper clip retractor in the midline pulling cranially the fatty layer of the superficial fascia, platysma and the submandibular glands, are performed as described above for the external jugular vein (see I.B).

As for the common carotid artery, dissection of the superficial fascia aims at cleaning the sternohyoid muscles, coursing parallel to the midline, and the sternal part of the sternocleidomastoid muscle. It is performed with two saturated gauzes moving in opposite directions cranio-caudally, as carried out for the external jugular vein (see above).

When the external jugular vein is found, the surgeon must have decided whether the access to the common carotid artery will be performed by midline separation of the sternohyoid muscles or by transection of the sternal part of the sternocleidomastoid muscle (see below). In the first case, no dissection of the external jugular vein is required. In the second case, as the external jugular vein courses on top of the sternal part of the sternocleidomastoid muscle, it is evident that the vein should be moved laterally before transection of the sternal part of the muscle. The vein should be retracted laterally together with the fatty tissue that most likely has remained from the cranio-caudal dissection of the superficial fascia. An extra paper clip retractor may be required to pull laterally the fatty tissue together with the external jugular vein. The retractor should not be placed directly on the external jugular vein, because of the risk of traumatizing it.

Note: The above preparation describes the procedure on the carotid artery to be performed separately from that on the external jugular vein. If the two procedures are performed in sequence, as usually happens, it is evident that the external jugular vein has already been dissected and mobilized. Then it is very easy to move it laterally in order to access the carotid artery with transection of sternal part of the sternocleidomastoid muscle. In the access of the carotid artery via separation of the sternohyoid muscles through the midline, the external jugular vein is not involved because it is found laterally, outside of the field.

1. Access to the common carotid artery by separation of sternohyoid muscles along the midline

a. Preparation of the surgical field

After removing the superficial fascia, the two sternohyoid muscles are recognized. It is reminded that internal to the sternohyoid muscles, the sternothyroid muscles are found; these are also strap muscles with the same cranio-caudal course, inserting in the thyroid cartilage. Both these layers of strap muscles are separated en mass from the counterparts of the other side, and moved laterally (**Fig. 9-10A**). The dissection is performed in the midline, which is avascular because it is formed by fusion of the investing fasciae of the muscles. Blunt dissection of the medial edge of sternohyoid and sternothyroid muscles from the trachea, and laterally moving the muscles will reveal the internal jugular vein (and the vagus nerve probably) found deep to these muscles, at small distance lateral to the trachea, on top of the prevertebral muscles (**Fig. 9-10B**). Then, a paper clip retractor can be placed to pull laterally the sternohyoid and sternothyroid muscles toward the surgeon. Dissection of the common carotid artery will follow.

b. Microsurgical dissection of the common carotid artery

It is necessary here to review some elements of surgical anatomy regarding the arrangement of the contents of the carotid sheath and the architecture of the deep fascia of the neck. The common carotid artery, internal jugular vein and the vagus nerve are all enveloped in the carotid sheath. In the carotid sheath, the internal jugular vein is found anterolaterally, the common carotid artery posteromedially, and the vagus nerve lies posteriorly, between the internal jugular vein and the carotid artery (medially to the vein).

These vessels and the nerve are ensheathed by a transparent elastic fascia. This is the deep fascia of the neck, which forms the so-called carotid sheath around the vessels and the vagus nerve; the fascia exists also between the vessels and nerve in the sheath. The deep fascia continues as investing fascia of the muscles and as pretracheal fascia around the trachea and the remaining viscera of the neck (esophagus, thyroid, etc.).

Resuming the dissection of the common carotid artery, the preparation of the surgical field so far, as expected from the above, revealed that the vessel found first is the internal jugular vein (**Fig. 9-10B**). The vagus nerve can be recognized at its medial edge. The common carotid artery is found deep to the internal jugular vein. The microsurgical dissection of the common carotid artery consists of opening the carotid sheath, lifting and cleaning of the artery, and preservation of the internal jugular vein and vagus nerve.

By using the microsurgical scissors and blunt dissection, the transparent carotid sheath can be easily opened. The common carotid artery is grasped from the adventitia with a microsurgical forceps and lifted up, leaving posteriorly the internal jugular vein and va-

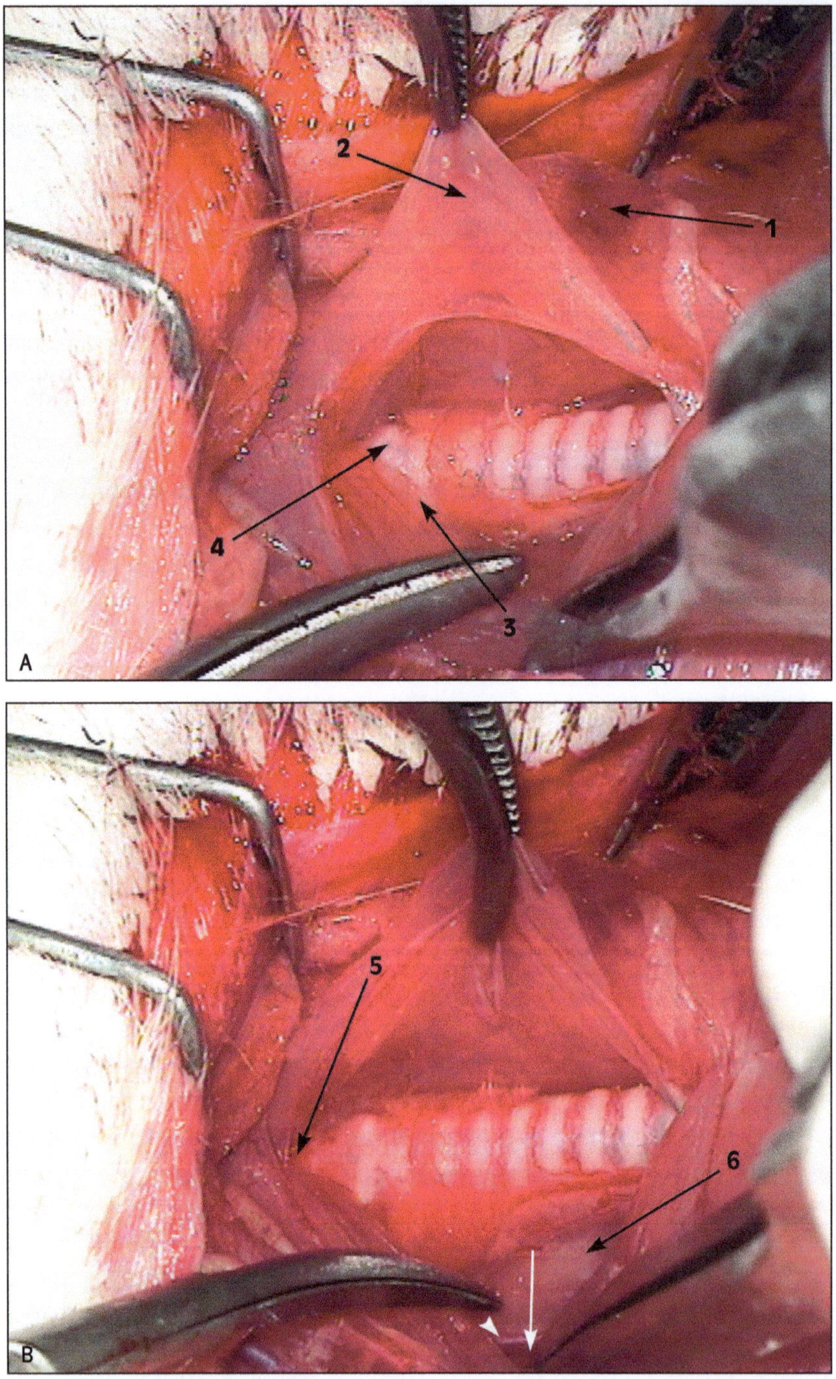

Figure 9-10

Access to the right common carotid artery through the midline. **A.** Anatomical forceps grasps and moves the sternohyoid and sternothyroid muscles away from the midline on either side, while the baby Metzenbaum scissors dissect the right sternothyroid muscle. **B.** The dissection continues deeper, lateral to the trachea, on the prevertebral muscles. The Dumont No. 3 forceps removes the sternohyoid and sternothyroid muscles to the right side, until the right internal jugular vein (white arrow) is found. The vagus nerve (white arrowhead) can be seen at the medial edge of the internal jugular vein. **1.** sternal part of the sternocleidomastoid muscle, **2.** left sternohyoid muscle, **3.** right sternothyroid muscle, **4.** cricoid cartilage, **5.** thyroid cartilage, **6.** prevertebral muscles. (From author's photo library)

gus nerve. The artery is cleaned from the deep fascia that surrounds it (as carotid sheath per se, and as 'packing' of the contents of the carotid sheath) (**Fig. 9-11A**).

It is reminded that the common carotid artery, in its course in the neck until the bifurcation to internal and external carotid arteries—i.e. the part of the vessel dissected here—, does not give any branches. The first branch of the external carotid artery is the superior thyroid artery, which, normally will not be encountered in this dissection. Small branches of the common carotid artery that supply the trachea or the muscles can be cauterized with impunity (**Fig. 9-11B**).

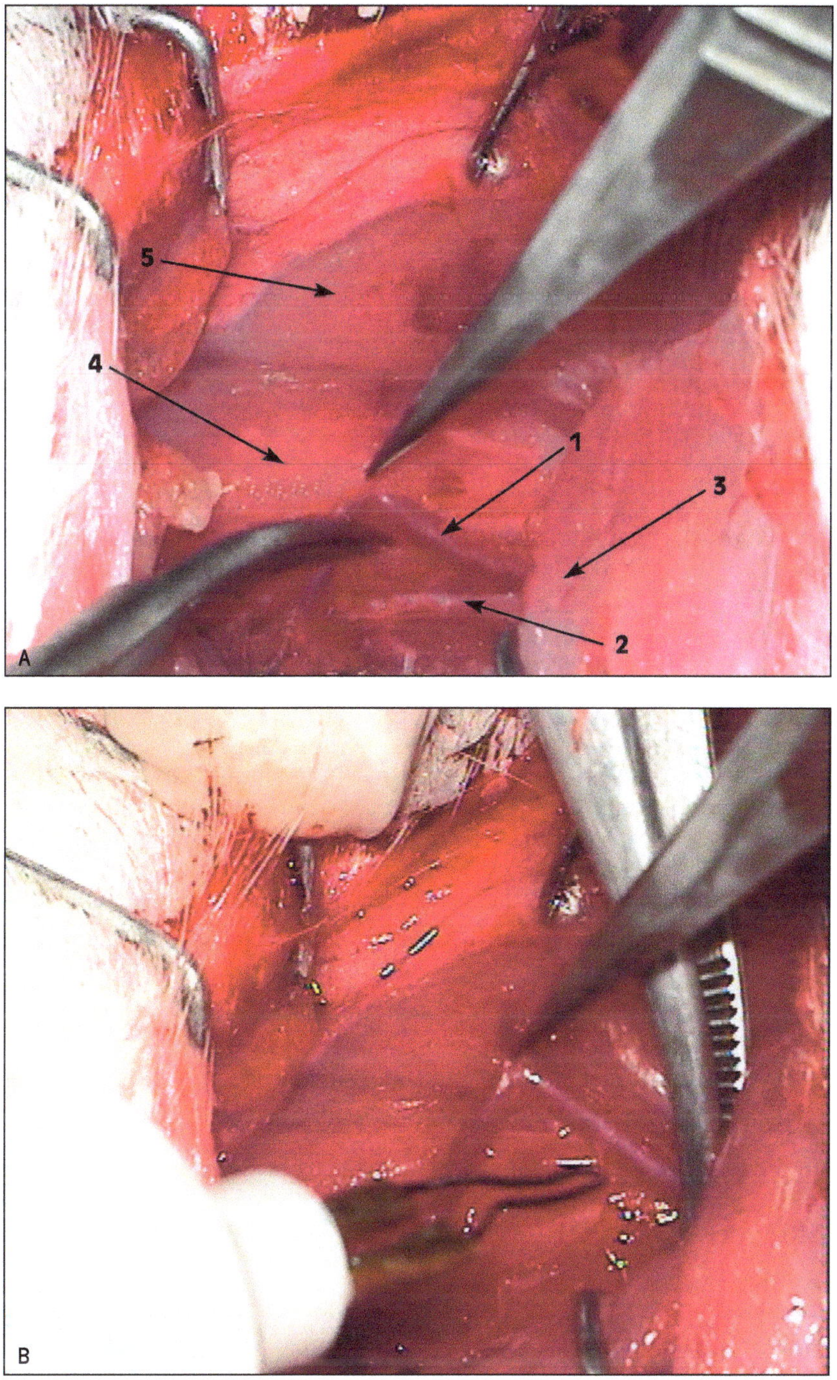

Figure 9-11

Microsurgical dissection of the common carotid artery. **A.** Dumont No. 3 forceps lifts the carotid artery from the adventitia. Thus, the carotid artery is found anterior to the internal jugular vein (reverse to the anatomical order). Microsurgical scissors dissect the deep fascia between the entities contained in the carotid sheath. **B.** Cauterization of a small branch of the common carotid artery. The carotid is elevated by Dumont No. 3 forceps and the single-use monopolar diathermy cauterizes the branch, which has also been freed from deep fascia. **1.** common carotid artery, **2.** internal jugular vein, **3.** right sternohyoid muscle (displaced by the retractor), **4.** left sternohyoid muscle, **5.** sternal part of the left sternocleidomastoid muscle. (From author's photo library)

2. Access to the common carotid artery by transection of the sternal part of the sternocleidomastoid muscle and deep dissection from the lateral border of the sternohyoid muscle

a. Preparation of the surgical field

A wider surgical field for dissection of the common carotid artery may be desired, especially for the trainee. Also, a wider surgical field may serve the expert microsurgeon for operations more complicated than simple anastomosis of the common carotid artery.

To obtain a wide access to the common carotid, the sternal part of the sternocleidomastoid muscle is transected with the monopolar diathermy (**Fig. 9-12**). If no diathermy is available, hemostatic sutures are placed and the muscle is transected with scissors between them. As said above (see II.B) it is evident that the exter-

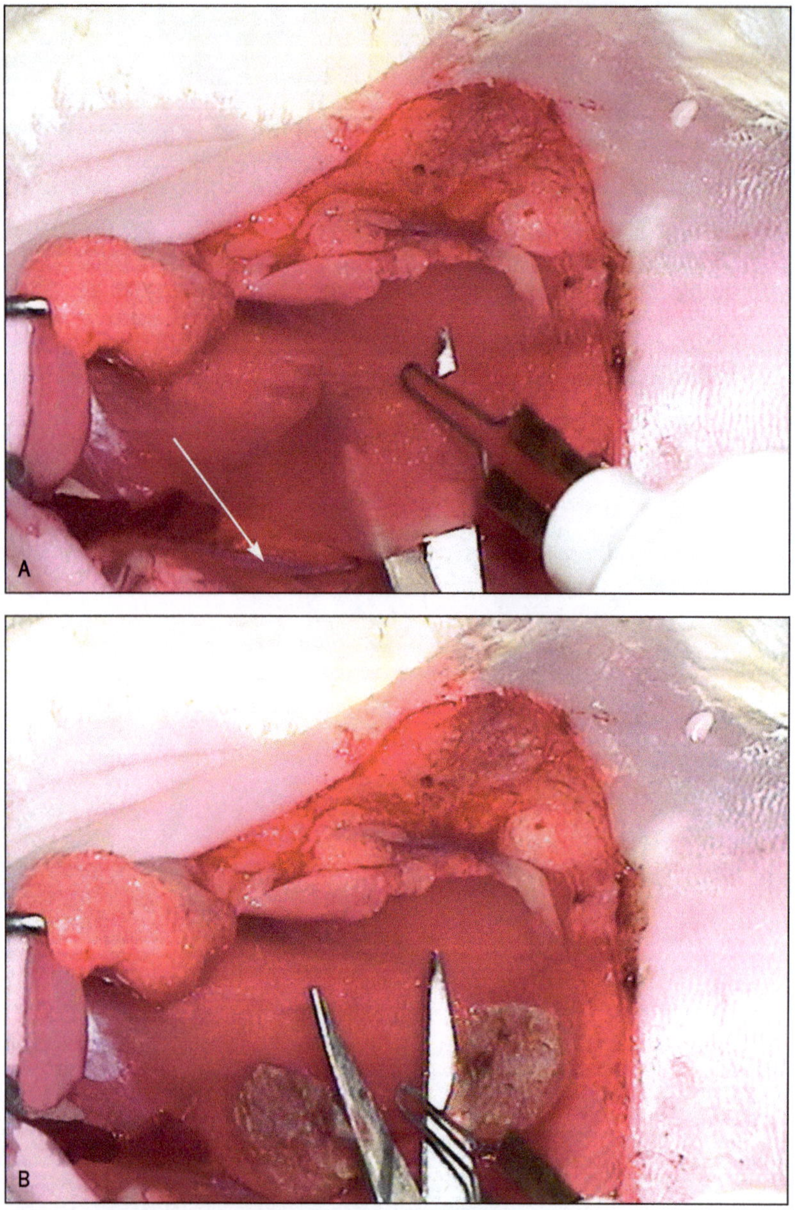

Figure 9-12

Transection of the sternal part of the right sternocleidomastoid muscle. **A.** The scissors lift the sternal part of the muscle. Transcection will be performed with the single-use monopolar diathermy between the scissors blades. Observe that under the scissors lies the external jugular vein (white arrow), which has been moved off the sternal part of the muscle. **B.** The stumps of the muscle after transection. (From author's photo library)

nal jugular vein, which courses on top of the sternal part of the sternocleidomastoid, has to be removed before transection of the muscle (**Fig 9-12A**). After the transection of the sternal part of the muscle, if a retractor had been used to remove the vein, it is withdrawn; the external jugular vein is not an obstacle to the following microsurgical dissection of the common carotid artery (**Fig. 9-13**).

After transection of the sternal part of the sternocleidomastoid muscle, the lateral edge of the sternohyoid muscle becomes evident along almost its whole length. By lifting the sternohyoid muscle and together the sternothyroid muscle from their lateral edges and moving them medially, the transparent carotid sheath and its contents become evident and accessible (**Fig. 9-13**). In order to realize the difference of the current access and the wider surgical field that it offers in relation to the midline access, compare the midline access in **Figure 9-10B** with the lateral access (from the lateral border of the strap muscles) in **Figure 9-13**.

The wide surgical field obtained with transection of the sternal part of the sternomastoid muscle and the deep access to the carotid sheath from the lateral border of the sternohyoid and sternothyroid muscles also offer a better view of the nerves to be protected, i.e. the vagus and the recurrent laryngeal nerve (see next paragraph).

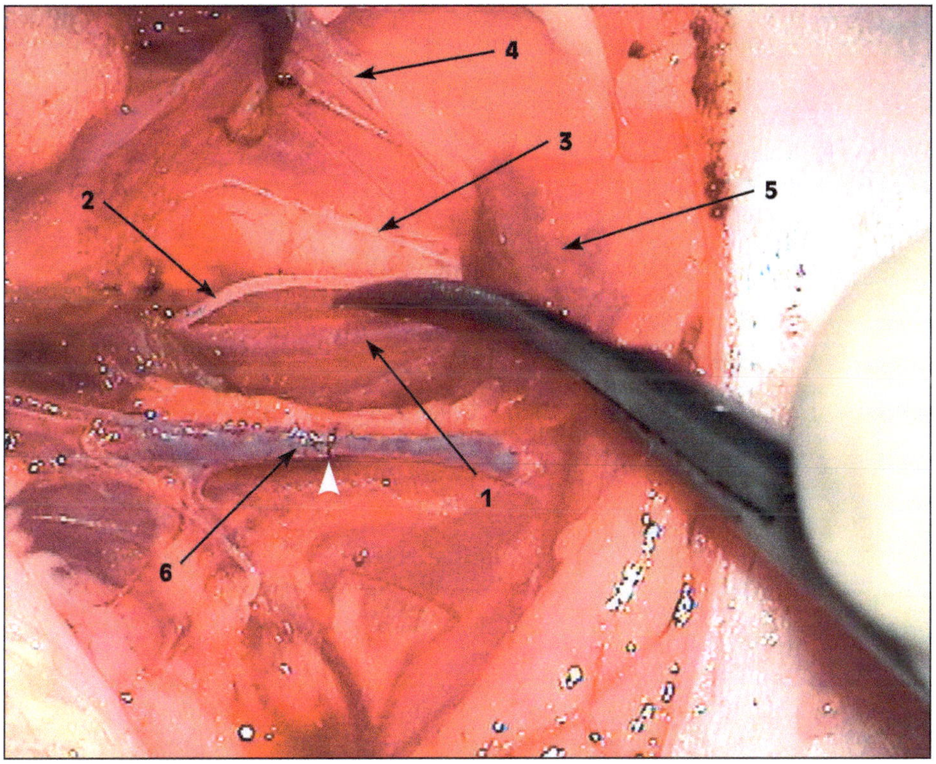

Figure 9-13

Micosurgical dissection of the right common carotid artery (transection of the sternal part of the sternocleidomastoid muscle, access from the lateral border of the sternotyroid muscle). The forceps lifts and moves medially the right sternohyoid and sternothyroid muscles. The carotid sheath has been opened and the scissors dissect the transparent deep fascia between the carotid artery and the vagus nerve (2). Observe the recurrent laryngeal nerve (3) that is lifted together with the muscles outside of its normal position in the paratracheal groove. **1.** common carotid artery, **2.** vagus nerve, **3.** recurrent laryngeal nerve, **4.** right sternohyoid muscle (underneath it is the sternothyroid muscle), **5.** stump of the transected sternal part of the sternocleidomastoid muscle, **6.** external jugular vein (the suture line of of the previous vein anastomosis during the same operation can be seen, white arrowhead). (From author's photo library)

The surgical field can be further broadened by transection of the omohyoid muscle that courses obliquely and covers the upper part of the carotid artery.

b. Microsurgical dissection of the common carotid artery

The reader will find the necessary elements of surgical anatomy in I.b, above.

By lifting and moving medially the sternohyoid and sternothyroid muscles (pulling their lateral borders), the contents of the carotid sheath can be easily accessed. The sheath is opened with blunt dissection using the microsurgical scissors, with repeated movements of the tip back and forth parallel to the long axis of the vessels. Then the common carotid artery can be lifted up with Dumont forceps holding it from the adventitia and comes in front of the internal jugular vein. The artery is fully dissected from the fascia surrounding it (as carotid sheath, but also as 'packing' between the artery, vein, and nerve in the sheath). Attention must be paid to the vagus nerve, which can be easily preserved due to the wide surgical field (**Fig 9-13**).

The recurrent laryngeal nerve can be also revealed. By lifting the sternohyoid and sternothyroid muscles, the nerve emerges from the paratracheal groove (it courses between trachea and esophagus) (**Fig. 9-13**). This happens because, as said above in 1.b, the investing fascia of the muscles and the pretracheal fascia, in which the nerve is packed, are essentially a continuous fascia (the deep fascia of the neck). Therefore, traction on the muscles is transferred to the nerve enveloped in their investing fascia, and the nerve is drawn upward on the trachea from the paratracheal groove.

As a reminder, the surgical field should be periodically irrigated with warm normal saline during the whole dissection. After dissection of the common carotid artery has been completed, a small plastic yellow background is placed under it (**Fig. 9-14**).

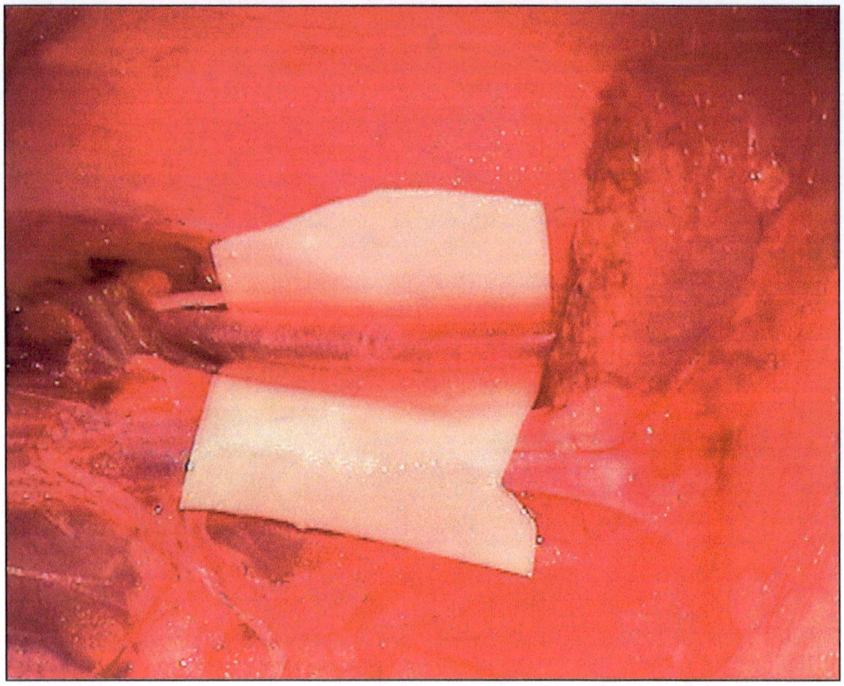

Figure 9-14

The right common carotid artery isolated on a yellow plastic background. (From author's photo library)

C. End-to-end anastomosis

The technique of the end-to-end anastomosis of vessels is described in full-length in Chapter 5.

- The anastomosis will be performed by placing **8 sutures 10/0**.

The steps of the process of the end-to-end anastomosis are as follows:

1. Placement of the double vascular clamp.
2. Transection of the vessel.
3. Irrigation of the lumen with normal saline. Warm normal saline is injected with a syringe attached to an angiocatheter 27G (**Fig. 9-15**).
4. Folding of the adventitia. Dumont No. 3 forceps immobilizes the vessel and Dumont No 5 forceps folds the adventitia.
5. Reapproximation of the clamps of the double clamp.
6. Placement of two corner sutures (12 o'clock and 6 o'clock) that will orient the artery stumps (**Fig. 9-16**).
7. Suturing of the anterior surface is completed. After placement of the corner sutures, there are 3 sutures remaining per surface, from which the first is placed in the middle of the semicircle, and each of the next two are placed in the middle of each quadrant on either side.
8. Rotation of the double clamp and checking that all sutures of the anterior surface have been placed correctly.
9. Suturing of the posterior surface is completed, using the same technique as in the anterior surface.
10. Release of the vessel from the double clamp.
11. Gauze (wet) placement on the anastomosis for 3 minutes.
12. Patency test.
    a. The classic patency test is described in Chapter 5.10 (**Fig. 5-4**). Very briefly, a forceps closes the lumen upstream, cranial to the anastomosis, and a second forceps placed next to it empties the lumen by moving 'half-closed' downstream (more cranially) and closes at a final position. The upstream forceps is withdrawn, and, if there is patency, the vessel is immediately filled up to the downstream forceps.
    b. Here is shown for the common carotid artery the alternative patency test described above, in paragraph I.D.10.b. In summary, an upstream forceps occludes the common carotid artery central to the anastomosis (towards the heart) and another forceps is placed initially immediately cranial to it and then moves 'half-closed' downstream (cranially) across the suture line to empty the lumen, and remains closed at a final position past the anastomosis (**Fig 9-17A**). The upstream forceps is

Figure 9-15

Irrigation of the lumen of the transected right common carotid artery. Dumont No 5 forceps holds the wall of the artery stump. With a fine Abbocath, warm normal saline is injected in the lumen. (From author's photo library)

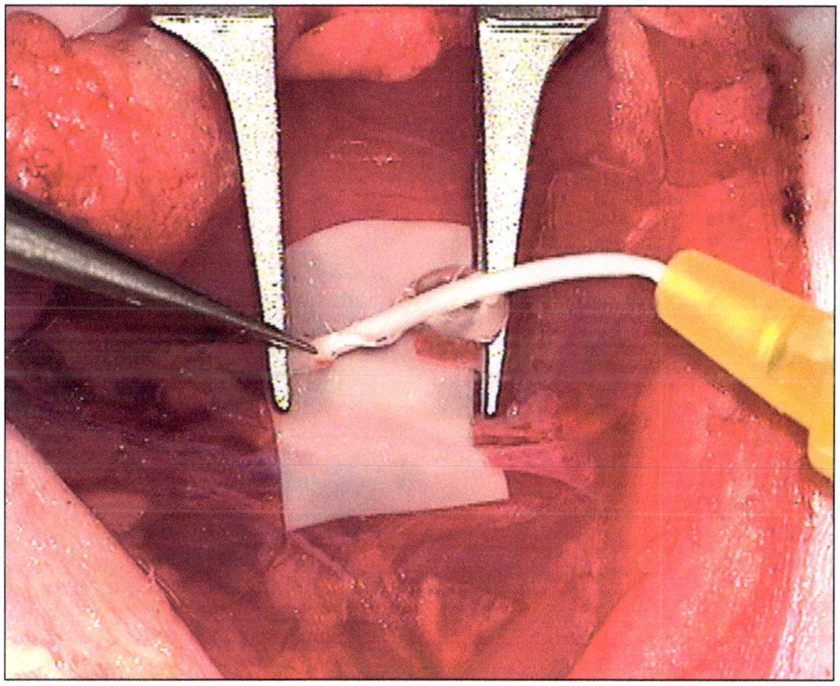

removed, and if there is patency, the vessel is immediately filled (**Fig 9-17B**). Of course, as mentioned above, this method has a risk because the second forceps slides over the suture line.

c. In order to avoid having the second forceps sliding over the suture line, there is the possibility to use two forceps emptying the vessel by moving in opposite directions on either side of the anastomosis. Then, as in b, the upstream forceps (towards the heart) is withdrawn, and if there is patency the vessel will be immediately filled up to the downstream (cranial) closed forceps. This alternate method is inferior to the classic patency test, because opposite forces are applied on the

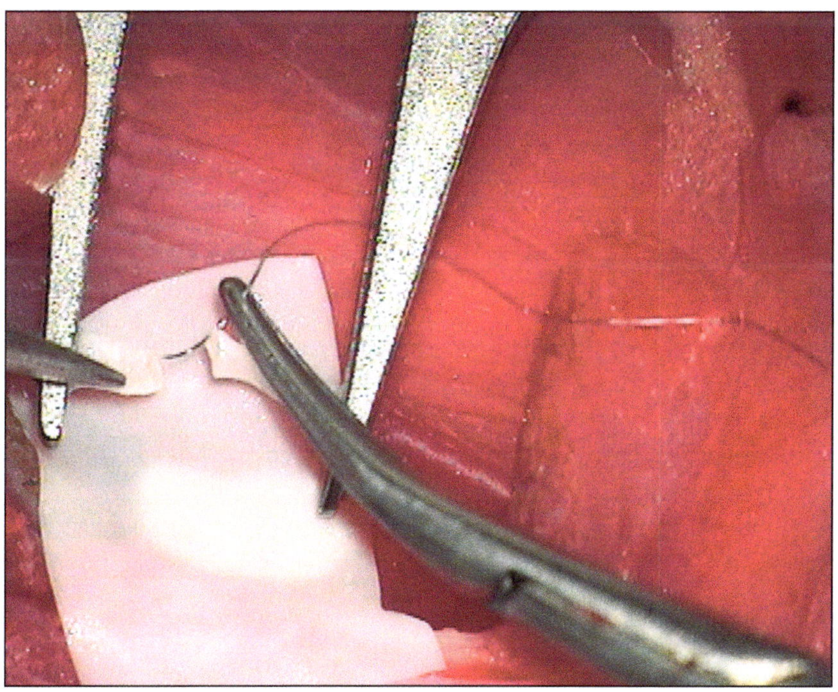

Figure 9-16

Placement of the first corner suture in one step, at 12 o'clock position. The needle holder holds the needle that has just passed through the wall of one stump of the right common carotid artery. Dumont No. 5 forceps grasps the folded adventitia of the other stump, to help the needle pass through it. The beginner should place the suture in two steps. (From author's photo library)

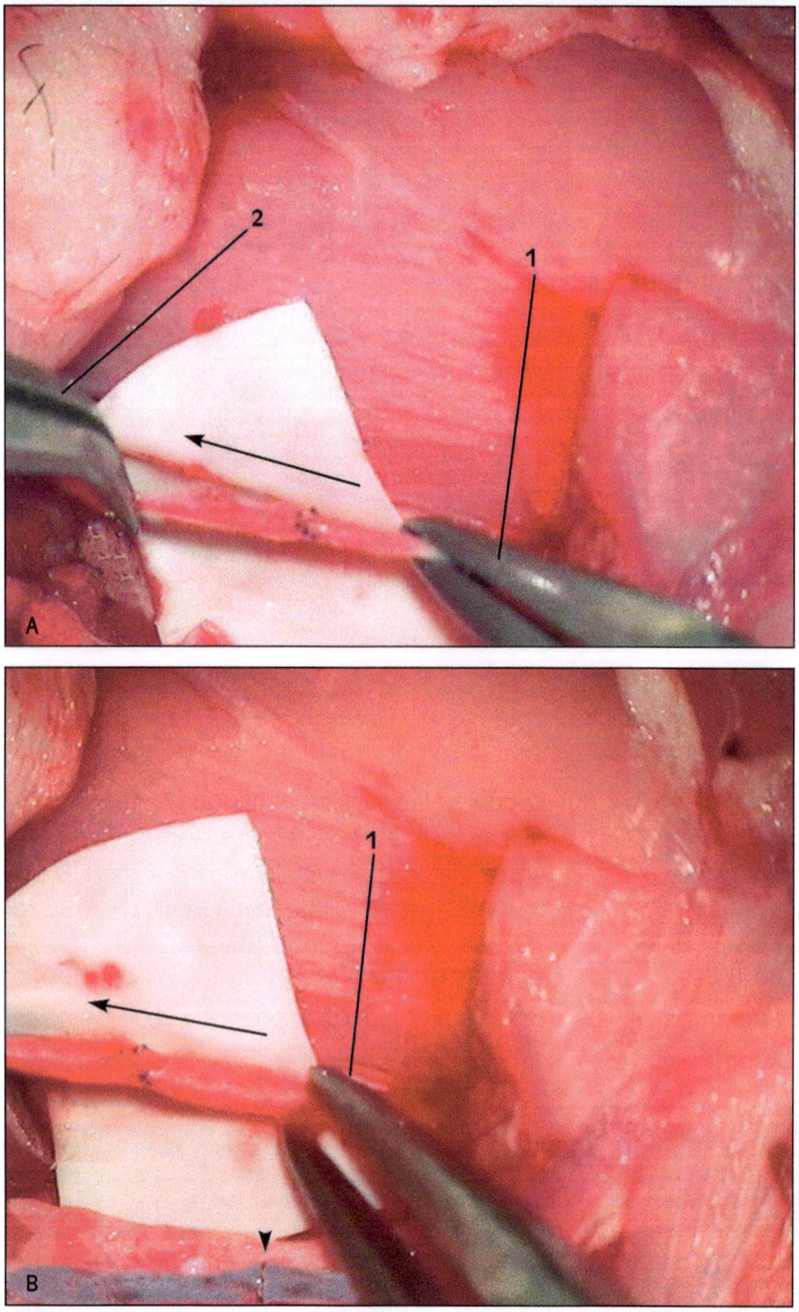

Figure 9-17

Alternative patency test of the end-to-end anastomosis of the right common carotid artery. **A.** The upstream (placed towards the heart) forceps **(1)** occludes the flow in the vessel central to the anastomosis. The downstream curved forceps **(2)** empties the lumen moving 'half-closed' cranially across the suture line (arrow), starting form a point next to forceps **(1)**; here forceps **(2)** is shown closed in terminal cranial position. **B.** Successful anastomosis. The upstream forceps **(1)** is shown here open and has released blood flow, which continues unobstructed cranially, past the anastomosis (while the downstream curved forceps, not shown here, stays closed in place). A previous anastomosis of the external jugular vein (arrowhead) can also be seen. (From author's photo library)

suture line, and if they are excessive, they could break the sutures. Also, note that this method cannot be applied to veins, because one of the forceps will move opposite to blood flow, and most likely against the action of a valve (this is the reason it is not suggested above for the external jugular vein).

13. Withdrawal of the yellow background.

D. Closure of surgical trauma

Closure of the surgical incision is done in one layer, suturing the skin and superficial fascia (platysma included)

... end-to-end anastomosis of the external jugular vein and of the common carotid artery

Synopsis...

Procedures refer to right vessels (can be identically be applied on left side)

A. **Position of the rat:** Laid on its back, head on the left of the surgeon. The limbs are immobilized on the working surface with adhesive tape.

B. **Preparation of the surgical field:** A transverse incision is performed at the base of the neck, from shoulder to shoulder. The fat of the superficial cervical fascia is dissected with two gauzes saturated in warm normal saline, moving in opposite directions cranio-caudally. A paper clip retractor pulls cranially pulls the skin, superficial fascia (platysma included), and submandibular salivary glands.

I. EXTERNAL JUGULAR VEIN

C. **Microsurgical dissection:** The external jugular vein is dissected from the upper edge of the pectoralis muscle to the trifurcation of the vein; small tributary veins are cut after double ligation or coagulation. A yellow plastic background is placed underneath it.

D. **End-to-end anastomosis: 8 or 10 sutures 10/0**

1. Placement of the double vascular clamp.
2. Transection of the vessel.
3. Irrigation of the lumen with normal saline.
4. Reapproximation of the clamps of the double clamp.
5. Placement of the two corner sutures (12 o'clock and 6 o'clock).
6. Suturing of the anterior surface is completed. If 8 sutures are placed, there are 3 remaining, put the first in the middle of the semicircle and the next two in the middle of each quadrant. If 10 sutures placed, there are 4 remaining, put at equal distances, first the 2 peripheral sutures (towards the corner sutures).
7. Rotation of the clamp and checking of sutures of the anterior surface.
8. Suturing of the posterior surface, similar to anterior.
9. Release of the double clamp.
10. Placement of a wet gauze on the anastomosis for 3 minutes.
11. Patency test.
12. Withdrawal of the yellow plastic background.

II. COMMON CAROTID ARTERY

B. **Continuation of preparation of the surgical field and microsurgical dissection:** Access to the common carotid artery is gained in 2 ways: 1) The sternohyoid and sternothyroid muscles are separated in the midline 2) The sternal part of the sternocleidomastoid muscle is transected and the sternohyoid and sternothyroid muscles are moved together medially lifted from their lateral edges.

The carotid sheath is opened, and the common carotid artery is lifted superficial to the internal jugular vein and cleaned from the fascia. The vagus and the recurrent laryngeal nerves are preserved (the latter is evident in access No. 2). The right common carotid artery is isolated on a yellow plastic background.

... end-to-end anastomosis of the external jugular vein and of the common carotid artery

Synopsis...

C. End-to-end anastomosis: 8 sutures 10/0

1. Placement of the double vascular clamp.
2. Transection of the vessel.
3. Irrigation of the lumen with normal saline.
4. Removal (folding) of the adventitia.
5. Reapproximation of the clamps of the double clamp.
6. Placement of the two corner sutures (12 o'clock and 6 o'clock).
7. Suturing of the anterior surface is completed. There are there are 3 remaining sutures, put the first in the middle of the semicircle and the next two in the middle of each quadrant.
8. Rotation of the clamp and checking of sutures of the anterior surface
9. Suturing of the posterior surface, similar to anterior.
10. Release of the double clamp.
11. Placement of a wet gauze on the anastomosis for 3 minutes.
12. Patency test.
13. Withdrawal of the yellow plastic background.

Closure of surgical trauma: The skin and the superficial fascia (including the platysma) are sutured in one layer with interrupted, non-absorbable 2/0 sutures.

10

Interposition of external jugular vein graft in the abdominal aorta

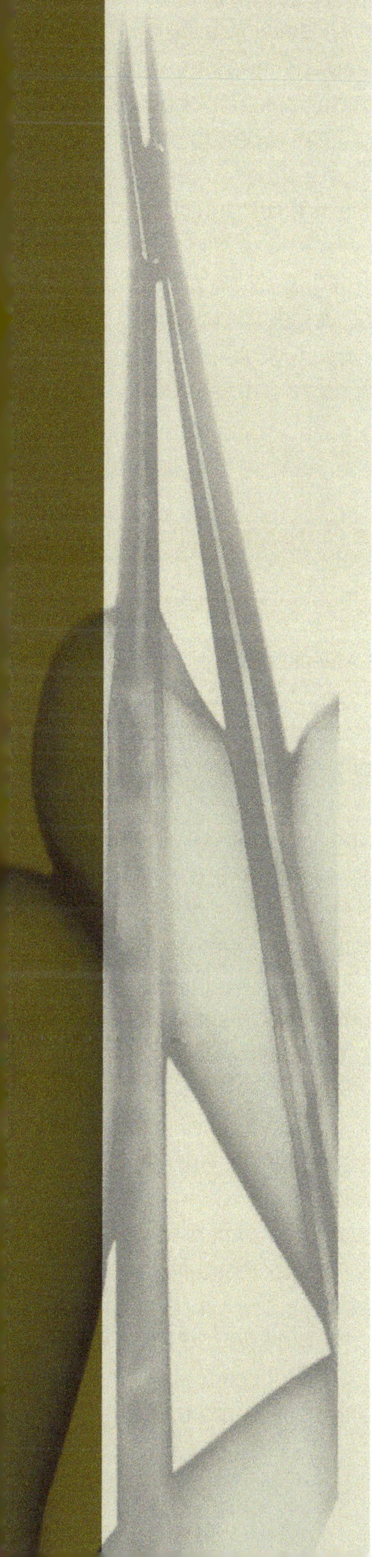

In this Chapter, the graft is taken form the right external jugular vein. The left external jugualr vein can also be similarly used.

A. Positioning of the rat

The rat is placed in supine position (dorsal decubitus) on the working surface. The long axis of the body of the rat is parallel to the frontal (coronal) plane of the surgeon's body, and the rat's head is placed on the surgeon's left. The limbs of the rat are immobilized on the working surface with adhesive tape.

The rat remains in the same position from throughout the operation, since the graft is taken from the right external jugular vein. If the left external jugural vein is going to be harvested, the head of the rat should be placed on the right for taking the graft, and then on the left for placement of the graft in the aorta (the rat's long axis is always kept parallel to the surgeon's frontal plane).

B. Preparation of the surgical field in the neck

For a detailed presentation and imaging, the reader is invited to read the respective preparation in Chapter 9.I.B. Here only a summary is given.

A transverse incision is performed at the base of the neck, extending from shoulder to shoulder. The superficial fascia is dissected to find the right external jugular vein. This is done with two gauzes saturated in warm normal saline, using light pressure to pull in opposite directions cranio-caudally. A paper clip retractor is placed in the middle of the incision, parallel to the midline, and pulls cranially the skin, superficial fascia and platysma, and the submandibular salivary glands. This preparation of the field reveals the right external jugular vein and tributaries, as it travels across the ipsilateral sternocleidomastoid muscle, from the edge of the pectoralis muscle to the mandible.

C. Microsurgical dissection of the external jugular vein

For a detailed presentation and imaging, the reader is invited to read the respective dissection in Chapter 9.I.C. Here only a summary is given.

Dissection of the right external jugular vein starts at the upper border of the pectoralis major muscle and continues past its trifurcation, until the mandible (see **Figure 9-3**). The vein and the three tributaries are carefully cleaned from the fat and the adventita is removed. The more meticulous dissection is focused on the major tributary vein. The smaller tributaries of the external jugular vein found between the pectoralis muscle and the trifurcation are also dissected and cut after cauterization, or preferably, after suture ligations.

➢ The two lesser tributary veins emptying at the trifurcation of the external jugular vein are ligated with 9/0 suture and cut between two ligations.

The major tributary vein is kept intact at this point of the operation. A gauze saturated in warm normal saline is placed on the surgical field of the neck.

D. Preparation of the surgical field in the abdomen

For a detailed presetnation and imaging, the reader is invited to read the respective preparation in Chapter 8.B. Here only a summary is given.

A median incision is performed starting 5 mm below the xiphoid cartilage and ending 5 mm above the pubic symphisis. The aponeuroses of the rectus abdominis muscles are separated in the linea alba with scalpel or scissors (baby Metzenbaum). Two paper clip retractors are placed symmetrically, each on either side.

The liver lobes projecting in the surgical field are removed with a paper clip retractor enveloped with gauze. The small intestine is fully mobilized, and then, grasped gently with wide anatomical forceps starting with the cecum, the intestines (small and large) are placed on a wet gauze on the right side of the rat. All the intestines are covered with a gauze pad saturated in warm normal saline. The intestines and the peritoneal cavity are periodically irrigated with warm normal saline. The spleen, if it is an obstacle in the surgical field, is moved to the left and cranially with a retractor enveloped with gauze.

E. Microsurgical dissection of the aorta

For a detailed presentation and imaging, the reader is invited to read the respective preparation in Chapter 8.C. Here only a summary is given.

The retroperitoneum is opened with two gauzes saturated with warm normal saline, drawn laterally away from each other, starting from the midline.

Dissection of the aorta starts just above the bifurcation into iliac arteries, and aims to develop a plane of separation between the aorta and the inferior vena cava. Microsurgical dissection of the aorta is continued cranially, up to the left renal vein. When expanding the plane of separation, the lumbar arteries must be double ligated with 9/0 suture or cauterized and cut.

After the aorta has been fully freed, a yellow plastic blackground is put underneath the vessel. Microsurgical dissection of the aorta stops here. A gauze saturated in warm normal saline is placed on the surgical field.

F. Harvest the graft from the external jugular vein

➢ The vein graft length should be at least 1 cm.

➢ The graft comprises the whole length of the external jugular vein and a part of the major tributary vein cranial to the trifurcation of the external jugular vein.

Both ends of the vein graft are ligated with 9/0 suture: the first ligation is placed at the inflow end near the mandible, and the second ligation is placed at the outflow end near the edge of the pectoralis muscle (**Fig. 10-1**). This order of ligations avoids entrapment of blood in the graft lumen. The vein graft is transected at both ends (**Fig. 10-2**), very close to the ligations.

The graft is placed aside in the surgical field of the neck with specific attention **not to be reversed.** Holding the inflow (cranial) end of the graft by the adventitia with No. 3 Dumont forceps, we wash the lumen with warm normal saline using a fine 27G angiocatheter attched to a syringe (**Fig. 10-3**). Irrigation of the lumen of the graft must be performed in the direction of the blood flow, i.e. from inflow to outflow, because it is probable that the vein graft contains a valve. The tip of

Figure 10-1

Ligation of the outflow end of the right external jugular vein with 9/0 suture, just above the edge of the pectoralis major muscle. (From author's photo library)

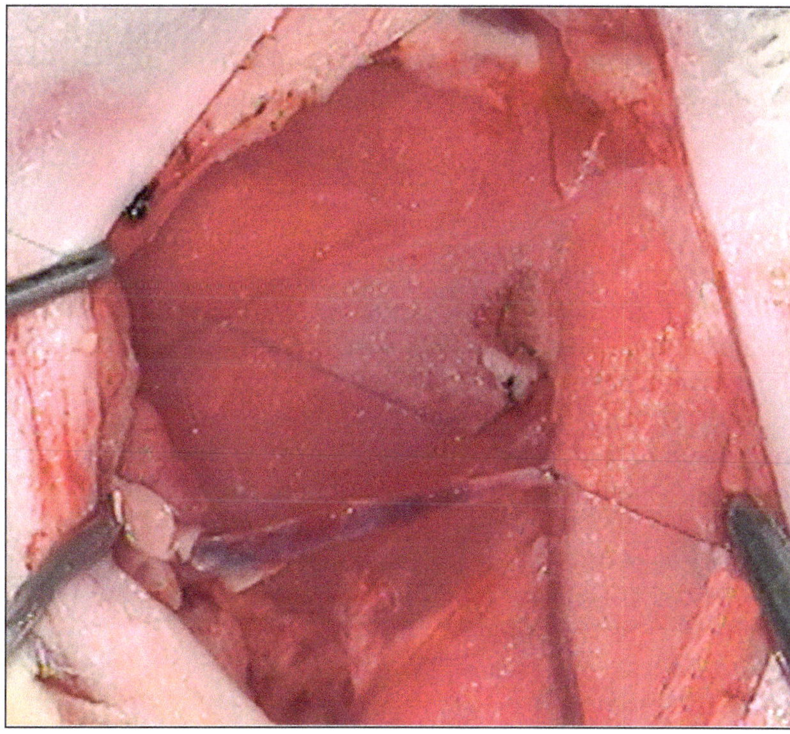

the catheter should not enter the lumen, to avoid trauma to the endothelium. The vein graft is placed on a wet gauze to be transferred into the surgical field of the aorta.

G. Transfer of the graft – Transection of the aorta

The graft is transferred into the abdomen and positioned on the yellow background, parallel and to the side

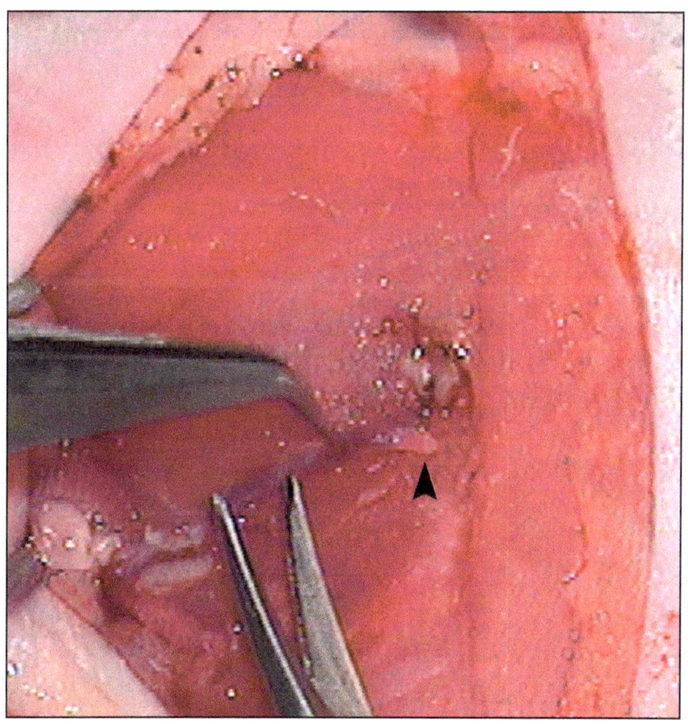

Figure 10-2

Transection of the vein graft. The curved microsurgical forceps lifts the right external jugular vein; transection at the outflow end (arrowhead) has been performed and the microsurgical scissors move cranially to make the transection at the inflow end of the graft. (From author's photo library)

of the aorta, on a wet gauze. Attention must be paid to retain the proper flow direction of the graft. This **should not be reversed** in any case, because, as said, a valve may be contained in the graft. In its final position, the graft should retain the same direction of blood flow as in the neck.

The lumen of the aorta is obstructed with the double vasular clamp. The aorta is transected and the lumens of both stumps are irrigated. A segment of aorta, at least 5 mm in length, is cut away from one of the stump edges and removed. The more mobilized stump is selected to have the segment removed. This maneuver prevents kinking of the vessel after placement of the graft. Then, the adventitia of the aorta is folded back.

Placement of the graft parallel to the aorta in the space between the edges of the aortic stumps (**Fig. 10-4**) shows if the two clamps have to be reapproximated so that the edges of the stumps come in contact with the edges of the graft. The anatomoses should not be performed under tension.

H. End-to-end anastomoses

The reader will find a detailed description of end-to-end vascular anastomosis in Chapter 5.

- **10 sutures 10/0 will be placed in each anastomosis**

The two anastomoses between the aortic stumps and the vein graft are performed **simultaneously,** as follows:

1. First the two upper corner sutures are placed at the 12 o'clock position in both anastomoses, and then the two lower corner sutures placed at 6 o'clock (**Fig. 10-5**). Placement of the sutures in this order permits the correct orientation of the vessels.
2. Suturing of the anterior surfaces of the anastomoses is completed. There are 4 sutures remaining per surface, which are placed at equal distances (from the corner sutures and between themselves), starting first with the two lateral (toward the corner sutures) and then the two more central sutures in the semicircle (technique 'de proche en proche', see Chapter 5) (**Fig. 10-6**).

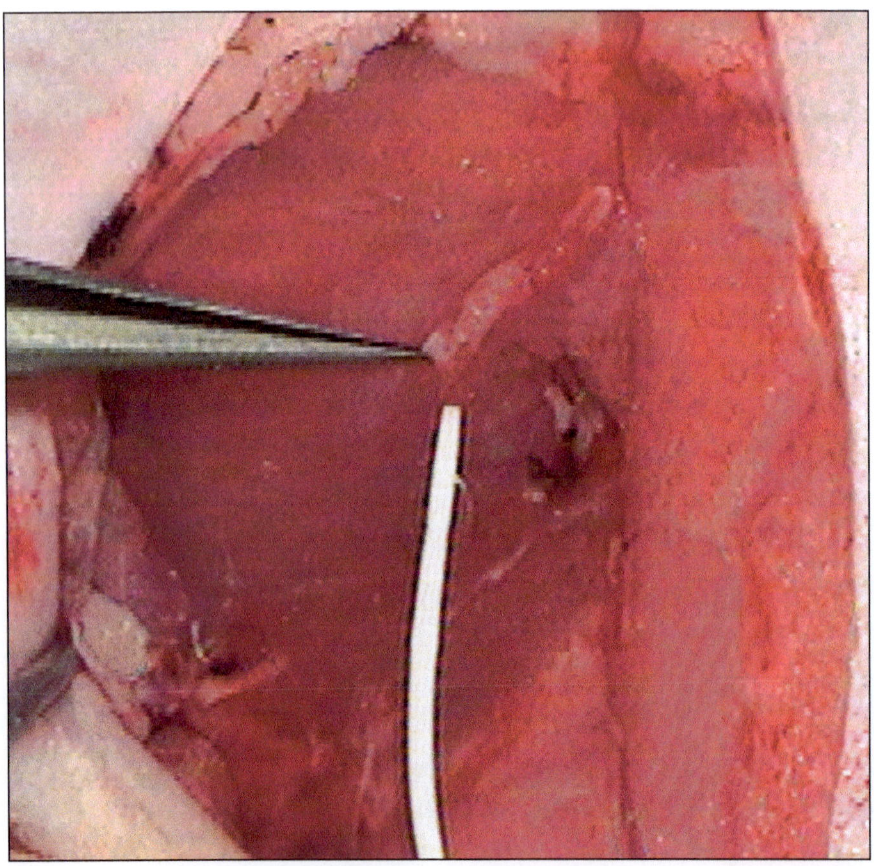

Figure 10-3

Irrigation of the vein graft (from the right external jugular vein). Dumont No. 3 forceps holds the graft from the outer surface, and warm normal saline is injected under pressure into the lumen from an angiocatheter 27G. The tip of the catheter does not enter the lumen. Irrigation is performed in the direction of blood flow in the graft at its initial position. (From author's photo library)

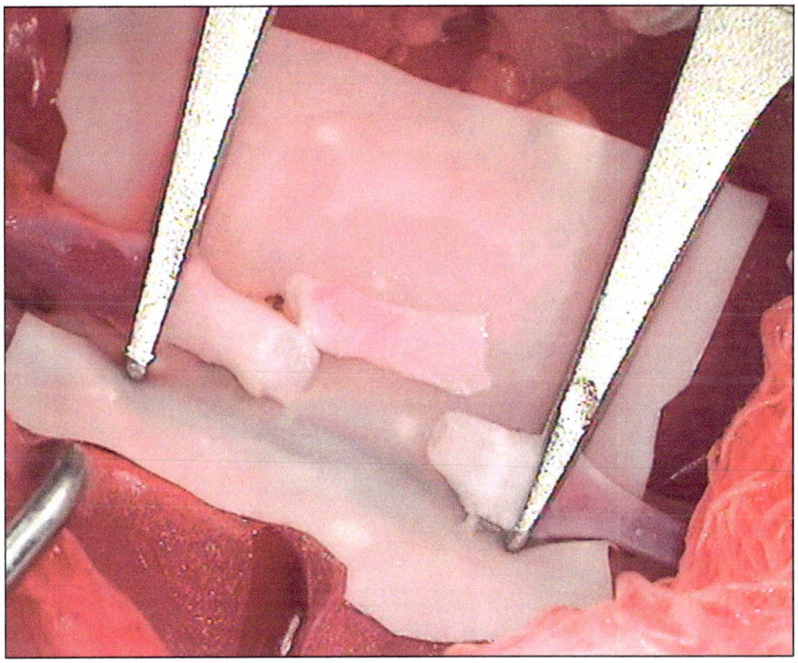

Figure 10-4

The vein graft has been transferred into the abdomen with care to retain the correct direction of flow. It is placed aside and parallel to the aorta, edge to edge with the aortic stumps. The correct distance of the arms of the double clamp is checked in order to avoid creating anastomoses under tension. (From author's photo library)

3. Rotation of the double clamp and checking that all sutures of the anterior surfaces have been placed correctly.
4. Suturing of the posterior surfaces similar to the anterior surfaces.
5. Release of the vessel from the double clamp.
6. Gauze (wet) placement on the anastomoses for 3 minutes.
7. Patency test.

   The patency test is performed as in a sole end-to-end anastomosis, as described in Chapter 5.10 (**Fig. 5-4**). Distal to the graft and before the aortic bifurcation, a first, upstream forceps occludes the aorta and a second, downstream forceps is placed initially next to the first forceps, and then moves distally while half-closed, milking the vessel and finally remains closed. The upstream forcpes is removed, and if there is patency, the vessel is immediately filled up to the downstream forceps. This test examines the patency of both anastomoses. Successful anastomo-

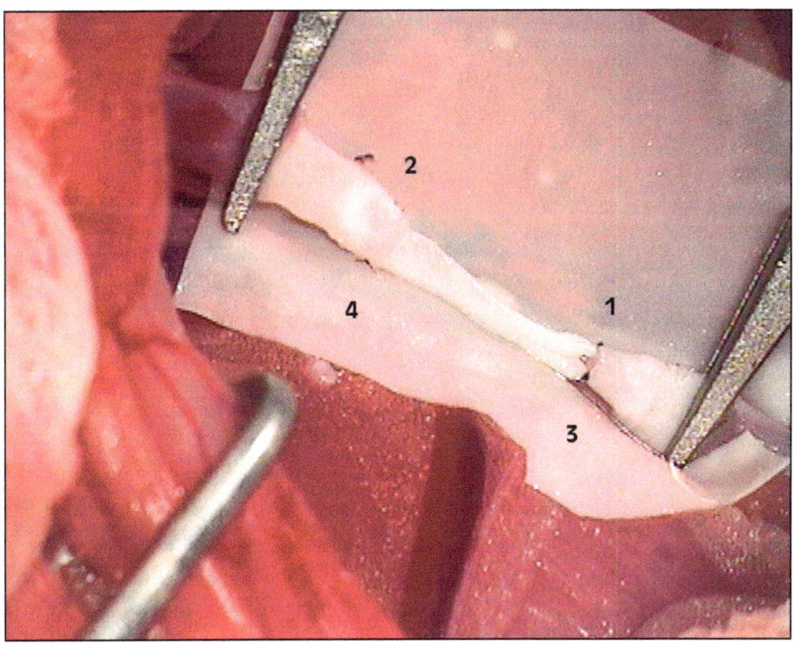

Figure 10-5

Placement of corner sutures between the aortic stumps and the external jugular vein graft. The numbers show the order of suture placement. (From author's photo library)

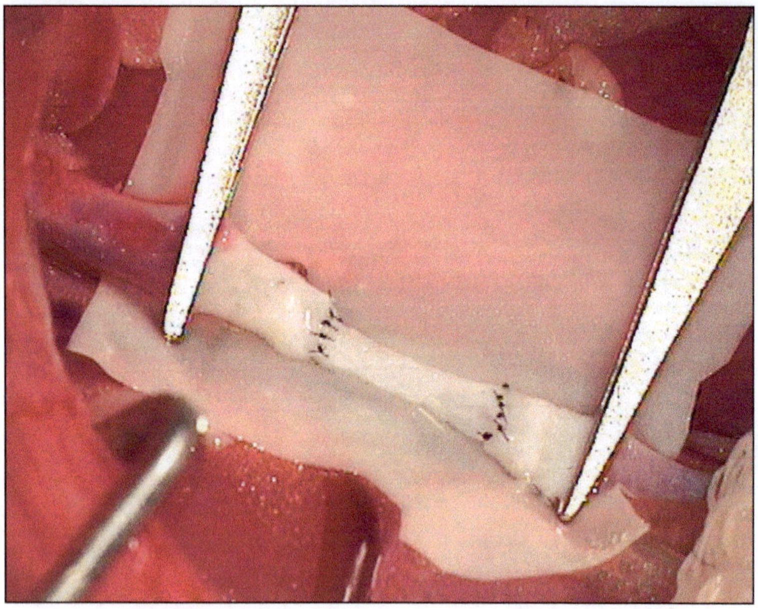

Figure 10-6

Completed suturing of the anterior surfaces of the anastomoses between the aortic stumps and the external jugular vein graft. (From author's photo library)

ses between aortic stumps and vein graft are shown in **Figure 10-7**.

If there is no patency, in order to find out which anastomosis failed and has to be redone, the first (cranial) anastomosis can be tested following the same technique. In this case, the forceps are applied on the vein graft, and the downstream forceps moves on it. Specific care must be taken, because of the fragile nature of the vein graft. If the first anastomosis is patent, it is evident that the second (caudal) anastomosis is responsible for the failure of the graft patency.

8. Withdrawal of the yellow background.

H. Closure of surgical traumas

After the splanchna have been returned to the abdomen, the abdominal wall is closed in two layers (muscles, subcutaneous-skin) with interrupted non-absorbable 2/0 sutures. Closure of the neck incision is performed in one layer including skin and superficial fascia (and plastysma) with interrupted, non-absorbable 2/0 sutures.

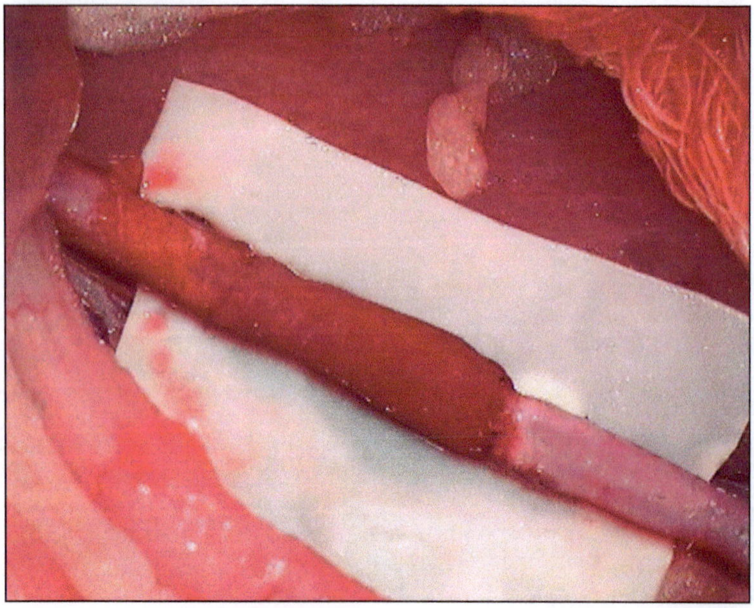

Figure 10-7

Placement of the external jugular vein graft in the aorta has been completed. The double clamp has been removed and blood flow has returned. The vein graft appears more distended than the aorta, because it receives a greater blood volume than in its original position, which exerts a higher pressure on the less rigid vein wall. (From author's photo library)

... of interposition of external jugular vein in the abdominal aorta

Synopsis...

A. **Position of the rat: Laid on its back, head on the surgeon's left.** The limbs are immobilized on the working surface with adhesive tape.

B. **Preparation of the surgical field in the neck:** Transverse incision at the base of the neck, from shoulder to shoulder. The superficial cervical fascia is dissected with two gauzes saturated in warm normal saline, moving in opposite directions cranio-caudally. A paper clip retractor pulls cranially, drawing the skin, superficial fascia (platysma included), and submandibular salivary glands out of the surgical field.

C. **Microsurgical dissection of the external jugular vein:** The vein is dissected from the remaining fat of the superficial fascia and the adventitia is removed, from the edge of the pectoralis major muscle to the mandible. The 3 tributary veins of the trifurcation are dissected, especially the major one. The small tributaries between the trifurcation and the pectoralis major are dissected, double-ligated or cauterized and cut. The two lesser tributaries of the trifurcation are double-ligated and cut.

D. **Preparation of the surgical field in the abdomen:** Median incision, from xiphoid process to pubic symphisis and placement of paper clip retractors. The lobes of the liver protruding in the field are packed with another retractor. The small intestine is mobilized and the intestines are moved out and packed in gauze, to the right side of the rat.

E. **Microsurgical dissection of the aorta:** The retroperitoneum is opened with two wet gauzes. The aorta is dissected from the iliac bifurcation to the left renal vein. A plane of separation between aorta and inferior vena cava is created. The lumbar arteries are dissected and divided between two ligations (9/) or after cauterization. A yellow plastic background is placed under the aorta.

F. **Harvest of the graft from the external jugular vein:** The graft comprises the external jugular vein and part of the major tributary vein, and should be at least 1 cm long. A 9/0 suture is placed at both ends of the graft. The graft ends are cut and the lumen is irrigated in the same direction as normal blood flow.

G. **Transfer of the graft – Transection of the aorta:** The graft is transferred into the abdomen, next to the aorta. The initial direction of blood flow must be kept (*attention not to inverse the graft*). The double clamp is applied to the aorta, the vessel is transected, the lumen irrigated, and a 5 mm piece is removed from one of the stumps. The adventitia is folded back at both stump edges. The graft is placed between the edges of the aortic stumps. Reapproximation of the clamps of the double clamp (if necessary).

H. **End-to-end anastomoses: 10 sutures 10/0 in each anastomosis**

1. Placement of the corner sutures, first those at the 12 o'clock position (upper) in both anastomoses, then the 6 o'clock (lower).
2. Suturing of the anterior surfaces is completed: 4 sutures in each, all at equal distances, starting by those toward the corner sutures.
3. Rotation of the double clamp and checking of anterior surfaces.

... of interposition of external jugular vein in the abdominal aorta

Synopsis...

4. Suturing of the posterior surfaces, similar to anterior surfaces.
5. Release of the vessel from the double clamp.
6. Gauze (wet) placement on the anastomoses for 3 minutes.
7. Patency test.
8. Withdrawal of the yellow background.

I. **Closure of surgical incisions:** In the neck, the skin and the superficial fascia (and platysma) are sutured in one layer with interrupted, non-absorbable 2/0 sutures. The same sutures are placed in the abdominal wall (2 layers) after return of the splanchna.

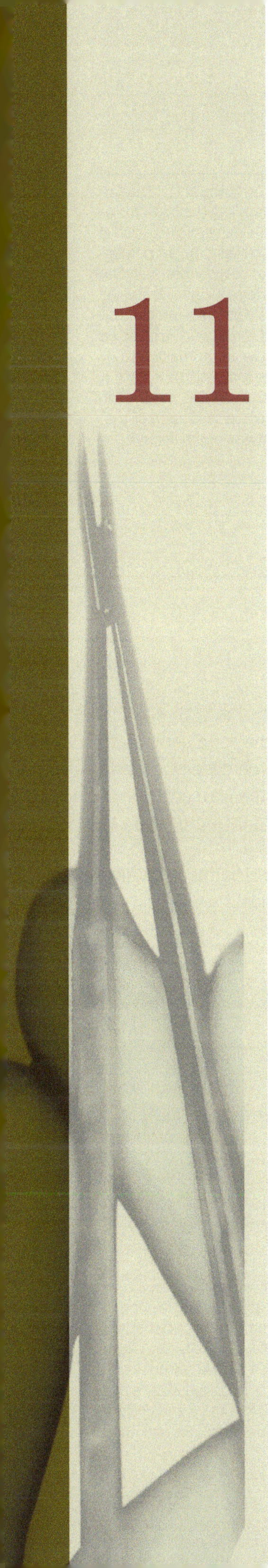

11 Abdominal aorta bypass graft using the external jugular vein

In this Chapter the vein graft is taken from the right external jugular vein. It can similarly be taken from the left external jugular vein.

The aim of the operation is to bypass an obstructed (ligated) area of the aorta using a vein graft taken from the external jugular vein. The graft will be anastomosed on the aorta in an end-to-side fashion, therefore the reader is invited to read Chapter 6, where the end-to-side vascular anastomosis is described in detail.

The following paragraphs are identical to Chapter 10:

A. **Positioning of the rat**
B. **Preparation of the surgical field in the neck**
C. **Microsurgical dissection of the external jugular vein**
D. **Preparation of the surgical field in the abdomen**
E. **Microsurgical dissection of the aorta**
F. **Taking the graft from the external jugular vein**

G. Transfer of the graft –Transverse incisions of the aorta

The graft is transferred to the abdomen and positioned parallel to the aorta. Attention must be paid to **not inverse the graft.** The graft is left to lie in the surgical field, either on the yellow plastic background of the aorta or next to it on a gauze, in such a way that the initial direction of blood flow in the neck is maintained, because a valve may exist in the graft. If placed in the reverse direction, the valve will obstruct the blood flow.

The lumen of the aorta is occluded with the double vascular clamp. In order to create an exit from the aorta to the graft, and an entrance from the graft to the aorta after the segment of the aorta to be bypassed, two transverse incisions are made on the aorta. As described in detail in Chapter 6.3.A, holding the aorta with Dumont forceps, a transverse incision is created in the vessel wall with microsurgical scissors (**Fig. 11-1**). The adventitia is dissected around the perimeter of the aortic incisions. It is generally easier to dissect the adventitia away from this area befo-

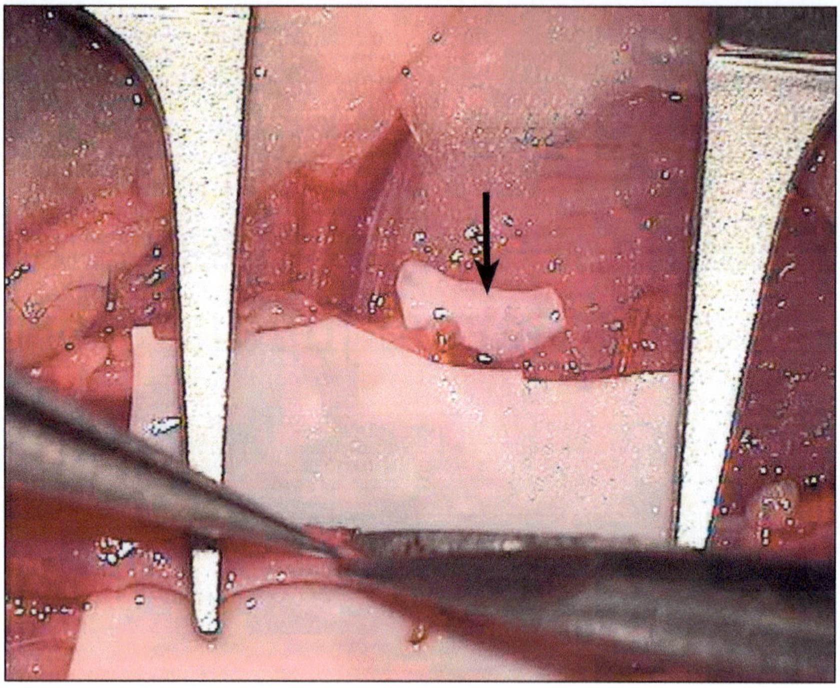

Figure 11-1

Transverse incision of the aorta. The Dumont No. 5 forceps lifts the aorta from the adventitia, while the microsurgical scissors–with the blades brought perpendicular to the axis of the vessel–perform the cranial transverse incision. The vein graft (arrow) has been transferred into the surgical field without being inversed, lying parallel to the aorta. The graft length will define the distance length between the cranial incision and the following caudal transverse incision of the aorta. (From author's photo library)

re the transverse incison is made. The lumen of the aorta is irrigated through the incision using a syringe attached to a fine angiocatheter, injecting warm normal saline. In the same way the second incision is performed more distally (caudally), after the adventitia has been removed from this site. The distance between the two incisions is dictated by the graft length. Again, the lumen of the aorta is irrigated through the caudal incision (**Fig. 11-2**). The warm normal saline exits through the first incision, so the segment of the aorta between the two incisions is totally cleaned. If there is any indication that the lumen was not appropriately cleaned, the wash can be performed in reverse, by flushing through the first incision and allowing saline to exit the second incision. The surgeon may choose to start the irrigation in this direction (first to second incision).

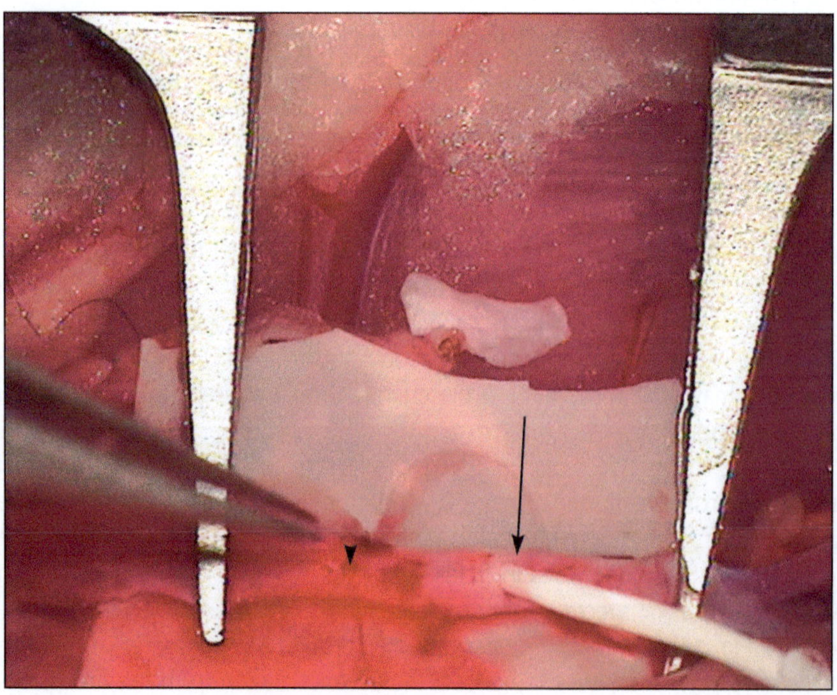

Figure 11-2

Irrigation of the aorta lumen through the caudal incision. The angiocatheter 27G injects normal saline into the caudal transverse incision (arrow), without entering the lumen; the saline washes the lumen and exits from the cranial incision of the aorta (arrowhead). (From author's photo library)

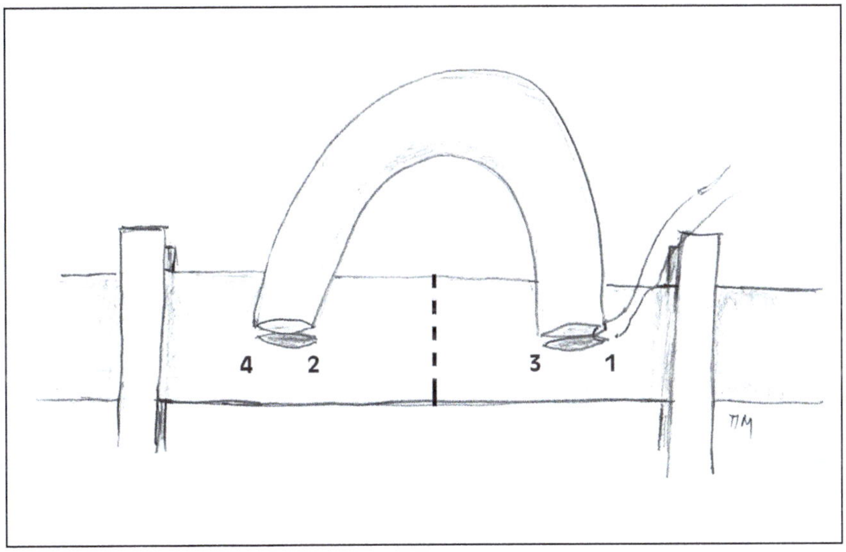

Figure 11-3

Placement of the corner sutures in the anastomoses between aorta and vein graft (aorta bypass). Numbers show the order of placement of corner sutures. The vertical dashed line shows the site where the aorta is ligated after the anastomoses are completed. (Drawing by the author)

H. End-to-side anastomoses – Intermediate ligation of the aorta

The reader is referred to Chapter 6.1 for details on the end-to-side anastomosis where the end-anastomosed vessel can be rotated.

- **10 or 12 sutures 10/0 will be placed in each anastomosis**

The two end-to-side anastomoses between the aorta (at the sites of incisions) and the vein graft are performed simultaenously, as follows:

1. Placement of the 4 corner sutures, first the right suture (toward the right hand of the surgeon) in each anastomosis starting from the right anastomosis, then the two left, starting again from the right anastomosis (**Fig. 11-3**).
2. Placement of the remaining sutures to complete the anterior surfaces of the anastomoses. If 10 sutures are placed in total, there are 4 sutures remaining in each surface, which are equally spaced from the corner sutures and between themselves, starting first with the two lateral (toward the corner sutures) and then the two central sutures. If 12 sutures are placed, there are 5 remaining, from which the median is put first in the middle of the semicircle, and 2 in each quadrant, all at equal distances (between themselves, from the corner sutures and median suture).
3. Flexion of the arch of the vein graft toward the right side of the rat (toward the surgeon) so that the posterior aspects of the edges of the graft and the semi-circles of the aortic incisions become accessible.
4. Check that the sutures of the anterior surfaces have been placed correctly.
5. Placement of the remaining sutures to complete the posterior surfaces of the anastomoses, using the same technique as described for the anterior surfaces (**Fig. 11-4**).
6. Ligation of the aorta with 9/0 suture in the middle of the distance between the two anastomoses (**Fig. 11-5**).
7. Release of the aorta from the double clamp.
8. Gauze (wet) placement on the anastomoses for 3 minutes.
9. Patency test.
   The patency test is performed in the same manner as for a single end-to-end anastomosis, as described in Chapter 5.10 (**Fig. 5-4**). Distal to the graft, toward the aortic bifurcation, a forceps placed upstream occludes the blood flow, and a second, downstream forceps initially placed next to the first moves further distally while half-closed, thus milking the vessel, until a final position where it remains closed. The upstream forceps is released, and if there is patency, the vessel is immediately filled up to the downstream forceps. This test evaluates the patency of both anastomoses simultaneously. However, a valid indication that the proximal anastomosis is patent is the filling of the graft when the upstream forceps is not yet released (**Fig. 11-6**).
10. Withdrawal of the yellow background.

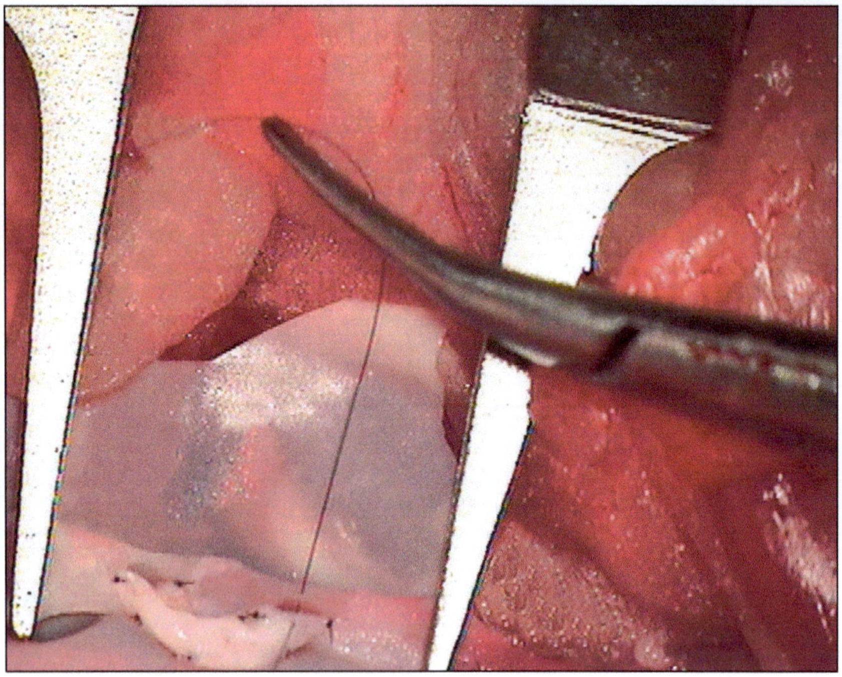

Figure 11-4

The vein graft has been bent toward the surgeon so that the posterior surfaces of the anastomoses can be accessible. The central suture of the posterior surface of the right-hand (caudal) anastomosis is being placed. Here 12 sutures are placed in each anastomosis, i.e. 5 in the posterior surface: first the middle, and then 2 at equal distances in each semi-circle. (From author's photo library)

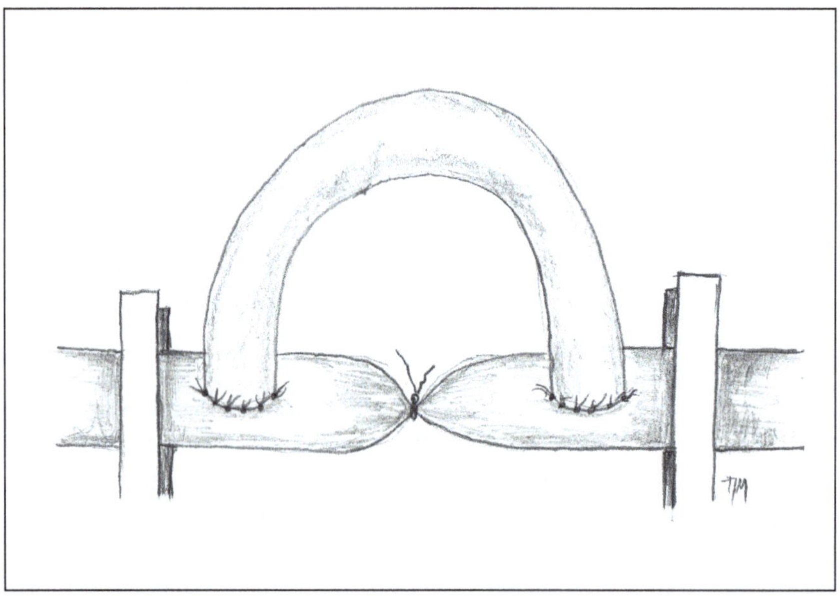

Figure 11-5

Ligation of the aorta between the end-to-side anastomoses with the vein graft. The ligation obstructs the aorta and blood flow is diverted to the graft. (Drawing by the author)

J. Closure of surgical traumas

After the splanchna have returned to the abdomen, the abdominal wall is closed in two layers (muscles, subcutaneous-skin) with interrupted non-absorbable sutures 2/0. Closure of the neck trauma is performed in one layer including skin and superficial fascia (and plastysma) with interrupted non-absorbable sutures.

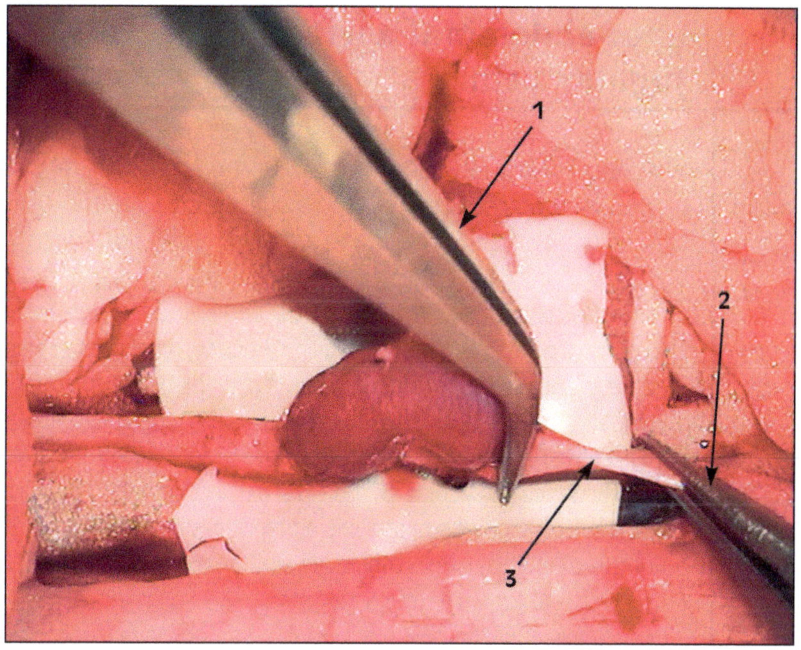

Figure 11-6

Patency test, distal to the vein graft. The upstream forceps **(1)** occludes the blood flow after the caudal (right-hand) anastomosis. The downstream forceps **(2)** empties the aorta lumen **(3)**. The graft is already filled, which indicates a patent cranial (left-hand) anastomosis. The full patency test will be successful if the vessel is filled up to the peripheral forceps after the first forceps has been released. (From author's photo library)

... of abdominal aorta bypass graft using the external jugular vein

Synopsis...

A. Position of the rat: Laid on its back, head on the left of the surgeon. The limbs are immobilized on the working surface with adhesive tape.

B. Preparation of the surgical field in the neck: Transverse incision at the base of the neck, from shoulder to shoulder. The superficial cervical fascia is dissected off with two gauzes saturated in warm normal saline, moving in opposite directions cranio-caudally. A paper clip retractor pulls cranially the skin, superficial fascia (platysma included), and submandibular salivary glands.

C. Microsurgical dissection of the external jugular vein: The wall of the vein is dissected from fat of the superficial fascia and the adventitia is removed, from the edge of pectoralis muscle until the mandible. The 3 tributary veins of the trifurcation of the external jugular vein are dissected, especially the major tributary. The small tributaries between the trifurcation and the pectoralis are dissected, then double-ligated or cauterized and cut. The two lesser tributaries of the trifurcation are ligated and cut.

D. Preparation of the surgical field in the abdomen: Median incision, from the xiphoid to pubic symphisis and placement of paper clip retractors. The lobes of the liver protruding in the field are packed with another retractor. The small intestine is mobilized and the intestines are moved out and packed in a gauze, on the right side of the rat.

E. Microsurgical dissection of the aorta: The retroperitoneum is opened with two wet gauzes. The aorta is dissected from the bifurcation to the left renal vein. A plane of separation between aorta - inferior vena cava is created and the lumbar arteries are dissected, cleaned, and divided after double ligation or cauterization. A yellow plastic background is placed under the aorta.

F. Taking the graft from the external jugular vein: The graft comprises the external jugular vein and part of the major tributary vein, and should be at least 1 cm long. A 9/0 suture is placed at both ends of the graft. The graft ends are cut and the lumen is irrigated in the same direction as native blood flow.

G. Transfer of the graft – Transverse incisions of the aorta: The graft is transferred into the abdomen, next to the aorta. The initial direction of blood must be kept (*attention not to inverse the graft*). The double clamp is placed on the aorta, and two transverse incisions are created. The lumen is irrigated through the incisions, and the adventitia is cleaned around the perimeter of the openings.

H. End-to-side anastomoses – Intermediate ligation of the aorta

Put **10 or 12 sutures 10/0 in each anastomosis**

1. Placement of the 4 corner sutures, first the right suture in each anastomosis, then the left suture, always starting from the right anastomosis.
2. Placement of the remaining sutures to complete the anterior surfaces of the anastomoses. If 10 sutures placed, there are 4 remaining, put at equal distances, starting with the 2 peripheral. If 12 sutures are placed, there are 5 remaining, 1 in the middle, and 2 in each quadrant, at equal distances.

... of abdominal aorta bypass graft using the external jugular vein

Synopsis...

3. Flexion of the vein graft toward the surgeon.
4. Check of the sutures of the anterior surfaces.
5. Placement of the remaining sutures to complete the posterior surfaces of the anastomoses, similar to the anterior surfaces.
6. Ligation of the aorta (9/0 suture) in the middle between the two anastomoses.
7. Release of aorta from the double clamp.
8. Gauze (wet) placement on the anastomoses for 3 minutes.
9. Patency test.
10. Withdrawal of the yellow background.

I. **Closure of surgical traumas:** In the neck, skin and the superficial fascia (and platysma) are sutured in one layer with interrupted, non-absorbable 2/0 sutures. The same sutures are used for a two layer closure of the abdominal wall after return of splanchna.

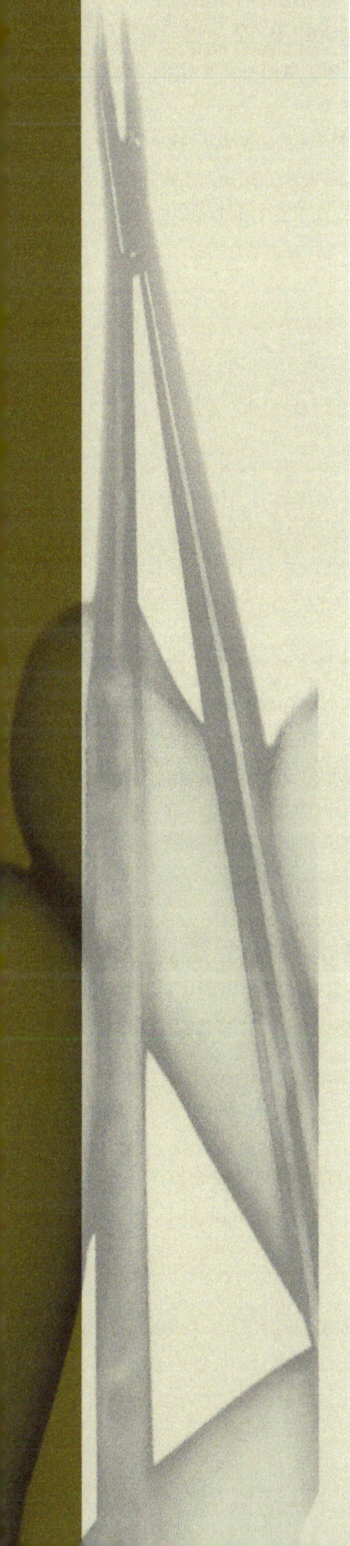

12 Interposition of external jugular (deep tributary) vein into the common carotid artery

The procedure is described for the vessels of the right side of the neck. It can identically be performed in the left side.

A. Positioning of the rat

The rat is positioned in supine position (dorsal decubitus) on the working surface. The long axis of the body of the rat is parallel to the frontal plane of the surgeon's body, and the rat's head is placed to the left of the surgeon. The limbs of the rat are immobilized on the working surface with adhesive tape.

B. Preparation of the surgical field in the neck for exposure of the external jugular vein

For a detailed presentation and imaging, the reader is invited to read the respective preparation in Chapter 9.I.B. Here only a summary is given.

A transverse incision is made at the base of the neck, extending from shoulder to shoulder. The superficial fascia is dissected to find the external jugular vein, using two gauzes saturated in warm normal saline, drawn under light pressure in opposite directions cranio-caudally. A paper clip retractor is placed in the middle of the incision, parallel to the midline, and pulls cranially the skin, superficial fascia, platysma, and the submandibular salivary glands. Thus, the external jugular vein (and its tributaries) is revealed, along its course on the ipsilateral sternocleidomastoid muscle, from the edge of the pectoralis major muscle to the mandible.

C. Microsurgical dissection of the external jugular vein and its deep tributary vein

For a detailed presentation and imaging, the reader is invited to read the respective dissection in Chapter 9.I.C. Here only a summary is given.

The microsurgical dissection aims to fully mobilize the external jugular vein and the tributaries at its trifurcation, to prepare the graft consisting of a major part of the deep tributary vein, and to save the vein axis of the external jugular vein.

- External jugular vein: Dissection starts at the upper border of the pectoralis major muscle and continues past the trifurcation of the external jugular vein, until the mandible (see **Figure 9-3**). The external jugular vein and the three tributary veins of its trifurcation are carefully cleaned from fat and the adventitia is removed. The smaller tributaries of the external jugular vein that are found between the edge of pectoralis muscle and the trifurcation are also dissected and cut after cauterization, or better, after ligation. The external jugular vein needs to be fully dissected and mobilized because during the access to the common carotid artery, it will be required to move the vein in order to transect the sternal part of the sternocleidomastoid muscle, on which the external jugular vein lies (see paragraph D)
- Deep tributary vein (lingual vein) of the trifurcation of the external jugular vein: Microsurgical dissection (mobilization and removal of the adventitia) focuses on the deepest of tributaries, the lingual vein (**Fig. 12-1**). The lingual vein courses deep to the mandible and accepts no tributaries in its course to the trifurcation. From this vein the graft will be taken (see below).
- Facial vein: cauterized or ligated, and transected (**Fig. 12-1**).
- Mandibular vein: fully dissected from the trifurcation to the mandible and preserved (**Fig. 12-1**). After ligation of the deep tributary vein that will follow (see below), the mandibular vein will be the unique tributary to the external jugular vein, to form with the latter the venous axis to be preserved.

D. Preparation of the surgical field in the neck for exposure of the common carotid artery

For a detailed presentation and imaging, the reader is invited to read the respective dissection in Chapter 9.II.B.2.a. Here only a summary is given.

Dissection of the superficial cervical fascia of the neck has been performed (see above). The sternohyoid muscles and the sternocleiodomastoid muscles are recognized. The vein axis "external jugular vein-mandibular vein" is moved laterally and the sternal part of the right sternocleidomastoid muscle is transected using diathermy. The sternohyoid muscle (and together the underlying sternothyroid muscle) is moved medially, lifted by its lateral border (see **Figures 9-12** and **9-13**). This access provides a surgical field wide enough for grafting the common carotid artery.

Access to the common carotid artery by moving the right sternohyoid lateral to the midline (midline access) is not recommended for placement of graft, because the obtained exposure of the vessel in the field is not adequate.

E. Microsurgical dissection of the common carotid artery

For a detailed presentation and imaging, the reader is invited to read the respective dissection in Chapter 9.II.B.2.b (and 1.b). Here only a summary is given.

The carotid sheath is opened, and the common carotid artery is mobilized and separated from the internal jugular vein and the vagus nerve. Attention must be paid not to traumatize the vagus nerve (found behind the internal jugular vein, between the internal jugular vein and the carotid artery) or the recurrent laryngeal nerve (found normally in the paratracheal groove between the trachea and esophagus, or moved on the trachea side during the dissection) (see **Figure 9-13**). A yellow plastic background is put under the common carotid artery after the surgical field has been irrigated with warm normal saline.

F. Taking the graft from the deep tributary of the external jugular vein

The ends of the deep tributary vein of the external jugular vein are ligated with 9/0 suture, first the peripheral (upstream) and then the central (downstre-

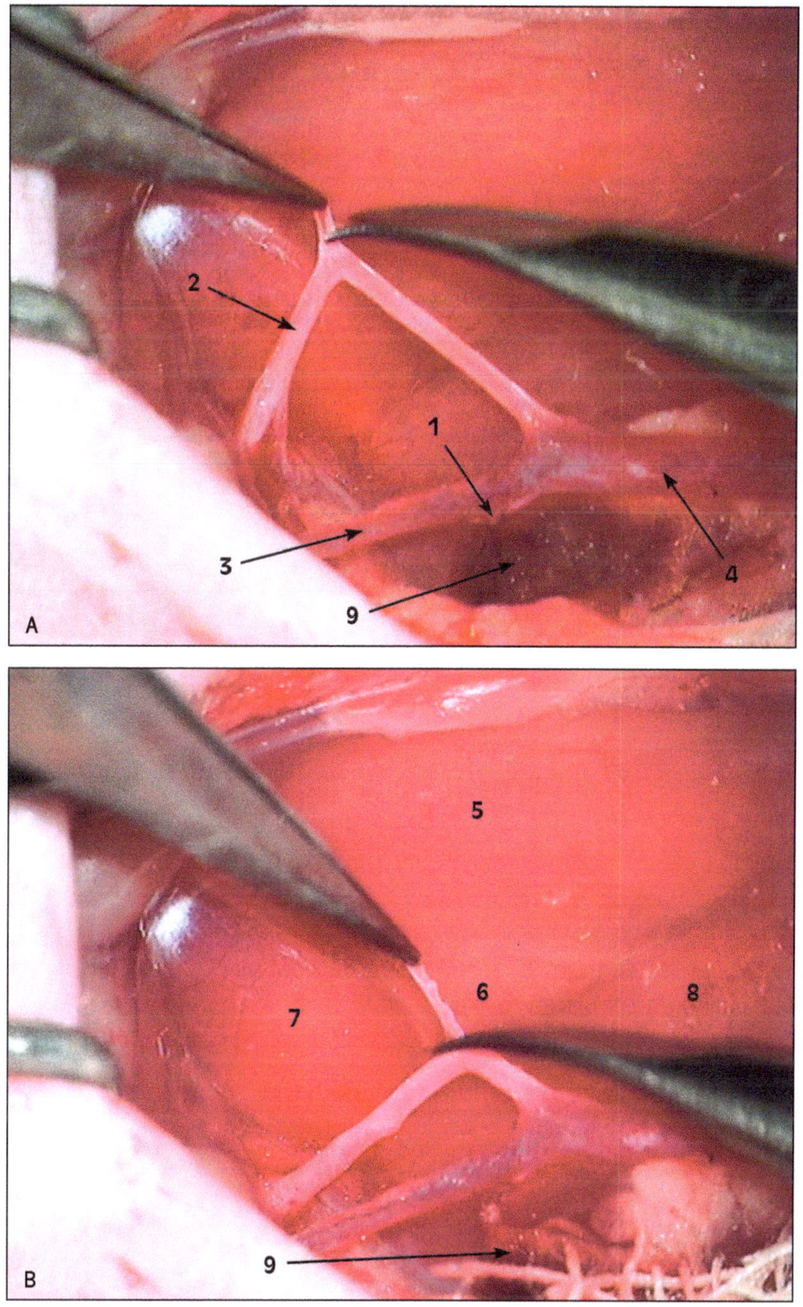

Figure 12-1

Dissection of the deep tributary vein of the right external jugular vein, the lingual vein **(2)**, cranial to the "trifurcation". The graft will be taken from the lingual vein. The facial vein **(1)** has been ligated and cut, while the mandibular vein **(3)** is preserved so that the vein axis of the external jugular vein is maintained. **A.** Dumont No. 5 forceps lifts and the scissors cut the adventitia of the lingual vein. **B.** Continuation of the dissection. Here it is clear that the lingual vein is deeper than the mandibular vein (underlined, because in **Figure 9-3**, where all three tributaries are shown, the false impression is given that the deepest vein is the mandibular). Also, here the neck muscles in the rat are very well seen (right side). **1.** facial vein (ligated and cut), **2.** lingual vein, **3.** mandibular vein, **4.** external jugular vein, **5.** sternohyoid muscle, **6.** sternothyroid muscle, **7.** omohyoid muscle, **8.** sternocleidomastoid muscle (sternal part), **9.** lymph node, indicating the trifurcation before dissection, here moved aside. (From author's photo library)

am), in order not to trap blood in the lumen (**Fig. 12-2**). The vein is transected at both ends, close to the ligations.

The lumen of the graft is irrigated with normal saline using a syringe with a 27G angiocatheter (**Fig. 12-3**). While holding the graft with a Dumnont No. 5 forceps, normal saline is injected in the lumen. The tip of the catheter does not enter the lumen, as not to traumatize the endothelium. Irrigation must be performed in the same direction with blood flow through the graft as it was in its initial position because it is possible that there is a valve in the graft.

G. Transfer of the graft – Transection of the common carotid artery

The graft is initially placed in the surgical field next to the common carotid artery, so that the direction of blood flow in the graft should be the same as in its in-

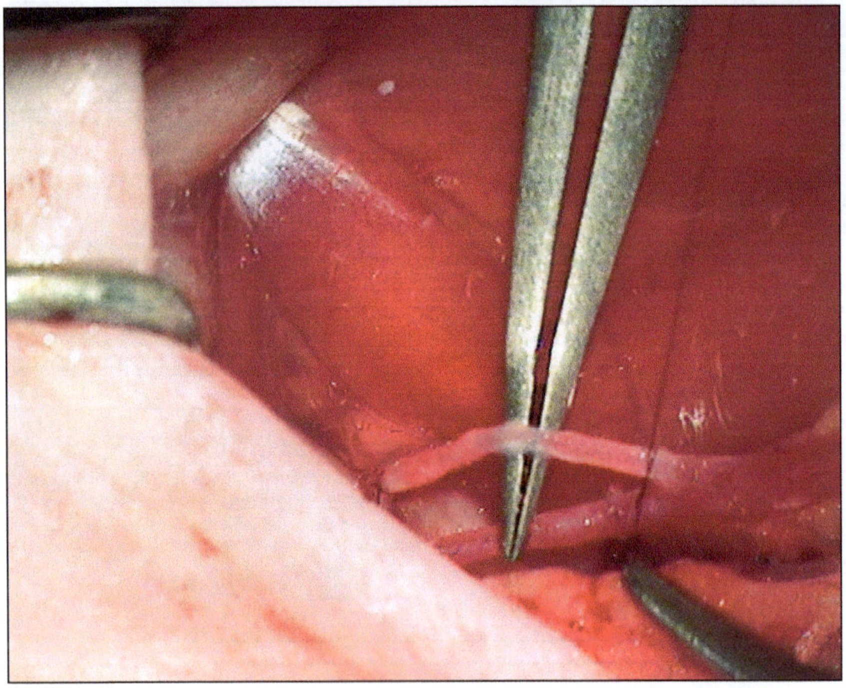

Figure 2-2

Ligation of the ends of the deep tributary vein of the right external jugular vein with 9/0 suture. The peripheral ligature has been placed, the Dumont No. 3 forceps lifts the vein, and here the first simple knot of the central ligature is tied. (From author's photo library)

tial position. Then, given that the blood flow in the common carotid artery, that will receive the graft, is opposite to the blood flow of the external jugular vein, from which the graft was taken, **the graft has to be reversed:** in the common carotid artery, the peripheral end of the graft is placed centrally, and the central end is placed peripherally. This is necessary because the vein graft may contain a valve that will obstruct the flow if the graft is placed in the common carotid artery in the same direction of its original flow.

The double clamp is applied to the common carotid artery (**Fig. 12-4**). The common carotid artery is transected

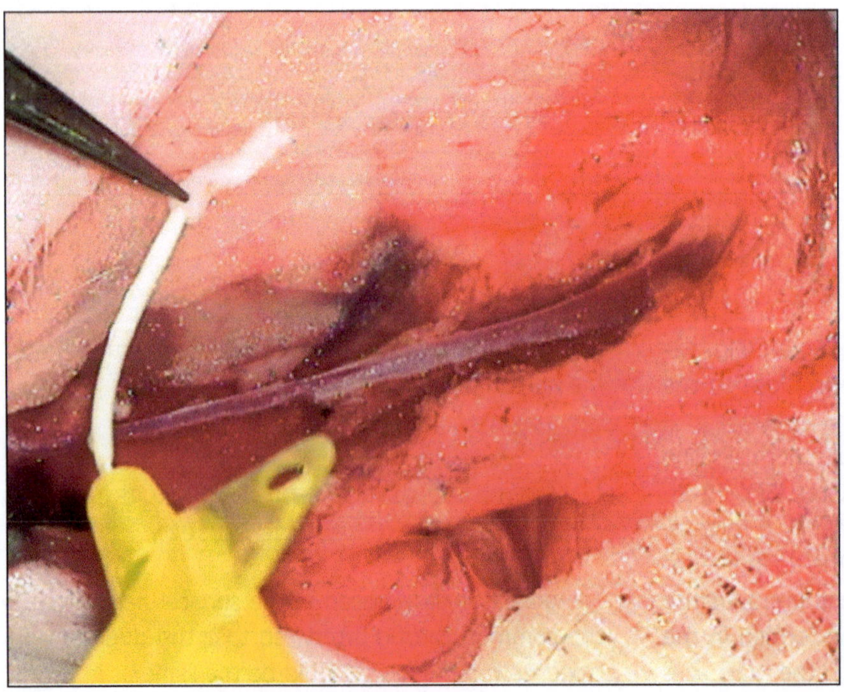

Figure 12-3

Irrigation of the lumen of the graft taken from the deep tributary of the external jugular vein. Dumont No. 5 forceps holds the graft and the 27G angiocatheter injects normal saline without entering the lumen. (From author's photo library)

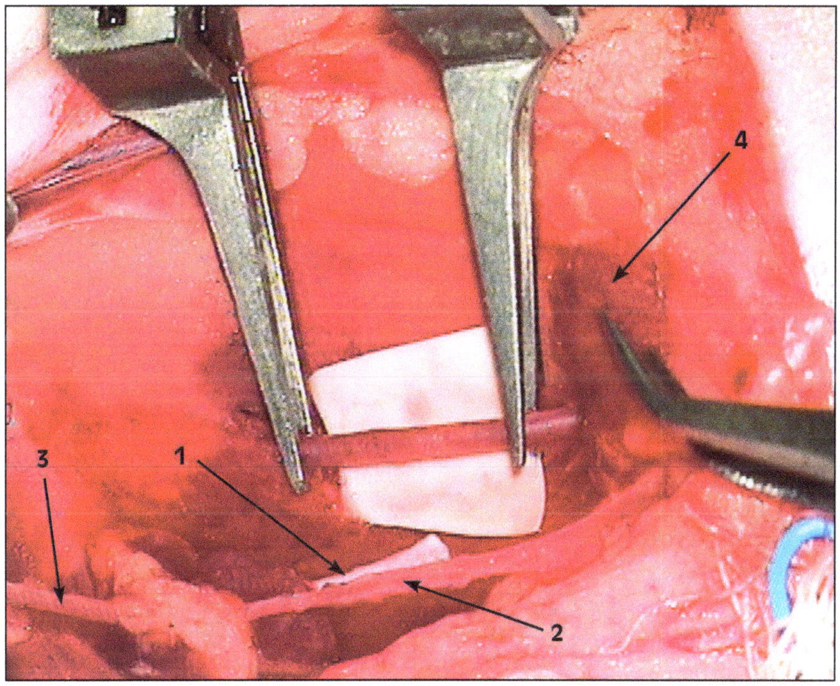

Figure 12-4

Placement of the common carotid artery in the double clamp (right side). Here the double clamp is not closed yet. The vessel should be placed near the edge within each clamp so that the double clamp can be rotated. The vein graft has been reversed, to retain the direction of blood flow it had in its initial position in the neck. **1.** graft (lingual vein, the deep tributary of the external jugular vein), **2.** external jugular vein, **3.** mandibular vein, as continuation of the external jugular vein after transection of the other two tributaries at the trifurcation of the external jugular vein, **4.** s-tump of the sternal part of the sternocleidomastoid muscle. (From author's photo library)

with sharp microsurgical scissors. The vessel is immediately irrigated with warm normal saline using a 27G angiochatheter to wash away blood and clots. A small piece—no greater than 2 mm—is cut and removed from one of the stumps. This will eliminate 'kinking'of the vessel after placement of the graft in case the graft length is longer than the gap between the carotid stumps. Then the adventitia of the artery is folded back in each stump (**Fig. 12-5**).

The vein graft is placed between the edges of the carotid stumps. It is possible that the two clamps of the double clamp may have to be reapproximated so that the anastomoses will not be performed under tension.

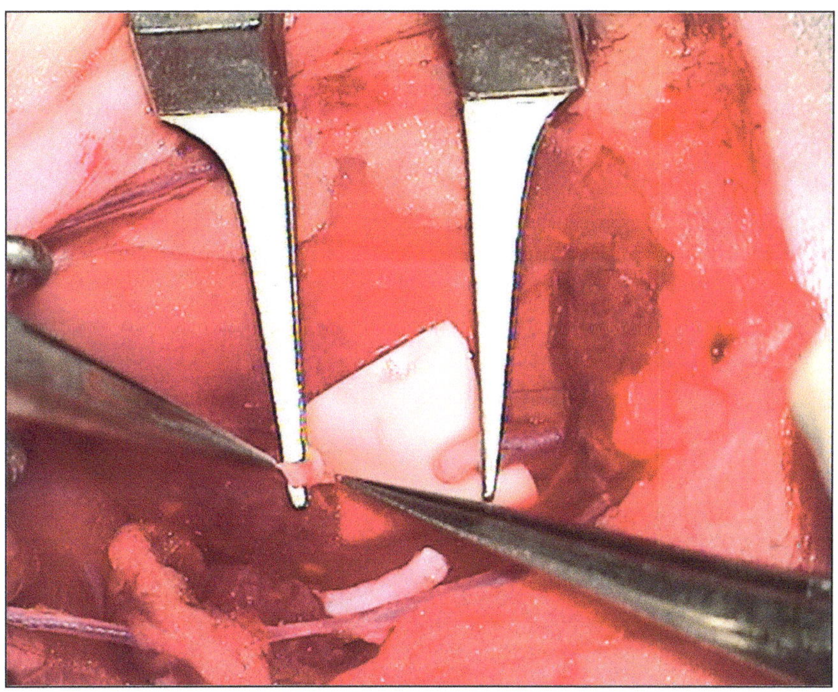

Figure 12-5

Folding of the adventitia of the right common carotid artery with two microsurgical forceps. Dumont No. 3 (left) immobilizes the vessel by holding the outer surface near the edge of the stump, and Dumont No. 5 (right) folds the adventitia backward. (From author's photo library)

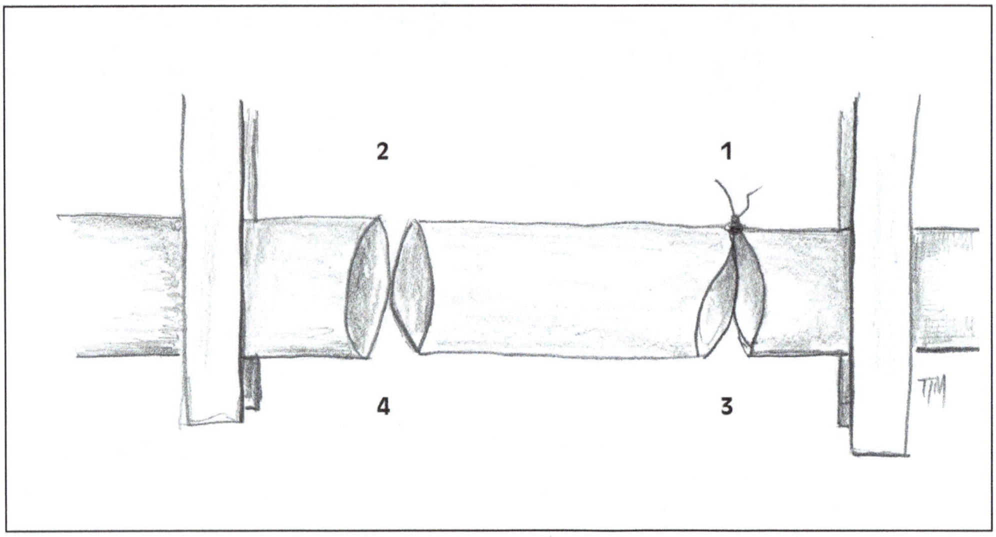

Figure 12-6

Schematic representation of the placement of the corner sutures between common carotid artery stumps and vein graft from the deep tributary of the external jugular vein. Numbers show the order of placement of sutures. The 1st suture has been placed. (Drawing by the author)

H. End-to-end anastomoses

The reader will find a detailed description of end-to-end vascular anastomosis in Chapter 5.

- **8 sutures 10/0 will be placed in each anastomosis**

The two end-to-end anastomoses between the common carotid artery stumps and the vein graft are performed simultaneously, as follows:

1. First the two upper corner sutures are placed at 12 o'clock positions in both anastomoses, and then the two lower corner sutures are placed at 6 o'clock positions (**Fig. 12-6**). Placement of the sutures in this order permits the correct orientation of the vessels.
2. Suturing the anterior surfaces of the anastomoses: from the 3 remaining sutures (per surface), the first is placed in the middle of the semicircle and each of the next two is placed in the middle of each quadrant (**Fig. 12-7**).

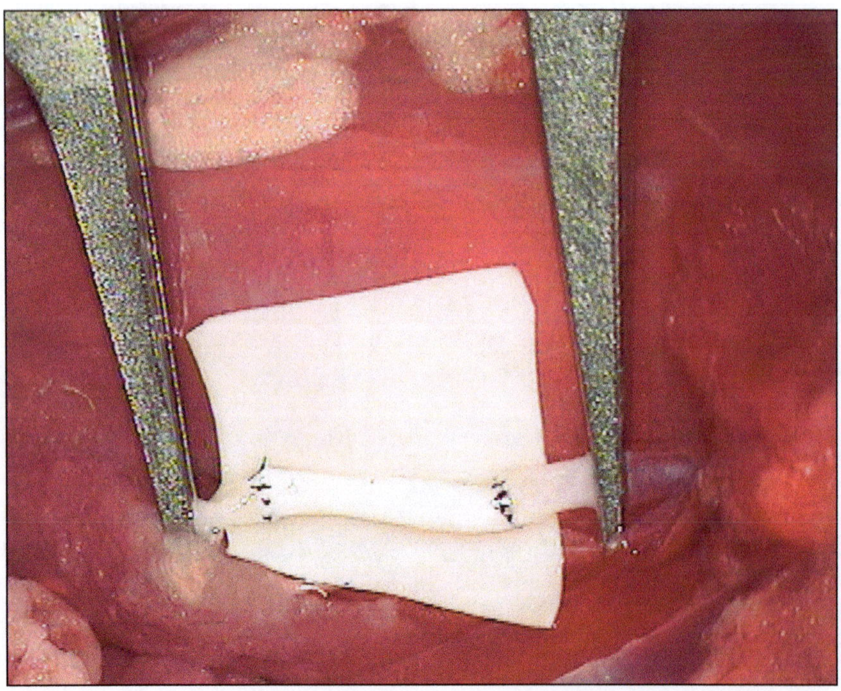

Figure 12-7

Completed suturing of the anterior surfaces of the anastomoses between the common carotid artery stumps and the vein graft taken from the deep tributary of the external jugular vein (right side). (From author's photo library)

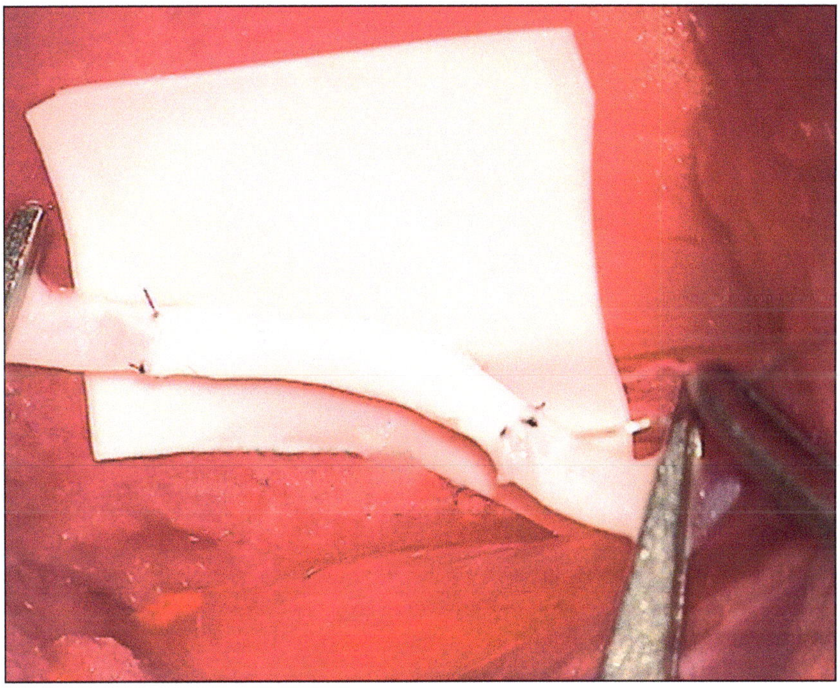

Figure 12-8

The double clamp has been rotated and suturing of the posterior surface of the central anastomosis between the common carotid artery and the vein graft has been completed (right side). The three sutures placed on the posterior surface can be seen (the corner sutures of 12 o'clock and 6 o'clock are not seen here). The posterior surface of the peripheral anastomosis has not been done, only the corner sutures of 12 o'clock and 6 o'clock can be seen. (From author's photo library)

3. Rotation of the double clamp and check that all sutures of the anterior surfaces have been placed correctly.
4. Suturing of the posterior surfaces similar to the anterior surfaces (**Fig. 12-8**).
5. Release of the vessel from the double clamp.
6. Gauze pad (wet) placement on the anastomoses for 3 minutes.
7. Patency test.

   The patency test is performed in an end-to-end anastomosis, as described in Chapter 5.10 (**Fig. 5-4**). Briefly, peripheral (cranial) to the graft a first forceps occludes the common carotid artery upstream and a second forceps is placed initially cranial to the first and then moves downstream (cranially), "half-closed", thus "milking" the vessel and then remains closed at its final position. The upstream forceps is removed, and if there is patency, the vessel is immediately filled up to the downstream forceps. This test examines the patency of both anastomoses. If there is no patency, each of the two anastomoses can be tested separately following the same technique, to find which one failed and has to be redone.

   Another technique for the patency test is shown **Figure 12-9**. A forceps is placed on the common carotid artery, upstream to the central anastomosis, and occludes the blood flow. Another forceps is placed immediatelly cranial to the first forceps, and moves downstream "half-closed" past the graft to close in final position. This maneuver empties the lumen. The upstream forceps is removed while the downstream stays in place. If the vessel is patent, the lumen before the remaining forceps is filled immediately. This technique tests both anastomoses simultaneously. It is more disadvantageous for the beginner compared to the classic technique because a half-closed forceps is drawn over the anastomoses and can traumatize them. For the more expert surgeon, this technique is simple and safe. It can be done in two steps to control each anastomosis separately: first the central if the downstream forceps stops between the two anastomoses; then the peripheral anastomosis if the forceps stops downstream (cranial) to it.
8. Withdrawal of the yellow background.

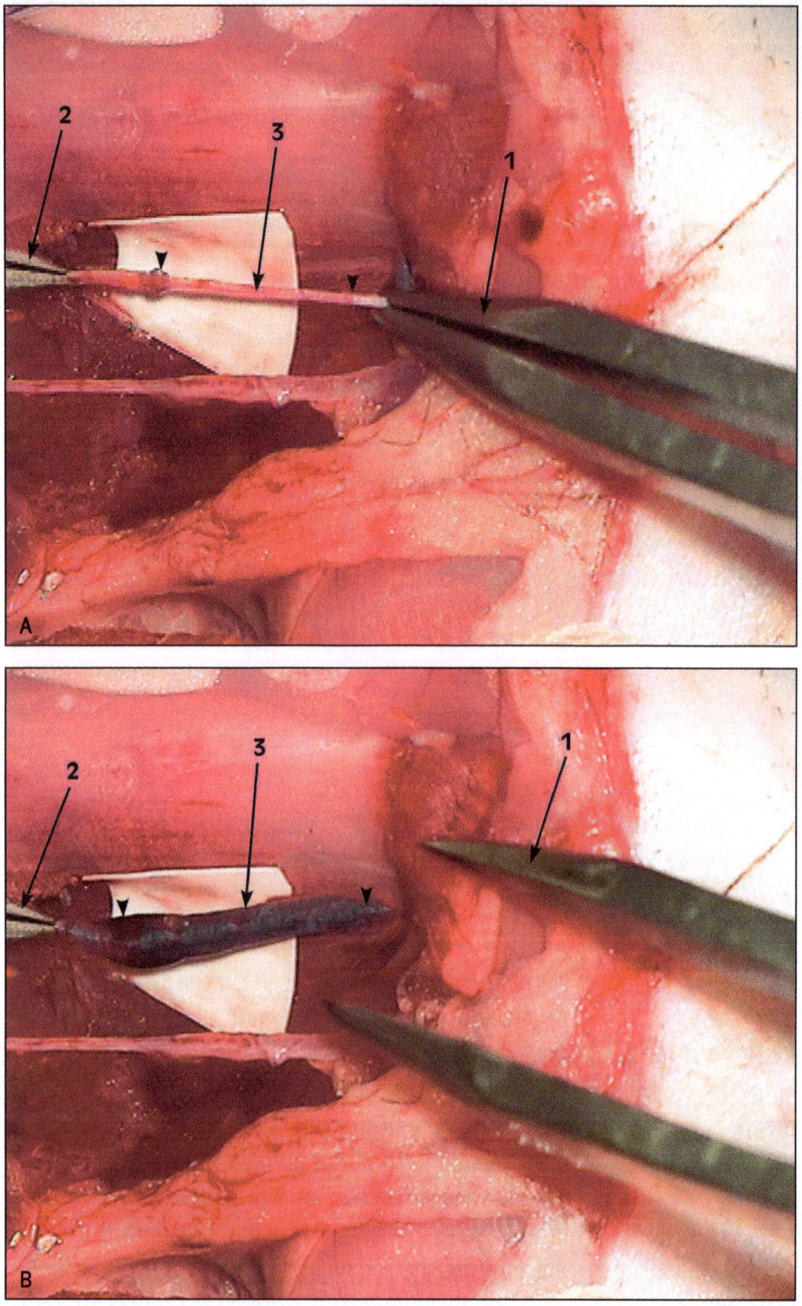

Figure 12-9

Patency test, alternative technique (right side). **A.** The central forceps occludes upstream the blood flow in the carotid artery. The peripheral forceps is placed cranial and next to it, and moves downstream, half-closed, past the graft, to close at a final position cranial to the peripheral anastomosis. **B.** The central forceps opens. The graft is patent and the vessel is immediately filled up to the peripheral forceps. **1.** central forceps, **2.** peripheral forceps, **3.** vein graft. Arrowheads show the sites of anastomoses. (From author's photo library)

J. Closure of surgical trauma

Closure of the surgical trauma is done in one layer, suturing the skin and superficial fascia (platysma included) with interrupted, non-absorbable 2/0 sutures.

... of interposition of external jugular (deep tributary) vein into the common carotid artery

Synopsis...

A. **Positioning of the rat:** Laid on its back with the head to the left of the surgeon. The limbs are immobilized on the working surface with adhesive tape.

B. **Preparation of the surgical field in the neck:** A transverse incision is made at the base of the neck, from shoulder to shoulder. The superficial cervical fascia is dissected with two gauzes saturated in warm normal saline, moving in opposite directions cranio-caudally. A paper clip retractor pulls the skin, superficial fascia (platysma included), and submandibular salivary glands cranially out of the surgical field.

C. **Microsurgical dissection of the external jugular vein and its deep tributary vein:** The external jugular vein is meticulously dissected from the edge of pectoralis muscle to the mandible. All three tributary veins of the trifurcation of the external jugular vein are dissected. The small tributaries between the trifurcation and pectoralis are dissected, ligated/cauterized, and cut. The deep tributary vein of the trifurcation (lingual vein) is preserved (graft will be taken from it). The facial vein of the trifurcation is cut after ligation or cauterization. To maintain the vein axis of the external jugular vein, the mandibular vein is dissected and preserved.

D. **Preparation of the surgical field in the neck for exposure of the common carotid artery:** The 'external jugular vein-mandibular vein' axis is moved laterally and the sternal portion of the sternocleidomastoid muscle is transected using bipolar cautery. The sternohyoid muscle and the underlying sternothyroid muscle are moved medially, elevated along their lateral border.

E. **Microsurgical dissection of the common carotid artery:** The carotid sheath is opened and the common carotid artery is separated from the internal jurgular vein and the vagus nerve. The vagus and recurrent laryngeal nerves are preserved. A yellow plastic background is placed under the carotid artery.

F. **Taking the graft from the deep tributary of the external jugular vein:** The ends of the deep tributary vein are ligated using 9/0 suture. The vein is cut near the sutures and irrigated with normal saline through a 27G angiocatheter.

G. **Transfer of the graft – Transection of the common carotid artery:** The graft is transfered and placed in a reversed position alongside the common carotid artery. The double clamp is applied on the common carotid artery, which is then transected and irrigated. A small piece (maximum 2 mm) is removed from one of the stumps. The adventitia is folded in both stumps and the graft is then placed between the edges of the carotid stumps. The clamps of the double clamp are reapproximated if necessary.

H. **End-to-end anastomoses: 8 sutures 10/0 on each anastomosis**

1. Placement of the corner sutures, first the two upper at 12 o'clock position in both anastomoses, then the two lower at 6 o'clock position in both anastomoses.
2. Suturing of the anterior surfaces is completed: 3 sutures on each, first in the middle of the semicircle, then one in the middle of each quadrant.

... of interposition of external jugular (deep tributary) vein into the common carotid artery

Synopsis...

3. Rotation of the double clamp and check of anterior surfaces.
4. Suturing of the posterior surfaces, similar to anterior surfaces.
5. Release of the vessel from the double clamp.
6. Gauze (wet) placement on the anastomoses for 3 minutes.
7. Patency test.
8. Withdrawal of the yellow background.

I. **Closure of surgical trauma:** skin and superficial fascia (and platysma) are sutured in one layer with 2/0 interrupted, non-absorbable sutures.

13 Common carotid artery bypass graft using the external jugular (deep tributary) vein

The procedure is described for the vessels of the right side of the neck. It can identically be performed in the left side.

The vein graft will be anastomosed end-to-side at at its edges to the artery, therefore the reader is invited to read Chapter 6, where the end-to-side vascular anastomosis is described in detail.

The following paragraphs are identical to the respective ones of Chapter 12:

A. **Positioning of the rat**

B. **Preparation of the surgical field in the neck for exposure of the external jugular vein**

C. **Microsurgical dissection of the external jugular vein and deep tributary vein**

D. **Preparation of the surgical field in the neck for exposure of the common carotid artery**

E. **Microsurgical dissection of the common carotid artery**

F. **Taking the graft from the deep tributary of the external jugular vein.**

G. Transfer of the graft - Transverse incisions of the carotid artery

As in Chapter 12, it is emphasized hat the vein graft is positioned in the surgical field of the common carotid artery so that the direction of blood flow (after anastomoses) should be the same as in its initial position because it is possible that it contains a valve. Therefore, taking into account that the flow in the external jugular vein is the opposite to that of the carotid artery, it is evident that **the vein graft should be reversed.** The graft is placed parallel, next to the common carotid artery (**Fig. 13-1**).

The lumen of the common carotid artery is obstructed with the double vasular clamp. In order to create an exit from the artery to the graft and an entrance from the graft into the artery after the part to be bypassed, two transverse incisions are performed in the common carotid artery. The central (upstream) incision is suggested to be made first. The distance between the two incisions is defined by the length of the graft.

Technically, the common carotid artery is lifted with a Dumont No. 5 forceps and the microsurgical scissors are brought vertically to the vessel and make the 1st transverse incision (**Fig. 13-1**). The adventitia is dissected around the incision and removed, or it is dissected and removed before the incision is made. The lumen of the common carotid artery is irrigated with normal saline using a syringe attached to 27G angiocatheter. The 2nd transverse incision is performed in the same way, and is followed by dissection and removal of the adventitia. It is also possible to remove the adventitia around the sites of the incisions before the incisions are made. Irrigation of the lumen is repeated through the 2nd incision.

H. End-to-side anastomoses – Intermediate ligation of the carotid artery

The reader is referred to Chapter 6.1 for details on the end-to-side anastomosis where the end-anastomosed vessel can be rotated.

- **8 sutures 10/0 will placed in in each anastomosis**

The two end-to-side anastomoses between the common carotid artery (at the sites of incisions) and the vein graft are performed **simultaneously,** as follows:

1. Placement of the 4 corner sutures, first the two right (toward the right hand of the surgeon) starting from the right anastomosis, then the two left starting again from the right anastomosis (see **Figure 11-3**).
   Once you have gained enough experience, you can break this order and place the two corner sutures in one anastomosis and then the two corner sutures of the other (**Fig. 13-2**). Thus, however, there is the risk that the graft is not aligned correctly and rotates around its long axis, which will disturb blood flow and lead to failure of the procedure. If there evidence or suspicion that this is the case, cut all sutures and come back to the classic method of **Figure 11-3**.
2. Placement of the rest of the sutures to complete the anterior surfaces of the anastomoses. After placement of the 2 corner sutures, there are 3 sutures remaining per surface in each anastomosis; the first suture is placed in the middle of the semicircle and each of the next two in the middle of each quadrant, on either side.
3. Flexion of the arch of the vein graft toward the right side of the rat (toward the surgeon) so that both the posterior surfaces of the edges of the vein graft and the semicircles of the incisions of the commnon carotid artery become accesible.
4. Check that the sutures of the anterior surfaces have been placed correctly.
5. Placement of the rest of the sutures to complete the posterior surfaces of the anastomoses, using the same technique as in the anterior surfaces.
6. Ligation of the common carotid artery with 9/0 suture in the middle of the distance of the anastomoses (see **Figure 11-5**).

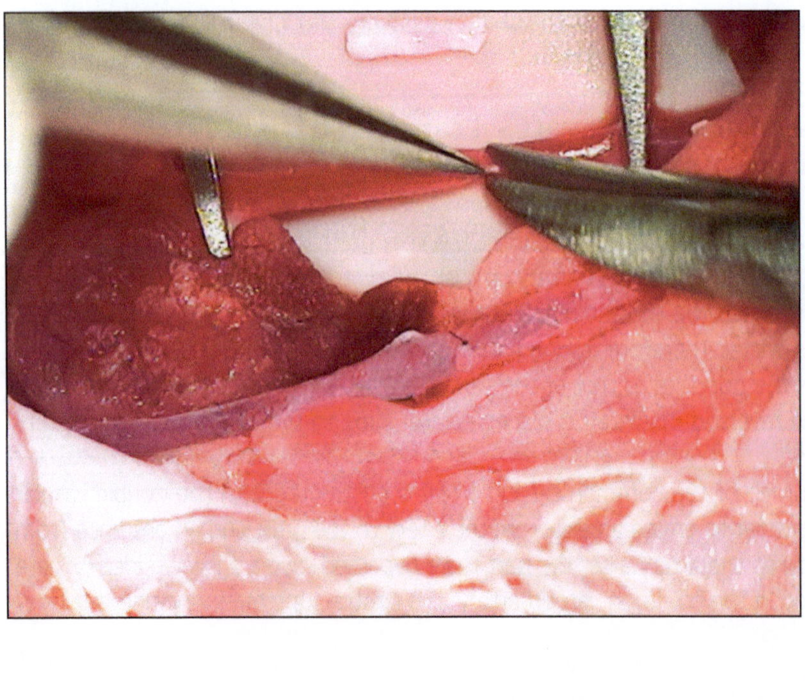

Figure 13-1

First transverse incision of the right common carotid artery for placement of bypass graft. The 1st incision is made centrally (upstream). Dumont No 5. forceps lifts the carotid wall and the scissors are brought perpendicular to the long axis of the vessel and make the incision. Observe the vein graft medially to the common carotid artery, on the yellow plastic background. The length of the graft will define the site of the 2nd arteriotomy. (From author's photo library)

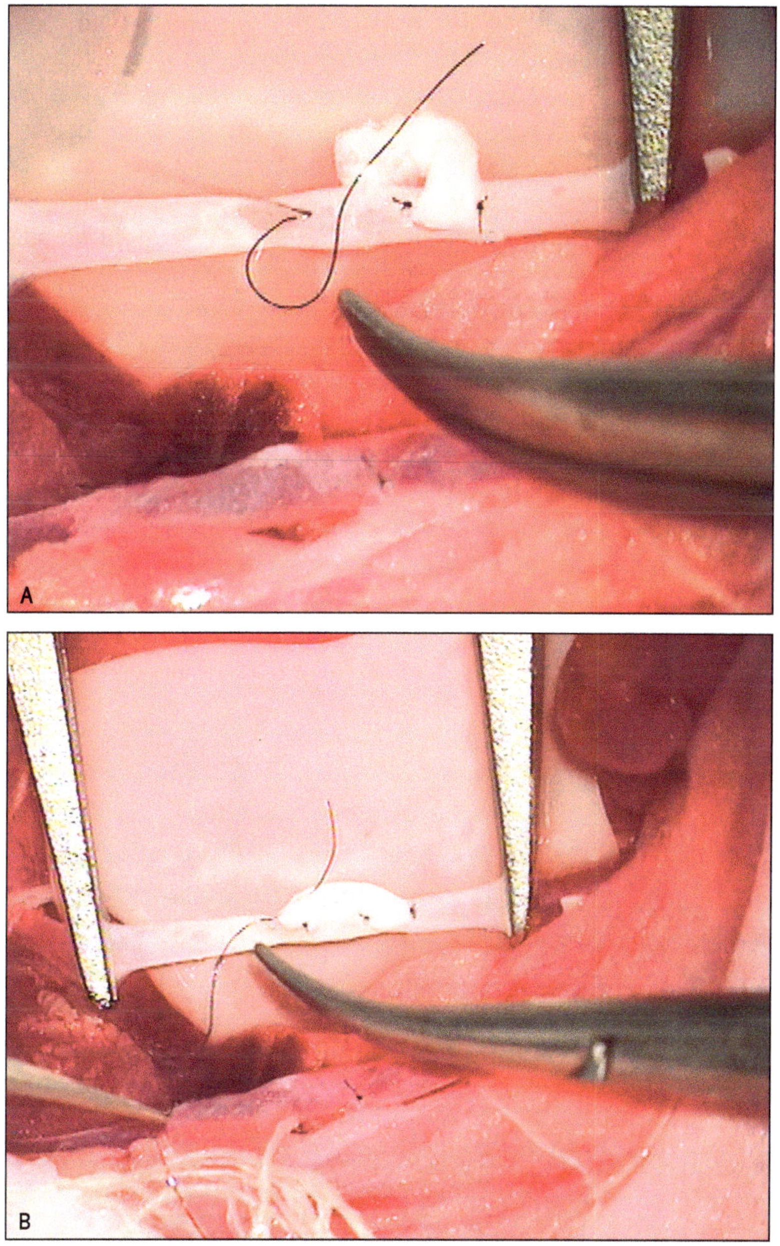

Figure 13-2

Alternative technique of placement of the corner sutures in the end-to-side anastomoses between common carotid artery and vein graft (right side). Here the generally applied order of sutures shown in **Figure 11-3** is not followed, and first the two corner sutures of the right (central) anastomosis and then the two corner sutures of the left (peripheral) are placed. **A.** The corner sutures of the right anastomosis have been placed, and now the first corner suture of the left anastomosis is placed. **B.** Placement of the second suture of the left anastomosis. (From author's photo library)

7. Release of the common carotid artery from the double clamp.
8. Placement of a wet gauze on the anastomoses for 3 minutes.
9. Patency test.

   The patency test is performed as in a sole end-to-end anastomosis, as described in Chapter 5.10 (**Fig. 5-4**). Briefly, upstream to the graft, a first forceps occludes the common carotid artery and a second forceps is placed initially just cranial to the first forceps. The second forceps moves downstream (cranially) "half-closed", to empty the vessel and then remains closed at a final position after a short distance. The upstream forceps is removed, and if there is patency, the vessel is immediately filled up to the downstream forceps. This test checks the patencey of the two anastomoses in toto.

   Another method is applied in **Figure 13-3**. A forceps is placed centrally on the common carotid artery and occludes the blood flow. This forceps is drawn "half-closed" upstream (centrally), empties the common carotid artery, and closes. A second forceps is placed peripherally after the graft, is also drawn "half-closed" downstream (cranially) to empty the lumen, and closes. The movement of the two forceps must be simultaneous, and with the same tension applied on the common carotid artery (each forceps provides resistence for the movement of the other). The upstream forceps is withdrawn, if there patency in both anastomoses, the artery is filled immediately up to the downstream forceps. As a variation of this techique, the central forceps can be immobile, just to occlude the common carotid artery, which is emptied only downstream by the movement of the peripheral forceps.

It is avoided, even by expert microsurgeons, to draw a 'half-closed' forceps over the graft in order to empty it (as applied on the graft from the external jugular vein put into the common carotid artery end-to-end, see **Figure 12-9**). In the current operation, the graft is not straight and application of this technique has a geat risk to traumatize it.

Before the above two suggested techiques of patency tests, a first indication that the central anastomosis is patent is the filling of the graft after release of the double clamp. This indication, however, does not replace the patency test. But, if this indication is absent, there are very few hopes that the vessel is patent.

10. Withdrawal of the yellow background.

I. Closure of surgical trauma

Closure of the surgical trauma is done in one layer, suturing the skin and superficial fascia (platysma included) with interrupted, non-absorbable 2/0 sutures.

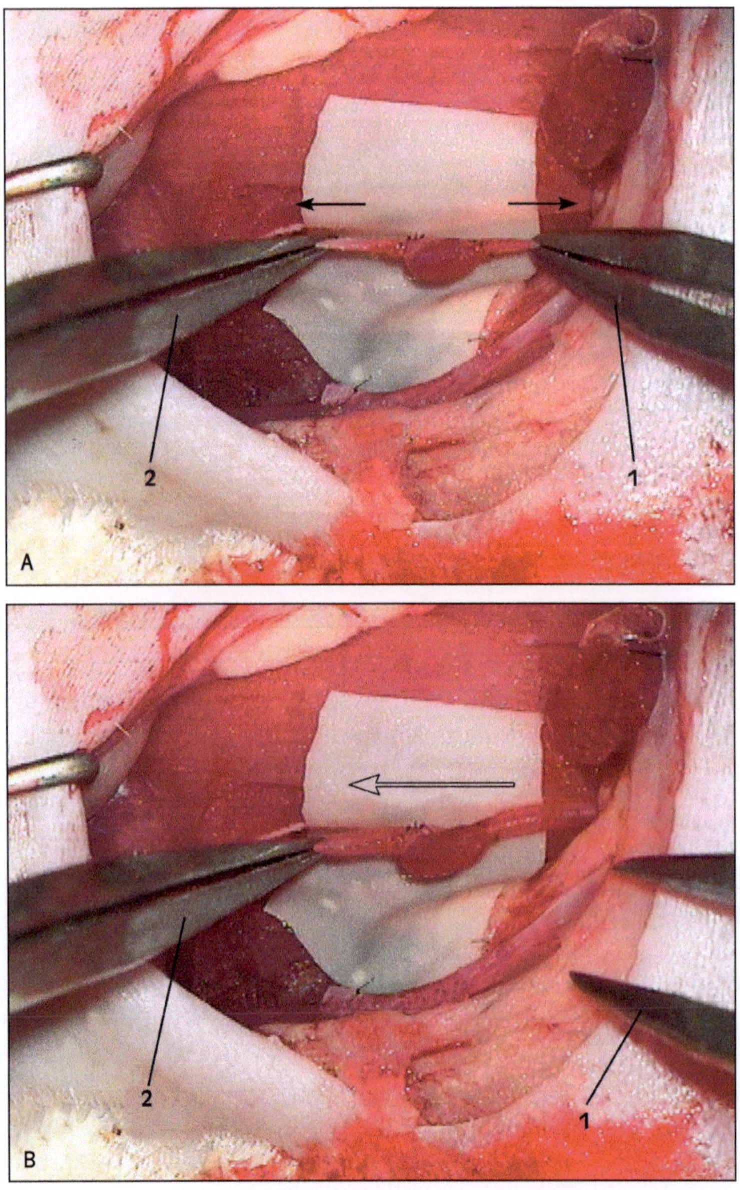

Figure 13-3

Alternative patency test of vein graft bypassing an area of the common carotid artery. **A.** An upstream forceps is placed central to the graft, moves 'half-closed' more centrally to empty the lumen, and stops closed. A downstream forceps is placed cranial to the graft and moves more cranially to empty the lumen, and stops closed. Here the two forceps are shown closed in final position. The black arrows show the direction of the simultaneous movement of the forceps. **B.** The upstream forceps is released, and filling of the graft and common carotid artery before the closed downstream forceps shows the patency of anastomoses. The empty arrow shows the direction of blood flow. **1.** upstream Dumont No. 3 forceps, **2.** downstream Dumont No. 3 forceps. (From author's photo library)

Synopsis... of common carotid artery bypass graf using the external jugular (deep tributary) vein

A. **Positioning of the rat:** Laid on its back with the head to the left of the surgeon . The limbs are immobilized on the working surface with adhesive tape.

B. **Preparation of the surgical field in the neck for exposure of the external jugular vein:** A transverse incision is performed at the base of the neck, from shoulder to shoulder. The superficial cervical fascia is dissected with two gauzes saturated in warm normal saline, moving in opposite directions cranio-caudally. A paper clip retractor pulls the skin, superficial fascia (platysma included), and submandibular salivary glands cranially out of the surgical field.

C. **Microsurgical dissection of the external jugular vein and its deep tributary vein:** The external jugular vein is meticulously dissected from the edge of pectoralis muscle until the mandible. All three tributary veins of the trifurcation of the external jugular vein are dissected. The small tributaries between trifurcation and pectoralis muscle are dissected, then ligated/cauterized and cut. The deep tributary vein of the trifurcation (lingual vein) is preserved (graft to be taken from this). The facial vein is cut after ligation/cauterization. To maintain the vein axis of the external jugular vein, the mandibular vein is dissected and preserved.

D. **Preparation of the surgical field in the neck for exposure of the common carotid artery:** The vein axis 'external jugular vein-mandibular vein' is moved laterally and the sternal part of the sternocleidomastoid muscle is transected using diathermy. The sternohyoid muscle (and together the underlying sternothyroid muscle) are moved medially, lifted by its lateral border.

E. **Microsurgical dissection of the common carotid artery:** The carotid sheath is opened, the common carotid artery is separated from the internal jugular vein and the vagus nerve. The vagus and recurrent laryngeal nerves are preserved. A yellow plastic background is put under the common carotid artery.

F. **Taking the graft from the deep tributary of the external jugular vein:** The ends of the deep tributary vein are ligated with 9/0 suture. The vein is cut near the sutures and irrigated with normal saline using an 27G angiocatheter.

G. **Transfer of the graft – Transverse incisions on the common carotid artery:** The graft is transferred and in a reversed position alongside the common carotid artery. The double clamp is applied on the artery, on which two transverse incisions are made. The adventitia is removed on their perimeters.

H. **End-to-side anastomoses – Intermediate ligation of the common carotid artery:**
8 sutures 10/0 in each anastomosis

1. Placement of the 4 corner sutures. First, the two right in each anastomosis, then the two left.
2. Placement of the rest of sutures to complete the anterior surfaces of the anastomoses: there are 3 sutures remaining in each, 1 placed in the middle of the semircle, and 1 in the middle of each quadrant.

... of common carotid artery bypass graf using the external jugular (deep tributary) vein

Synopsis...

3. Flexion of the vein graft toward the surgeon.
4. Check of the sutures of the anterior surfaces.
5. Placement of the rest of sutures to complete the posterior surfaces of the anastomoses, similar to the anterior surfaces.
6. Ligation of the common carotid artery (9/0 suture) between the anastomoses.
7. Release of the carotid artery from the double clamp.
8. Gauze (wet) placement on the anastomoses for 3 minutes.
9. Patency test.
10. Withdrawal of the yellow background.

I. **Closure of surgical trauma:** The skin and the superficial fascia (and platysma) are sutured in one layer with interrupted, non-absorbable 2/0 sutures.

14

End-to-side anastomosis of the common carotid artery to the external juglar vein

[model of arterio-venous fistula]

The procedure is described for the vessels of the right side. It can identically be performed on the left side; if so, the head of the rat has to be on right.

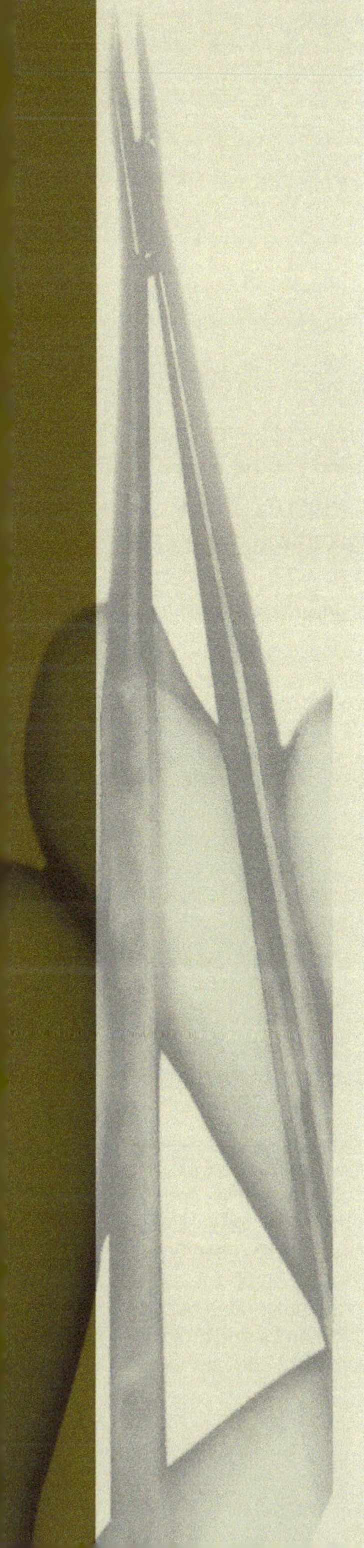

The anastomosis of the common carotid artery to the external jugular vein will be performed end-to-side. It is an exemplary case where the end-anastomosed vessel (common carotid artery) cannot be rotated. The reader is invited to read Chapter 6 where end-to-side vascular anastomosis is discussed in detail, and especially the section 6.2.I for the case where the end-anastomosed vessed cannot be rotated but the posterior surface is accessible.

The reader will find the following in Chapter 9.I:

A. **Positioning of the rat**

B. **Preparation of the surgical field for exposure of the external jugular vein**

C. **Microsurgical dissection of the external jugular vein.** The dissection of the external jugular vein in the current operation can stop at the trifurcation, without including the tributary veins. It is possible, however, that dissection of the tributaries becomes necessary in order to further mobilize the external jugular vein. The yellow plastic background is not placed under the external jugular vein in this phase.

As for the common carotid artery, the reader should refer to Chapter 9.II:

D. **Preparation of the surgical field for exposure of the common carotid artery:** (see Chapter 9.II.B.2.a).

E. **Microsurgical dissection of the common carotid artery:** (see Chapter 9.II B.2.b). Note that for the current procedure the yellow plastic background will be under the external jugular vein and not under the common carotid artery.

F. Central occlusion-peripheral ligation and transection of the common carotid artery

A single clamp is placed on the common carotid artery as centrally as possible to oc-

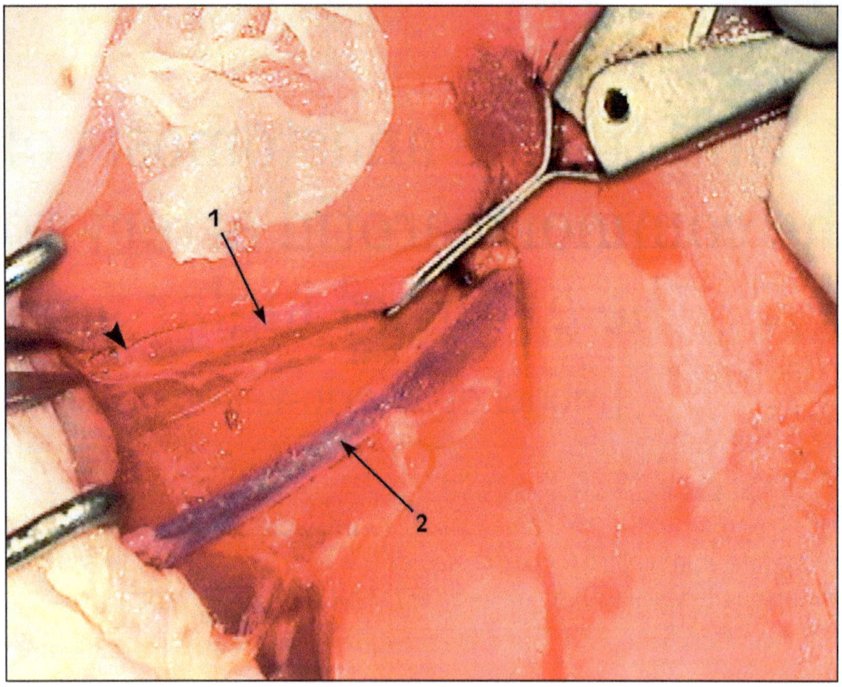

Figure 14-1

Preparation of the transection of the common carotid artery for end-to-side anastomosis to the external jugular vein (right side). The single clamp occludes the common carotid artery centrally, and a ligature with 9/0 suture is placed on it cranially (arrowhead). **1.** common carotid artery, **2.** external jugular vein. (From author's photo library)

clude the blood flow; then, peripherally, as cranially as possible in the surgical field, a ligature is placed on the common carotid artery (**Fig. 14-1**). The vessel is transected very close to the ligation (**Fig. 14-2**), in order to get advantage of the maximum available length so that the vessel can easily turn laterally to be anastomosed end-to side with the external jugular vein. It is a common observation that the stump of the common carotid artery retracts and becomes much shorter after transection. Then, the lumen of the stump is irrigated with warm normal saline using a syringe attached to a 27G angiocatheter, which injects saline without entering the lumen.

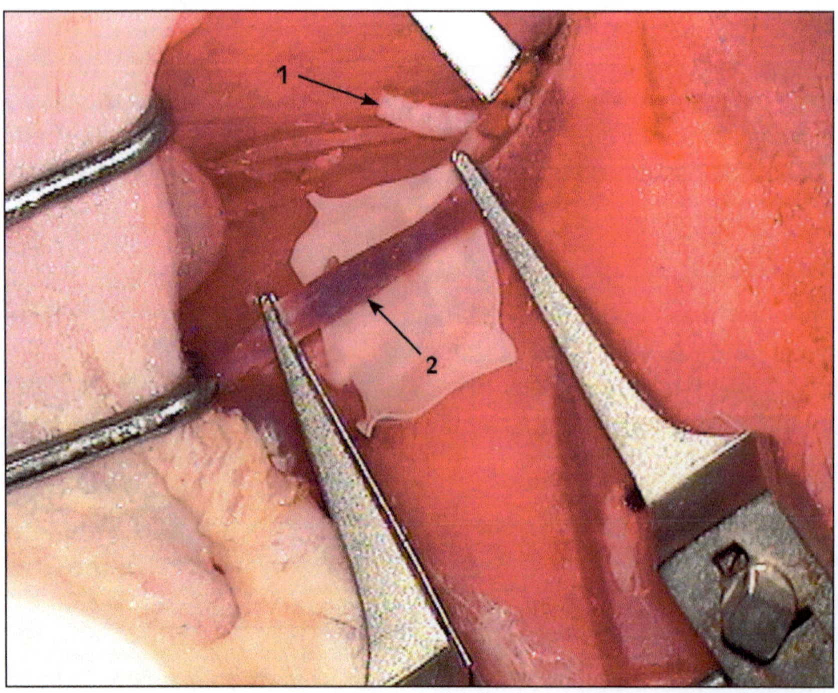

Figure 14-2

The right common carotid artery has been transected cranially, while centrally is occluded with the single clamp. The right external jugular vein has been occluded with the double clamp and a yellow plastic background has been put underneath it. **1.** common carotid artery, **2.** external jugular vein. (From author's photo library)

G. Occlusion-transverse incision of the external jugular vein

A yellow plastic background is placed underneath the external jugular vein, and the vein is occluded with the double clamp (**Fig. 14-2**). A transverse incision is made in the external jugular vein as described in detail in Chapter 6.3.A and in the same way as presented in **Figures 11-1** and **13-1** (transverse incision of aorta and common carotid artery respectively).

Immediately after the incision, the external jugular vein is irrigated with warm normal saline using a syringe attached to a 27G angiocatheter, which does not enter the lumen. The saline injection is performed with pressure to remove blood and clots from the lumen of the vein.

The adventitia is removed around the perimeter of the incision of the vein. The edges of the incision must be as clean as possible. This procedure is relatively easy in arteries. In veins, it needs specific attention and delicate handling. The beginner should pay attention not to remove excess tissues of the vein wall perceived as adventitia (in truth these can be deeper layers). If this mistake is made, the bare area of the vein will project outward after the anastomosis, risking aneurysm or rupture. Of course, removal of the adventitia is also required at the edge of the stump of the common carotid artery before the anastomosis (**Fig. 14-3**).

H. End-to-side anastomosis

The reader is referred to the Chapter 6.2.I for the case where the end-anastomosed vessel (common carotid artery here) cannot be rotated, but its posterior surface is accessible.

- **8 sutures 10/0** will be placed

The steps of the process of the end-to-side anastomosis are as follows:

1. The anastomosis starts from the middle of the posterior surface because the single clamp that occludes the common carotid artery cannot be rotated. The technique is described in Chapter 6.2.I (see **Figures 6-6** and **6-7B**). Briefly, the first suture is placed in the middle of the posterior surface. This suture (and all in the suite) is placed from external to internal (in the lumen) and then from internal to external; the knot is then tied outside the lumen. The sutures 2 and 3 are placed at equal distances on either side in the posterior surface. The sutures 4 and 5 are the corner sutures, and then on the anterior surface, sutures 6 and 7 are placed on either side, at equal distances from the corner sutures, and last, suture 8 in the middle of the distance between sutures 6 and 7.

   Another technique, but not for beginners, is presented here in **Figure 14-4**. The difference from the

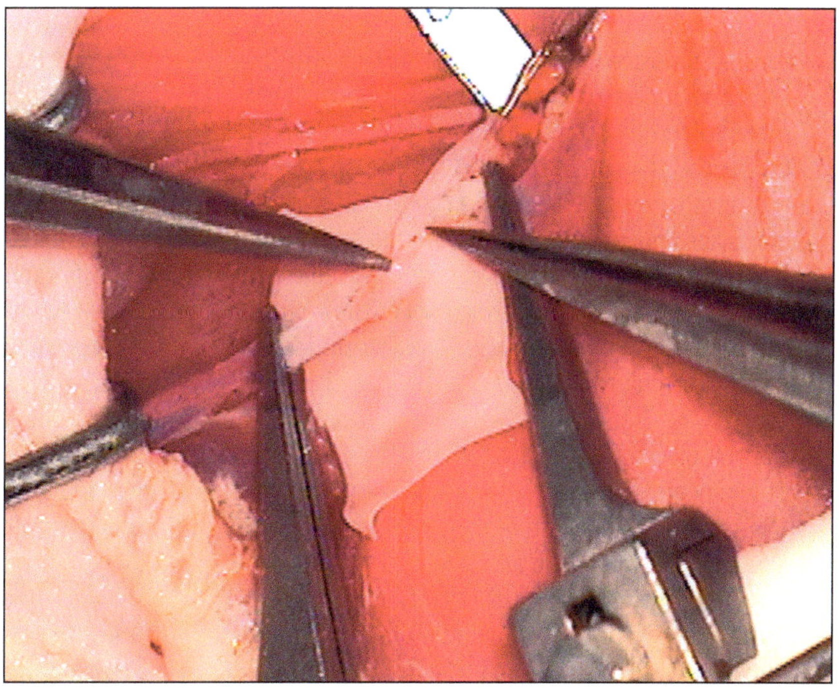

Figure 14-3

Removal of the adventitia at the edge of the stump of the common carotid artery (right side). Dumont No. 3 forceps (left) holds the vessel from the outer coatings and Dumont No. 5 forceps (right) folds the adventitia. (From author's photo library)

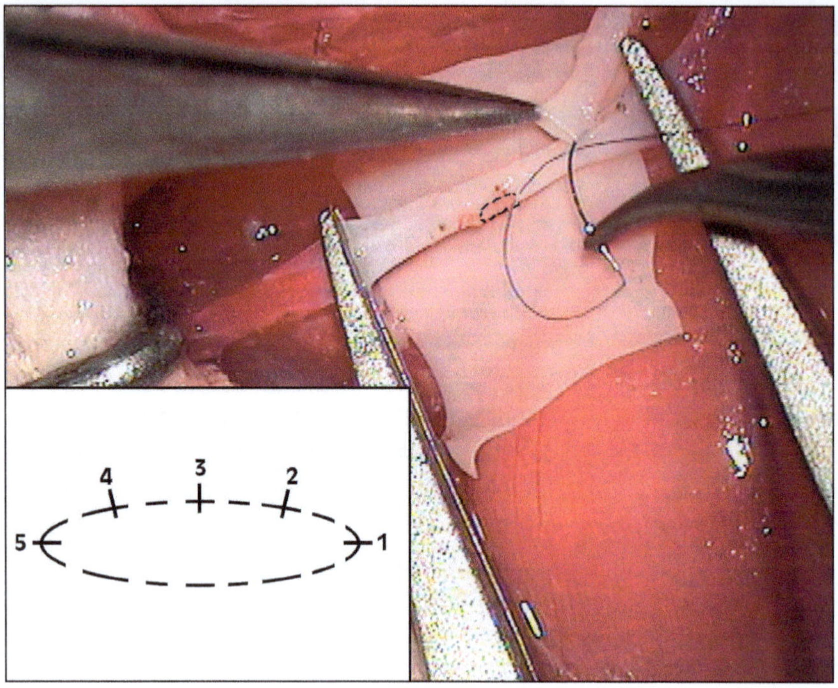

Figure 14-4

Alternative technique of suturing of the posterior wall of the end-to-side anastomosis between the stump of common carotid artery and external jugular vein. The 1st suture is placed as a corner suture in the acute angle of the anastomosis–and not in the middle of the posterior surface, as in the classic technique. Here the suture has passed into the lumen of the external jugular vein and now the needle passes through the wall of the stump of the common carotid artery. **Inset:** Numbers show the order of placement of sutures in the posterior surface. The 5th suture is placed diametric to the 1st, as corner suture in the obtuse angle. The 2nd, 3rd, and 4th sutures are placed at equal distances between themselves and from the corner sutures. (Photo from author's photo library, diagram by the author)

above-mentioned technique is that stitches in the posterior surface of the anastomosis are placed one next to the other, starting by the acute (right) angle between the stump of the right common carotid artery and external jugular vein, and continuing cranially toward the diametric point of the obtuse (left) angle between the two vessels. The 1st suture placed is the corner suture in the acute angle of the anastomosis. Then, taking into consideration that the 5th suture will be the diametric corner suture, 3 sutures are placed in the posterior surface after the 1st suture, one next to the other, all at equal distances. Last in the posterior surface, the 5th suture will be placed, as a corner suture in the obtuse angle of the anastomosis. It is essential that the surgeon marks (or figures out, if expert) the position of the 5th suture on the carotid stump after placement of the 1st suture, so that the distances of the rest of the sutures can be configured. On the anterior surface of the anastomosis, 3 sutures are placed in the classic way. This alternative technique comes with the risk of incorrect estimation of suture distances on the posterior surface.

2. The vascular clamps are removed, first the double clamp of the external jugular vein and then the single clamp of the common carotid artery.
3. A wet gauze is placed on the anastomosis for 3 minutes.
4. Patency test.

   The classic technique of patency test is described in Chapter 6.9.2. (see **Figure 6-10**). In brief, two forceps are applied on the external jugular vein and move half-closed in opposite directions, away from the anastomosis, and close; this maneuver empties the lumen. Then, they are brought closer to each other with a quick movement and if there is patency, the lumen between the forceps fills immediately.

   It is recommended that the beginner applies this classic technique. Since a vacuum may not be achieved in the external jugular vein with the two forceps, a single, supplement clamp may be placed on the carotid artery, which will be removed when the two forceps occluding the external jugular vein approach each other (assistance will be required to place and then remove the single clamp).

   An alternative patency test technique is shown in **Figure 14-5**. A forceps is applied on the common carotid artery and moves half-closed centrally to empty the lumen, and closes at a final position; this maneuver empties the lumen of the common carotid artery. Another forceps is applied on the external jugular vein cranial to the anastomosis, moves half-closed more cranially and stops closed. This forceps empties the external jugular vein cranial to the anastomosis. Emptying the part of the vein on the other side of

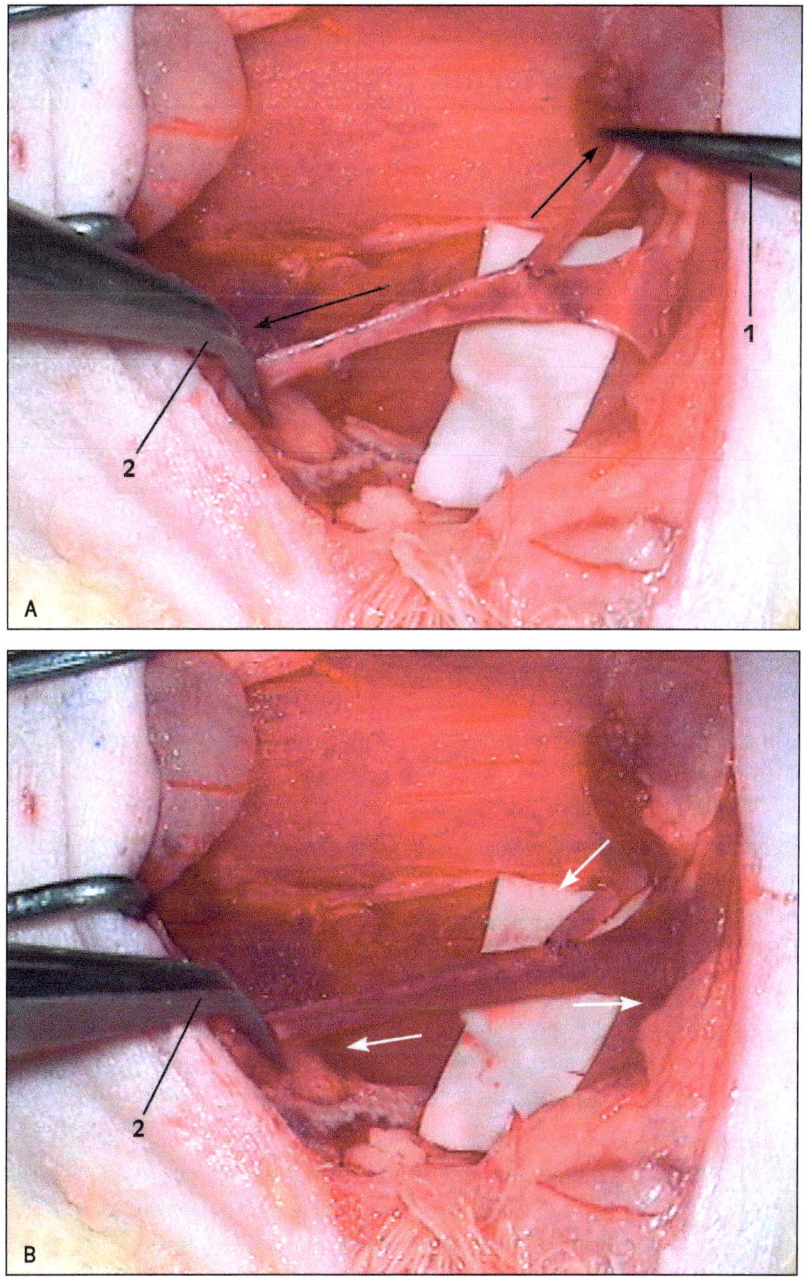

Figure 14-5

Alternative patency test for the end-to side anastomosis between the carotid artery-external jugular vein (right side). **A.** The forceps on the carotid artery **(1)** moves half-closed centrally and empties the artery. The forceps on the external jugular vein **(2)** moves cranially and empties the vein cranial to the anastomosis. The caudal part of the vein empties by tension of the forceps 2. Black arrows show the movements of the forceps. **B.** The carotid artery is released, while the forceps 2 on the external jugular vein stays closed. The vein fills (cranially and then caudally), which means that the anastomosis is patent. White arrows show the direction of blood flow. (From author's photo library)

the anastomosis (centrally) is achieved with tension on the vein by the forceps. Then, the forceps of the carotid artery is removed, while the forceps on the external jugular vein stays closed in place (without traction on the vein). If the anastomosis is successful, the vein will fill immediately, initially up to the forceps and then caudal to the anastomosis (the vein remains obstructed cranially).

5. Withdrawal of the yellow plastic background.

J. Closure of surgical trauma

Closure of the surgical trauma is done in one layer, suturing the skin and superficial fascia (platysma included) with interrupted non-absorbable 2/0 sutures.

Synopsis...

... of end-to-side anastomosis of the common carotid artery to the external jugular vein

A. **Positioning of the rat:** Dorsal decubitus (supine), with the head to the left of the surgeon. The limbs are immobilized on the working surface with adhesive tape.

B. **Preparation of the surgical field in the neck for exposure of the external jugular vein:** A transverse incision is performed at the base of the neck, from shoulder to shoulder. The superficial cervical fascia is dissected with two gauzes saturated in warm normal saline, moving in opposite directions cranio-caudally. A paper clip retractor pulls the skin, superficial fascia (platysma included) and the submandibular salivary glands cranially out of the surgical field.

C. **Microsurgical dissection of the external jugular vein:** The external jugular vein is meticulously dissected, from the edge of the pectoralis major muscle until the trifurcation. Small tributaries between the trifurcation and pectoralis are dissected and cut after double ligation or cauterization.

D. **Preparation of the surgical field in the neck for exposure of the common carotid artery:** The external jugular vein is moved laterally and the sternal part of the sternocleidomastoid muscle is transected using diathermy. The sternohyoid muscle (and together the underlying sternothyroid muscle) is moved medially, lifted by its lateral border.

E. **Microsurgical dissection of the common carotid artery:** The carotid sheath is opened, the common carotid artery is separated from the internal jugular vein and the vagus nerve. The vagus and recurrent laryngeal nerves are preserved.

F. **Central occlusion-peripheral ligation and transection of the common carotid artery:** Centrally, a single clamp and peripherally a 9/0 ligature are placed. The common carotid artery is transected close to the ligation. The lumen is irrigated with normal saline through an angiocatheter 27G. The adventitia is folded.

G. **Occlusion-transverse incision of the external jugular vein:** A yellow plastic background is placed underneath the vein, which is occluded with the double clamp. A transverse incision is performed in the vein. The lumen is irrigated and the adventitia is removed around the perimeter of the incision.

H. **End-to-side anastomosis. 8 sutures 10/0**

1. The first suture is placed in the middle of the posterior surface, sutures 2 and 3 on either side at equal distances, sutures 4 and 5 are the corner sutures, sutures 6 and 7 at equal distances from the corner sutures in the anterior surface, suture 8 in the middle of the distance between 6 and 7.
2. The double clamp of the vein is released first, then the single clamp of the artery.
3. Placement of a wet gauze on the anastomosis for 3 minutes.
4. Patency test.

I. **Closure of surgical trauma:** The skin and the superficial fascia (and platysma) are sutured in one layer with interrupted, non-absorbable 2/0 sutures.

15 End-to-end anastomosis between the aorta and right common iliac artery

(model of end-to-end anastomosis between vessels of different diameter)

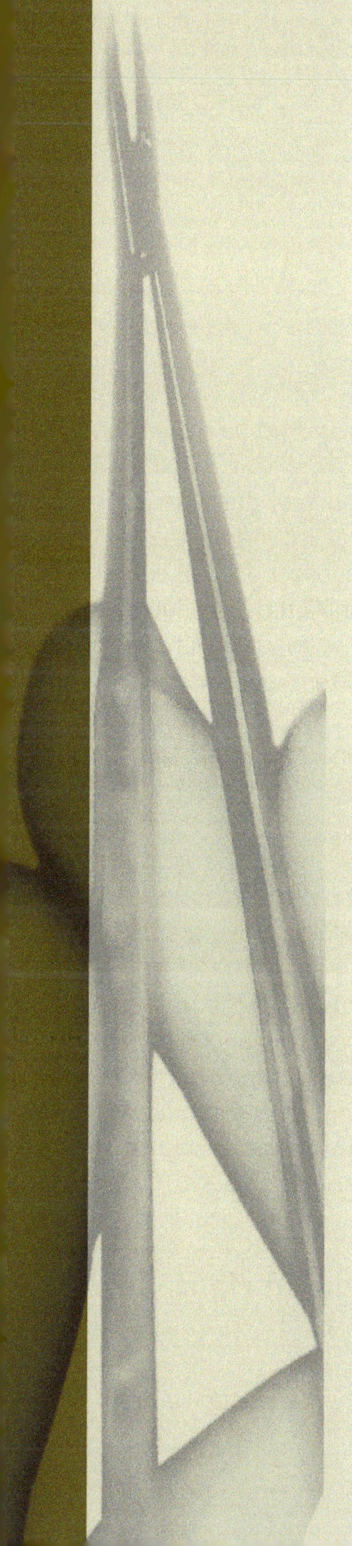

For the dissection and preparation of the aorta, the reader is asked to refer to Chapter 8 for the following paragraphs:

A. **Positioning of the rat**

B. **Preparation of the surgical field**

C. **Preparation of the microsurgical field and microsurgical dissection of the aorta.**
The only difference is that here the yellow plastic background is not put underneath the aorta at the end of the dissection, because the dissection is continued on the right common iliac artery (see below).

D. Microsurgical dissection of the right common iliac artery

The plane of separation between the aorta and the inferior vena cava is extended caudally following the right common iliac artery. At least 1 cm of the right common iliac artery must be fully dissected. It is advised to continue the dissection until the first branch of the right common iliac artery is met in the surgical field.

During the dissection of the right common iliac artery, specific attention must be given to the *middle sacral artery* (**Fig. 15-1**). This branch arises from the dorsal surface of the aorta bifurcation (into common iliac arteries). In the rat, the middle sacral artery is particularly well-developed, because it delivers blood to the vertebrae, the muscles attached to the sacrum, and muscles of the tail. The caudal artery, found in the middle of the ventral surface of the tail, is essentially the continuation of the middle sacral artery. During the dissection of the middle sacral artery, do not forget the smaller muscular branches that may arise from it; similar branches are also given by the caudal artery (No. 4, **Fig. 15-1**). These branches need specific attention to avoid bleeding during dissection. When met, they should be cauterized since there is no space there to put a double ligation. When the middle sacral artery is fully dissected, it is double ligated (9/0 suture) near its origin from the aorta, and cut between the two sutures.

The dissection of the right common iliac artery consists of separation from the companion vein (sometimes in the rat more than one common iliac vein is found) and continues until the first branch of the common iliac artery. Usually, this dissec-

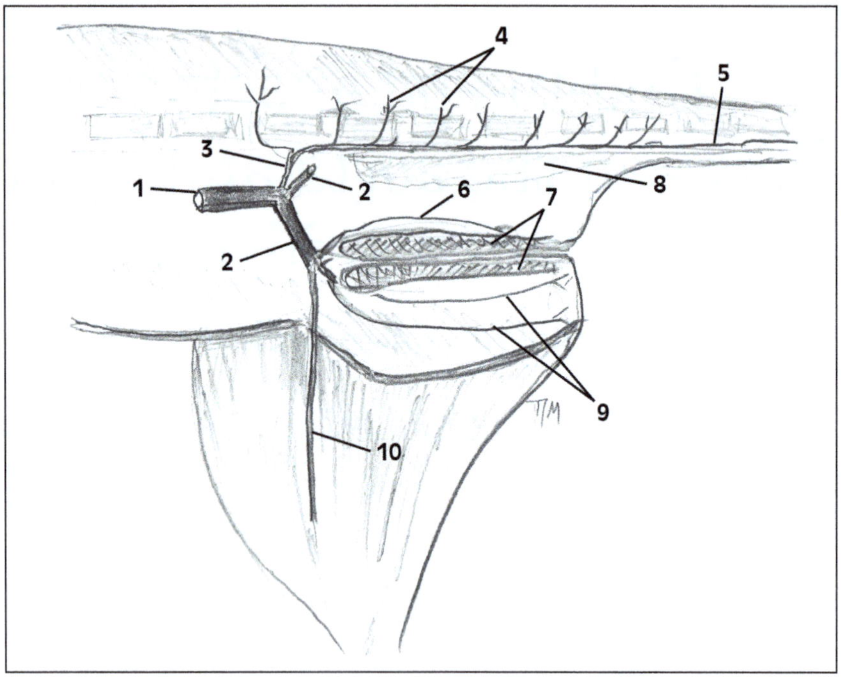

Figure 15-1

Branches of the aorta bifurcation and common iliac artery in the rat. **1.** aorta, **2.** common iliac artery, **3.** middle sacral artery, **4.** segmental branches for vertebrae and muscles, **5.** caudal artery, **6.** uterine artery, **7.** uterus, **8.** ovary, **9.** perineal branches, **10.** femoral artery. (Drawing by the author)

tion provides enough length for the anastomosis with the aorta.

The guideline for the dissection of the right common iliac artery is '*until the first branch*'. Sometimes this instruction will be violated, since a small early branch may be encountered and the length until this branch is not enough for rotation of the artery and anastomosis (see below). It may be necessary to ligate and cut this first small branch (and some small muscular branches too).

Understanding basic elements of surgical anatomy of the common iliac artery is important, so that the surgeon knows what is to be ligated if required, and understands the consequences of the ligation of the common iliac artery or a branch of it. In **Figure 15-1**, the branches of the aorta bifurcation and common iliac artery are shown in the rat. In this animal, there is much variation in the branching pattern of the common iliac artery to external and internal iliac arteries, while sometimes there is no bifurcation but continuation of the same artery. However, in our experience, the common iliac artery usually does bifurcate into external and internal iliac arteries. In these cases, the pelvic splanchnic and perineal branches are given by the internal iliac artery, which is recognizable in the surgical field.

The reader will find a detailed description of the branches of the internal iliac arteries in Chapter 29.C.I, which we recommend to be studied now, so that he/she will be aware of what is to be ligated if necessary.

In cases without typical bifurcation of the common iliac artery into internal and external iliac arteries, the iliac artery [the term 'common' no longer applies] continues and supplies the leg (femoral artery), abdominal wall (inferior epigastric artery), pelvic splanchna (uterine artery, umbilical artery, vesical artery, etc.) and perineum.

It is amazing that after ligation and transection of the common iliac artery in this procedure, vascular supply to the posterior limb will be given by collateral circulation. The non-existstent consequences of the ligation of a parietal branch of the common iliac artery, or of ligation of the internal or external iliac artery are discussed in detail in Chapter 29.C.III.4.

As a reminder, the vascular supply to the gonads (testes or ovaries) comes from branches of the aorta and not from the internal iliac arteries. Therefore, these vessels –assuming no gross mistake such as taking them in the vascular clamp—will not be involved in this dissection.

E. Ligation of the aorta and right common iliac artery

The aorta is ligated just above the bifurcation with a

Figure 15-2

Ligation of the aorta and right common iliac artery after they have been dissected. Ligation is placed on the aorta just proximal to the bifurcation; the common iliac artery is ligated proximal to branching (white arrowheads). **1.** aorta, **2.** right common iliac artery, **3.** left common iliac artery, **4.** cauterized lumbar arteries. (From author's photo library)

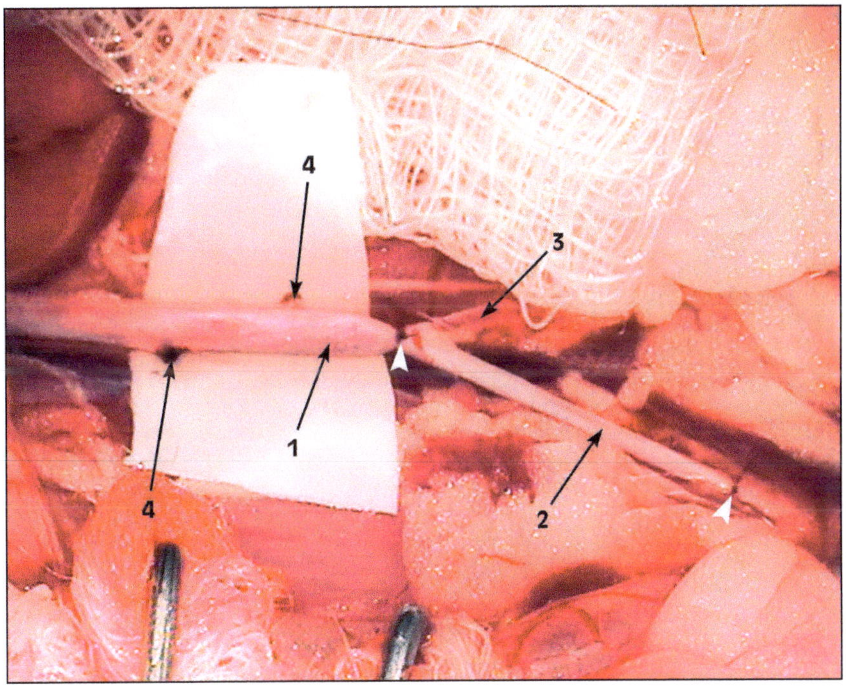

9/0 free suture. Take care to identify the inferior mesenteric artery, and place the ligation distal to it. The right common iliac artery is also ligated with 9/0 free suture just proximal to the bifurcation into external and internal iliac. In case there is no typical bifurcation, the ligation is placed at a point proximal to which there is at least 1 cm of dissected vessel. A yellow plastic background is placed underneath the aorta, cranial to the bifurcation, where the anastomosis will be done (**Fig. 15-2**).

F. Placement of clamps - transection of the aorta and right common iliac artery - rotation of the right common iliac artery

The design of the operation is shown in **Figure 15-3**. The aim is to rotate the right common iliac artery (around the point of aorta bifurcation) and anastomose it with the aortic stump. Finally, the right common iliac artery will be continued with the left common iliac artery. The continuation of the right common iliac artery is terminated. The details are as follows:

The proximal clamp of the double vascular clamp is placed on the aorta, caudal to the left renal artery; the distal clamp remains open waiting for the stump of the right common iliac artery. The aorta is transect-

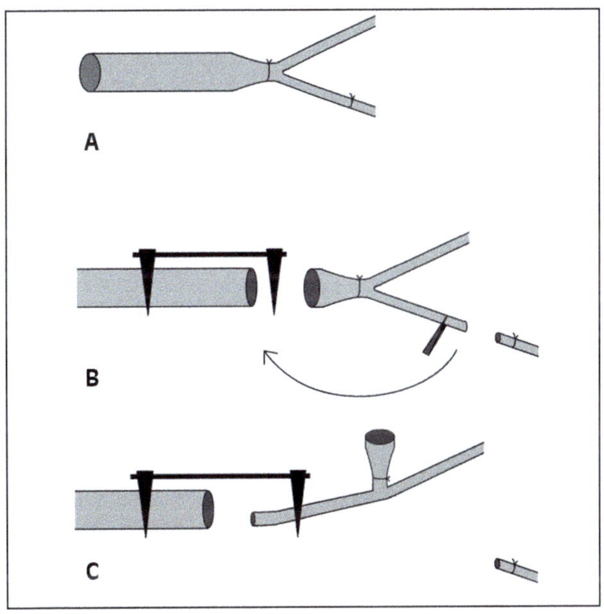

Figure 15-3

Anastomosis of the aorta with the right common iliac artery: design of the steps for mobilization and final positioning of the vessels. **A.** Ligation of the aorta and right common iliac artery. **B.** One of the two arms of the double clamp is placed on the aorta cranial to the ligation, and the aorta is transected between the clamp and the ligation, proximal to the ligation. A single clamp is placed on the right common iliac artery. The vessel is transected between the single clamp and the ligation, and the stump of the right common iliac artery is rotated cranially to face the central aortic stump. **C.** The inverted common iliac artery stump is placed in the free clamp of the double clamp. (Diagram: E. Kontis)

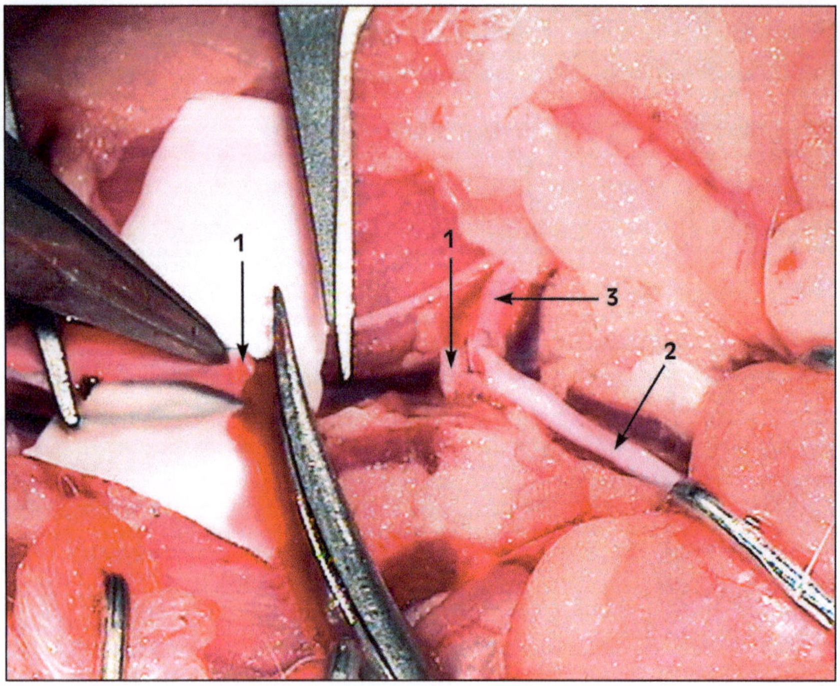

Figure 15-4

Transection of the aorta. Observe the open jaws of the free arm of the double clamp (next to the scissors) prepared to receive the right common iliac artery, which will be transected and rotated. **1.** aortic stumps, **2.** right common iliac artery, **3.** left common iliac artery. (From author's photo library)

ed with scissors, with a clean cut, cranial to the ligation (**Fig. 15-4**). The lumen of the aorta is irrigated with warm normal saline through a 27G catheter, which should not enter the lumen to avoid trauma of the endothelium. The adventitia of the aorta is folded (**Fig. 15-5**).

Next, the right common iliac artery is transected proximal to the ligation. Previously, this vessel has been obstructed with a small single clamp placed proximal, between the aorta bifurcation and site of the transection of the common iliac artery. After transection, the stump is inverted, using the single clamp

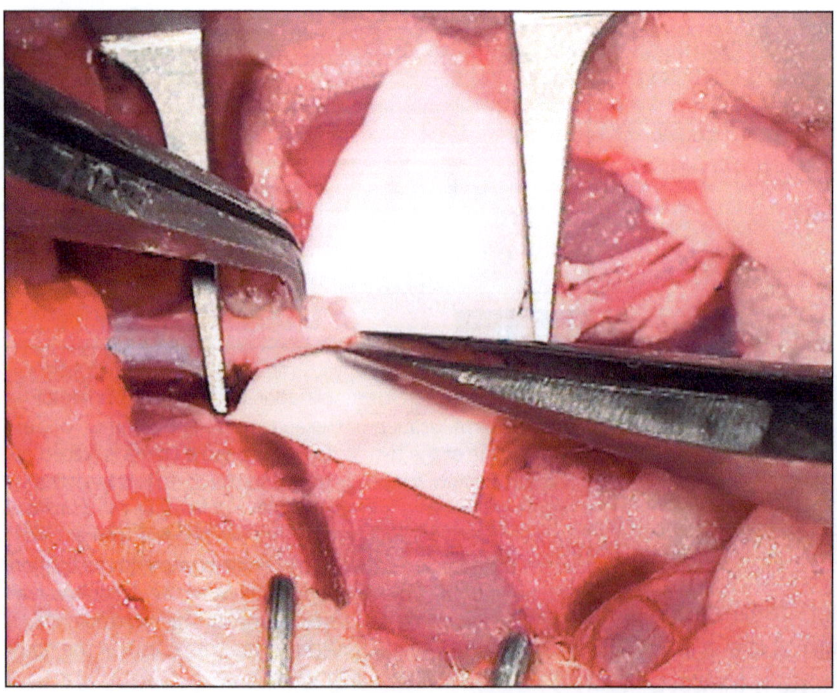

Figure 15-5

Folding of the adventitia of the aorta. The curved forceps holds the aorta, while the forceps Dumont No. 3 folds the adventitia. (From author's photo library)

(**Fig. 15-3B**). The lumen is irrigated with warm normal saline. The stump of the common iliac artery is placed in the free clamp of the double clamp, taking care to position the stump with enough length to allow anastomosis with the proximal aortic stump (**Fig. 15-3C**). The single clamp is then released from the common iliac artery and the lumen is again irrigated with normal saline. The adventitia of the common iliac artery is folded (**Fig. 15-6**).

G. Correction of the disproportion of lumen sizes (dilatation of the right common iliac artery)

The reader is invited to read the methods of correction of the disproportion of lumen size in end-to-end anastomoses of vessels in Chapter 5.

The two clamps of the double clamp are approximated so that the stumps of the aorta and inverted right common iliac artery come in contact. The difference of the lumen diameters is likely to be smaller than a 2:1 ratio. We underscore that the difference in lumen diameters depends on how far distally the dissection has been extended on the common iliac artery (the more distal, the smaller the lumen). According to our experience, the mechanical dilatation of the lumen of the iliac artery is effective, and rarely was another method used.

To dilate the lumen of the iliac artery, a Dumont No. 3 forceps is inserted closed into the lumen of the vessel, while another forceps stabilizes the wall of the vessel (**Fig. 15-7**). The forceps Dumont No. 3 is left to open gradually, in a slow controlled manner, because the sudden or extended opening of the legs of the forceps risks rupture (tear) to the vessel. For this maneuver, it is safer to use the Dumont No. 3 forceps as opposed to the finer No. 5 forceps, because the latter are too pointy and risk traumatizing or tearing the vessel wall. The dilation is not achieved with one movement but with repeated openings of the forceps, until we estimate that the width of the lumen of the common iliac artery is approximately equal to the aorta width.

In case the width of the lumen of the aorta appears to be almost double the width of the lumen of the inverted common iliac artery, this mechanical dilatation will not be effective. In such a case, it is indicated to perform an oblique transection of the lumen of the right common iliac artery (**Fig. 15-8**). A piece of the left side of the wall is removed. The removed piece is double layered (anterior and posterior surface) and has the shape of a right angle triangle. The vertical legs are: the lumen diameter before transection,

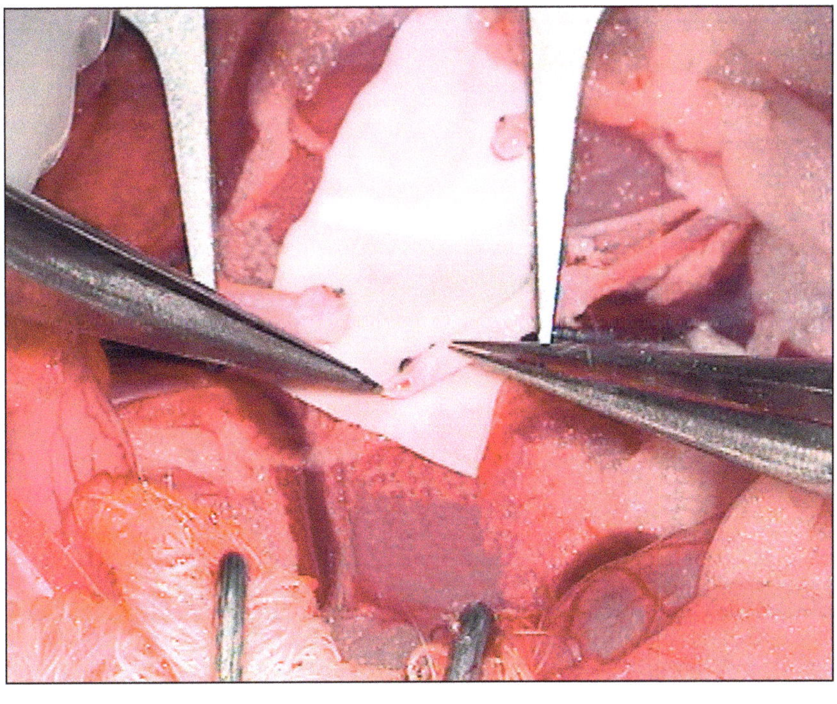

Figure 15-6

Folding of the adventitia of the iliac artery. The forceps No. 3 holds the artery from the outer surface of the wall, while the forceps No. 5 folds the adventitia. (From author's photo library)

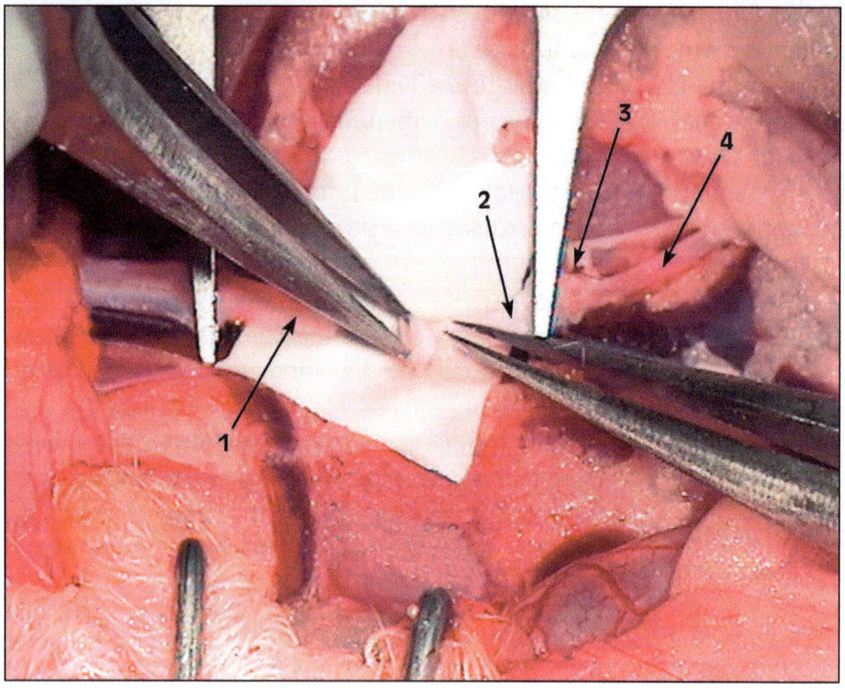

Figure 15-7

Dilatation of the lumen of the inverted stump of the right common iliac artery. Dumont No. 5 forceps (right hand) holds the artery from the outer surface of the wall. Dumont No. 3 forceps enters the lumen closed, and is left to open slowly to dilate the lumen. The maneuver is repeated until the width of the lumen of the stumps of the aorta and right common iliac artery become approximately equal. **1.** proximal stump of the aorta, **2.** inverted stump of the common iliac artery, **3.** distal stump of the aorta, **4.** left common iliac artery. (From author's photo library)

and the length of the vessel portion to be removed ; the hypotenuse is the line of transection. As an important reminder, as described in Chapter 5, the angle of transection should not be greater than 30°. This will be the angle of deviation between the axis of the aorta and the axis of the inverted right common iliac artery (see **Figure 5-6**).

The criteria to choose one of the two above methods are not absolute; the surgeon is not expected to measure exact diameters of the vessels and calculate

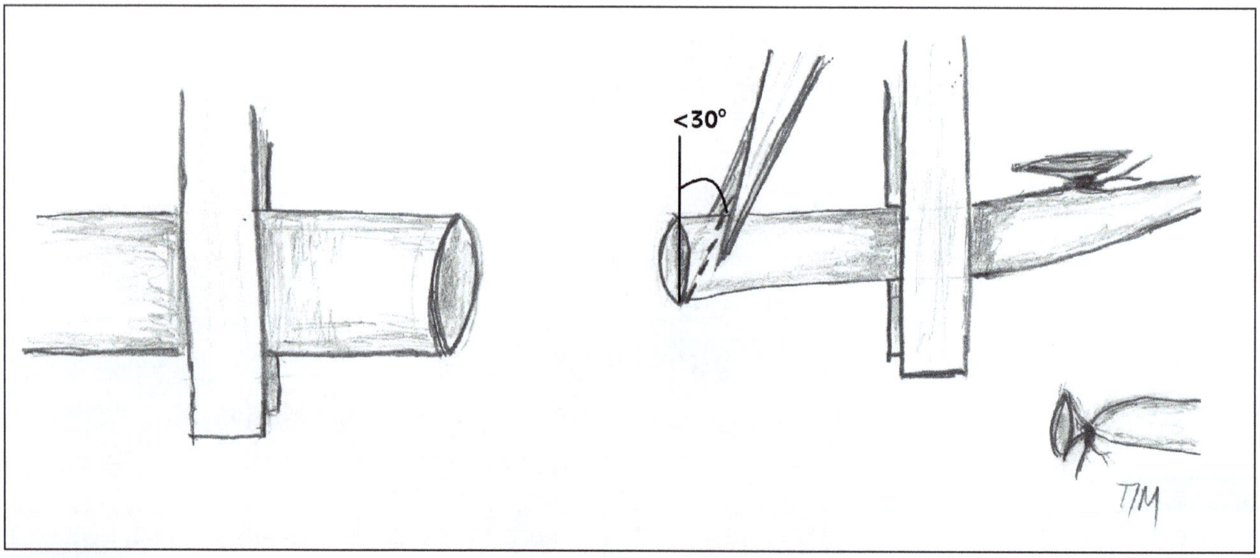

Figure 15-8

Oblique transection of the inverted right common iliac artery. The maximum permitted angle between the transection line (marked as dashed line) and the perpendicular of the vessel line is 30°. (Drawing by the author)

their ratio. In most cases, mechanical dilatation of the stump of the common iliac artery is sufficient. If adjustment is needed, a small wedge of the wall of the common iliac artery can be removed, always taking into consideration that the total angle of deviation to the left of the inverted right common iliac artery should not exceed 30°. In addition, it is reminded that a slight correction of disproportionate lumen sizes can be performed during suturing by taking longer 'steps' (distance between sutures) in the larger vessel and narrower steps in the smaller vessel.

H. End-to-end anastomosis

The technique of the end-to-end anastomosis of vessels is described in full-length in Chapter 5.

- The anastomosis will be performed by placing **10 sutures 10/0**.

  Alternatively, 8 sutures 9/0 can be placed. We recommend the use of 10/0 sutures.

The steps of the process of the end-to-end anastomosis are as follows:

1. Placement of the two corner sutures (12 o'clock and 6 o'clock) that will orient the vessel stumps.
2. Suturing of the anterior surface is completed. There are 4 sutures remaining per surface, from which the 2 lateral (toward the corner sutures) will be put first, then the 2 more central, all at equal distances from the corner sutures and between themselves.
3. Rotation of the double clamp and check that all sutures of the anterior surfaces have been placed correctly.
4. Suturing of the posterior surface is completed, using the same technique as described for the anterior surface.
5. Release of the vessels from the double clamp (**Fig. 15-9**).
6. Gauze (wet) placement on the anastomosis for 3 minutes.
7. Patency test.

   As described in Chapter 5.10, the patency test will be performed with two microsurgical forceps, initially placed on the vessel one next to the other, after the suture line, following the blood flow. The proximal forceps (close to the anastomosis) occludes the vessel, while the distal forceps empties the vessel and finally stays closed. The proximal forceps is withdrawn, and if there is patency across the suture line, the vessel will immediately fill to the distal forceps (**Fig. 15-10**).
8. Withdrawal of the yellow plastic background.

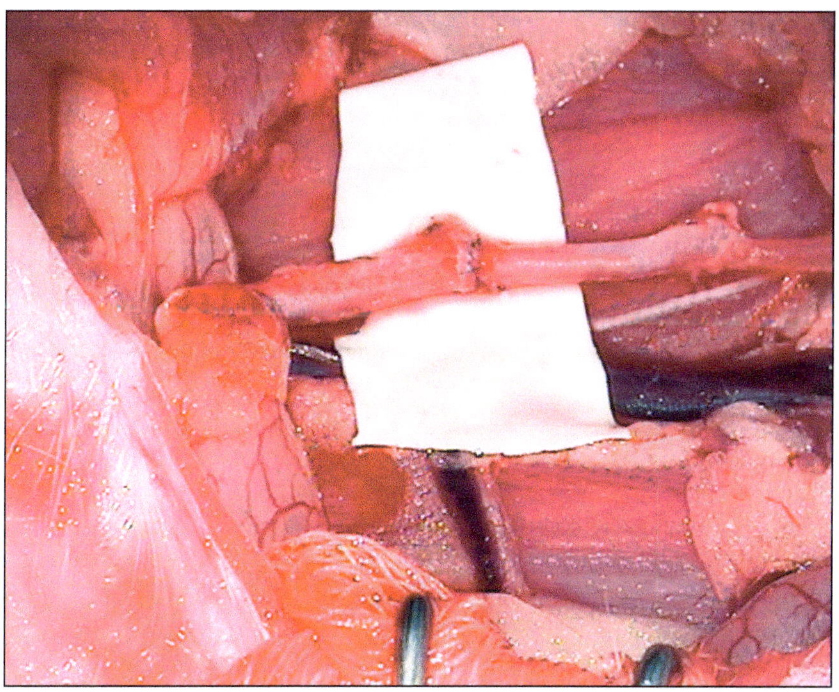

Figure 15-9

The anastomosis of the aorta with the inverted right common iliac artery after removal of the double vascular clamp. (From author's photo library)

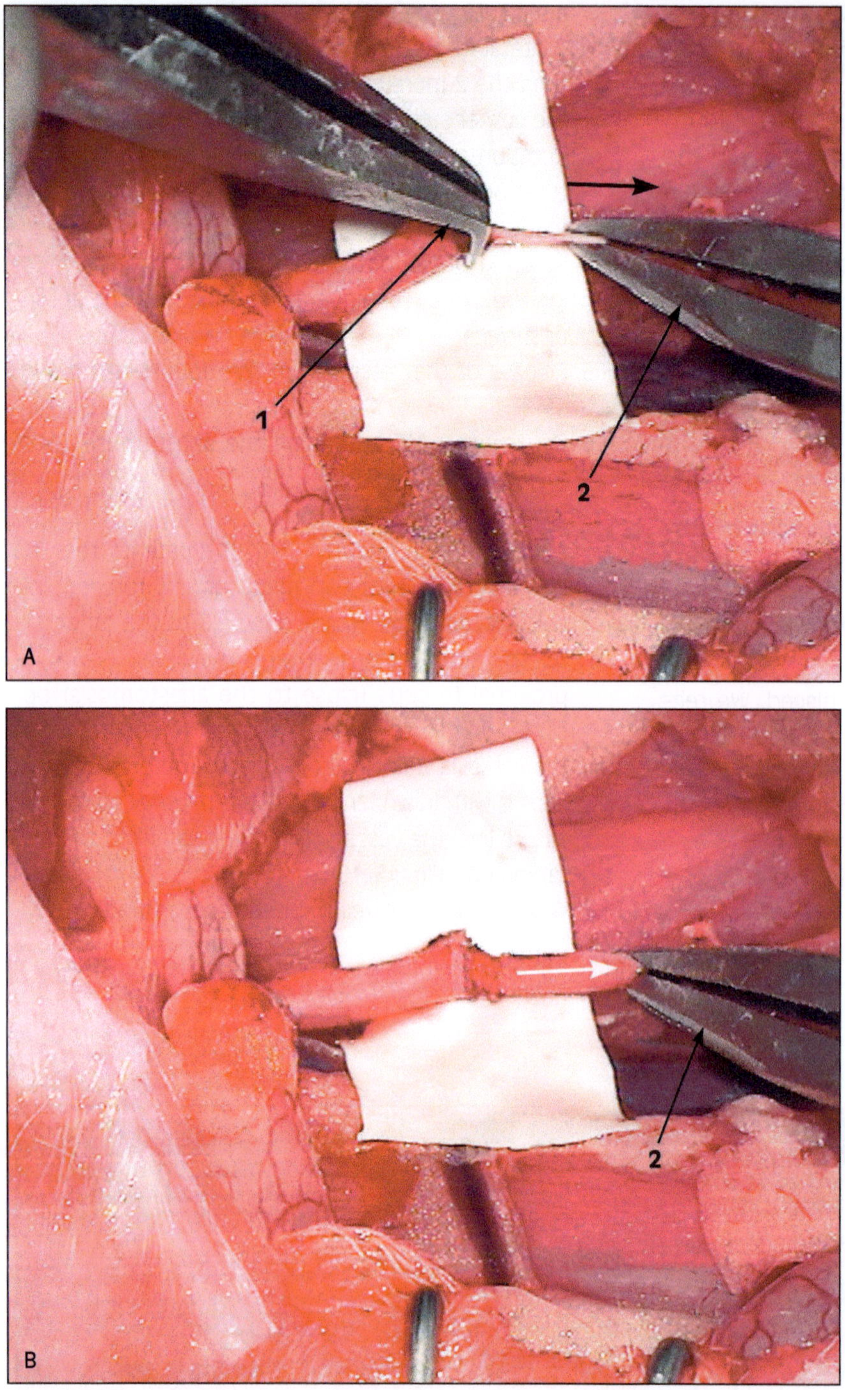

Figure 15-10

Patency test of the anastomosis of the aorta with the inverted right iliac artery. **A.** The proximal forceps **(1)** occludes the blood flow distal to the anastomosis. The distal forceps **(2)** then moves 'half-closed' caudally and empties the lumen (the black arrow shows the movement of the forceps). Here, the forceps has stopped, totally closed. **B.** The proximal forceps has been removed from the field, the distal forceps **(2)** remains in place. The immediate filling of the vessel shows that the anastomosis was successful (the white arrow shows the blood flow). (From author's photo library)

J. Closure of the surgical trauma

After the splanchna have been returned in the abdomen, the abdominal wall is closed in two layers (muscles, subcutaneous-skin) with interrupted, non-absorbable sutures 2/0.

Synopsis...

... of end-to-end anastomosis between the aorta and right common iliac artery

A. **Position of the rat:** Laid on its back, head on the surgeon's left). The limbs are immobilized on the working surface with adhesive tape.

B. **Preparation of the surgical field:** Median incision, from the xiphoid process to the pubic symphisis. Paper clip retractors are placed at the edges of the incision. The lobes of the liver protruding in the field are packed with another retractor. The small intestine is mobilized and the intestines are moved out of the abdomen and packed in a wet gauze, placed to the right of the rat.

C. **Preparation of the microsurgical field and microsurgical dissection of the aorta:** The retroperitoneum is opened with two wet gauzes. A plane of separation between aorta and inferior vena cava is created and the aorta is completely cleaned, from the bifurcation to the height of the left renal vein. All lumbar arteries are dissected, cleaned and divided either between two ligations (9/0 suture) or using monopolar diathermy.

D. **Microsurgical dissection of the right common iliac artery:** Dissection of the right common iliac artery continues as distal as possible. The aorta bifurcation is also dissected, and the middle sacral artery is double-ligated (9/0) and cut in between. A yellow plastic background is placed underneath the aorta.

E. **Ligation of the aorta and right common iliac artery:** The aorta is ligated just above its bifurcation (9/0 suture). The right common iliac artery is also ligated (9/0 suture) just above its bifurcation, or allowing at least 1 cm of available artery if there is no apparent bifurcation.

F. **Placement of clamps - transection of the aorta and right common iliac artery - rotation of the right common iliac artery:** The aorta is placed in the proximal arm of the double clamp, and is transected cranial to the ligation. A single clamp is placed proximal on the right common iliac artery (between the aorta bifurcation and the common iliac artery ligation), and the artery is transected proximal to the ligation; the stump is inversed and placed in the free clamp of the double clamp. The single clamp is removed and the lumens of the vessels are irrigated with normal saline. The adventitia of both vessels are folded.

G. **Correction of the disproportion of lumens sizes:** Re-approximation of the clamps of the double clamp. **Dilatation of the right common iliac artery** with a Dumont No. 3 forceps inserted into the lumen, which is repeatedly left to open gradually.

H. **End-to-end anastomosis: placement of 10 sutures 10/0**
1. Placement of the two corner sutures (12 o'clock and 6 o'clock).
2. Suturing of the anterior surface is completed: 4 remaining, put at equal distances, starting with the 2 peripheral.
3. Rotation of the clamp and check of sutures on the anterior surface.
4. Suturing of the posterior surface, similar to anterior.
5. Release of the double clamp.
6. Placement of a wet gauze on the anastomosis for 3 minutes.
7. Patency test.
8. Withdrawal of the yellow plastic background.

J. **Closure of surgical trauma:** The abdominal wall is closed in two layers (muscles, subcutaneous-skin) with interrupted non-absorbable sutures 2/0.

16

End-to-side anastomosis of the portal vein to the inferior vena cava

(portocaval anastomosis)

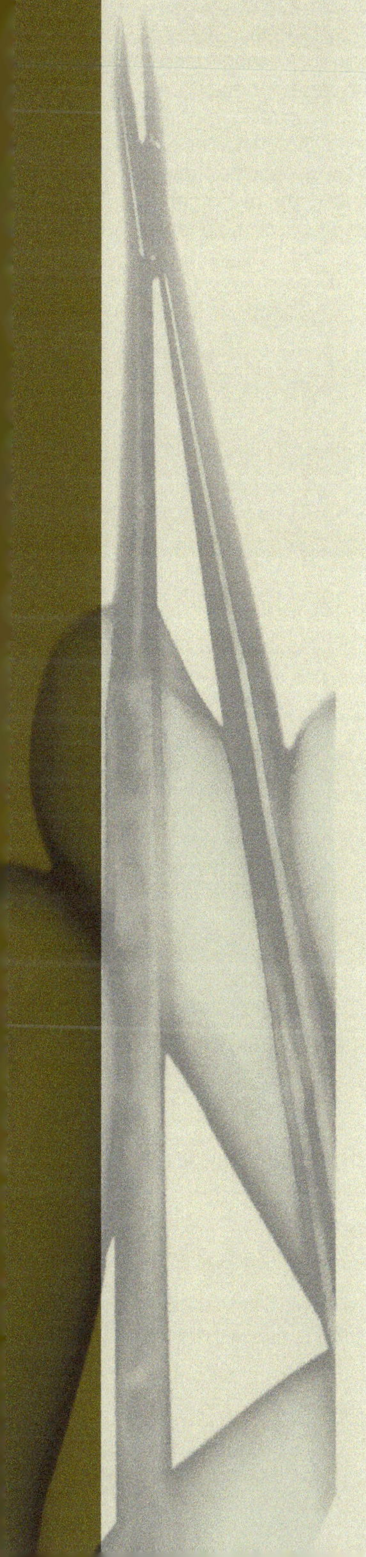

The strategy of the operation is shown in **Figure 16-1**. The beginning steps are dissection of the inferior vena cava in the area of the the confuences of the renal veins as well as dissection of the portal vein. Next, the first tributary vein of the portal vein, the gastroduodenal vein, is ligated. Following this, the portal vein is ligated centrally, toward the liver, and divided. Lastly, the portal vein is anastomosed end-to-side with the inferior vena cava (after a transverse incision on the latter) starting with the posterior surface as there is no possibility for the end-anastomosed portal vein to rotate.

Remember

- For this procedure, anesthesia with ether is necessary
- The total time of portal vein occlusion cannot surpass 30 minutes

A. Positioning of the rat

The rat is positioned in supine position (dorsal decubitus) on the working surface. The long axis of the body of the rat is parallel to the frontal (coronal) plane of the surgeon's body, and the rat's head is placed on the surgeon's left. The limbs of the rat are immobilized on the working surface with adhesive tape.

B. Anesthesia

Anesthesia is achieved with ether administered to the rat with a mask. The usual intramuscular injection of ketamine-chloropromazine should not be used in portocaval anastomosis because in this operation circulation of the liver, where these agents are metabolized, is disturbed.

Technically, a gauze moistured with ether will be used, placed in the bottom of the cylinder of a 50 ml syringe with the plunger removed. For younger rats, a 20 ml syringe is used. It is very likely that additional ether will need to be used during the operation, so the bottle of ether should be nearby on the bench. Pay attention to

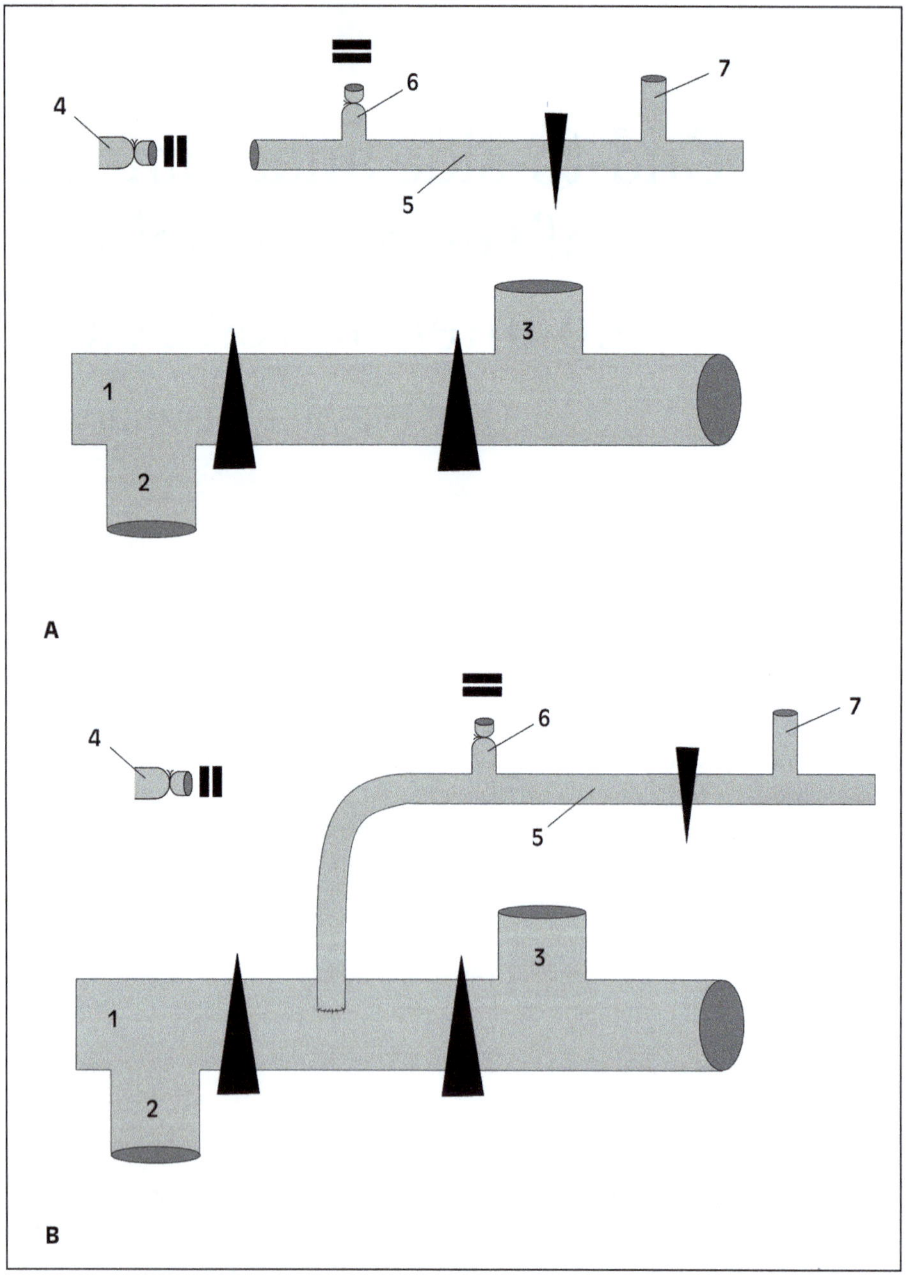

Figure 16-1

Design of the portocaval anastomosis. **A.** Ligation and transection of the gastroduodenal vein; central ligation and transection of the portal vein. **B.** Following transverse incision of the interior vena cava, end-to side portocaval anastomosis. **1.** inferior vena cava, **2.** right renal vein, **3.** left renal vein, **4.** hepatic stump of the portal vein, **5.** peripheral part of the portal vein, **6.** gastroduodenal vein, **7.** splenic vein. The two parallel bold lines denote transection of the vessel and the black triangles the vascular clamps (the small triangle shows the single clamp on the peripheral stump of the portal vein, the two larger triangles the double clamp on the inferior vena cava. (Diagram: E. Kontis)

keep the bottle closed to prevent inhaling any ether vapor. Additionally, remain cognizant of the flammability of ether.

C. Preparation of the surgical field

Preparation of the surgical field has much in common with the respective preparation of the field of the aorta, presented in detail and with rich imaging in Chapter 8.B. To avoid repetition, the common steps are summarized here; emphasis is given to the differences regarding the portal vein and inferior vena cava.

A median incision is performed from 5 mm inferior to the xiphoid process to 5 mm superior to the pubic symphisis. A small incision is then performed in the linea alba with baby-Metzenbaum scissors; the incision is extended cranially and caudally and the aponeuroses of the recti abdomini muscles are pulled apart with a paper clip retractor on each side.

Handling the lobes of the liver

To work with the portal vein, the surgeon requires detailed knowledge of liver anatomy (in Chapter 8.B.2, in which the reader is referred, the liver lobes were just moved away from the surgical field). Because the portal vein will be dissected toward the hilum of the liver, exact recognition and then cephalad rotation of the lobes of the liver is necessary.

In the rat, the liver consists of more lobes than in human: the right, middle, left, and caudate lobes (**Fig. 16-2**). The lobes are separated by true deep fissures (in contrast to human), and are therefore mobile. The left lobe comprises two segments, one large lateral segment and a smaller medial segment. The left lobe segments are also separated by a deep fissure and can move independently. The left lobe has a relatively long stalk in which course the blood vessels addressed to it (left branch of the portal vein and hepatic artery) and the left hepatic duct running from it, all wrapped in connective tissue. The stalk itself, however, is mobile and can undergo torsion and strangulation if caution is not taken (see below). In most cases, the right lobe is not segmented, although the trace of a fissure can be sometimes seen on its surface.

The lobes of the liver will have to be moved to obtain visualization of and access to the entire portal vein. Following the midline incision, the middle lobe and the lateral segment of the left lobe often protrude through the opening in the abdominal wall with little to no pressure (**Fig. 16-3**). The medial segment of the left lobe is posterior to the lateral segment and usually does not protrude through the incision. However, the lobes protruding from the incision are not the exact lobes that need to be moved from the surgical field for exposure of the portal vein.

The right and middle lobes of the liver should be rotated to the right and cranially with a retractor that has been wrapped with a wet gauze. In general, rotation of the left lobe is avoided because of the risk of strangulation of its stalk. If necessary, it is safer to rotate the medial segment of the left lobe out of the way. If the lateral segment must also be rotated, attention is needed to avoid strangulation of its stalk. Following mobilization of any segment of the left lobe, be sure that no color change occurs as compared with the right and middle lobes. If this is suspected, immediately release the left lobe from the retractor. Once complete, the bed of the surgical field will contain the rest of the lobes and segments of the visceral surface of the liver—the remainder of the right lobe (if not divided in segments) or the medial segment (if divided), the caudate lobe, and the lateral

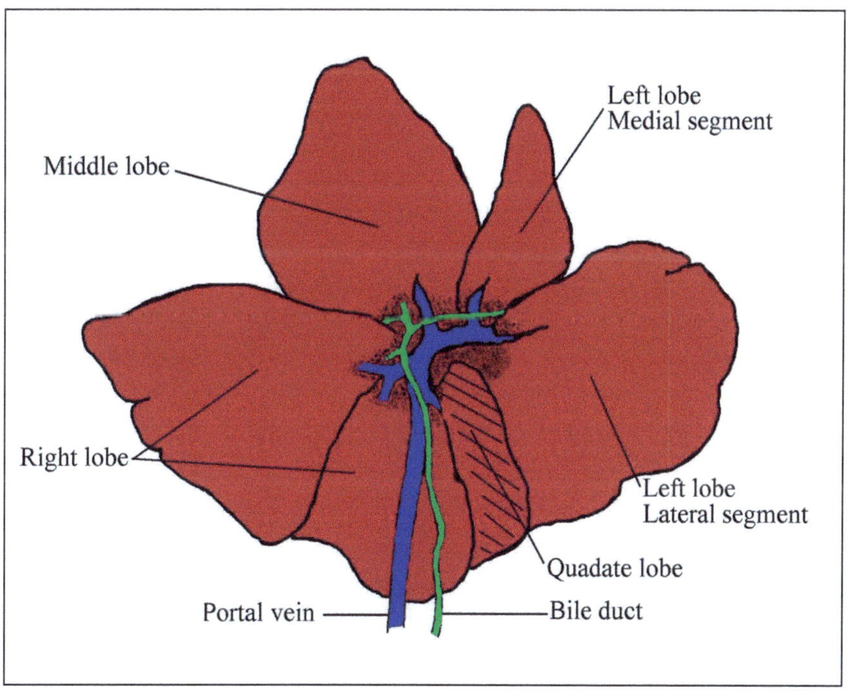

Figure 16-2

Lobes of the liver in the rat as seen from the visceral surface. Observe the 1st and 2nd order branching of the portal vein toward the lobes and segments respectively. Also, see the relatively long stalk of the vessels addressed to the left lobe, as marked here with a white ring around the left branch of the portal vein and the left hepatic duct. Note that although not shown here, the ring also comprises the left branch of the hepatic artery. (Modified from Waynforth H. B. Experimental and Surgical Technique in the Rat. London: Academic Press Inc, 1980)

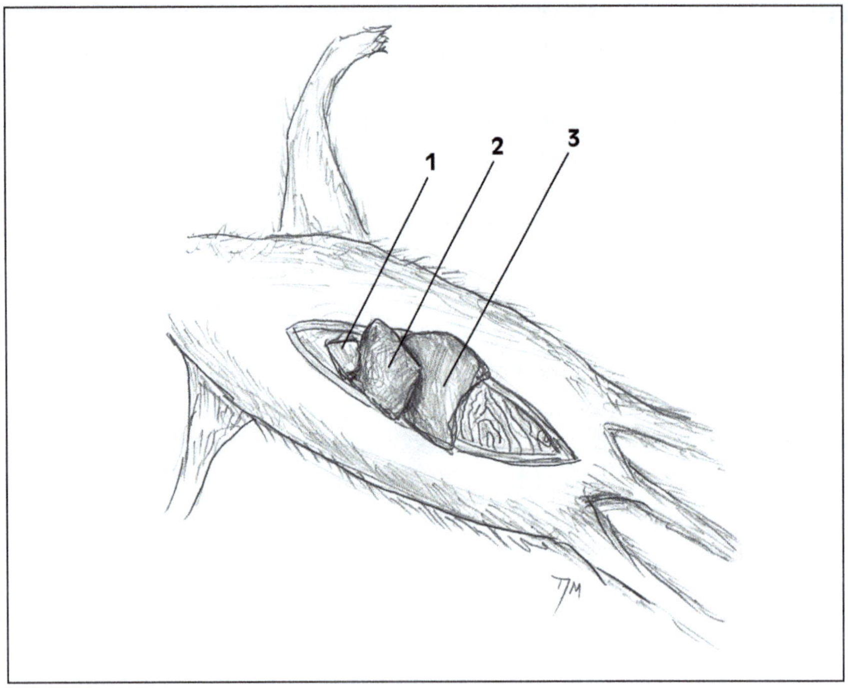

Figure 16-3

After median incision the middle lobe and the lateral segment of the left lobe of the liver can protrude through the opening of the abdominal wall. **1.** xyphoid process (cartilaginous), **2.** middle lobe, **3.** lateral segment of the left lobe. (Drawing by the author)

segment of the left lobe (if the medial segment has been rotated) (**Fig. 16-2**).

Mobilization of the intestine

Beginning at the cecum, the intestine is grasped with broad anatomical forceps and pulled out of the abdomen. The transparent distal part of the mesentery of the small intestine (attached to the posterior peritoneum next to the rectum) is divided in order to attain adequate mobilization (see **Figure 8-3**). The intestines should be wrapped in wet gauze and placed *on the left side of the rat* in order to obtain a satisfactory view of the portal vein and inferior vena cava in the surgical field. This is different from operations described in previous chapters, where the intestine was placed on the right side of the rat. The intestine and the opened peritoneal cavity should be periodically irrigated with warm normal saline.

Note that placement of the intestine on the left side does not require any handling of the spleen (which was necessary in Chapter 8.B.2) because the spleen will be 'packed' under the left subcostal arch together with the intestines moved to the left.

Dissection of the retroperitoneum

The posterior peritoneum should be opened with two gauzes saturated in warm normal saline, which are drawn laterally, on either side, moving away from the midline (see **Figure 8-5A**).This maneuver permits the blunt dissection of the retroperitoneum. If performed correctly, it exposes the microsurgical field of the inferior vena cava and aorta.

Knowledge of the topographic relation between the aorta and the inferior vena cava along the retroperitoneum is of major importance to the dissection that will follow. After opening the retroperitoneum, it can be seen that caudally the aorta runs anteriorly to the interior vena cava. For this reason, dissection of the aorta should begin just proximal to its bifurcation and extend cranially, as alluded to in Chapter 8.C.2. Gradually, the relation of the two vessels changes (see **Figure 8-5B**). At the level of the first lumbar vessesls, the inferior vena cava is found lateral to the aorta on its right side. At the level of the left renal vein, the inferior vena cava is clearly anterior to the aorta. This is the relationship between the inferior vena cava and aorta that will be seen in the surgical field during dissection of the inferior vena cava for portocaval anastomosis, which takes place for the most part in the area between the exits of the two renal veins.

The portal vein

Opening the retroperitoneum with the two gauzes will

also expose the portal vein. The portal vein is in close relation with the pancreas, which is almost gelatinous and very friable in the rat. For this reason, repeated gentle movements of the gauzes are required for the exposure of the portal vein.

The portal vein courses in the retroperitoneum until it enters the hepatoduodenal ligament and then the porta hepatis, as in humans. The portal vein carries the venous outflow of the abdominal viscera. In the human, the portal vein runs along the dorsal surface of the pancreas; in most cases, the uncinate process extends posteriorly behind the portal vein in the area of the neck of the pancreas. In the rat, the portal vein seems to course mainly 'within' the pancreas after opening the retroperitoneum or 'superficially' to the pancreas after further dissection with the two gauzes (**Fig. 16-4**). This is due to changes in anatomical relations after moving the intestines and opening of the retroperitoneum, as well as to the gelatinous structure of the pancreas, which permits the portal vein to be found more superficially.

The first tributary of the portal vein that can be found distally is the gastroduodenal vein (No. 7, **Fig. 16-4**). The next large tributary is the *splenic vein*—in the current positioning of the splanchna in the surgical field, it gives the impression that it courses vertical to the portal vein 'inside' the pancreas (No. 9, **Fig. 16-4**, and No. 3, **Fig. 16-8**). Of course, the portal vein of the rat also accepts large tributary (superior and inferior mesenteric) veins from the small and large intestine, which are not involved in the current dissection.

Proximally towards the liver, the portal vein is in close relation with the hepatic artery and trie bile duct. The duct in the rat is very small and thin and courses parallel to the portal vein. Close to the hilum of the liver the two structures cross each other, bringing the bile duct anterior to the portal vein (with the visceral surface of the liver rotated cranially, see **Figure 16-2**).

D. Microsurgical dissection of the inferior vena cava

The inferior vena cava should be dissected between the renal veins, which join the inferior vena cava at a different height. The left renal vein is found more caudally as compared to the right renal vein.

In order to proceed with this part of the dissection, a plane should be created between the inferior vena cava and the aorta. As the dissection is performed, the aorta should be preferentially handled as it has a strong wall and can be lifted by the adventitia in a safer and easier way than the inferior vena cava. This plane of separation can start caudal to the left renal vein, where

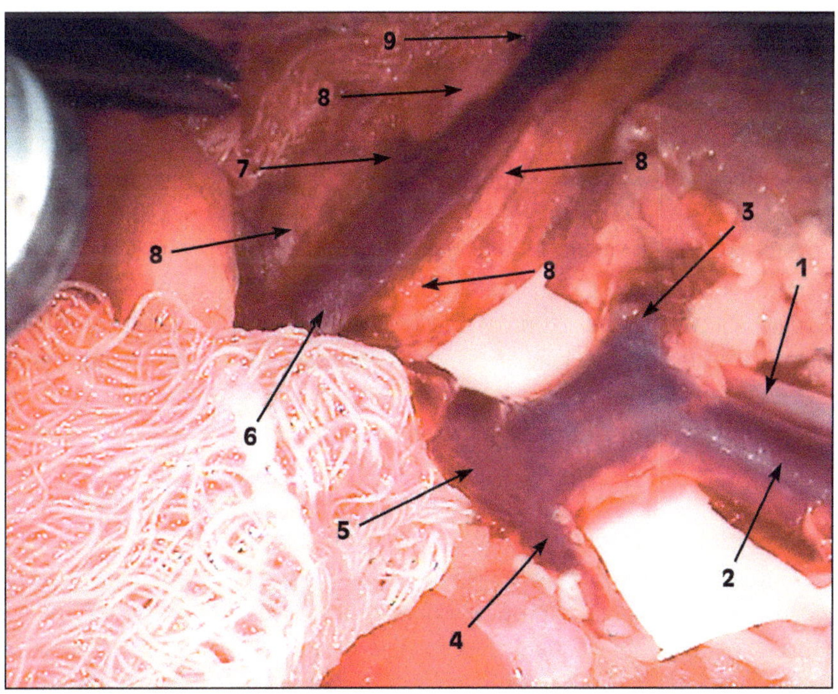

Figure 16-4

View of the surgical field after microsurgical dissection of the inferior vena cava and portal vein. Observe the position of the aorta in relation to the inferior vena cava, as well as the course of the portal vein in relation to the pancreas. The dissection results in a 'winding' course of the inferior vena cava. **1.** aorta, **2.** inferior vena cava, caudal to the confluence of renal veins, **3.** left renal vein, **4.** right renal vein, **5.** inferior vena cava, cranial to the renal veins, 6. portal vein, **7.** gastroduodenal vein, **8.** pancreas, **9.** splenic vein. (From author's photo library) the aorta is lateral to the the inferior vena cava, or even more caudally, where the aorta is anterior to the inferior vena cava.

For development of the plane between the aorta and the inferior vena and the aorta, blunt dissection is the proper way to approach because of the fragile wall of the inferior vena cava. Using the blunt scissors closed, try, with repeated movements, to create a 'window' and enter between the two vessels. If necessary, your dissection should be performed at the expense of the aortic wall. The 'window' in the connective tissue between the vessels is extended on either direction, cephalad and caudal, with repeated movements.

➢ Pay extreme attention not to traumatize the inferior vena cava. If the inferior vena ruptures, especially in an area not perfectly dissected and with a poor view, then the hemorrhage will be massive and the result likely fatal for the small animal. If this happens, place immediately, even blindly, a single vascular clamp caudal to the rupture and another cranial to it. When you manage to stop the bleeding, clean the blood and irrigate the field with normal saline under pressure to try and find the rupture. Repair the laceration with a running 10/0 suture. Of course, after repair, this area is no longer suitable for anastomosis, and you will have to extend your dissection.
The author remembers very well the first time he inadvertently opened the inferior vena cava, despite the many years that have passed since then. He also remembers his satisfaction after he managed, with agony, to save the near-fatal situation following his mistake. You will almost certainly come across similar ranges of emotions in your microsurgical career.

After the inferior vena cava has been fully dissected between the renal veins, dissection may be extended caudally for better mobilization of the inferior vena cava. During this process, lumbar tributary veins will be encountered. They should be dissected, cleaned, double ligated with 9/0 suture, and divided between the ligations. The use of diathermy is very risky on these veins.

The wall of the inferior vena cava must be totally stripped of remnants of peritoneum, fat, or connective tissue. This cleaning must be done as bluntly as possible, using broader anatomical forceps or a small cotton wool stick moistured in normal saline. The cleaner the wall of the inferior vena cava is, especially anteriorly, the easier the anastomosis with the portal vein.

When the inferior vena cava is fully dissected and cleaned, a yellow plastic background is placed underneath it, in the space between the confluence of the renal veins (**Fig. 16-4**).

E. Microsurgical dissection of the portal vein

The microsurgical dissection of the portal vein is more complicated and difficult. Near the hilum of the liver, the portal vein should be separated from the hepatic artery. This dissection is difficult, because the outer layers of the vessels are closely attached to each other as they course in the hepatoduodenal ligament towards the hilum of the liver. Additionally, the gastroduodenal artery may be encountered in the inferior part of the ligament; this artery is small and not easily visualized.

The dissection of the portal vein is performed with both a straight and a curved atraumatic forceps. Using the the straight forceps the portal vein is pulled caudally and to the left, while the curved forceps is used to free it from the hepatic artery. The same maneuver should be used for the gastroduodenal artery if it is encountered. Attention is needed during this dissection as these arteries are easily traumatized and can spasm. If this happens to the hepatic artery, blood supply to the liver will be disturbed. Moreover, given the significant contribution of the portal vein to the blood supply of the liver, the straight forceps that pulls the portal vein, if it obstructs its lumen, should also be removed periodically during this part of the dissection.

As the dissection of the portal vein is progressed distally, the pancreas will be encountered. While stripping the portal vein of fat or connective tissue, the pancreatic tissue may erroneously be perceived as fat or connective tissue given its gelatinous nature, and small pancreatic pieces may be excised in the attempt to clean the portal vein from fat. The small hemorrhage that will occur from inadvertantly removing pancreatic tissue may mistakenly be attributed to trauma of adipose tissue vessels. A piece of advice on how to avoid the gross mistake of removing pieces of pancreatic tissue is to continue your dissection staying strictly on the wall of the portal vein. The pancreas should be gently detached and pushed posteriorly from the posterolateral surfaces of the vein. There should be minimal problems along the anterior surface of the portal vein as the opening of the retroperitoneum should have provided an adequate exposure.

The gastroduodenal vein appears to perpendicularly enter the portal vein at the cranial side of the lumen (**Fig. 16-4**). Similarly to the portal vein, the gastroduodenal vein seems to course 'through' the pancreas. Despite the fact that the space between the pancreas and the final part of the gastroduodenal vein is very narrow, the vein should be dissected, double ligated with 9/0 suture and transected between the ligatures. Cauterization of this vein is too risky.

It is important to continue the dissection of the portal vein as distally as possible in order to obtain enough length for the portal vein to be mobilized caudally and anastomosed with the inferior vena cava. The dissection should continue until the splenic vein is reached (No 3, **Fig. 16-8**).

F. Microsurgical dissection and occlusion of the aorta cranial to the celiac artery (optional)

The goal of this exposure of the aorta, which is not associated with the dissection for the portocaval anastomosis, is to create a 'window' so that a single vascular clamp can be applied on the aorta, cranial to the origin of the celiac artery. This proximal occlusion of the aorta is done to prevent congestion of the splanchnic vasculature that will occur following obstruction of the portal vein.

➢ Proximal clamping of the aorta is not routinely performed in the portocaval anastomosis; this maneuver is not necessary when the microsurgeon is experienced enough to perform the portocaval anastomosis while occluding the portal vein for less than 10 minutes

Note that in this Chapter, 30 minutes of portal vein occlusion are generously allowed to the trainne; nevertheless, occlusion of the aorta is not performed. The surgeon, however, should know how and why to perform this maneuver. If kept in place for too long, proximal clamping of the aorta (cranial to the origin of the renal arteries) can have serious consequences in the blood supply of the kidneys, and, theoretically, of the lower limbs. For these reasons, this maneuver cannot be performed for an extended period of time.

Of course, to access the aorta at this height, rearrangement of the surgical field will be required. The stomach should be rotated cranially and the retroperitoneum opened with gauzes cranial to the celiac artery.

Cranially to the origin of the celiac artery, the aorta runs posteriorly to the inferior vena cava. The aorta should be grasped and gently pulled up by the adventitia, and with blunt dissection a window of 5 mm width will be created behind the vessel to provide space for placement of the vascular clamp.

In order to avoid congestion of the splanchnic vasculature of the abdomen without the consequences of the proximal occlusion of the aorta, the surgeon could selectively occlude the celiac artery and the superior and inferior mesenteric arteries. Of course, broader preparation and dissection are needed to even locate and identify each of these branches. In principle, however, this might be the best solution.

G. Placement of the double vascular clamp on the inferior vena cava – Incision - Irrigation

The inferior vena cava should be lifted to allow the double vascular clamp to be applied to the vessel such that the two clamps are placed *between the confluences of the renal veins*. The distal clamp should be placed cranially to the confluence of the left renal vein, and the proximal clamp should be placed caudally to the confluence of the right renal vein, which is found higher (**Fig. 16-5**).

After the double vascular clamp has been placed, the anterior wall of the inferior vena cava should be lifted gently with a Dumont forceps. A transverse incision is then performed with sharp microsurgical scissors (see details in Chapter 6). Irrigation of the lumen of the vein follows using a syringe with a 27G angiocatheter attached to it (**Fig. 16-6**).

H. Proximal ligation of the portal vein - Distal single clamp placement - Transection - Irrigation

A proximal ligation using 9/0 suture should be placed on the portal vein, as close as possible to the hilum of

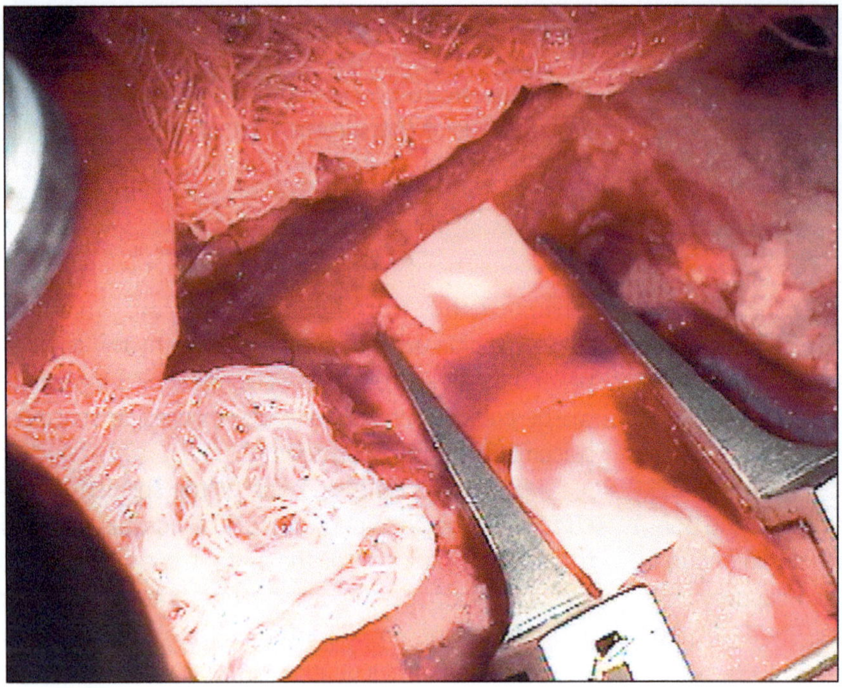

Figure 16-5

Placement of the double vascular clamp on the inferior vena cava between the confluence of the left renal vein, which is located caudally, and the confluence of the right renal vein, which is located cranially (see Nos. 3 and 4, **Fig. 16-4**). (From author's photo library)

the liver (**Fig. 16-7**). Immediately after that, a single clamp is applied on the portal vein as distal as possible, past the transected gastroduodenal vein (**Fig. 16-8**).

Transection of the portal vein should be performed as close to its ligation as possible, thus ensuring enough length for the stump to reach the site of transverse incision on the inferior vena cava. Before transecting the portal vein, make sure that the length available is sufficient. If not, release and move the single clamp distally as there should be room until the splenic vein is reached. Any additional dissection of the portal vein that is required must be quick, since the portal vein has already been ligated and a risk of thrombosis is present. Again, remember that the total time that the portal vein

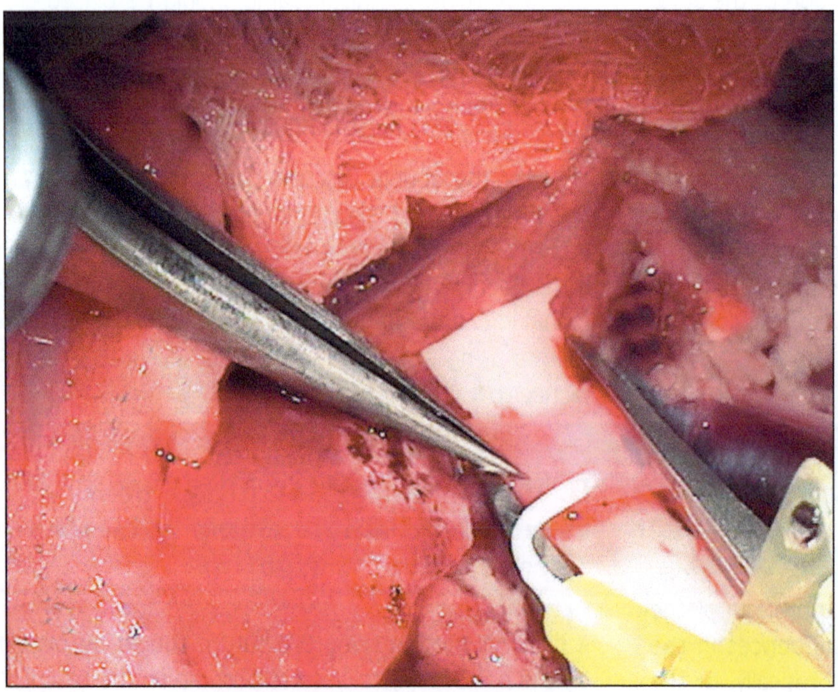

Figure 16-6

Irrigation of the inferior vena cava through the opening of the transverse incision. The Dumont No. 3 forceps lifts the anterior wall to open the lumen. Injection is done under pressure—the angiocatheter is passed just into the opening so that the lumen is not traumatized. Note the traumas on the surface of the right lobe of the liver, which (wrongly) here is not rotated with a retractor. (From author's photo library)

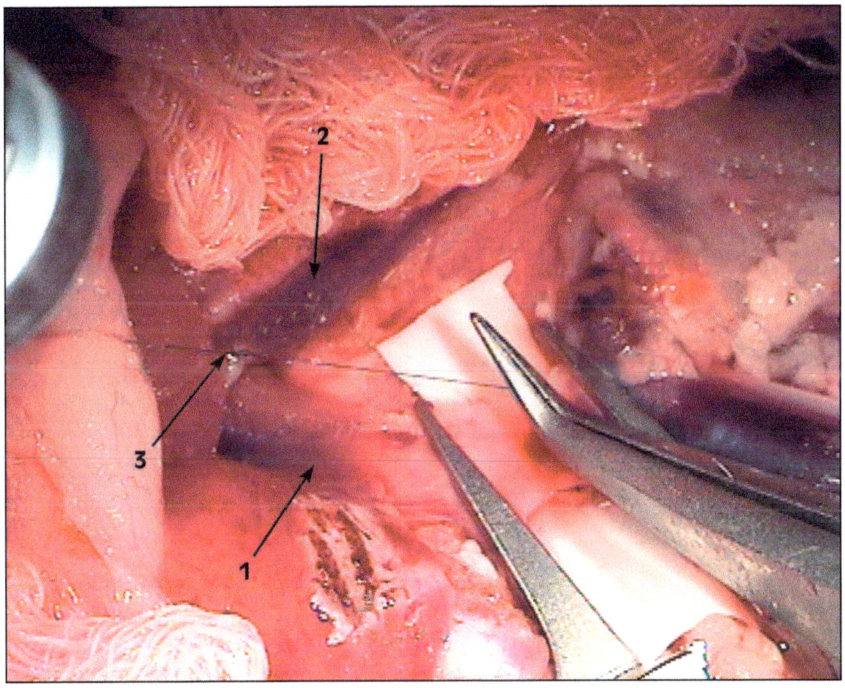

Figure 16-7

Ligation of the portal vein with 9/0 suture, close to the hilum of the liver. **1.** inferior vena cava, **2.** portal vein, **3.** descent of the 2nd knot. (From author's photo library)

is occluded in this operation should not exceed 30 minutes.

To perform the transection, the microsurgical scissors should be placed perpendicular to the long axis of the vessel, 2-3 mm before the ligation of the portal vein. The cut is done with one clean movement to prevent any debris in the lumen that will be involved in the portocaval anastomosis (**Fig. 16-9**). The suture of the ligation on the proximal stump of the gastroduodenal vein may be used to maneuver the portal vein; however, it can slip from the stump, so avoid pulling hard.

Irrigation of the portal vein follows with warm normal saline injected with pressure from a 27G angiocatheter attached to a syringe.

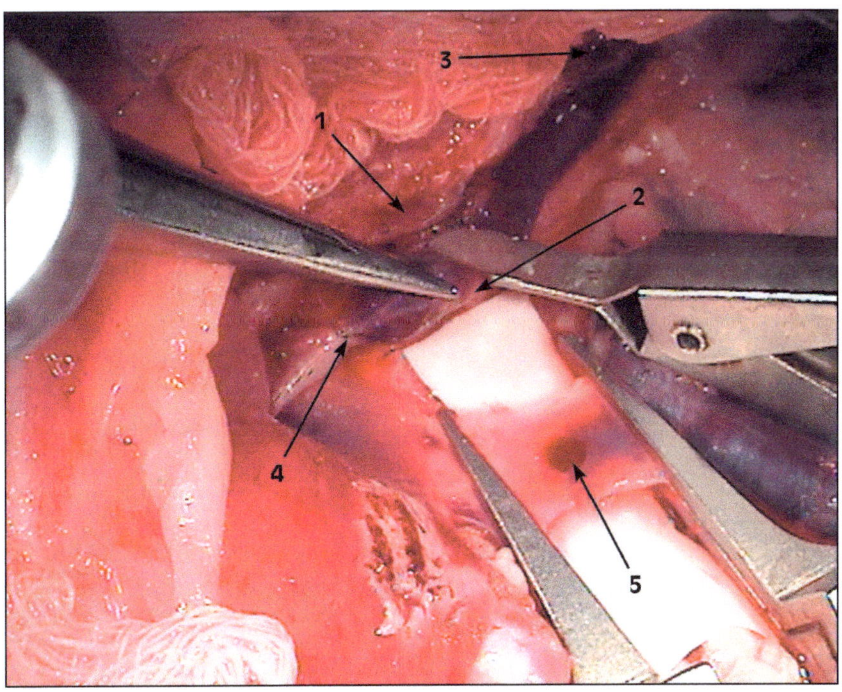

Figure 16-8

Placement of the single clamp distally on the portal vein. The Dumont No. 3 forceps holds the suture around the proximal stump of the gastroduodenal vein. **1.** distal stump of the gastroduodenal vein (toward the pancreas), **2.** proximal stump of the gastroduodenal vein (on the portal vein), **3.** splenic vein, **4.** ligation of the portal vein near the hilum of the liver, **5.** opening of the transverse incision of the inferior vena cava. (From author's photo library)

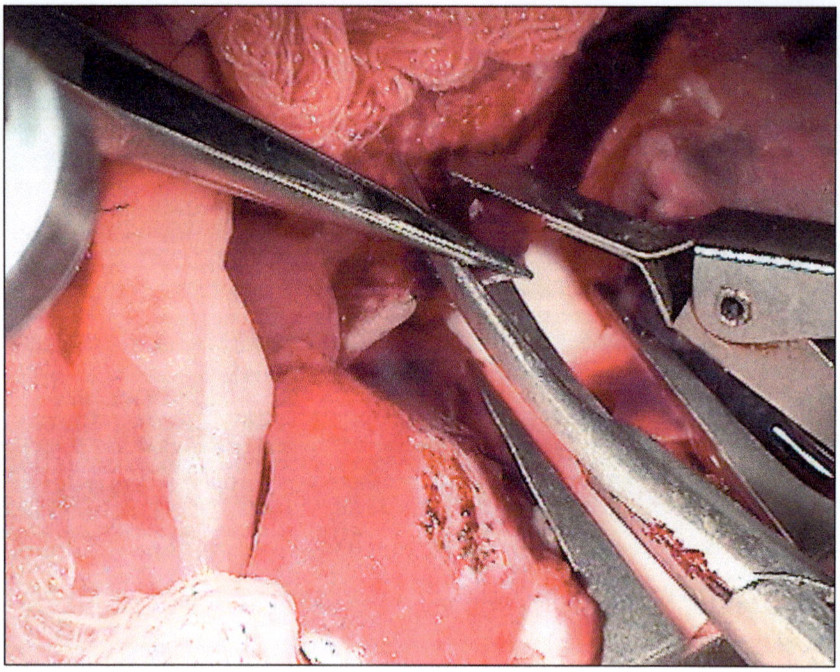

Figure 16-9

Transection of the portal vein at a distance of 2-3 mm from the ligation placed near the hilum of the liver. The single vascular clamp has already been applied distally. The scissors are brought perpendicular to the vessel, and the portal vein is cut with one clean movement. The Dumont No. 3 forceps holds the suture of the ligation on the stump of the gastroduodenal vein in order to maneuver the portal vein. (From author's photo library)

I. End-to-side anastomosis

The reader is invited to read the technique of the end-to-side anastomosis for the case where the end-anastomosed vessel cannot be rotated, as described in detail in Chapter 6.2.I (see ***Figures 6-7 C and D****).*

- ➢ The anastomosis will be performed with **10 or 12 sutures 10/0.**

The steps of the process of the end-to-side portocaval anastomosis, given that the portal vein cannot be rotated, are as follows:

1. The anastomosis starts with placement of the 1st suture in the middle of the posterior surface. The suture passes the wall of the portal vein from external to internal, and then the wall of the inferior vena cava from internal to external, resulting in the placement

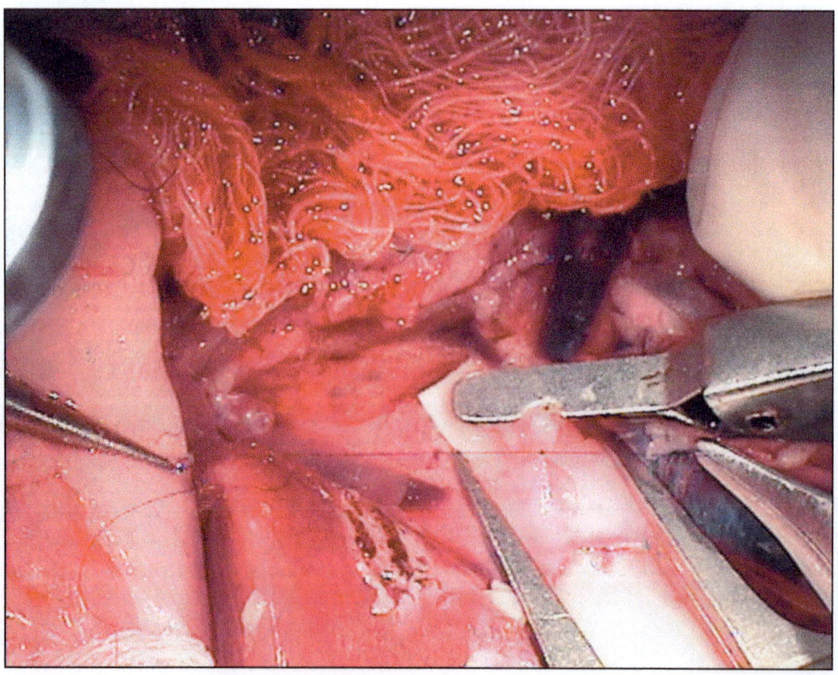

Figure 16-10

Placement of the first suture in the portocaval anastomosis. Since the portal vein cannot be rotated, the first suture is placed in the middle of the posterior surface of the anastomosis. (From author's photo library)

Figure 16-11

Complete portocaval anastomosis. (From author's photo library)

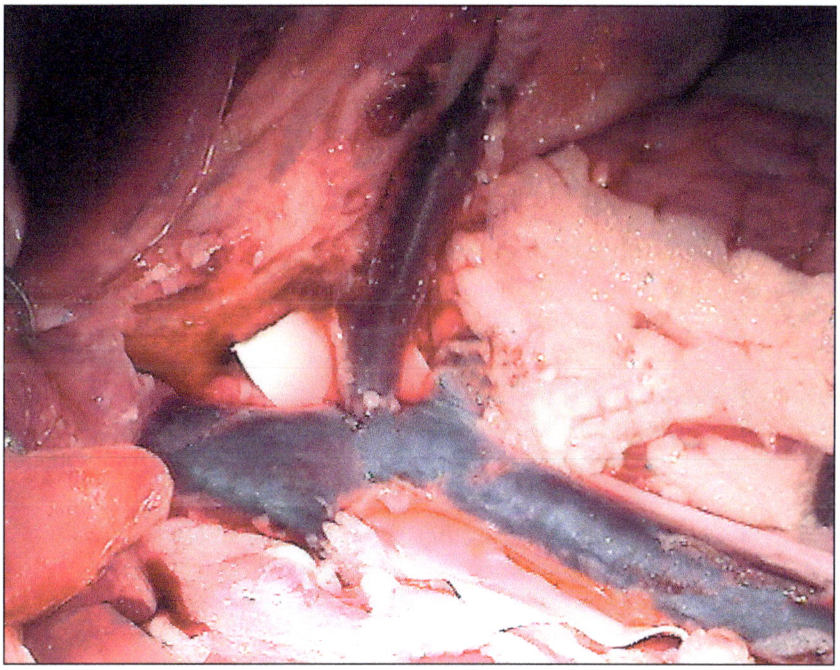

of knot outside the lumen (**Fig. 16-10**). The rest of the sutures of the posterior surface are placed at equal distances, on either side. According to the total number of sutures, corner sutures may or may not be placed, as described in Chapter 6. We continue in the anterior surface by similarly placing sutures at equal distances; the last suture will placed in its middle.

2. The clamps are released, first the double clamp from the inferior vena cava, then the single clamp from the portal vein. **Figure 16-11** shows the complete portocaval anastomosis.
3. Placement of a wet gauze on the anastomosis for 3 minutes.

   Patency test. The reader is refered to Chapter 6.9.2 (**Fig. 6-10**) for a detailed description. In brief, two forceps are applied on the inferior vena cava and move half-closed in opposite directions, away from the anastomosis, and close; this maneuver empties the lumen. Then, they are brought closer to each other with a quick movement and if there is patency, the lumen between the forceps fills immediately. Of course the space of opposite movements of the two forceps is resticted by the exits of the renal veins (see **Figure 16-11**). If the forcpes surpass the confluene of the renal veins, it is evident that the inferior vena cava will be filled by renal vein blood and the patency test cannot be performed, unless a signle vascular clamp is applied on each renal vein to obstruct it.
4. Removal of the yellow background.

J. Closure of surgical trauma

After the splanchna have returned in the abdomen, the abdominal wall is closed in two layers (muscles, and subcutaneous tissue/skin) with interrupted 2/0 non-absorbable sutures.

Synopsis...

... of end-to-side anastomosis of the portal vein to the inferior vena cava

Attention

➤ ***Anesthesia must be delivered with ether mask only***

➤ ***The duration of occlusion of the portal vein must be less than 30 minutes***

A. **Position of the rat:** Laid on its back, left to right of the surgeon (head on the surgeon's left). The limbs are immobilized on the working surface with adhesive tape.

B. **Anesthesia:** Make an ether mask with gauze moistened in ether placed in the bottom of a syringe. Be wary of the risk of ether overdose.

C. **Preparation of the surgical field:** Median incision, from the xiphoid process to the pubic symphysis. Paper clip retractors are placed at the edges of the incision. The small intestine is mobilized, and all intestines (cecum, transverse colon, small intestine) are packed in a wet gauze, and placed to *the left* of the rat. The middle and right lobes of the liver are rotated cephalad and packed with another retractor. The retroperitoneum is opened with two wet gauzes.

D. **Microsurgical dissection of the inferior vena cava:** The inferior vena cava is fully dissected between the left and right renal veins (the confluence of the left renal vein is located more caudally than the right). A 'window' is created with blunt dissection between the inferior vena cava and the aorta (which is posterior to the inferior vena cava at this level). The inferior vena cava is stripped of fat; lumbar veins are transected between two ligations. A yellow plastic background is put under the vessel.

E. **Microsurgical dissection of the portal vein:** Dissection of the portal vein, separation from the hepatic artery, double ligation and transection of the gastroduodenal vein. Separation of the portal vein from the pancreas continues up to the splenic vein.

F. **Microsurgical dissection and occlusion of the aorta cranial to the celiac artery (optional):** opening of a 'window' between the inferior vena cava and the aorta, placement of a single clamp on the aorta in order to prevent congestion of splanchna following obstruction of the portal vein.

G. **Placement of the double clamp on the inferior vena cava between the confluences of the renal veins - Transverse incision - Irrigation of the lumen.**

H. **Proximal ligation of the portal vein - Distal single clamp placement - Transection - Irrigation:** The portal vein is ligated with a 9/0 suture as close as possible to the hilum of the liver, and the single clamp is placed close to the splenic vein. The transection is performed 2-3 mm from the central ligation.

I. **End-to-side anastomosis: 10 or 12 10/0 sutures**

The portal vein cannot be rotated.

1. The first suture is placed in the middle of the posterior surface, and the rest of the sutures at equal distances on either side until the middle of the anterior surface.

... of end-to-side anastomosis of the portal vein to the inferior vena cava

Synopsis...

2. The vessels are released from the clamps (first the double clamp from the inferior vena cava, then the single clamp from the portal vein).
3. Placement of a wet gauze on the anastomosis for 3 minutes.
4. Patency test.
5. Removal of the yellow background.

J. **Closure of surgical trauma:** the abdominal wall is closed in two layers (muscles, and subcutaneous tissue/skin) with interrupted non-absorbable 2/0 sutures.

17 Anastomosis of the sciatic nerve & Grafting of the sciatic nerve

Microsurgical suturing technique for nerves and the relevant nerve microanatomy are described in detail in Chapter 7.

I. ANASTOMOSIS OF THE SCIATIC NERVE

A. Positioning the rat

The rat is placed in ventral decubitus position on the working surface, with the head away from the surgeon. Two folded gauze pads are placed on the dorsal surface of the rat under the inguinal crease of the operative leg (**Fig. 17-1**). Finally, the limbs of the rat are immobilized on the working surface with adhesive tape.

B. Preparation of the surgical field and microsurgical dissection of the sciatic nerve

A transverse incision, 4 cm in length, is performed in the middle of the thigh (**Fig 17-1**). The superficial fascia is dissected. The superficial fascia in the thigh, similar to that of the anterior abdominal wall, includes a superficial fatty and a deep membranous layer. In the thigh, this deep membranous layer attaches to the investing fascia of the underlying muscles.

Using small surgcical forceps and Metzenbaum scissors, a plane of separation is developed between the tensor fasciae latae muscle and the biceps femoris muscle (**Fig. 17-2**). These muscles are then separated with a retractor placed on the tensor fasciae latae muscle, revealing the sciatic nerve in the surgical field (**Fig. 17-3**). Ensure adequate exposure to fully dissect 1 cm of nerve from the investing fasciae of the surrounding muscles (neurolysis). Then, a yellow plastic background is placed under the nerve (**Fig. 17-4**). During the dissection of the nerve, the surgical field is regularly irrigated with xylocaine solution 2%. Irrigation with normal saline (as performed in all other operations in this book) can not be used due to the edema its use causes in nerves.

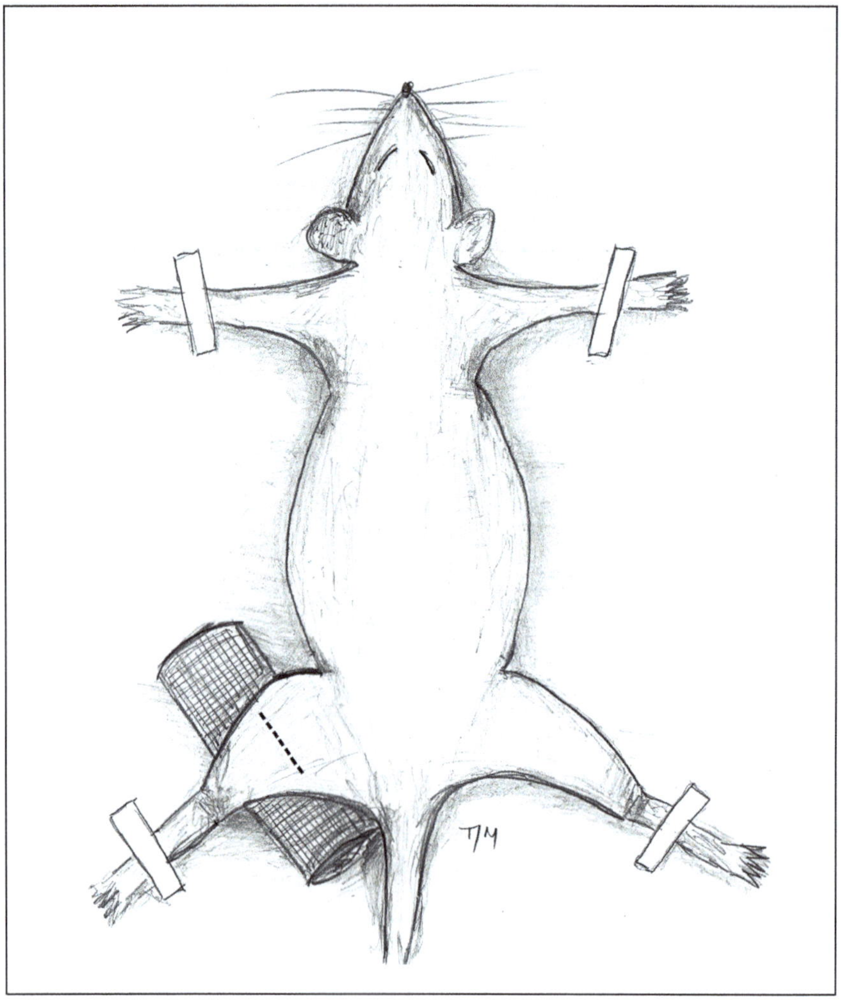

Figure 17-1

Positioning the rat for anastomosis of the sciatic nerve (or grafting the sciatic nerve). Two folded gauzes are placed under the leg. A transverse incision is performed in the mid-thigh (dashed-line). (Drawing by the author)

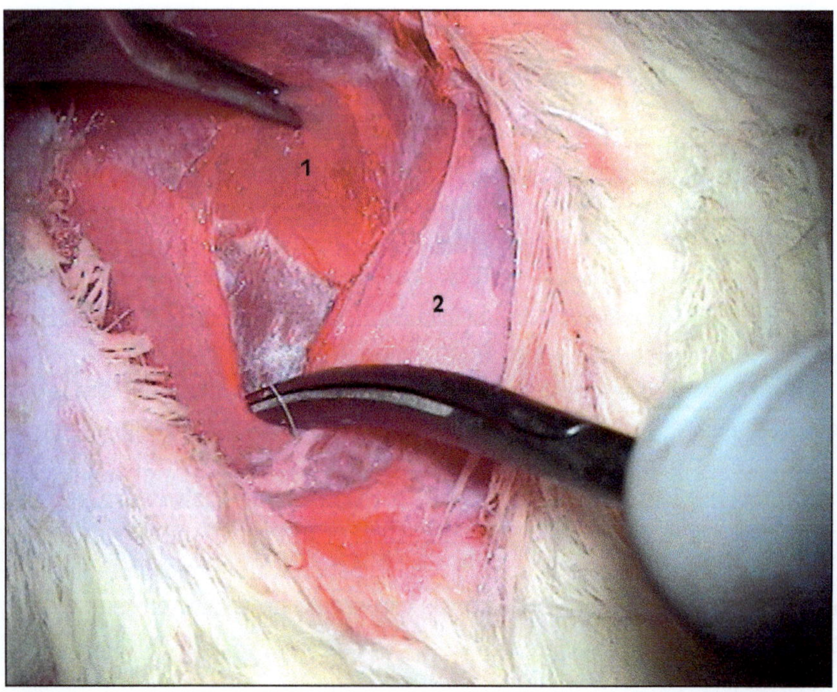

Figure 17-2

Development of the plane of separation between the biceps femoris muscle **(1)** and the tensor fasciae latae muscle **(2)**. (From author's photo library)

Figure 17-3

The sciatic nerve (arrowhead) is revealed and lifted by a Dumont forceps. (From author's photo library)

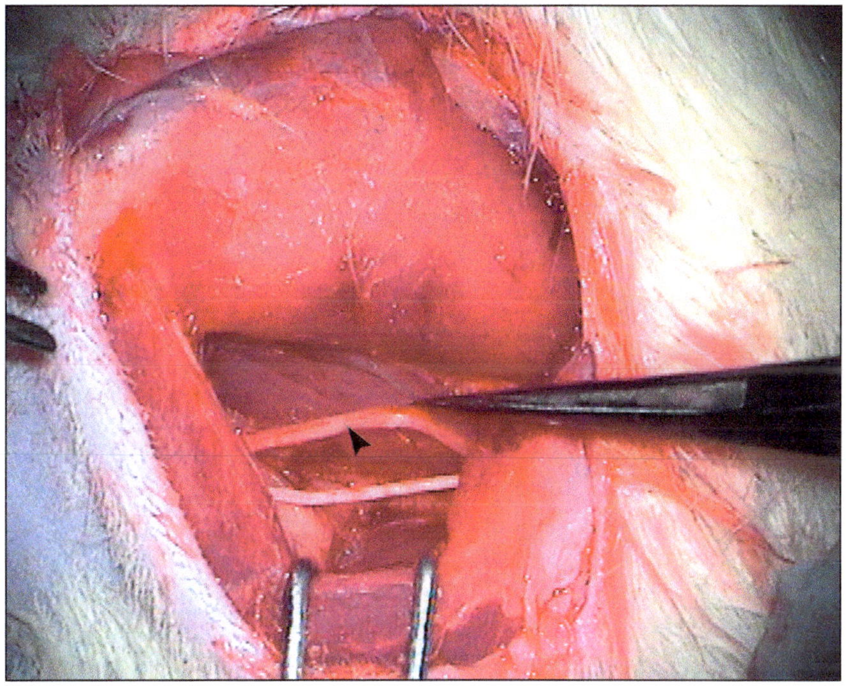

C. Transection of the sciatic nerve

The nerve is held using Dumont No. 5 forceps and scissors are brought perpendicular to the nerve. The transection is performed with a single movement, ensuring a 'clean' cut of the nerve. After transection, the two stumps of the nerve retract along the longitudinal axis and seperation of the nerve edges occurs (**Fig. 17-5**).

D. Microsurgical dissection of the epi-perineurium

For a detailed review of the microanatomy of nerves, refer to Chapter 7.

In the rat, the sciatic nerve is comprised of a single bundle of axons. The epineurium (the outer covering of the nerve) is in direct contact with the perineurium (the

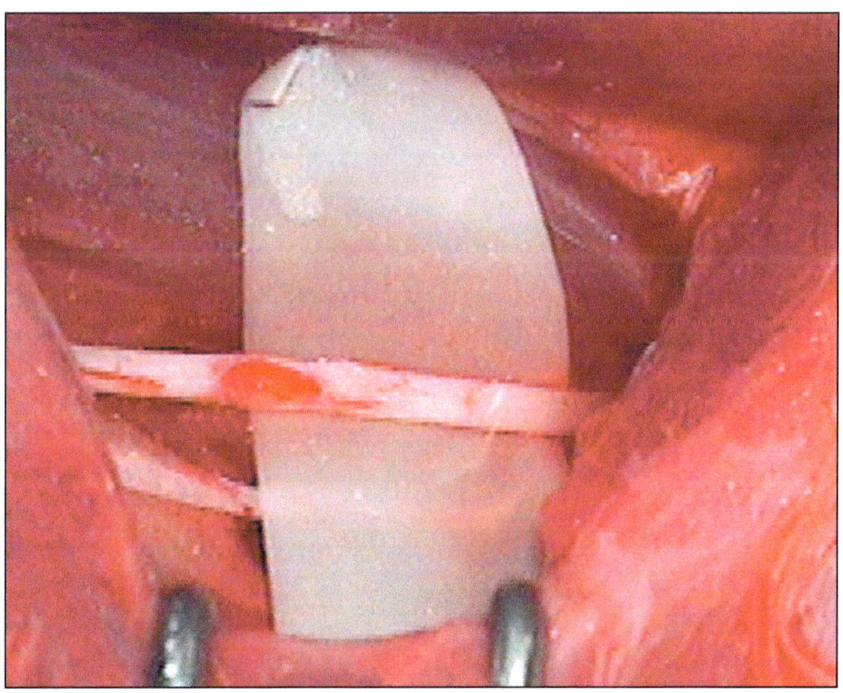

Figure 17-4

The sciatic nerve isolated on a yellow plastic background. (From author's photo library)

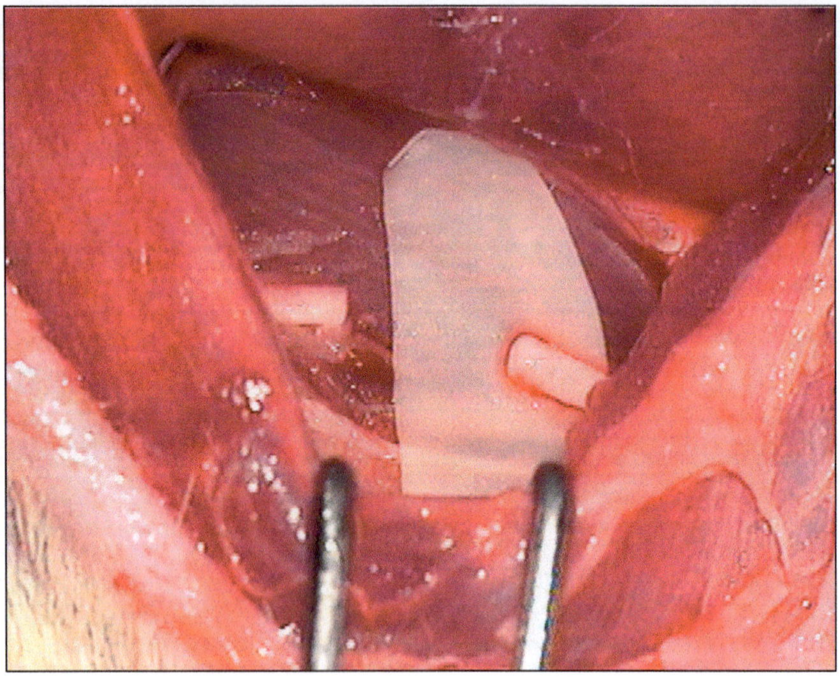

Figure 17-5

The stumps of the sciatic nerve retract after transection of the nerve. (From author's photo library)

covering of the nerve bundle) and the two appear to exist as a single outer covering of the nerve. After transection of the nerve, the nerve fibers may spontaneously exceed the border of the cut and 'overflow' (analogous to toothpaste as it is extruted from its tube, as mentioned in Chapter 7).

The sciatic nerve is embedded in the investing fasciae of the muscles (deep fascia). Using two microsurgical forceps, Dumont No. 3 and No. 5, the epineurium is meticulously dissected. Any vestigies of muscle investing fascia adhering to the nerve should be detached from the fibrous epineurium (**Fig. 17-6**). This dissection should be performed gently so that the nerve fibers contained within the epi-perineurium retain their pristine edge. If the fibers overflow, the borders of the edge of the nerve stumps are lost and suturing becomes extremely difficult. In such a case, the sciatic nerve may be transected again at a distance of 1 to 2 mm from

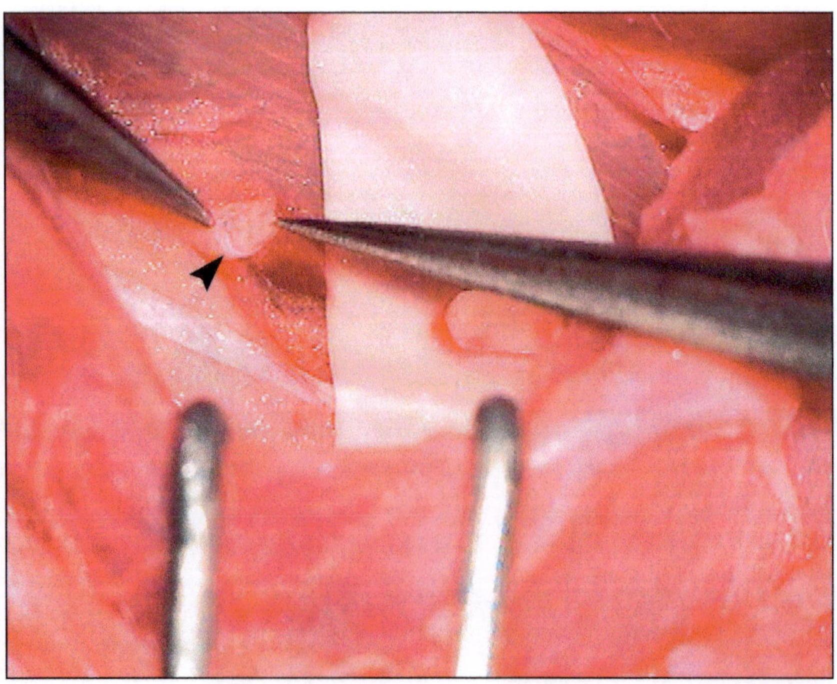

Figure 17-6

Dissection of the epineurium of the sciatic nerve with two forceps (Dumont No. 3 and No. 5). The sciatic nerve of the rat is comprised of a single bundle of nerve fibers, causing the epineurium to be internally fused with the single perineurum in one layer (arrow). Observe the gelatinous consistency of the nerve fibers, which are ready to outflow from the epi-perineurim. (From author's photo library) the damaged edge to create a new pristine edge for suturing. Avoid cutting too far from the nerve edge as there are limits to the elastictity of the nerve along the longitudinal axis. Repeated cutting of the nerve, or cutting too far from the edge, may necessitate nerve grafting. For instance, in the adult human, a gap of 2 cm can be sutured while gaps between 2 and 4 cm are more tenuous. Any gap greater than 4 cm must have a nerve graft placed for repair. It is also important to remember that nerve anastomoses should never be performed under tension.

E. End-to-end anastomosis of the nerve

The anastomosis will be performed with **9/0 sutures** placed on the epi-perineurium (**Fig. 17-7A**). Care should be taken to prevent torsion of the nerve after the anastomosis by maintaing the correct orientation of the nerve ends during the procedure. As discussed in Chapter 7, alignment can be obtained by following the course of the vasa nervorum on the epineurium (see **Figure 7-1**).

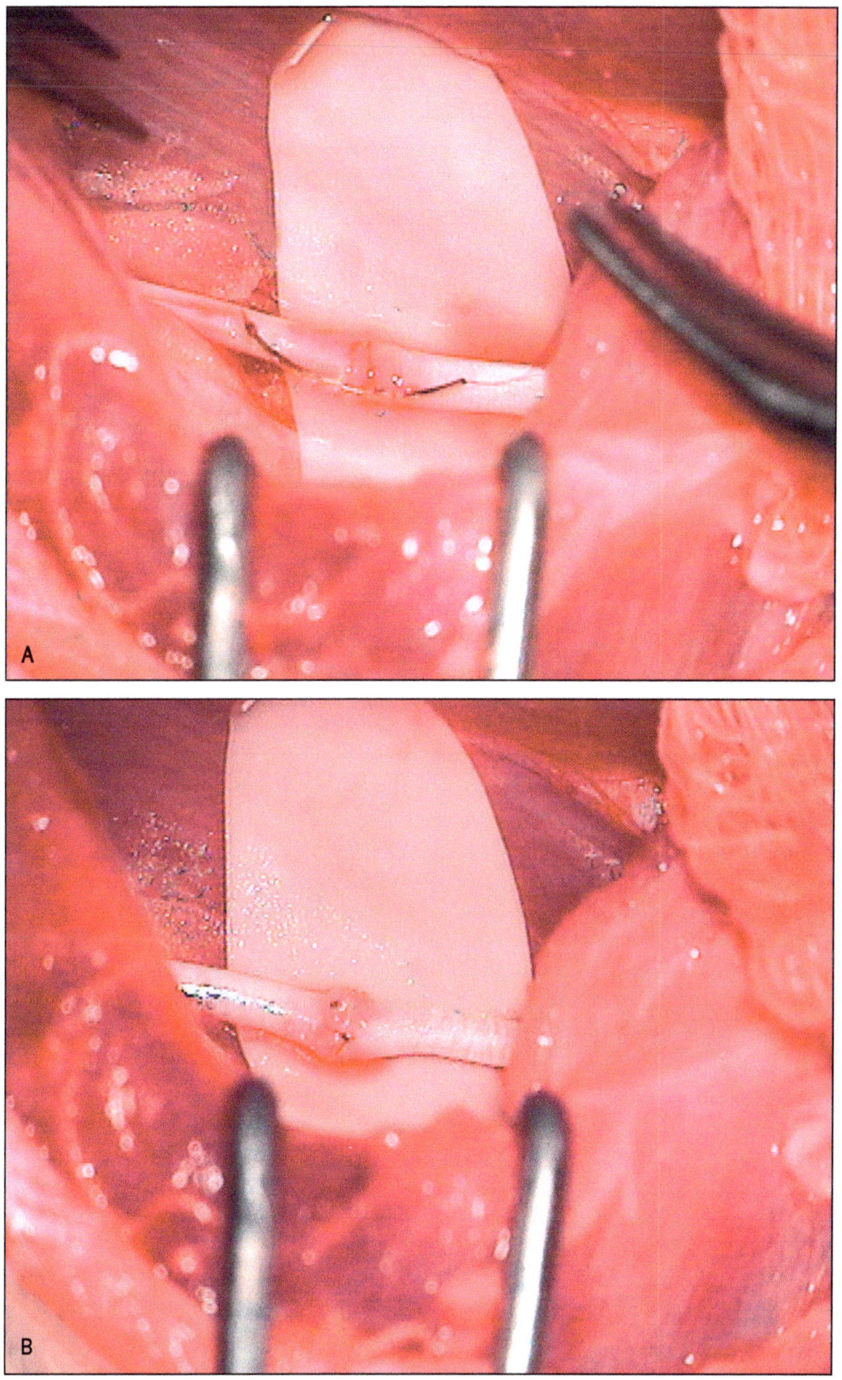

Figure 17-7

Suturing of the epi-perineurium, **A.** The needle of a 9/0 suture is seen passing through the epi-perineurium at 6 o'-clock; a suture at the 12 o'clock position has been placed previously. **B.** End-to-end anastomosis using 2 interrupted sutures. Notice the protrusion of the nerve fibers from the edges of the approximated stumps on the anterior surface of the nerve. To prevent this, placement of 4 sutures is recommended. (From author's photo library)

Other texts suggest **2 sutures** are enough to bring the nerve fibers into contact, however, since the jelly nerve fibers protrude through the gaps when end-to-end anastomoses are completed using two sutures placed 180° apart (**Figure 17-7B**), it is the author's opinion that **4 sutures** should be used to prevent this. After the placement of the initial two sutures at 12 and 6 o'clock, two additional sutures are placed, first at 3 o'clock (middle of the anterior surface), then at 9 o'clock (middle of the posterior surface).No vascular clamp is applied and the nerve remains free to rotate around the longitudinal axis, making placement of these additional sutures straightforward.

F. Closure of the surgical trauma

Upon completion, the skin and the superficial fascia are closed in a single layer using interrupted, non absorbable 2/0 sutures.

II. GRAFTING OF THE SCIATIC NERVE

A. Positioning the rat

The rat is positioned in the same manner as described in section I.A with the addition of two rolled gauze pads placed under the contralateral inguinal crease.

B. Preparation of the bilateral surgical fields and microsurgical dissection of the sciatic nerves

The graft will be taken from the contralateral sciatic nerve, which must be exposed. Therefore, the preparation of the surgical field and the microsurgical dissection of the sciatic nerve is performed on both posterior limbs, as described in section I.B.

C. Harvesting the nerve graft from one side

At least 1 cm of nerve is harvested from the donor nerve and placed adjacent to the contralateral sciatic nerve recipent site where it will be anastomsed (**Fig. 17-8**). **Ensure the correct direction and orientation** of the nerve graft is maintained during transfer from donor site to recipent site.

D. Transection of the contralateral sciatic nerve

As described in section I.C.

E. Microsurgical dissection of the epi-perineurium of the contralateral sciatic nerve

As described in section I.D.

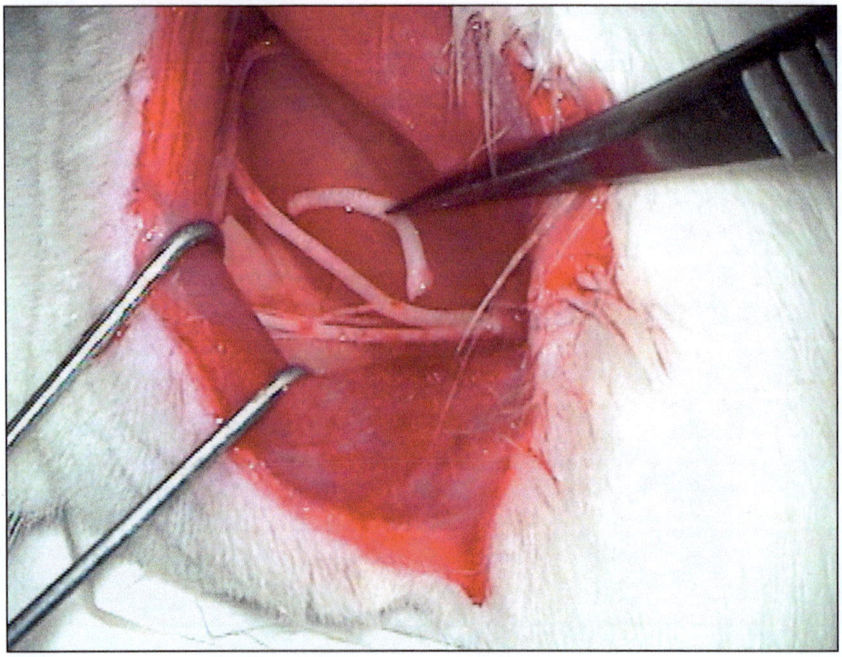

Figure 17-8

Transfer of the nerve graft. The graft is lifted from the donor site by grasping the epineurium with a Dumont No. 5 forceps and transferred to the contralateral recipient site. The correct direction and orientation of the nerve graft must be maintained during the transfer (From author's photo library)

F. Positioning of the graft and end-to-end anastomoses

The graft is aligned with the stumps of the transected sciatic nerve. Each edge of the graft is anastomosed with the ipsilateral edge of the stump of the sciatic nerve. On each anastomosis **2, or better 4, sutures 9/0** are placed (**Fig. 17-9**). The 12 o'clock sutures are placed first in both anastomoses, followed by the 6 o'clock sutures. Placing the sutures in this order helps maintain proper orientation of the graft and prevents torsion. If four sutures are being placed, the additional sutures are placed at the 3 o'clock and 9 o'clock positions in each anastomosis (see details in Chapter 7).

G. Closure of the surgical trauma

As described in section I.F.

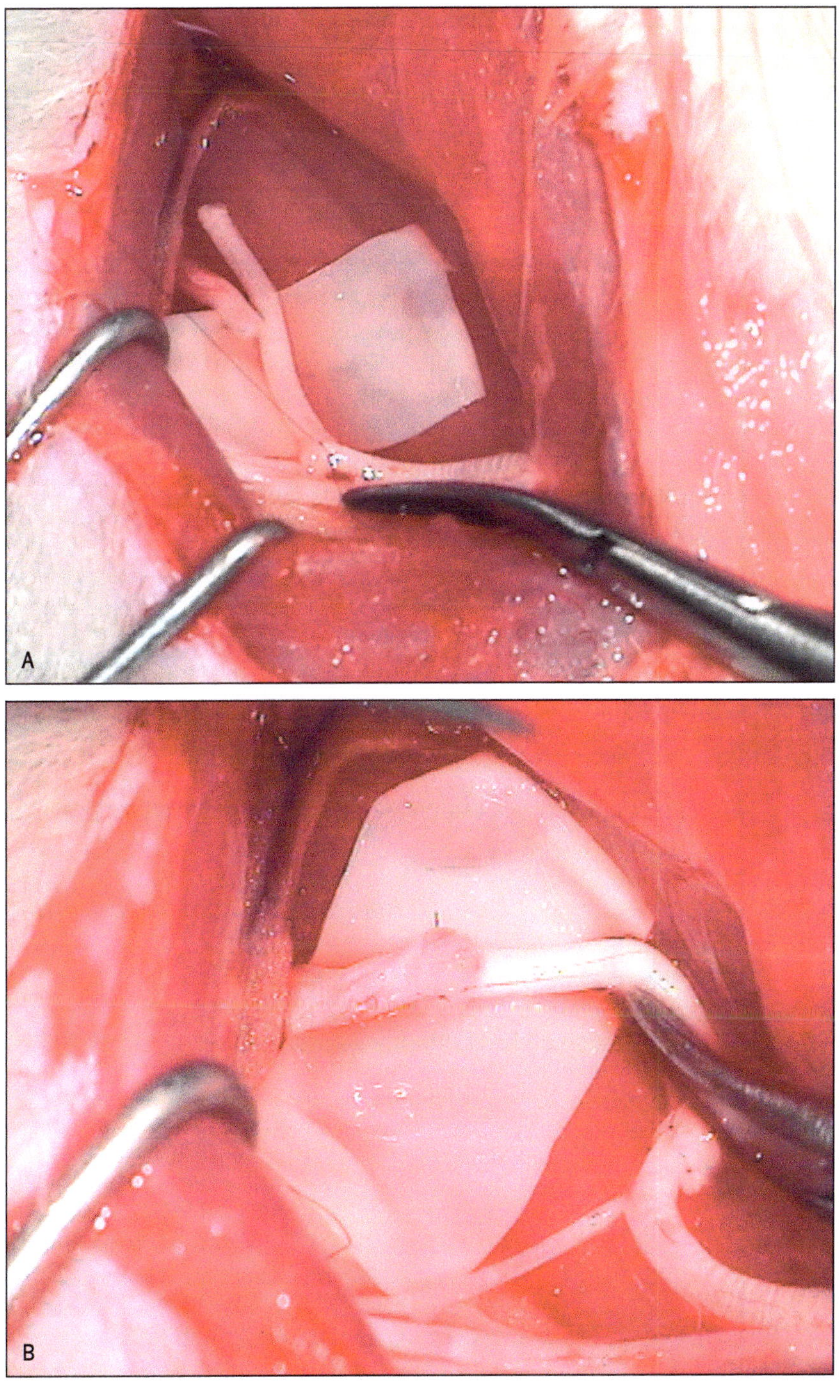

Figure 17-9

Suturing the sciatic nerve graft. **A.** Placement of the 1st suture at 12 o'clock position, caudally. **B.** The sutures at 12 o'clock and 6 o'clock have been placed on both anastomoses. Since nerve fibers are seen protruding from the gaps between sutures, two additional sutures should be added at the 3 o'clock and 9 o'clock positions. (From author's photo library)

... of anastomosis of the sciatic nerve & grafting of the sciatic nerve

Synopsis...

I. ANASTOMOSIS OF THE SCIATIC NERVE

A. **Positioning of the rat:** Ventral decubitus (prone) with the head away from the surgeon. Two folded gauze pads are placed under the inguinal crease of the posterior leg. The limbs are immobilized with adhesive tape.

B. **Preparation of the surgical field and microsurgical dissection of the sciatic nerve:** A transverse incision, 4 cm in length, is made in the middle of the thigh. The superficial fascia is dissected from the investing fascia of the underlying muscles. The tensor fasciae latae muscle is separated from the biceps femoris muscle, and a retractor is placed in the former. The sciatic nerve is revealed and 1 cm is dissected free of muscle fasciae. A yellow plastic background is placed under the nerve.

C. **Transection of the sciatic nerve:** The sciatic nerve is transected with one clean cut.

D. **Microsurgical dissection of the epi-perineurium** [the sciatic nerve of the rat is comprised of a single bundle of axons]: Any remaining investing muscle fascia is gently dissected from the fused epi-perineurium of the nerve.

E. **End-to-end anastomoses of the nerve: 4 sutures (9/0):** Sutures are placed on the epi-perineurium at 12 o'clock and 6 o'clock, followed by 3 o'clock and 9 o'clock.

F. **Closure of the surgical trauma:** The skin and superficial fascia are closed in a single layer with 2/0 interrupted, non-absorbable sutures.

II. GRAFTING OF THE SCIATIC NERVE

A. **Positioning of the rat:** As described in I.A. with the addition of two folded gauzes under the contralateral inguinal crease.

B. **Preparation of the bilateral surgical fields and microsurgical dissection of the sciatic nerves:** As described in I.B.

C. **Harvesting the nerve graft from one side:** A graft at least 1 cm in length is harvested from the donor site and transferred to the recipient site while maintaining the correct orientation and direction.

D. **Transection of the contralateral sciatic nerve:** As described in I.C.

E. **Microsurgical dissection of the epi-perineurium of the contralateral sciatic nerve:** As described in I.D.

F. **Positioning of the graft and end-to-end anastomoses:** 4 sutures (9/0) are placed in each anastomosis starting with the 12 o'clock sutures in both anastomoses, then the 6 o'clock sutures in both anastomoses, and finally the remaining 3 o'clock and 9 o'clock sutures in each anastomosis.

G. **Closure of the surgical trauma:** As described in I.F.

18

End-to-end anastomoses of the femoral vessels

Remember that the anastomoses will be performed using 11/0 suture.

A. Position of the rat

The rat is placed in dorsal decubitus (supine) position on the working surface. The long axis of the body of the rat is positioned perpendicular to the frontal plane of the surgeon's body with the rat's head directed away from the surgeon. The limbs of the rat are immobilized on the working surface with adhesive tape (**Fig. 18-1**).

B. Preparation of the surgical field

1. Necessary elements of surgical anatomy

Prior to dissection, the surgeon should be familiar with the branches of the femoral vessels that will be encountered in the surgical field, as depicted in **Figure 18-2**.

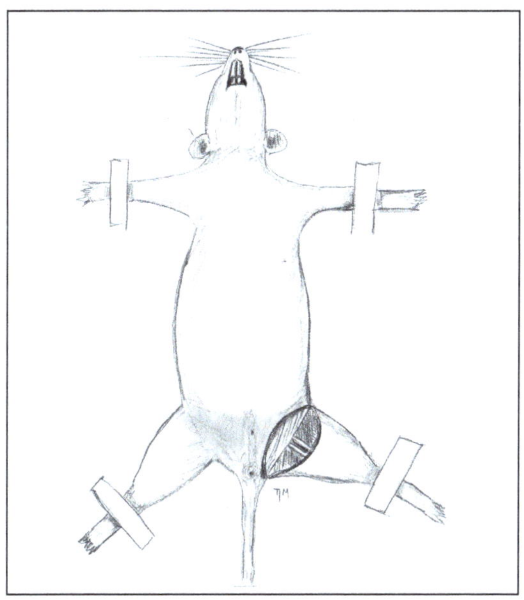

Figure 18-1

Positioning of the rat on the working surface. The incision has been made below the inguinal crease and the femoral vessels are seen in the surgical field. (Drawing by the author)

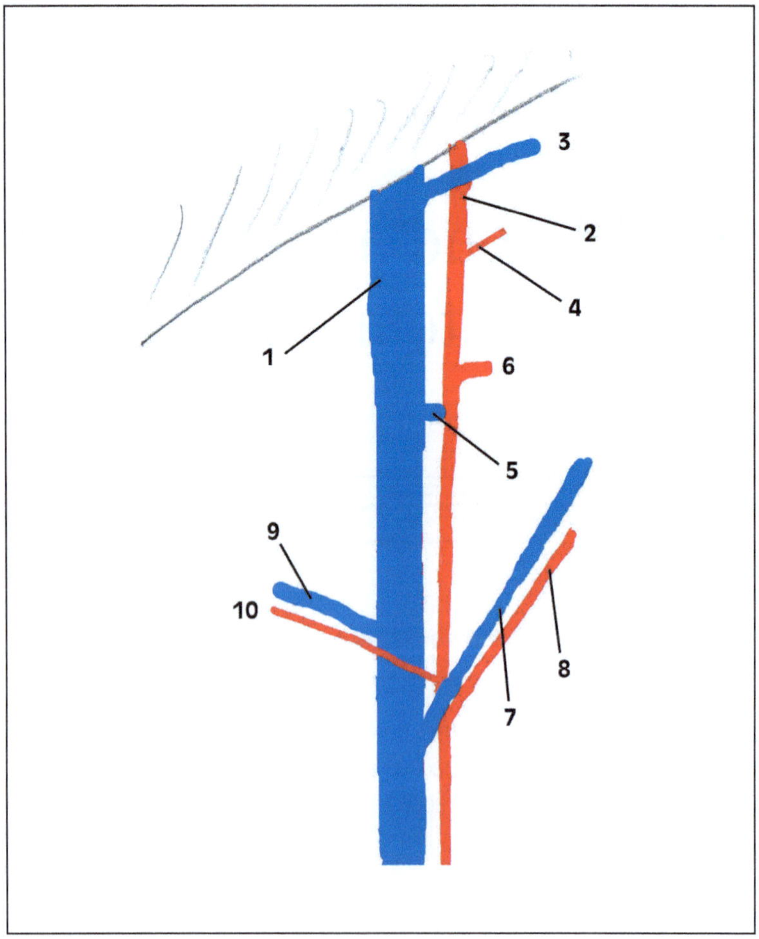

Figure 18-2

Diagrammatic representation of the branches of the femoral vessels encountered during the dissection of the femoral vessels, left side. Veins are shown in blue, arteries in red. **1.** femoral vein, **2.** femoral artery, **3.** superficial circumflex vein, **4.** arterial muscular branch, **5.** deep tributary of the femoral vein, **6.** deep branch of the femoral artery, **7.** superficial inferior epigastric vein, **8.** superficial inferior epigastric artery, **9.** vein from the adductor muscle, **10.** artery for the adductor muscle. (Diagram by the author)

The branches of the femoral artery and the tributaries of the femoral vein include vessels that are probably well known to the reader such as the superficial epigastric vessels and the superficial circumflex vein, as well as other less known that the reader will study here, such as the deep branch/tributary of the femoral artery/vein and muscular branches/tributaries of the artery and vein (for the adductor muscle and other muscles).

To appreciate the location and relationship of these branches, one must understand the surgical layers that contain these vessels:

- The superficial fascia, comprised of a superficial fatty layer and a deeper membranous layer, can be easily separated from the deep fascia. The fatty layer contains the 'superficial' vessels, i.e. the superficial circumflex vein and the superficial inferior epigastric vessels.
- The deep fascia is the fascia enveloping the muscles (investing fascia), which also surrounds the deeper vessels and forms a sheath around them. The femoral vessels along with the muscular branches feeding the adductor muscle and the saphenous vessels are enclosed within the deep fascia and can be seen through this transparent investing fascia.

Another two basic things are important: In general,

- In the vessel sheaths there is an artery, a vein and a nerve. Their arrangement, from medially to laterally, is 'VAN': vein, artery, nerve.
- The veins are in front of the arteries and are larger than the arteries.

2. Access to the femoral vessels

A 2 cm incision is made 1 cm below the inguinal crease (**Fig. 18-1**). The superficial fascia is dissected using fine surgical forceps and Baby-Metzenbaum scissors. A retractor is placed in the middle of the incision to bring the flap of skin and superficial fascia medially and upward (toward the abdomen).

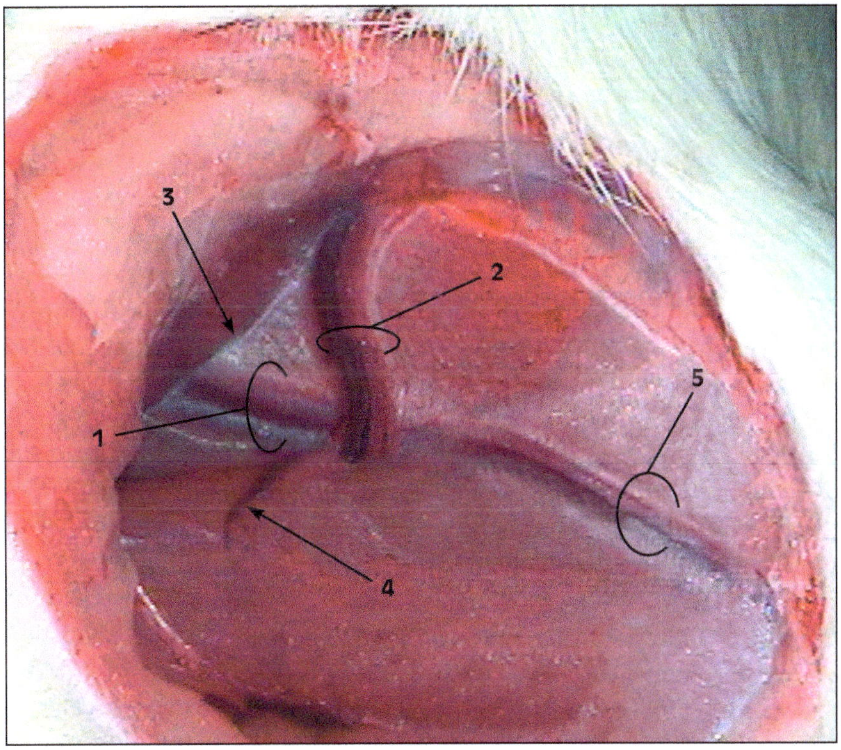

Figure 18-3

View of the surgical field following subinguinal incision and dissection of the superficial fascia. The vessels are visible through the transparent deep fascia. The vessels that are visualized include both those that arise from a deep plane and course subcutaneously (called 'superficial') and those that arise deep and continue to course deep. **1.** femoral vessels, **2.** superficial inferior epigastric vessels, **3.** superficial circumflex vein, **4.** vein from the adductor muscle. **5.** saphenous vessels. (From author's photo library)

If the incision is made within the correct surgical layer, the femoral vessels and most of their branches will be easily viewable (**Fig. 18-3**). The femoral vessels can be seen under the transparent deep fascia. Also, the superficial inferior epigastric vessels, which originate from the femoral vessels and then course towards the superficial fascia, can be easily visualized under the deep fascia. The vessels on the muscles, such as the vein from the adductor muscle and the saphenous vessels can also be seen under the investing fascia of the muscles (deep fascia). The superficial circumflex vein can be visualized as well, but more dissection of the superficial fascia may be needed (see below).

The next step in the dissection is to spread the deep fascia apart using two gauze pads moistened in warm normal saline. This step is similar to the process of opening the retroperitoneum during dissection of the aorta. In the surgical field (**Fig. 18-4**), the femoral artery and vein will begin to separate from each other, and the origin of the deep branch of the femoral artery (No. 4, **Fig. 18-4**), coming from its postero-lateral surface, will become apparent. In order to reveal the deep tributary vein of the femoral vein, microsurgical dissection is needed. Dissection of the deep fascia may also separate the superficial inferior epigastric artery (No. 6, **Fig 18-4**) from its corresponding vein (No 5,

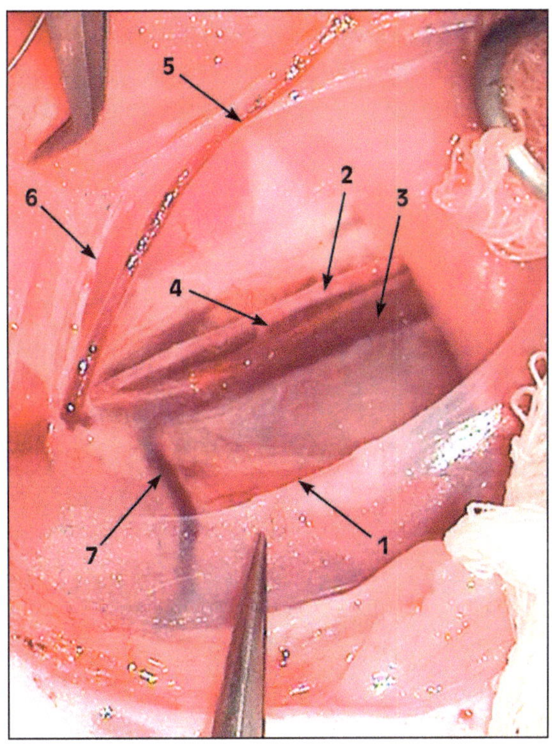

Figure 18-4

View of the surgical field upon opening the deep fascia, right side. **1.** membranous layer of the superficial fascia, **2.** femoral artery, **3.** femoral vein, **4.** deep branch of femoral artery, **5.** superficial inferior epigastric vein, **6.** superficial inferior epigastric artery, **7.** vein from the adductor muscle. (From author's photo library)

Fig. 18-4), which will make the muscular vein from the adductor muscle (No. 7, **Fig. 18-4**) more prominent as it arises from the muscle on the medial portion of the thigh.

C. Microsurgical dissection of the femoral vessels

Microsurgical dissection of the femoral vessels requires further dissection of the deep fascia to separate completely the two femoral vessels from each other, which will allow successful double ligation and in between transection of the arterial branches and tributary veins. Dissection of the deep fascia is performed with blunt dissection (without the use of cutting) or with a combination of blunt and sharp dissection.

Microsurgical dissection of the femoral vessels starts with the femoral artery, which is found laterally and slightly posterior to the femoral vein. The robust wall of the artery allows for more gross manipulation at the start of the dissection, which would not be possible with the vein. Dissection of the artery begins just cranially to the superficial inferior epigastric vessels. Using Dumont No. 3 forceps, the artery is lifted by the adventitia to develop the surgical plane between the femoral artery and vein and the posterior attachments of the deep fascia are obliterated (**Fig. 18-5**). If the dissection continues cranially to isolate the deep branch of the artery, care must be taken to avoid damaging the superficial circumflex vein (No. 3, **Fig. 18-6**), which crosses over the femoral artery. Therefore, this step of the dissection is delayed and we continue with dissection of the femoral vein.

Dissection of the anterior surface of the femoral vein (without lifting it) will reveal the superficial circumflex vein, which will be found just caudal to the inguinal ligament (**Fig. 18-6**). Of note, in contrast to that seen in a human, the inguinal ligament of a rat is more muscular than aponeurotic. As stated above, the superficial circumflex vein courses over the femoral artery while proximal to the inguinal ligament. The superficial circumflex vein should be double-ligated and transected between ligations, in order to continue the dissection of the femoral artery (see below). Cranially, just under the inguinal ligament, there is often another small vein that needs attention, which, due to its small size, can be cauterized.

Then, dissection of the posterior surface of the femoral vein is performed (**Fig. 18-7**). Following this dissection, the femoral vein is freed and lifted. This provides adequate visualization of the deep branch of the

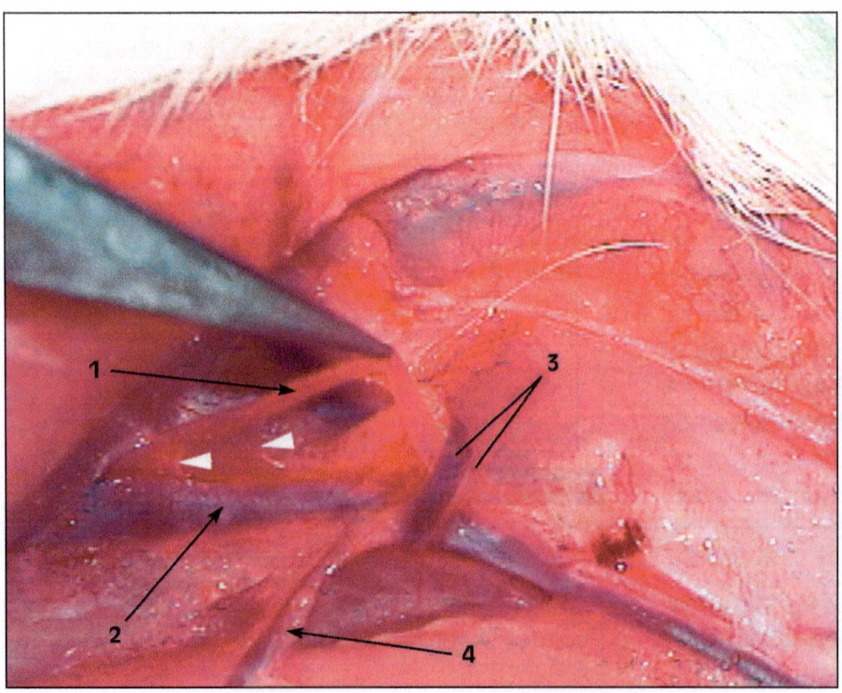

Figure 18-5

Microsurgical dissection of the femoral artery. Dumont No. 3 forceps lifts the artery, holding the adventitia. In this position, both the attachment of the deep fascia behind the artery and the attachment between the femoral artery and vein, created by the same fascia (white arrowheads), can be seen once the sheath of the femoral vessels is opened. **1.** femoral artery, **2.** femoral vein, **3.** superficial inferior epigastric vessels, **4.** vein from the adductor muscle. (From author's photo library)

Figure 18-6

Exposure and dissection of the superficial circumflex vein, tributary of the femoral vein. **A.** By lifting the femoral artery with the tips of the microsurgical s-cissors in the space between the deep branch (not yet dissected, but found behind the scissors) and the inguinal ligament, one can see that the superficial circumflex vein crosses over the femoral artery. **B.** The superficial circumflex vein is freed from the deep fascia with Dumont No. 3 forceps and microsurgical s-cissors. **1.** femoral artery, **2.** femoral vein, **3.** superficial circumflex vein, **4.** superficial inferior epigastric vessels, **5.** vein from the adductor muscle. (From author's photo library)

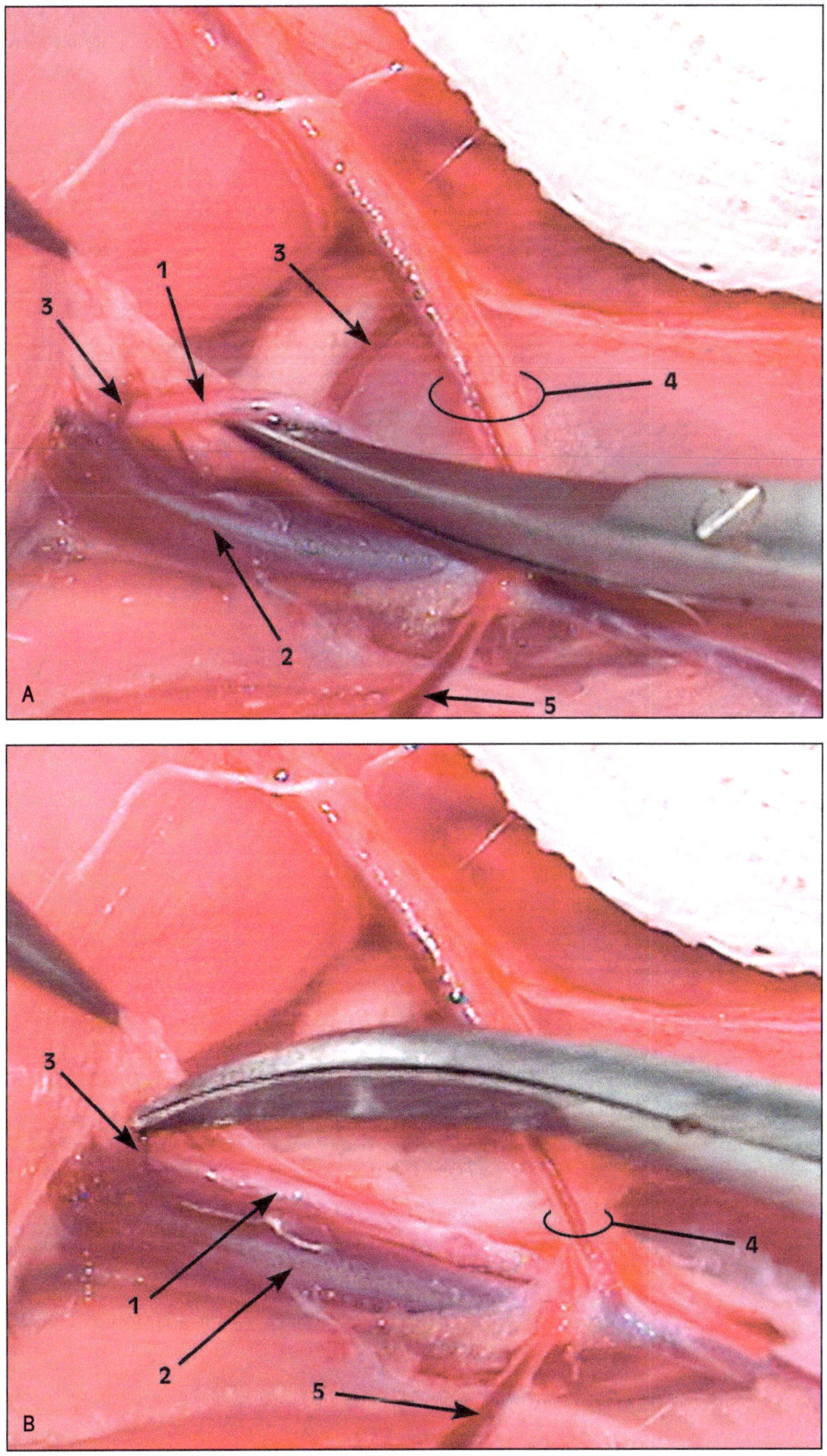

femoral vein for blunt dissection (**Fig. 18-8**). Once the deep tributary of the femoral vein is isolated from the deep fascia, the vein is ligated, first distally and then proximally. The proximal ligation is placed as close as possible to its confluence with the femoral vein so that the vein can then be transected between the two ligations with ease (**Fig. 18-9**). Cauterization of the deep tributary vein should not be utilized.

The dissection then returns to the femoral artery. Once the superficial circumflex vein has been transec-

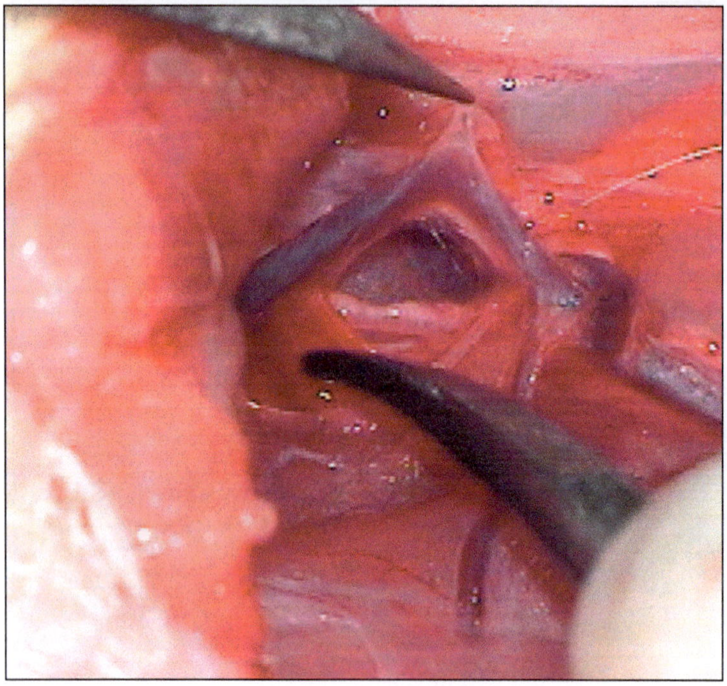

Figure 18-7

Dissection of the femoral vein. Dumont No. 3 forceps lifts the femoral vein from a residue of deep fascia left on the vein, and the microsurgical scissor tips (with the legs closed) open the posterior attachment of the vein. Through the developed window, the femoral artery can be seen, located laterally to the vein. (From author's photo library)

ted, the femoral artery can be lifted in order to visualize and dissect the deep branch of the femoral artery. This branch can be cauterized and transected by the experienced surgeon (**Fig. 18-10A**). During cauterization, caution must be used to prevent the transmission of heat to the adjacent femoral vein or its tributaries as hemorrhage from the femoral vein can be massive. Therefore, for the novice, it is recommended to ligate the artery using 9/0 suture and then transect between the proximal and distal ligations.

During this dissection, a small arterial branch may be found cranially to the deep branch of the femoral arte-

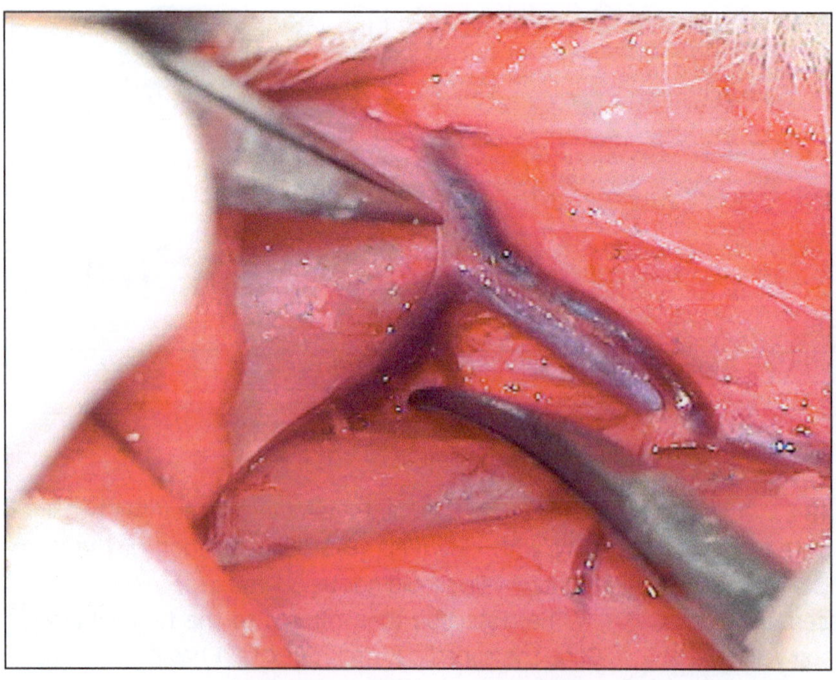

Figure 18-8

Dissection of the deep tributary of the femoral vein. Dumont No. 3 forceps lifts the femoral vein from a residue of the deep fascia left on the vein and the microsurgical scissor tips (with the legs closed) open the deep fascia in the angle between the femoral vein and the deep tributary vein. (From author's photo library)

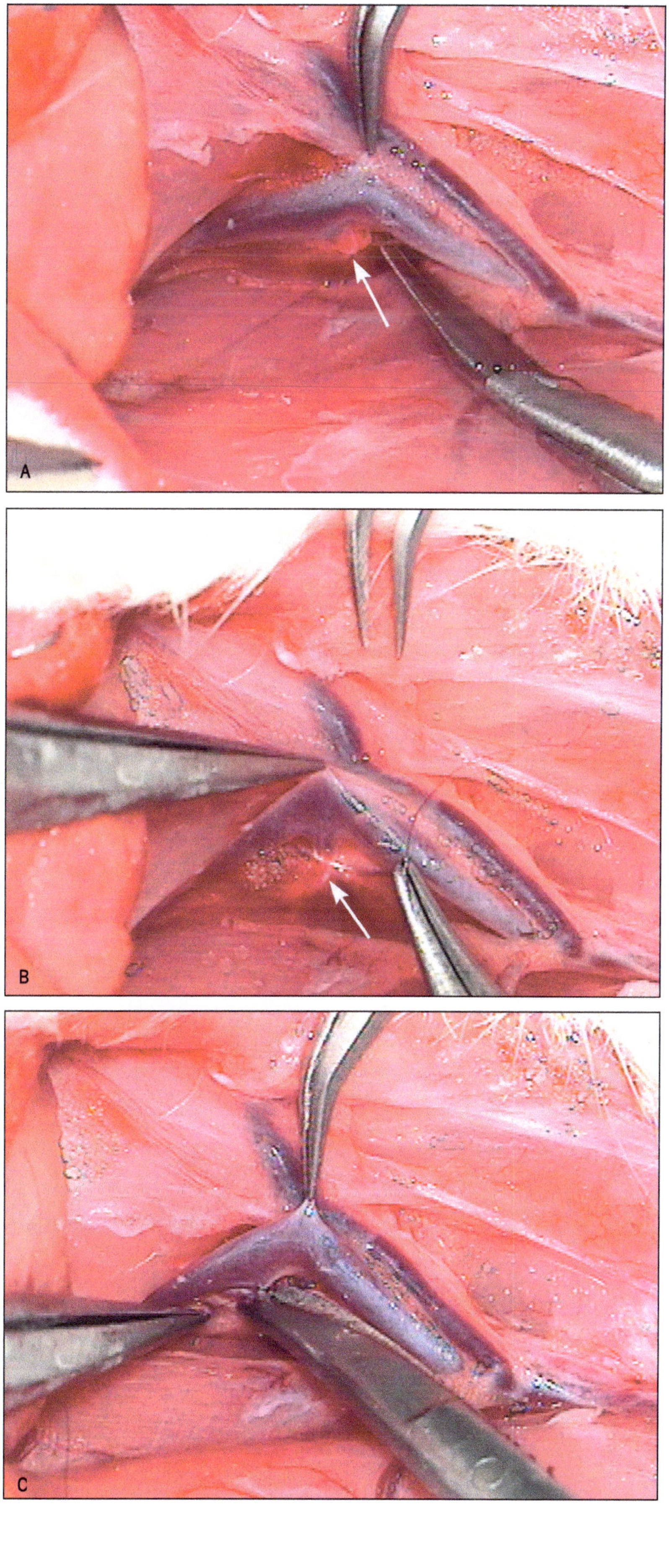

Figure 18-9

Ligations and transection of the deep tributary vein of the femoral vein. **A.** The distal ligation is placed first (white arrow). The curved forceps pulls the femoral vein from a residue of the deep fascia, while the needle holder and the Dumont No. 3 forceps tie the knot. **B.** The proximal ligation is placed next. The Dumont No. 3 forceps pulls the femoral vein, while the needle holder directs the needle to pass behind the deep tributary vein. The proximal suture should be placed as close as possible to the femoral vein, so that the vein can be transected between the two ligations with ease. **C.** The vein is transected between ligations. The proximal suture has been left long for traction and is pulled by the Dumont No. 3 forceps, the curved forceps lifts the femoral vein and the scissors transect the deep tributary vein. (From author's photo library) ry (as depicted by the arrow in **Figure 18-10B**). This branch (No. 4, **Fig. 18-2**) is the first branch of the femoral artery distal to the inguinal ligament. Other authors argue that in the rat, the first branch of the femoral artery distal to the inguinal ligament is the superficial circumflex artery. In our opinion, the location of this small branch is deep and not superficial, which shows that this is a muscular branch. During our dissections, we found that the superficial circumflex vein (No. 3, **Fig. 18-3**) is not accompanied by a superficial circumflex artery in the majority of cases. This topic is a subject of debate and not within the scope of this book. However, based on our findings, a superficial circumflex artery is not expected within the surgical field. In con-

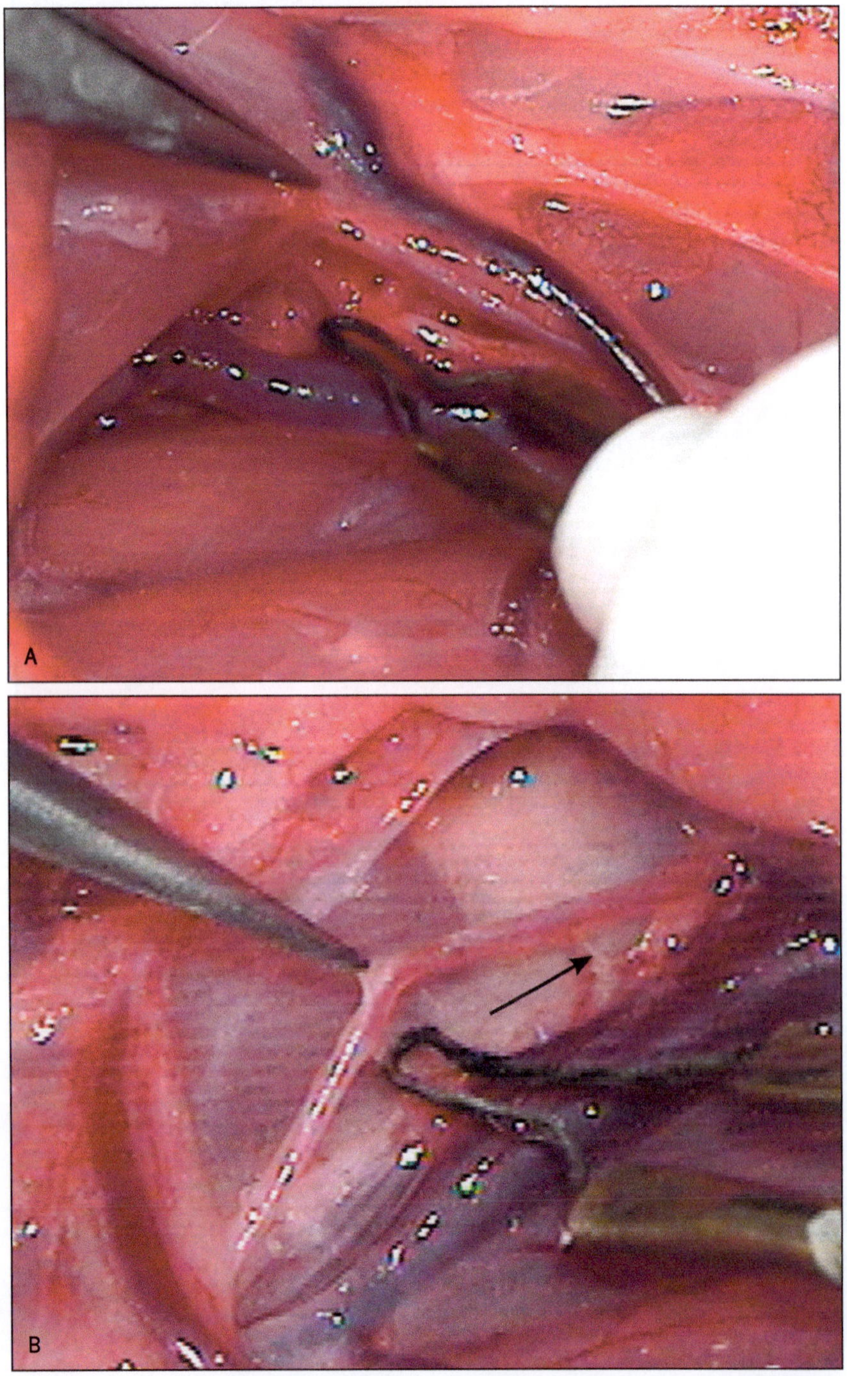

Figure 18-10

Cauterization of the deep branch of the femoral artery. **A.** Left side. Dumont No. 3 forceps lifts the femoral artery from a residue of the deep fascia, while the monopolar diathermy is ready to cauterize the deep branch. **B.** Right side. Same as in A. Notice the presence of a muscular branch cranial to the deep branch of the femoral artery (black arrow). [This photo is from another dissection, which is why the femoral vein has not been dissected.] (From author's photo library) clusion, if you encounter an arterial branch cranial to the deep branch of the femoral artery, mo matter its name, it can be cauterized.

Next, the artery and vein of the adductor muscle are dissected. The vein is very prominent and consistently seen in our dissections. The size of the vein is rather large, may be similar to that of the superficial inferior epigastric vein. The size of the accompanying artery, however, is very small, and thus the artery can be cauterized. Notice that this artery, near its origin from the femoral artery, courses in front of the vein, but it is then found caudal to the vein at the adductor muscle (**Fig. 18-11A**). Following dissection, the vein can potentially be cauterized (**Fig. 18-11B**); however, double ligation and transection is the safer option.

➢ At least 1 cm of the femoral artery and vein must be fully dissected for easy anastomoses of the femoral vessels.

This can hardly be achieved without transection of the deep branches (artery and vein) of the femoral vessels; however, transecting the vessels of the adductor muscle will provide more space and freedom for anastomoses of the femoral vessels. While optional for this dissection, transection of the deep branches will be re-

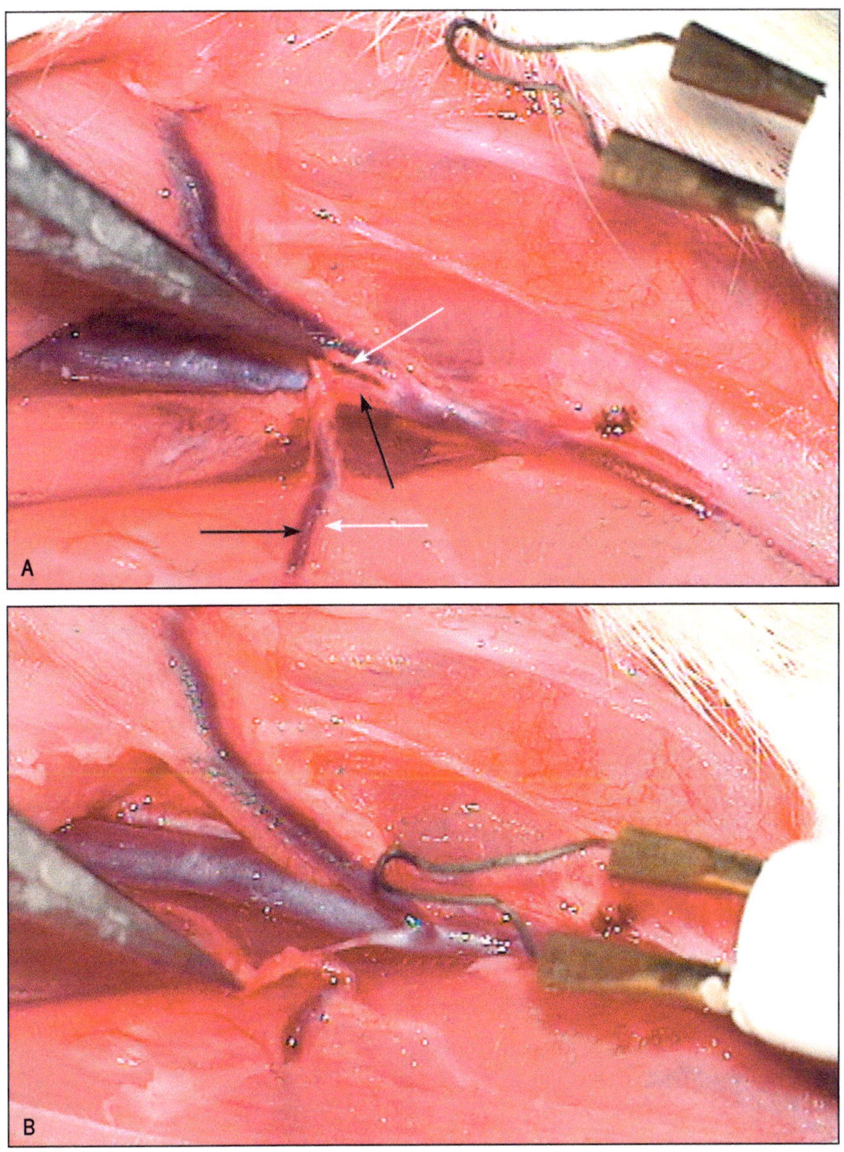

Figure 18-11

Cauterization and transection of the vessels of the adductor muscle. **A.** Dumont No. 3 forceps lifts the artery (white arrow) and pulls it cranially. The normal position of the artery is caudal to the vein (black arrow), as seen on the muscle [also shown by Nos. 9 and 10 in Figure 18-2]. The monopolar diathermy is in the field, ready to cauterize the artery. **B.** The forceps stays still, holding the artery as seen in A. The vein from the adductor muscle is exposed and ready to be cauterized. (From author's photo library) quired for more technically involved dissections of the femoral vessels, as in Chapters 22 to 24.

After dissection is completed, a yellow plastic background is placed beneath each vessel. The femoral artery will be transected and sutured first, so the plastic background should be located below the artery and above the vein (**Fig. 18-12**).

D. End-to-end anastomoses

The reader can find details about end-to-side anastomoses in Chapter 5. A brief description is given here.

Femoral artery

- The anastomosis will be performed by placing **6 sutures 11/0.**

The steps of the process of the end-to-end anastomosis are as follows:

1. Placement of the double clamp (**Fig. 18-13**).
2. Transection of the vessel.
3. Irrigation of the lumen with warm normal saline.
4. Folding of the adventitia (**Fig. 18-14**).
5. Reapproximation of the two clamps of the double clamp.
6. First are placed the 12 o'clock and 6 o' clock sutures that will orientate the two stumps of the vessel.
7. The anterior surface is completed with the placement of 2 sutures, at equal distances between themselves and from the corner sutures (**Fig. 18-15**).
8. Rotation of the double clamp and check of the sutures of the anterior surface.
9. Suturing of the posterior surface, similar to the anterior.
10. Release the double clamp.
11. Placement of a wet gauze pad on the anastomosis for 3 minutes.
12. Patency test. The reader is referred to Chapter 5.10 (**Fig. 5-4**) for a detailed description. In brief, a first microsurgical forceps is applied upstream, distal to the anastomosis, to occlude the femoral artery. A second forceps is applied next to the first and then moved downstream while 'half-closed' to empty the vessel. After a short distance, the second forceps is closed and remains in this position. The upstream forceps is then removed, and if the anastomosis is patent, the artery will immediately fill to the downstream forceps.
13. Withdrawal of the yellow plastic background.

Femoral vein

- The anastomosis will be performed by placing **6 or 8 sutures 11/0.**

The steps of the process of the end-to-end anastomosis are as follows:

1. Placement of the double clamp.
2. Transection of the vessel.

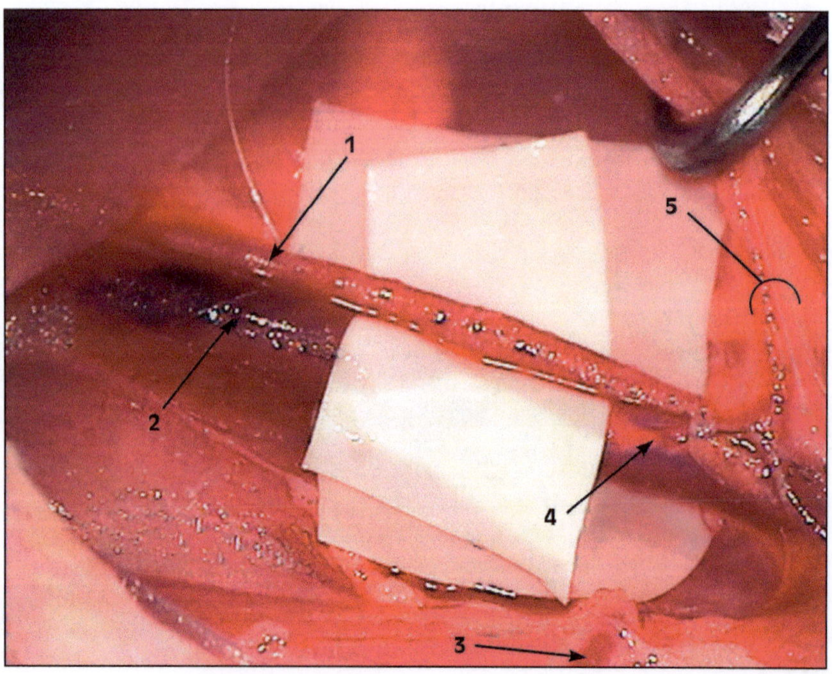

Figure 18-12

Completed dissection of the femoral vessels. Since each anastomosis will be performed separately, a piece of yellow plastic background is put under each vessel. Notice how much space is obtained in the surgical field with the transection of the artery and vein of the adductor muscle. **1.** femoral artery, **2.** femoral vein, **3.** distal stump of the vein of the adductor muscle, **4.** proximal stump of the vein of the adductor muscle, **5.** superficial inferior epigastric vessels. (From author's photo library)

Figure 18-13

Placement of the double clamp on the femoral artery. (From author's photo library)

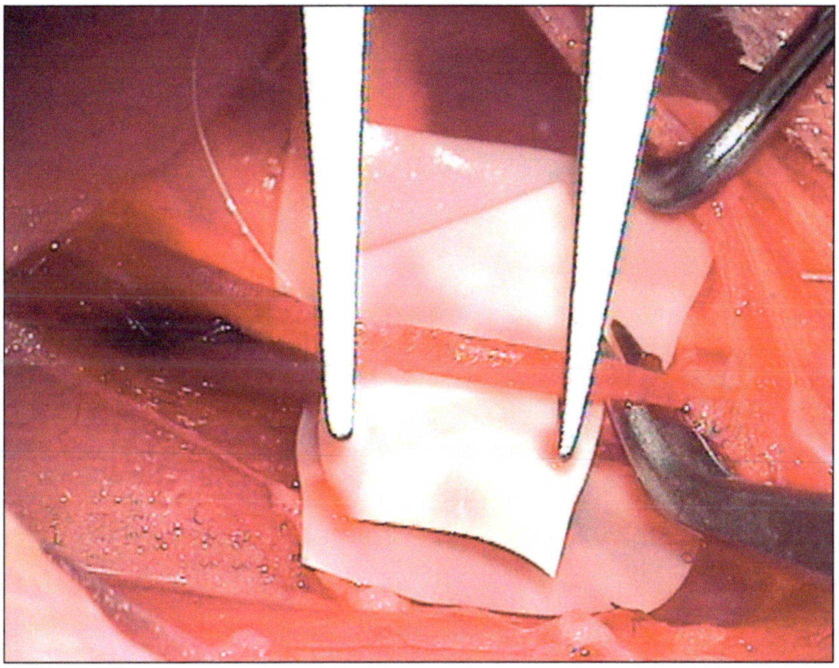

3. Irrigation of the lumen with warm normal saline.
4. Folding of the adventitia.
5. Reapproximation of the two clamps of the double clamp.
6. First are placed the 12 o'clock and 6 o' clock sutures that will orientate the two stumps if the vessel.
7. The anterior surface is completed with the placement of 2 sutures, at equal distances between themselves and from the corner sutures.
8. Rotation of the double clamp and check of the sutures of the anterior surface.
9. Suturing of the posterior surface, similar to the anterior (**Fig. 18-16**).
10. Release of the double clamp.

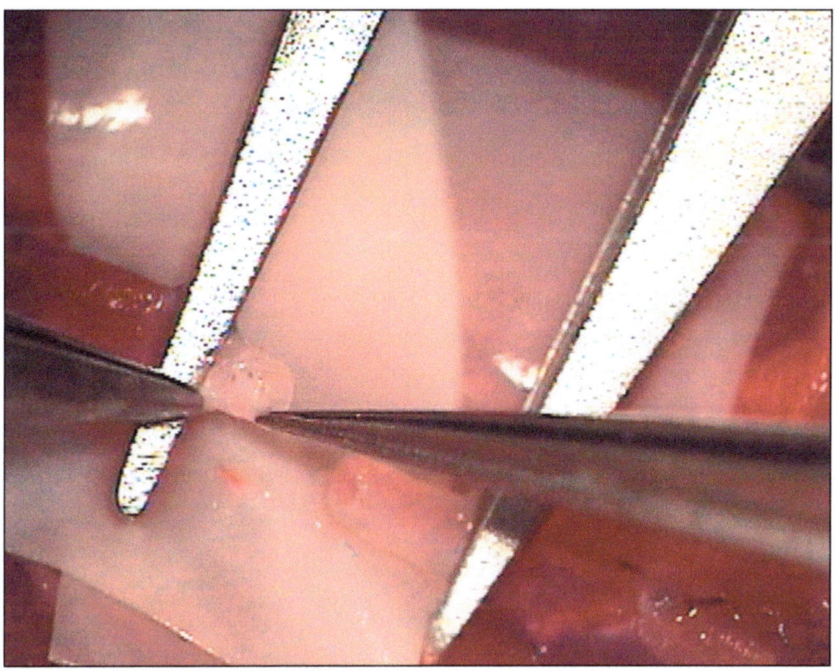

Figure 18-14

Folding of the adventitia of the femoral artery using two Dumont forceps, No. 3 and No. 5. (From author's photo library)

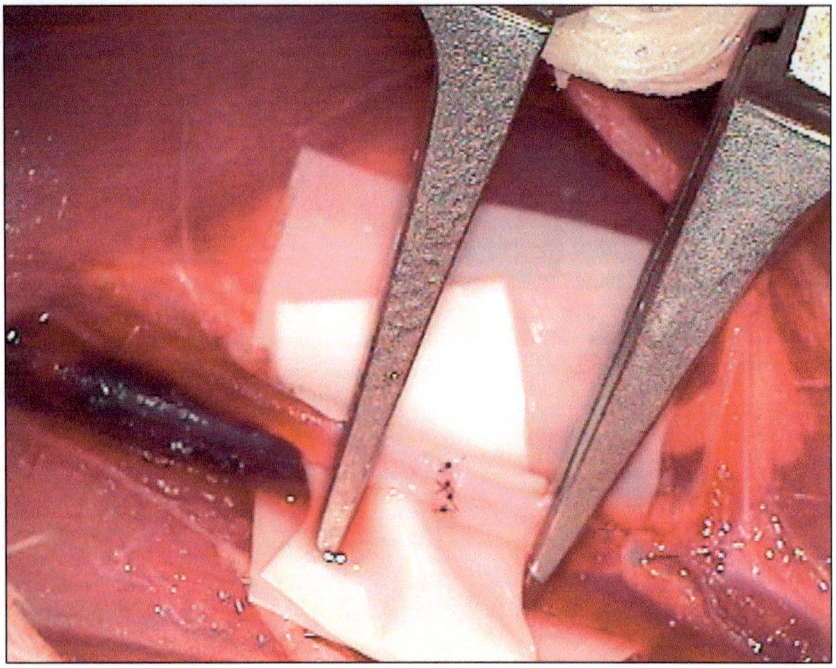

Figure 18-15

Completed suturing of the anterior surface of the femoral artery. (From author's photo library)

11. Placement of a wet gauze pad on the anastomosis for 3 minutes.
12. Patency test. It is performed as for the femoral artery (see above), but both forceps are placed proximal to the anastomosis and the downstream forceps moves cranially.
13. Withdrawal of the yellow plastic background.

E. Closure of the surgical trauma

The skin and superficial fascia are closed as a single layer with interrupted, non-absorbable 2/0 sutures.

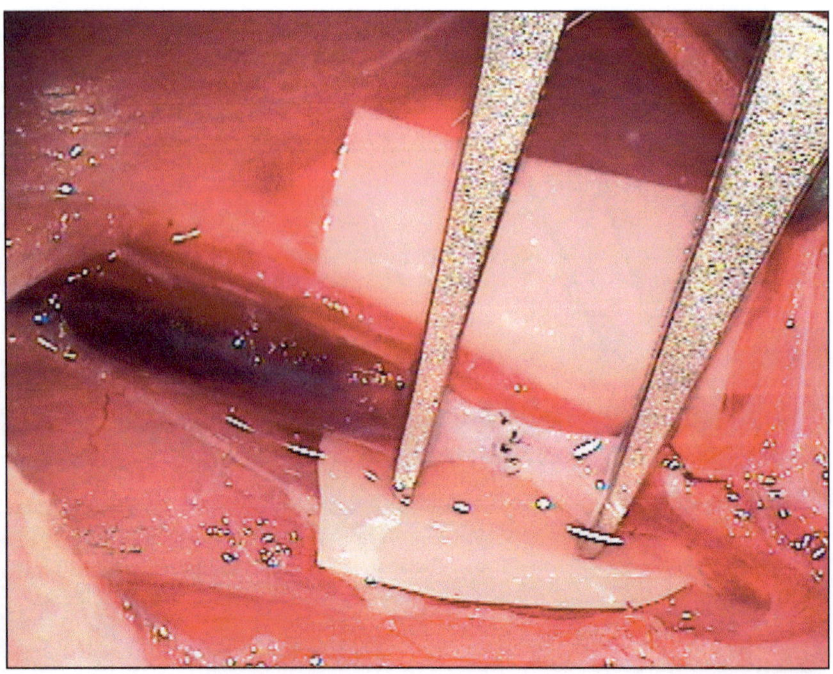

Figure 18-16

Completed suturing of the posterior surface of the femoral vein. (From author's photo library)

... of end-to-end anastomoses of the femoral vessels

Synopsis...

A. **Positioning of the rat:** Supine with its head away from the surgeon (the longitudinal axis of the rat is perpendicular to surgeon's frontal level). The limbs are immobilized on the working surface with adhesive tape.

B. **Preparation of the surgical field:** A 2 cm incision is made 1 cm below the inguinal crease. The superficial fascia is dissected and then the deep fascia by spreading it with two gauze pads moistened in warm, normal saline. This exposes the femoral vessels, the superficial inferior epigastric vessels, the vein from the adductor muscle (accompanied by a small artery) and the saphenous vessels. A retractor is placed in the middle of the incision and pulled toward the abdomen.

C. **Microsurgical dissection of the femoral vessels:** The femoral vessels are dissected from the superficial inferior epigastric vessels up to the inguinal ligament. The femoral artery is separated from the femoral vein and both are isolated from their deep fascia attachments. Next, the branches, or tributaries, of the femoral vessels, which can be found distal to the inguinal ligament, are transected between two ligations in the following order: the superficial circumflex vein, the deep branch and the deep tributary vein (found on the posterior surface of the femoral vessels), possibly a muscular arterial branch cranial to the deep branch of the femoral artery, and then the vessels of the adductor muscle.

D. **End-to-end anastomoses**

Femoral artery

1. Placement of the double clamp.
2. Transection of the vessel.
3. Irrigation of the lumen with warm normal saline.
4. Folding of the adventitia.
5. Re-approximation of the two clamps of the double clamp.
6. The anastomosis of the vessel is performed with placement of **6 sutures 11/0**. The first sutures are placed in the 12 o'clock and 6 o' clock position.
7. The anterior surface is completed with the placement of 2 sutures, at equal distances between themselves and from the corner sutures.
8. Rotation of the double clamp and check of the sutures of the anterior surface.
9. Suturing of the posterior surface, similar to the anterior.
10. Release of the double clamp.
11. Placement of a wet gauze on the anastomosis for 3 minutes.
12. Patency test.
13. Withdrawal of the yellow plastic background.

Femoral vein

1. Placement of the double clamp.
2. Transcection of the vessel.
3. Irrigation of the lumen with warm normal saline.
4. Folding of the adventitia.
5. Reapproximation of the two clamps of the double clamp.
6. The anastomosis of the vessel is performed with placement of **6 or 8 sutures 11/0**. First are placed the 12 o'clock and 6 o' clock sutures.

... of end-to-end anastomoses of the femoral vessels

Synopsis...

7. The anterior surface is completed with the placement of 2 sutures, at equal distances between themselves and from the corner sutures.
8. Rotation of the double clamp and check of the sutures of the anterior surface.
9. Suturing of the posterior surface, similar to the anterior.
10. Release of the double clamp.
11. Placement of a wet gauze on the anastomosis for 3 minutes.
12. Patency test.
13. Withdrawal of the yellow plastic background.

E. Closure of the surgical trauma: The skin and superficial fascia are closed as a single layer with interrupted, non-absorbable 2/0 sutures.

19

Interposition of superficial inferior epigastric vein graft in the femoral artery

The following paragraphs are identical to Chapter 18:

A. **Positioning of the rat**

B. **Preparation of the surgical field**

C. Microsurgical dissection

1. Femoral artery

The reader will find a detailed description of the micosurgical dissection of the femoral vessels in Chapter 18.C. With regard to the femoral artery, we emphasize the following:

- Dissection of the femoral artery begins at the branching point of the superficial epigastric artery and continues cranially.
- At a minimum, a 1 cm segment of the femoral artery should be dissected.
- In general, the dissection of the femoral artery can be performed without dissection of the femoral vein. Be mindful of the superficial circumflex vein as it crosses over the femoral artery near the inguinal ligament (**Fig. 18-6**). If the dissection of the femoral artery is continued in the cranial direction to a point in which the superficial circumflex vein is exposed, double ligation and transection (for the beginner) or cauterization and transection (for the more experienced surgeon) of the vein will minimize the risk of rupture during manipulation.
- For easy placement of the double clamp, the deep branch of the femoral artery must be double-ligated and transected or cauterized and transected (**Fig. 18-10**).
- For this operation, dissection of the vein and small artery of the adductor muscle is not necessary.
- Once the dissection has been completed, a yellow plastic background is placed under the femoral artery (**Fig. 19-1**).

2. Superficial inferior epigastric vein

Using blunt dissection, the superficial inferior epigastric vein is separated from the corresponding artery (**Fig. 19-2**). Next, the adventitia is gently removed from the wall of the vessel (**Fig. 19-3**). Dissection of the superficial inferior epigastric vein be-

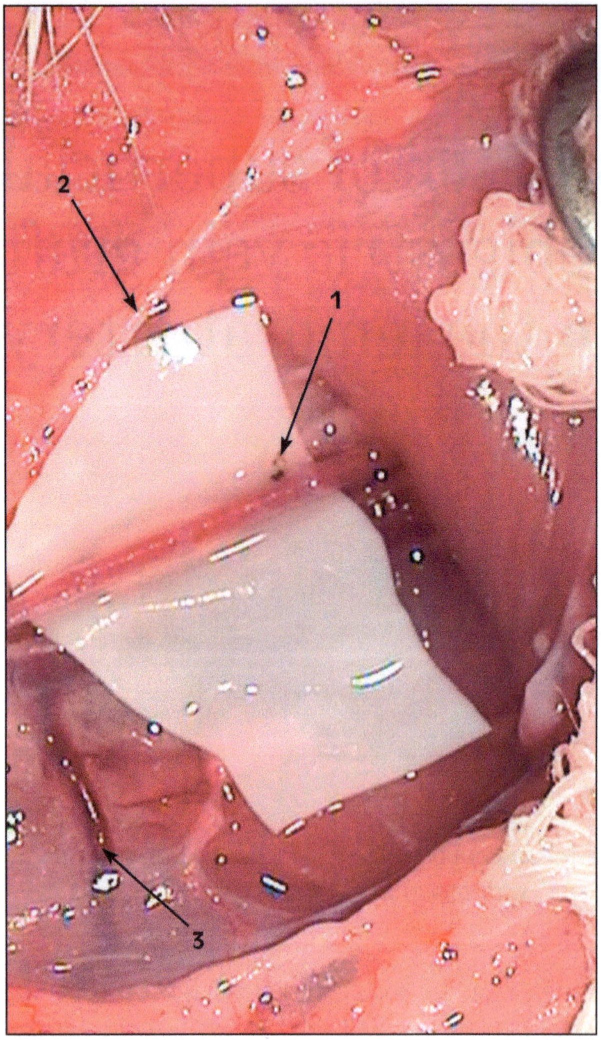

Figure 19-1

Completed dissection of the femoral artery, right side. Under the artery, a yellow piece of plastic has been placed as a background. **1.** cauterized deep branch (the femoral artery has been rotated with the placement of the background and therefore the stump of the deep branch is seen laterally), **2.** superficial inferior epigastric vessels, **3.** vein from the adductor muscle. (From author's photo library)

gins at its confluence with the femoral vein and extends for 1 cm along its course toward the muscles of the anterior abdominal wall.

D. Harvesting the graft from the superificial inferior epigastric vein

Using 9/0 suture, two ligations are placed on the superficial inferior epigastric vein; the first as close as possible to its conflunce with the femoral vein and the second as far as possible from the first ligation (**Fig. 19-4**). The length of the graft to be harvested from the superficial inferior epigastric vein (between the two ligations) should be at least 1 cm.

The graft is transected close to the ligations. Holding the graft from the outer surface of the vein wall with

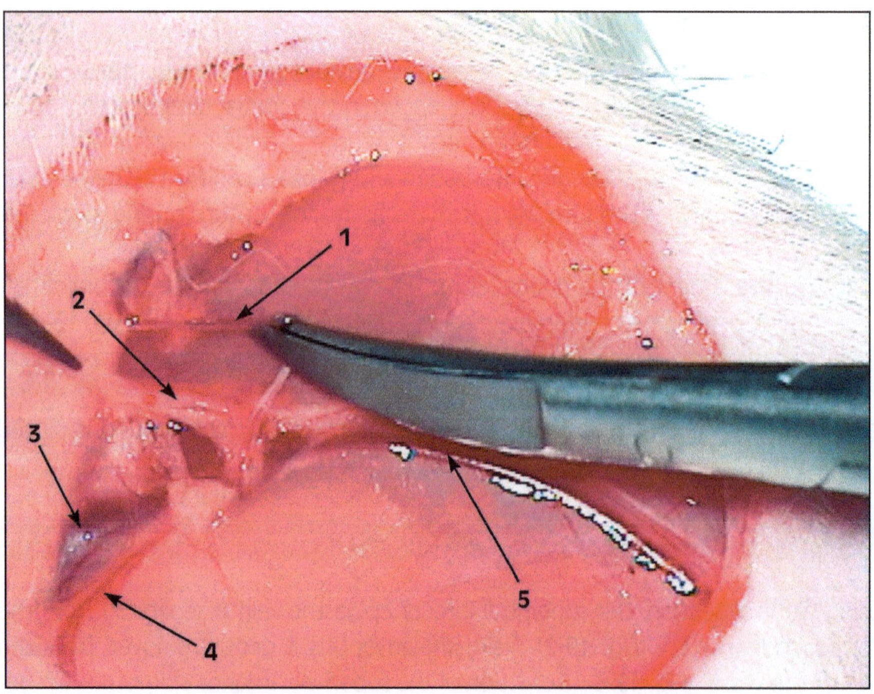

Figure 19-2

Separation of the superficial inferior epigastric vein from its corresponding artery, left side. Microsurgical forceps holds the artery, while the scissors bluntly dissect the vein. **1.** superficial inferior epigastric vein, **2.** superficial inferior epigastric artery, **3.** femoral vein, **4.** vein from the adductor muscle, **5.** saphenous vein. (From author's photo library)

Figure 19-3

Removal of the adventitia from the superficial inferior epigastric vein using two micosurgical forceps. The lower forceps stabilizes the vein, while the upper forceps removes the adventitia. (From author's photo library)

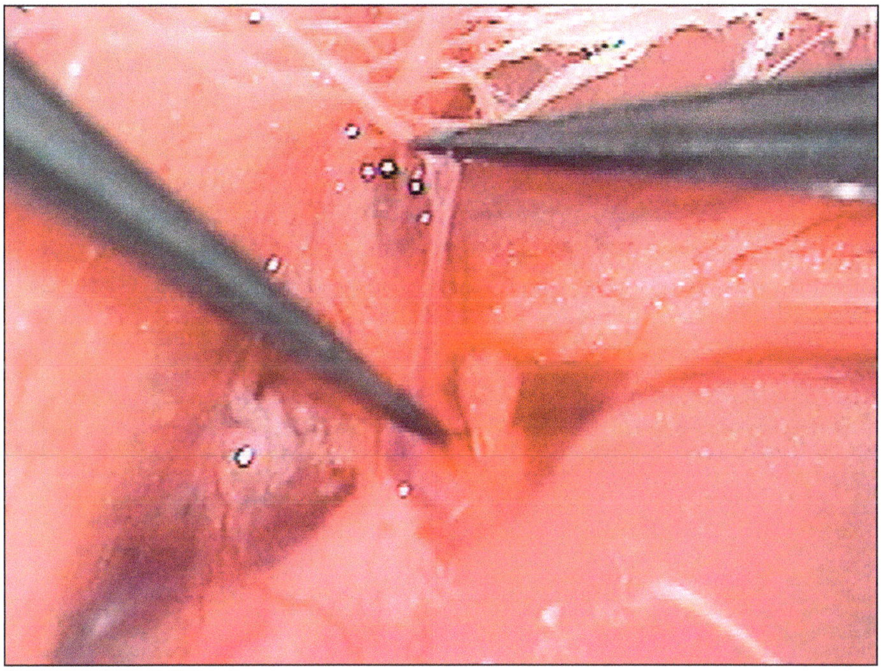

Dumont No. 3 forceps, the lumen of the graft is irrigated with warm, normal saline using a syringe attached to a 27G angiocatheter (as in **Figure 10-3**). The irrigation must be performed in the direction of blood flow through the vein (from distal to proximal) because the venous graft may contain a valve. To avoid traumatizing the endothelium, the tip of the angiocatheter must not enter the lumen of the venous graft.

The above instructions outline the most common method used for irrigation of a vein graft. However, because the superficial inferior epigastric vein is very small (the smallest vein handled so far in this book) and will likely have collapsed walls, it may be difficult to keep the lumen open and irrigate in the correct direction. Therefore, the irrigation of the superficial inferior epigastric vein can be performed in a retrograde direction (opposite to blood flow) with a smaller angiocatheter once the vein has been cut from the femoral vein near the proximal ligation (**Fig. 19-5**). With an intact catheter tip (not cut diagonally, as usally done to enter a small vessel), gently insert the catheter into the lumen. This will reduce the risk of traumatizing the endothelium of the graft. The irrigation should be performed very slowly and with low pressure because the saline will first flow

Figure 19-4

Placement of ligations on the dissected superficial inferior epigastric vein. The suture ends of the distal ligation are pulled taut with the needle-holder (seen towards the right hand of the reader) and forceps (not seen here). The proximal ligation has been placed previously, close to the femoral vein and is marked by the black arrow. (From author's photo library)

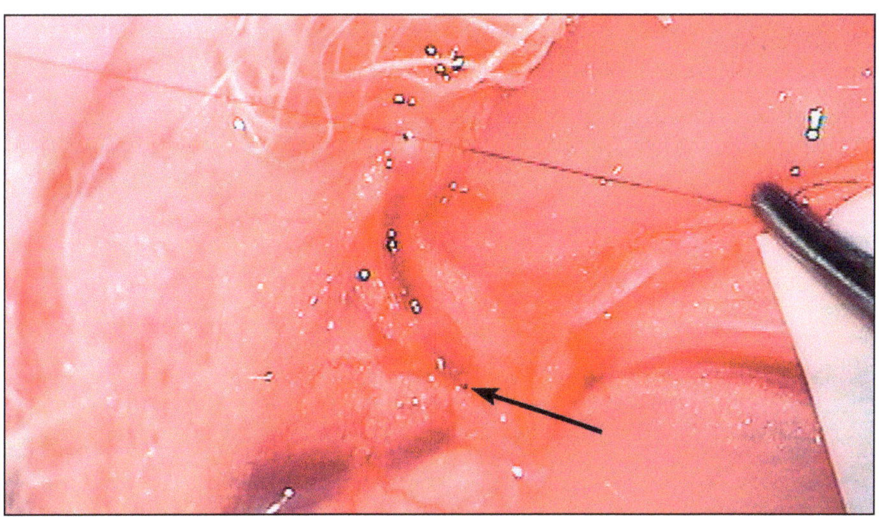

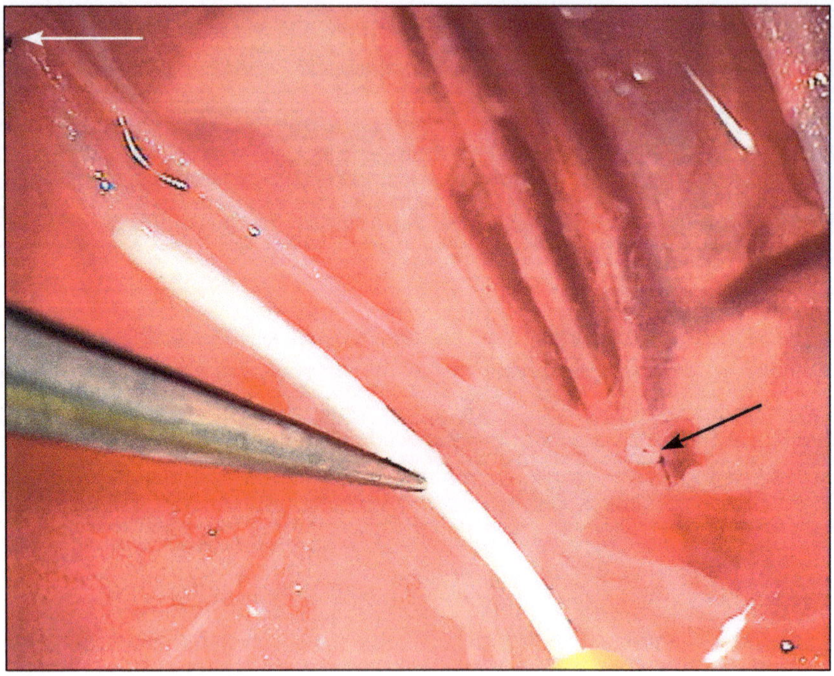

Figure 19-5

Retrograde irrigation of the superficial inferior epigastric vein. The vein has been cut at the proximal ligation (black arrow). The distal ligation is marked by the white arrow. The vein is gently lifted by Dumont No. 3 forceps and the intact tip of the catheter is seen within the lumen of the vein. Irrigation is performed with very low pressure. (From author's photo library)

in an antegrade and then retrograde direction once the saline reaches the distal ligation. If you apply high pressure, the catheter may abruptly exit from the vein, the vein may be damaged or both events may occur. In our experience, this method of retrograde irrigation is almost always successful, possibly indicating the absence of valves within the superficial inferior epigastric vein in the rat.

Following irrigation, the proximal opening of the graft (near the femoral vein) can be dilated (**Fig. 19-6**). The graft is then transected near the distal ligation (**Fig. 19-7**). The distal opening of the graft can then be dila-

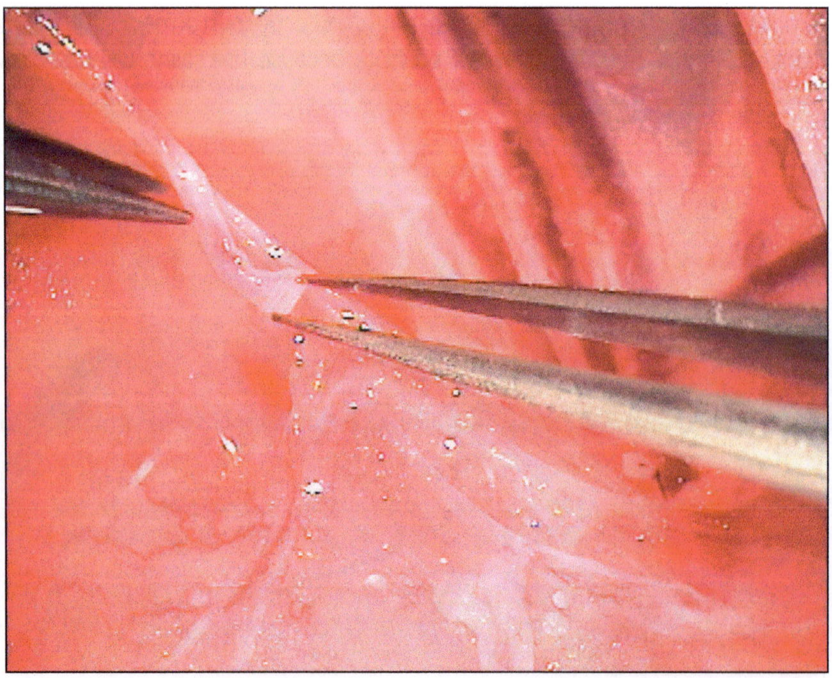

Figure 19-6

Dilation of the proximal opening of the graft taken from the superficial inferior epigastric vein. The vessel is lifted by Dumont No. 3 forceps (seen open here), while Dumont No. 5 forceps enters the lumen in the closed position and then is allowed to slowly open in order to dilate the lumen. (From author's photo library) ted in a fashion similar to the proximal end. Dilation of the graft is used to approximate the lumen width of the superficial inferior epigastric vein to the lumen width of the femoral artery.

E. Transfer of the graft

The graft taken from the superficial inferior epigastric vein is transferred to the field of the femoral artery and placed parallel to the artery. During the transfer, the venous graft should be placed in the proper direction so that blood flow through the graft follows that of the native venous flow. This rule applies to all venous grafts that may carry valves. For this procedure, the distal end of the superficial inferior epigastric vein graft must be placed at the proximal end of the femoral artery and the proximal end of the venous graft (the end originally near the femoral vein) is placed at the distal end of the femoral artery.

F. Preparation of the femoral artery

The femoral artery is placed in the arms of the double clamp and occluded. Using microsurgical scissors, the artery is transected in a direction perpendicular to the long axis of the vessel and cut in a single closure of the scissors (**Fig. 19-8**). Using an 27G angiocatheter attached to a syringe, the lumens of the stumps of the artery are irrigated with warm, normal saline (**Fig. 19-9**). As with all artery transections, the adventitia is folded in both stumps to obtain clean edges (**Fig. 19-10**).

G. End-to-end anastomoses

The reader will find a full description of the end-to-end anastomosis in Chapter 5.

- Each anastomosis will be performed by placing **6/0 sutures 11/0**

The two end-to-end anastomoses between the two edges of the venous graft and the two stumps of the femoral artery are performed **simultaneously**.

The steps of the process of the end-to-end anastomoses are as follows:

1. Placement of the corner sutures, first at the 12 o'clock positions of the anastomoses and then at the

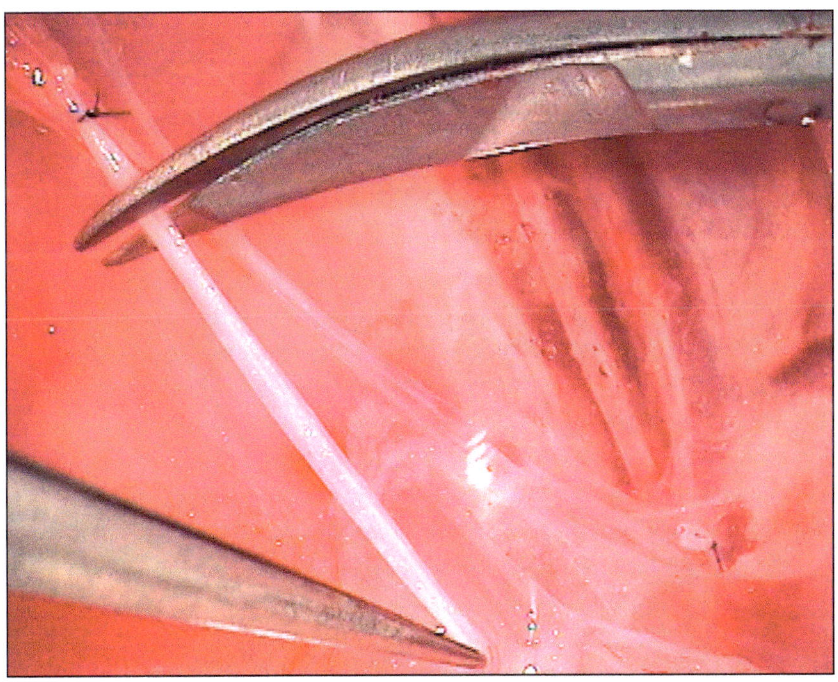

Figure 19-7

Transection of the distal end of the graft taken from the superficial inferior epigastric vein. The forceps Dumont No. 3 holds the proximal end of the graft. (From author's photo library)

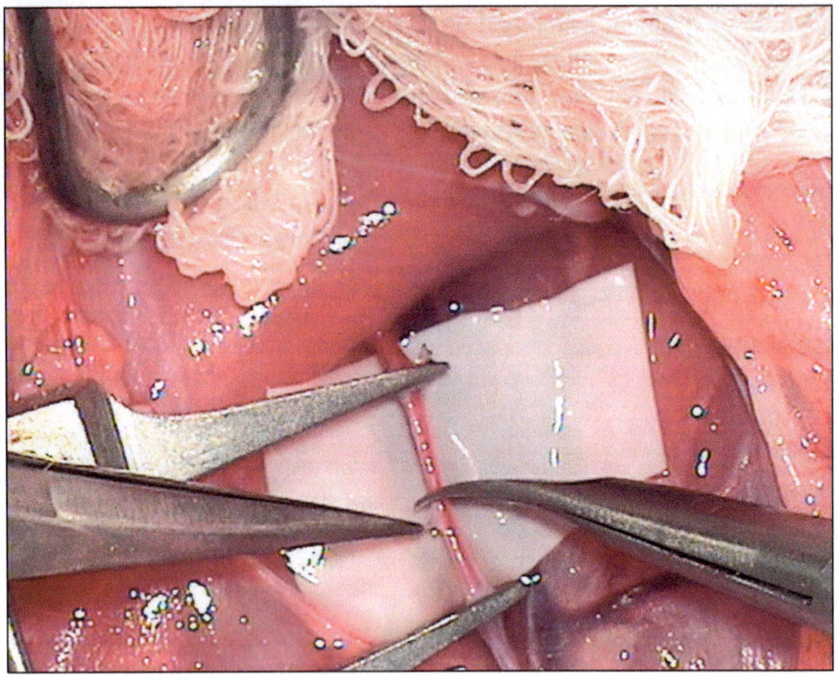

Figure 19-8

Transection of the femoral artery after it has been placed in the double clamp. Dumont No. 3 forceps holds the artery from the adventitia while scissors are seen perpendicular to the vessel and at an equidistant location to the clamp arms. (From author's photo library)

6 o'clock positions (**Fig. 19-11**). Placement of the corner sutures in this order helps orientate the vessels and provides support for subsequent suture placement.

2. Completion of the anterior surface of each anastomosis with the placement of 2 sutures, at equal distances between themselves and from the corner sutures.
3. Rotation of the double clamp to check the sutures along the anterior surface of each anastomosis.
4. Suturing of the posterior surfaces of the anastomoses in a fashion similar to the anterior surface anastomoses.
5. Release of the vessel from the double clamp.
6. Placement of a wet gauze on the anastomoses for 3 minutes.

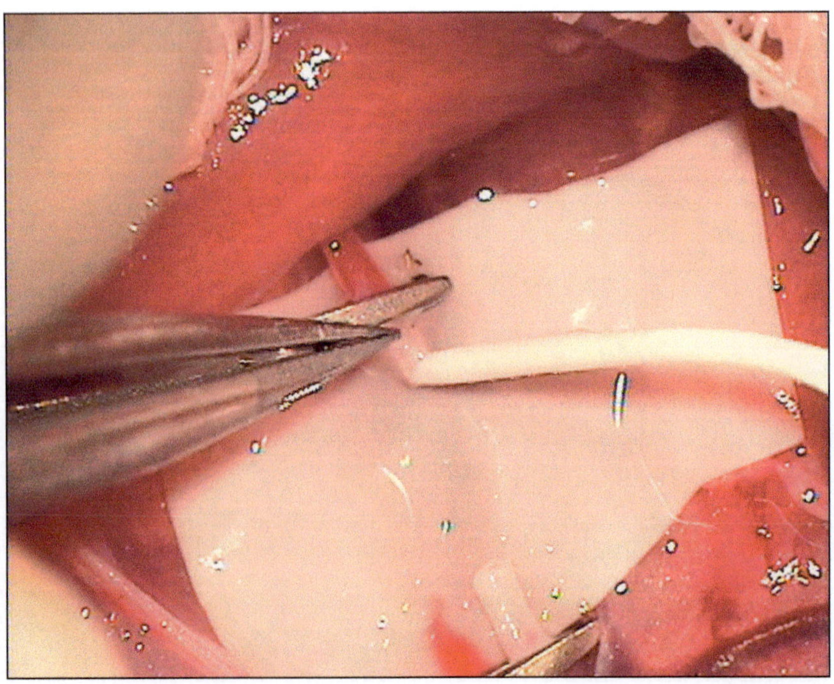

Figure 19-9

Irrigation of the lumen of the stumps of the femoral artery. Dumont No. 3 forceps holds the artery from the adventitia while the lumen is irrigated with warm, normal saline through the angiocatheter. (From author's photo library)

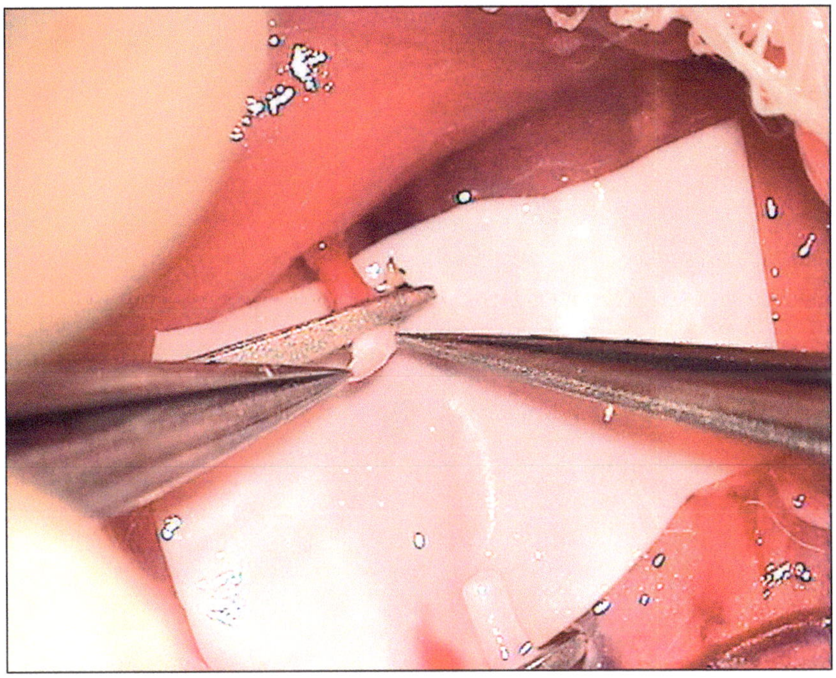

Figure 19-10

Folding of the adventitia of the stumps of the femoral artery. Dumont No. 3 forceps holds the artery from the edge while Dumont No. 5 forceps folds the adventitia. (From author's photo library)

7. Patency test.

The patency test is performed as in an end-to-end anastomosis, described in Chapter 5.10 (**Fig. 5-4**). In brief, an upstream forceps is applied on the femoral artery, at a point distal to the graft and between the distal anastomosis and the origin of the superficial epigastric vessels, to occlude the vessel. A second forceps is applied next to the first, then moved downstream while being held 'half-closed' to empty the vessel and then after a short distance, the forceps is closed and remains in this position. The upstream forceps is then released, and if the anastomosis is patent, the vessel will instantly fill up to the downstrem forceps. This procedure tests both anastomoses simultaneously. If there is no patency, then the same procedure can be performed distal to the

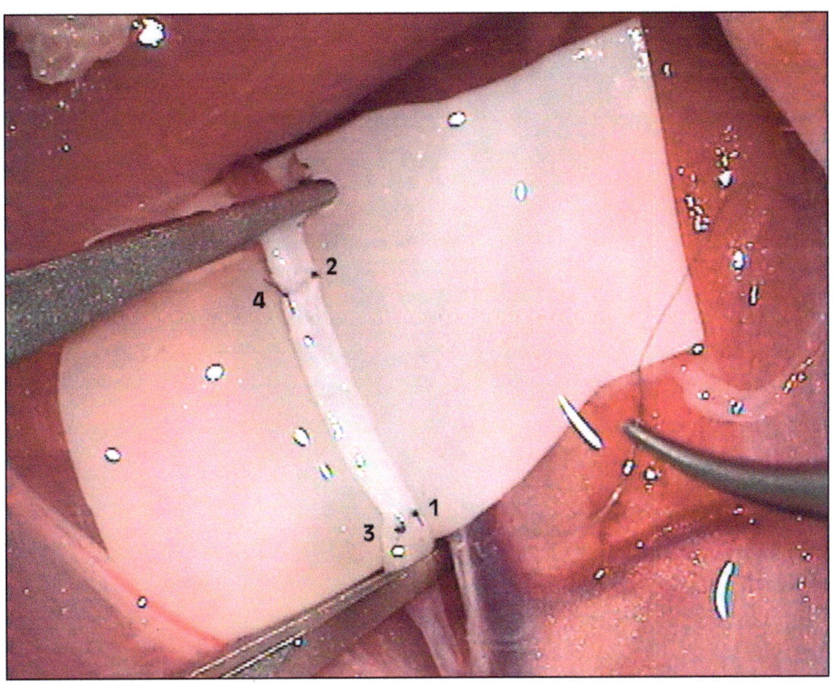

Figure 19-11

Placement of the four corner sutures in the anastomoses between the stumps of the femoral artery and the venous graft. Numbers depict the order of placement. (From author's photo library)

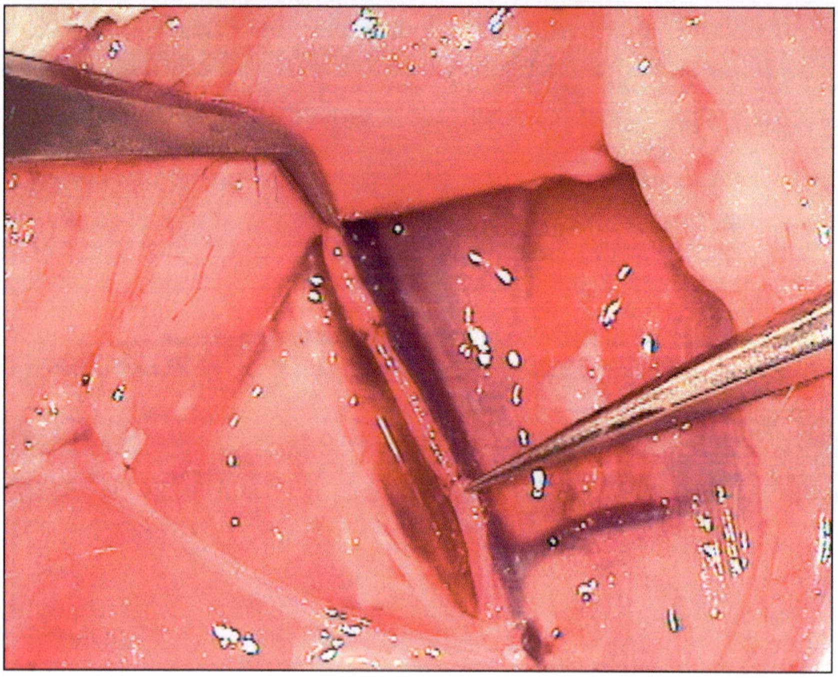

Figure 19-12

Placement of the graft from the superficial inferior epigastric vein into the femoral artery has been completed and the blood flow has been released. (From author's photo library)

proximal anastomosis. In this case, the two forceps are applied to the venous graft and the second forceps moves along the graft, requiring great care. This process will reveal which anastomosis is not patent and will therefore need to be redone. **Figure 19-12** shows successful anastomoses between the stumps of the femoral artery and the venous graft.

8. Withdrawal of the yellow plastic background.

H. Closure of the surgical trauma

The skin and the superficial fascia are closed in one layer with interrupted, non-absorbable 2/0 sutures.

Synopsis...

... of interposition of superficial inferior epigastric vein graft in the femoral artery

A. **Positioning of the rat:** Dorsal decubitus (supine) position with its head away from the surgeon (the longitudinal axis of the rat is perpendicular to surgeon's frontal level). The limbs are immobilized on the working surface with adhesive tape.

B. **Preparation of the surgical field:** A 2 cm incision is made 1 cm below the inguinal crease. The superficial fascia is dissected and then the deep fascia is opened by spreading it with two gauze pads moistened in warm, normal saline. This exposes the femoral vessels, the superficial inferior epigastric vessels, the vein from the adductor muscle (accompanied by a small artery) and the saphenous vessels. A retractor is placed in the middle of the incision and pulled toward the abdomen.

C. **Microsurgical dissection:** The femoral artery is dissected and mobilized from the origin of the superficial inferior epigastric artery to free at least a 1 cm segment of artery. This requires transection after double ligation, or cauterization, of the deep branch of the femoral artery, which arises from the posterior surface of the artery. The superficial inferior epigastric vein is dissected from its confluence with the femoral vein to free at least a 1 cm segment of vein. A yellow plastic background is placed under the femoral artery.

D. **Harvesting the graft:** A ligation (9/0) is placed at the each edge of the dissected portion of the superficial inferior epigastric vein. The vein is transected close to the proximal ligation (near the femoral vein), irrigated, and finally transected close to the distal ligation.

E. **Transfer of the graft:** The graft is transferred to the field of the femoral artery. It is placed parallel to the artery and, in the proper direction, so that blood flow through the graft follows that of the native venous flow.

F. **Preparation of the femoral artery:** The femoral artery is placed in the double clamp and transected. The lumen of the stumps are irrigated with warm, normal saline. The adeventitia is folded at the edges of the stumps.

G. **End-to-end anastomoses: 6 sutures 11/0** in each anastomosis.

1. Placement of the corner sutures, first at the 12 o'clock positions of the anastomoses (on the surgeon's right) and then at the 6 o'clock position (on the surgeon's left).
2. Completion of the anterior surface of each anastomosis with the placement of 2 sutures, at equal distances between themselves and from the corner sutures.
3. Rotation of the double clamp to check the sutures along the anterior surface of each anastomosis.
4. Suturing of the posterior surfaces of the anastomoses in a fashion similar to the anterior surface anastomoses.
5. Release of the vessel from the double clamp.
6. Placement of a wet gauze on the anastomoses for 3 minutes.
7. Patency test.
8. Withdrawal of the yellow background.

H. **Closure of the surgical trauma:** The skin and superficial fascia are closed in one layer with interrupted, non-absorbable 2/0 sutures.

20

Femoral artery bypass graft using the superficial inferior epigastric vein

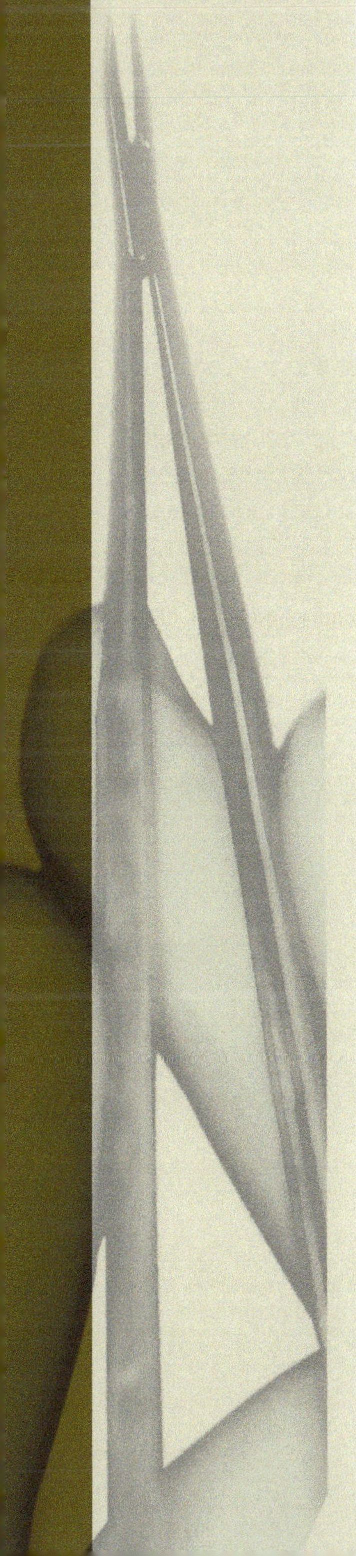

Refer to Chapter 19 for sections A-E:

A. Positioning of the rat

B. Preparation of the surgical field

C. Microsurgical dissection

  1. Femoral artery

  2. Superficial inferior epigastric vein

D. Taking the graft from the superificial inferior epigastric vein

E. Transfer of the graft

F. Preparation of the femoral artery

The femoral artery is occluded with the double clamp. Two, transverse arteriotomies are then made along the femoral artery. These openings provide an entrance and exit site for the bypass graft along the femoral artery. Of note, once the graft is placed, the femoral artery will be ligated, and therefore obstructed, between these entrance and exit sites.

A detailed decription of the transverse arteriotomy technique can be found in Chapter 6. In summary, the femoral artery is held using a Dumont forceps and a transverse incision is made along the arterial wall using microsurgical scissors (**Fig. 20-1**). The adventitia is dissected and removed from the perimeter of the incision site. The lumen is irrigated with warm, normal saline through the incision site using a fine angiocatheter (27G). Using the same technique, a second transvere incision is made distal to the first arteriotomy along the femoral artery. The distance between the two arteriotomies is dictated by the length of the vein graft (**Fig. 20-2**). The lumen is then irrigated and the adventitia is removed from the perimeter of the second arteriotomy site.

G. End-to-side anastomoses - Ligation of the femoral artery

Refer to Chapter 6.1 for an in-depth description of the technique used for an end-to-side anastomosis for the case that the end-anastomosed vessel can be rotated.

- Each anastomosis will be performed by placing **6 sutures 11/0.**

At each incision site, an end-to-side anastomoses is made between the superficial

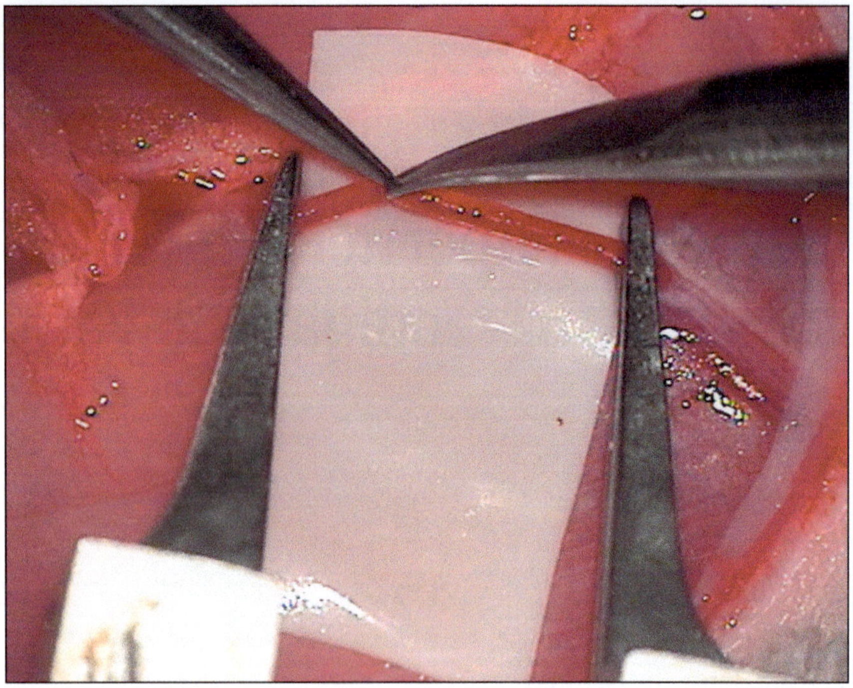

Figure 20-1

Transverse arteriotomy of the femoral artery (left side). Dumont No. 3 forceps holds the adventitia as microsurgical scissors are brought perpendicular to the vessel and make a transverse incision. (From author's photo library)

inferior epigastric vein graft and the femoral artery. The anastomoses are performed **simultaneously**, as follows:

1. A total of 4 corner sutures are placed, two per anastomosis. The first 2 corner sutures are made on the right hand side of each anastomosis, starting at the right anastomosis. The second 2 corner sutures are placed on the left hand side, again starting from the right anastomosis (**Fig. 11-3**).
2. The anterior surface of each anastomosis is completed with 2 additional sutures. These sutures should be equidistant from each other and the corner sutures (**Fig. 20-3**).
3. The vein graft is rotated to visualize the posterior surfaces of the edges of the graft and the posterior surfaces of the femoral artery at the incision sites.
4. Following rotation of the graft, the sutures on the anterior surface are checked.
5. The posterior surface of each anastomoses is completed with 2 additional sutures per anastomosis, as described in step 2 (**Fig. 20-4**).

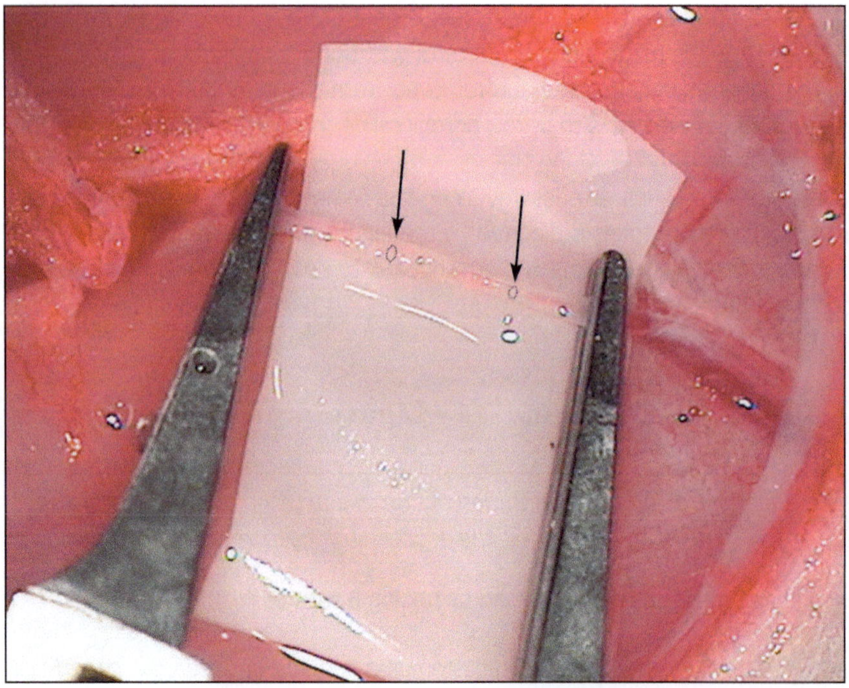

Figure 20-2

The left femoral artery following arteriotomy and irrigation of the lumen. The incisions are outlined by dotted lines and found below the black arrows. (From author's photo library)

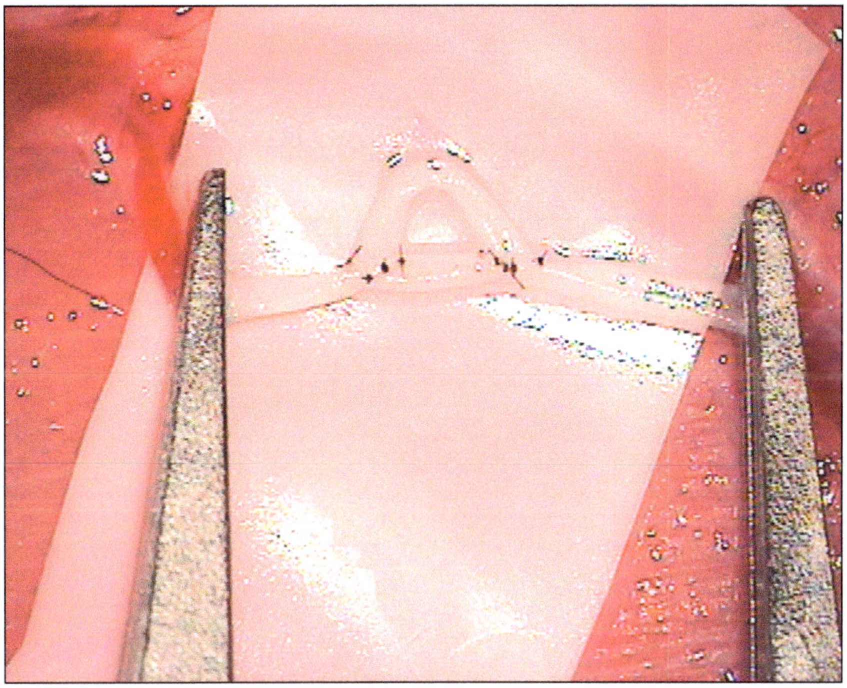

Figure 20-3

The anterior surfaces of the anastomoses between the bypass vein graft and the femoral artery, following placement of all sutures. (From author's photo library)

6. The femoral artery is ligated in the middle of the distance between the two anastomoses using a 9/0 suture (**Fig. 20-5**).
7. The femoral artery is released from the double clamp.
8. A wet gauze is lightly placed on the anastomoses for 3 minutes.
9. Perform a patency test.

   The patency test is performed in similar fashion as in a single end-to-end anastomosis, as described in Chapter 5.10 (**Fig. 5-4**). In brief, an upstream microsurgical forceps is applied distally to the graft, between the distal anastomosis and the junction of the superficial epigastric vessels, to occlude the femoral artery. A second forceps is applied next to the first forceps and then moved, while being held 'half-closed', downstream to empty the vessel. After a short distance, the forceps is closed and remains in this position. The upstream forceps is then released. If patent, the vessel will instantly fill towards the

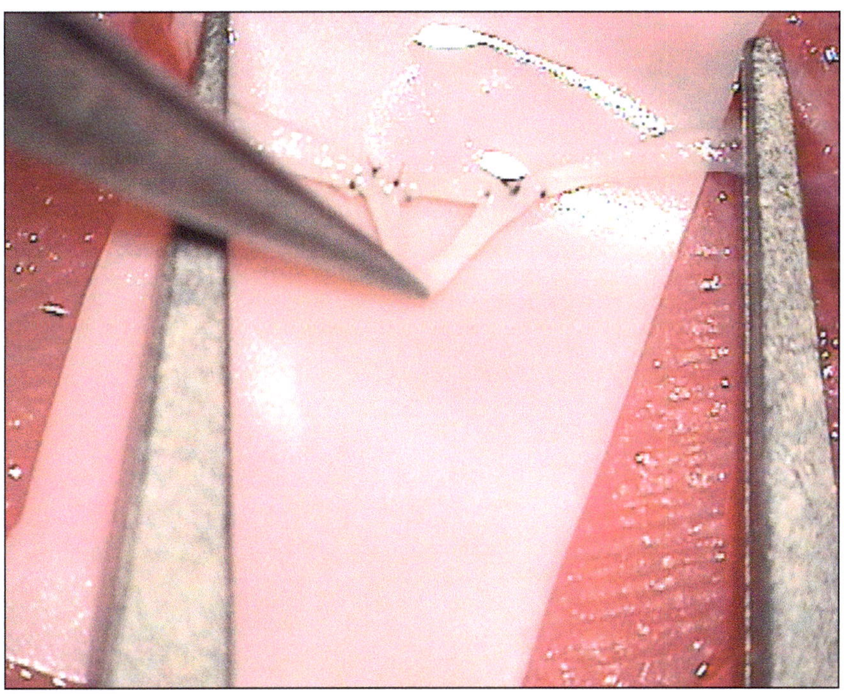

Figure 20-4

The posterior surfaces of the anastomoses between the bypass vein graft and the femoral artery, following placement of all sutures. Dumont No. 3 forceps reflects the graft towards the right side of the rat to show the posterior aspect of the anastomoses. (From author's photo library)

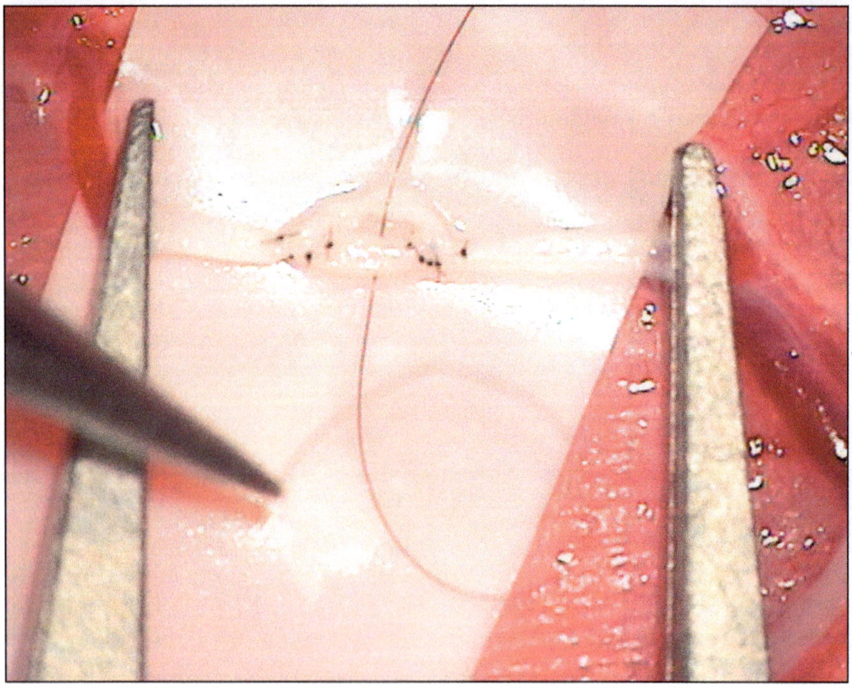

Figure 20-5

Ligation of the left femoral artery between the anastomoses of the graft. A 9/0 suture has been passed under the femoral artery. Once the suture is tied, the blood flow will be driven through the graft and bypass this portion of the femoral artery. (From author's photo library)

downstream forceps. This procedure tests both anastomoses. **Figure 20-6** shows successful anastomoses between the superficial inferior epigastric vein graft and the femoral artery.

If the patency test fails and the vessel does not instantly fill, then the same procedure can be performed to check the proximal anastomosis (as in Chapter 19.G.7). In this case, both forceps are applied on the venous graft and the second forceps moves along it, therefore great care is needed because of the fragile nature of the vein graft and the limited space available. This process will reveal which anastomosis is not patent and needs to be redone.

10. Withdraw the yellow background.

H. Closure of the surgical trauma

The skin and the superficial fascia are closed in one layer with interrupted, non-absorbable 2/0 sutures.

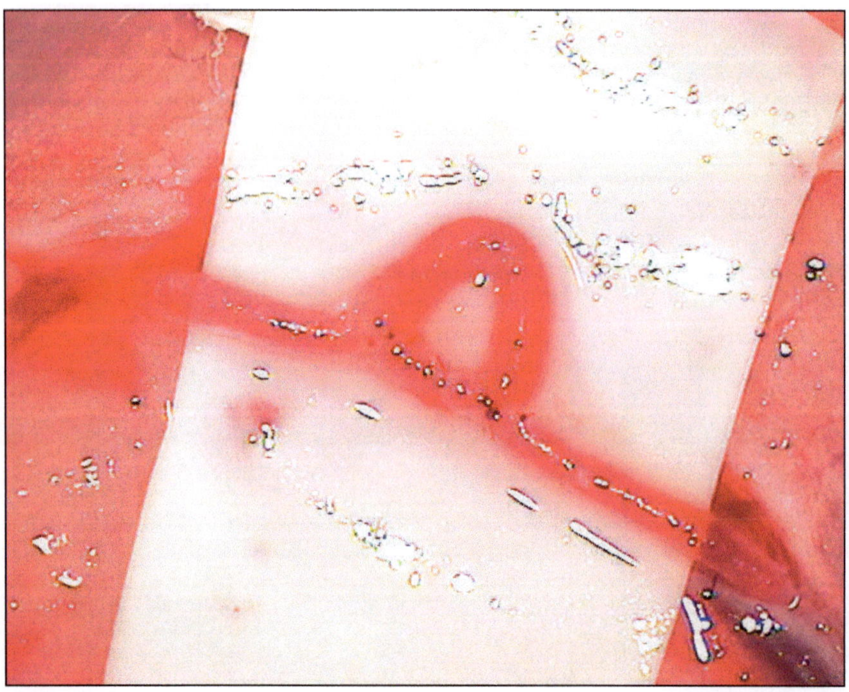

Figure 20-6

Completed left femoral artery bypass graft using the superficial inferior epigastric vein. The graft is seen arching over the obstructed part of the femoral artery. (From author's photo library)

Synopsis... of femoral artery bypass graft using the superficial inferior epigastric vein

A. **Positioning of the rat:** Dorsal decubitus (supine) position with its head away from the surgeon (the longitudinal axis of the rat is perpendicular to surgeon's frontal level). The limbs are immobilized on the working surface with adhesive tape.

B. **Preparation of the surgical field:** A 2 cm incision is made 1 cm below the inguinal crease. The superficial fascia is dissected and then the deep fascia by spreading it with two gauze pads moistened in warm, normal saline. This exposes the femoral vessels, the superficial inferior epigastric vessels, the vein from the adductor muscle (accompanied by a small artery) and the saphenous vessels. A retractor is placed in the middle of the incision and pulled toward the abdomen.

C. **Microsurgical dissection:** The femoral artery is dissected and mobilized from the origin of the superficial inferior epigastric artery to free at least a 1 cm segment of artery. This requires transection (between two ligations 9/0 or after cauterization) of the deep branch of the femoral artery, which arises from the posterior surface of the artery. The superficial inferior epigastric vein is dissected from its confluence with the femoral vein to free at least a 1 cm segment of vein. A yellow plastic background is placed under the femoral artery.

D. **Harvesting the graft:** A ligation (9/0) is placed at the each edge of the dissected portion of the superficial inferior epigastric vein. The vein is transected close to the proximal ligation (near the femoral vein), irrigated, and finally transected close to the distal ligation.

E. **Transfer of the graft** to the field of the femoral artery, parallel to it and in the proper direction so that blood flow through the graft follows that of the native venous flow.

F. **Preparation of the femoral artery:** The femoral artery is placed in the double clamp. Two transverse arteriotomies are made at a distance approximately equal to the length of the graft. The lumen is irrigated through each incision and the adventitia is removed from the perimeter of the incision sites.

G. **End-to-side anastomoses - Ligation of the femoral artery:**
6 sutures (11/0) are placed in each anastomosis
1. Placement of 2 corner sutures per anastomosis, first the right suture in each anastomosis, then the left suture, always starting from the right anastomosis.
2. Placement of 2 equidistant sutures in each of the anterior surfaces of the anastomoses.
3. Rotation of the vein graft.
4. Assessment of the sutures of the anterior surface in each anastomosis following rotation of the vein graft.
5. Placement of 2 equidistant sutures in each of the posterior surfaces of the anastomoses.
6. Ligation of the femoral artery between the two anastomoses using a 9/0 suture.
7. Release of the femoral artery from the double clamp.
8. Placement of a moist gauze on the anastomoses for 3 minutes.
9. Patency test.
10. Withdrawal of the yellow background.

H. **Closure of surgical trauma:** The skin and superficial fascia are closed in one layer with interrupted, non-absorbable 2/0 sutures.

21 End-to-end anastomoses of the superficial inferior epigastric vessels

A. Positioning of the rat

The rat is placed in the dorsal decubitus (supine) position on the working surface. The long axis of the body of the rat is perpendicular to the frontal plane of the surgeon's body, and the rat's head is placed away from the surgeon. The limbs of the rat are immobilized on the working surface with adhesive tape (**Fig 18-1**).

B. Preparation of the surgical field

The reader can find a more thorough presentation of the same operative field in the respective paragraph in Chapter 18.

A 2-cm long incision is made parallel to and 1 cm below the inguinal crease. After opening the skin and the fatty layer (Camper's fascia) of the superficial fascia, the membranous layer of the superficial fascia (Scarpa's fascia) can be observed if the incision is performed gently (No. 1, **Fig. 18-4**). The superficial inferior epigastric vessels are found in the superficial fascia, on the membranous layer (**Fig. 21-1**). When the membranous layer is detached from the deep fascia investing the muscles, the superficial epigastric vessels move along with it. Placement of a retractor usually is not necessary during the dissection of the superficial inferior epigastric vessels.

C. Microsurgical dissection of the vessels

Starting from the femoral vessels, a plane separating the superficial inferior epigastric artery from the homonymous vein is developed in the membranous layer of the superficial fascia (**Fig. 21-1**). Then, the membranous layer is removed from the vessels wall as much as possible. This dissection may be done sharply (forceps-scissors) or bluntly (forceps-forceps), or used interchangeably. Evidently, specific attention must be paid to the superficial inferior epigastric vein whose wall is more fragile (**Fig. 21-2**). The artery, however, also needs attention because it may easily spasm with manipulations due to its miniscule size. The aim of this dissection is to separate the superficial epigastric vessels and to clean them completely from the attaching fascia (**Fig. 21-3**).

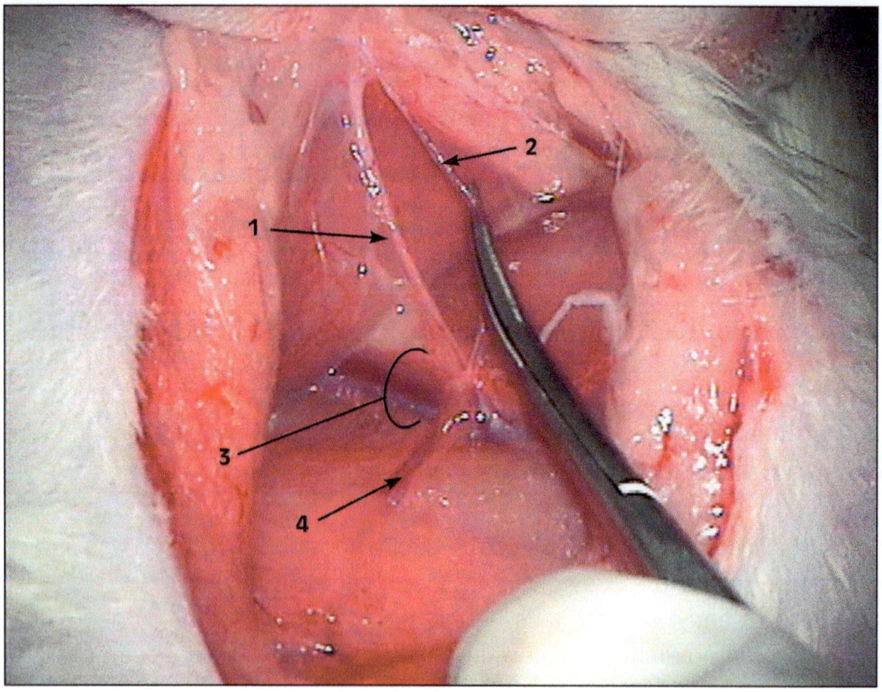

Figure 21-1

Preparation of the surgical field of the superficial inferior epigastric vessels. The vessels lie on the membranous layer of the superficial fascia of the lower abdominal wall. The membranous layer has been opened with microsurgical scissors between the artery and the vein. The tip of the microsurgical scissors is passed behind the membranous layer of the superficial fascia; this layer has been detached from the deep fascia that invests the abdominal wall muscles. **1.** superficial inferior epigastric artery, **2.** superficial inferior epigastric vein, **3.** femoral vessels, **4.** vein of the adductor muscle. (From author's photo library)

D. End-to-end anastomoses

The reader is invited to read the full description of end-to-end anastomosis in Chapter 5. A brief description is given here.

Superficial inferior epigastric artery

- The anastomosis will be performed by placing **4 sutures 11/0**.

The steps of the process of the end-to-end anastomosis are as follows:

1. Placement of a yellow plastic background under the artery.
2. Application of the double clamp on the artery.
3. Transection of the vessel.
4. Irrigation of the lumen with warm normal saline.
5. Folding of the adventitia in both stumps.
6. Approximation of the two clamps of the double clamp.

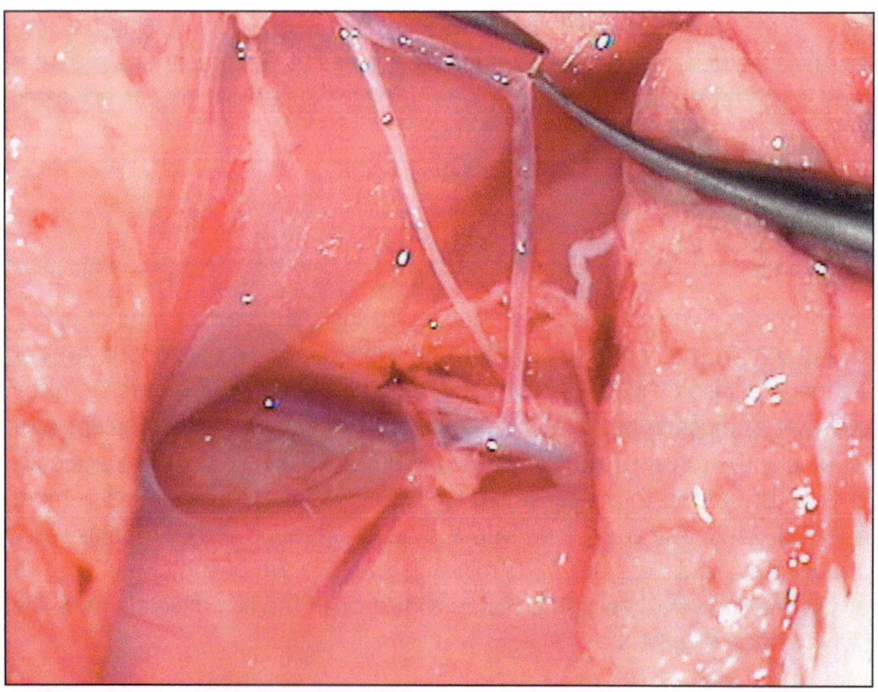

Figure 21-2

Dissection of the superficial inferior epigastric vein. Dumont No. 3 forceps holds and the scissors cut a residue of fascia attached to the vein. (From author's photo library)

Figure 21-3

Completely dissected superficial inferior epigastric vessels. **1.** superficial inferior epigastric artery, **2.** superficial inferior epigastric vein, **3.** femoral artery, **4.** femoral vein, **5.** vein from the adductor muscle. (From author's photo library)

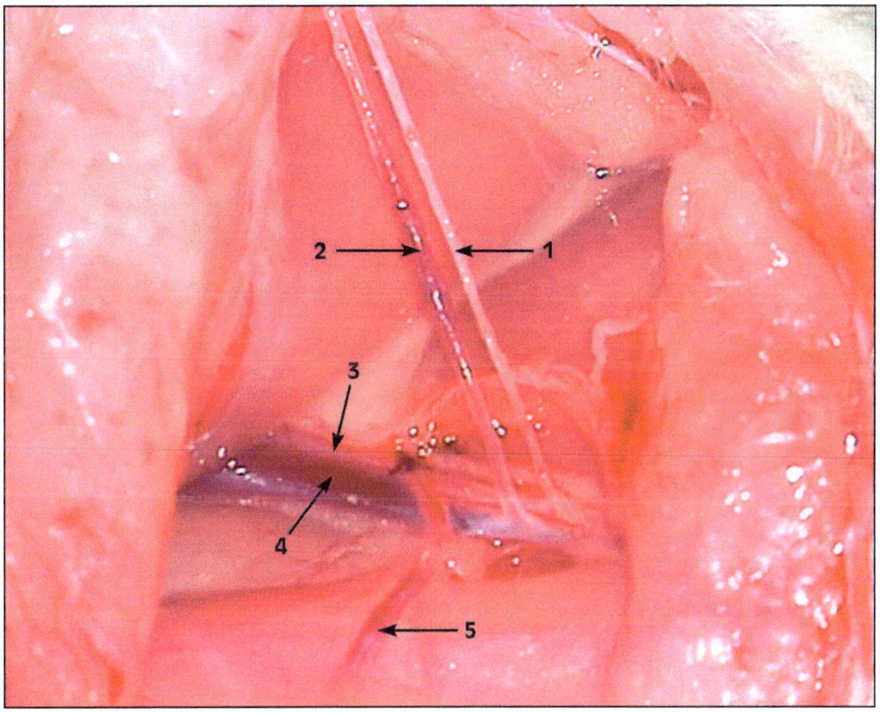

7. Anastomosis of the arterial stumps starts with placement of the 2 corner sutures that will orient the two stumps.
8. The anterior surface of the anastomosis is completed with the placement of one suture in the middle of the semicircle.
9. Rotation of the double clamp.
10. Check of the suture of the anterior surface.
11. The posterior surface is completed with one suture in the middle of the semicircle.
12. Release of the vessel from the double clamp.
13. Placement of a wet gauze on the anastomosis for 3 minutes.
14. Patency test, as described in Chapter 5.10 (**Fig. 5-4**). In brief, distal to the anastomosis, a first forceps is applied upstream to occlude the vessel. A second forceps is placed just next to the first, then moves 'half-closed' downstream to empty the vessel, and closes completely at some point. The first forceps is removed and the lumen is immediately filled up to the second forceps if there is patency.
    Due to its small size, the superficial inferior epigastric artery can easily spasm with the manipulations of the patency test. *In such a case, the vessel looks 'empty', and characteristically this happens central to the anastomosis* (**Fig. 21-4**). The spasm can be resolved with irrigation of the field with warm normal saline. If there is no response to this, irrigation with 1% papaverine follows. The patency test is repeated after resolution of the arterial spasm.
15. Withdrawal of the yellow plastic background.

Superficial inferior epigastric vein

- The anastomosis will be performed by placing **6 sutures 11/0**.

The steps of the process of the end-to-end anastomosis are as follows:

1. Placement of a yellow plastic background under the vein.
2. Application of the double clamp on the vein.
3. Transection of the vessel.
4. Irrigation of the lumen with warm normal saline.
5. Removal of the adventitia in both stumps.
6. Approximation of the two clamps of the double clamp.
7. Anastomosis of the venous stumps starts with placement of the corner sutures that will orient the two stumps (**Fig. 21-5**).
8. The anterior surface of the anastomosis is completed with the placement of 2 sutures equidistant from each other and from the corner sutures.
9. Rotation of the double clamp.
10. Checking of the sutures of the anterior surface.
11. The posterior surface is completed with 2 sutures equidistant from each other and from the corner sutures.

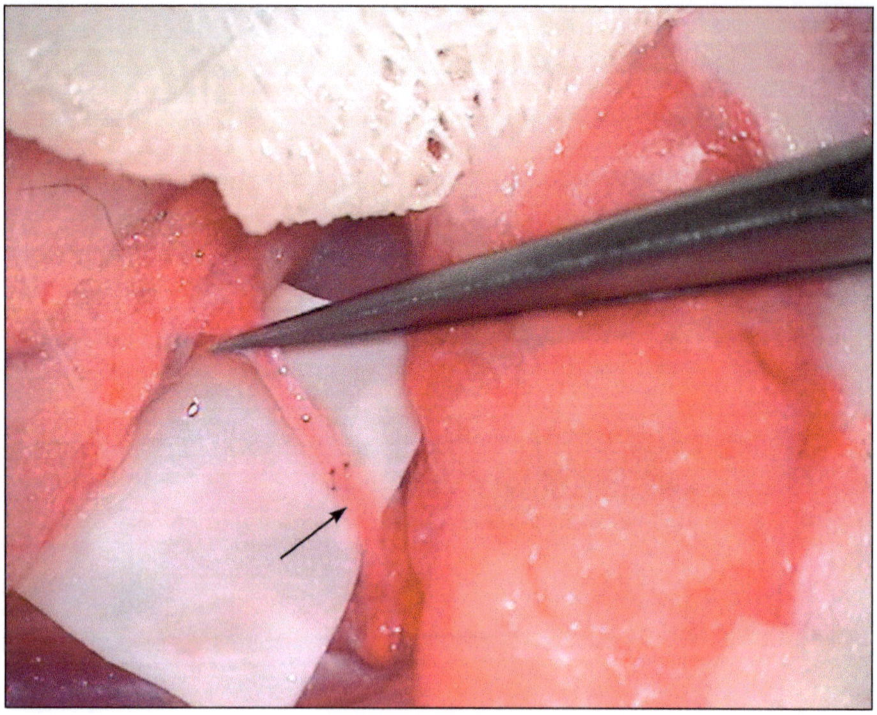

Figure 21-4

In the final step of the patency test (in the previous step the lumen has been emptied with two forceps, see Figure 5-4), the upstream (central) forceps has been removed and the superficial inferior epigastric artery looks empty up to the downstream remaining forceps. The fact that it looks empty central to the anastomosis means that this is due to spasm of the miniscule artery. The three sutures of the anterior surface of the anastomosis can be seen, and the arrow shows the empty central part of the vessel. The patency test will be repeated after resolution of the spasm by irrigation with normal saline or 1% papaverine. (From author's photo library)

12. Release of the vessel from the double clamp.
13. Placement of a wet gauze on the anastomosis for 3 minutes.
14. Patency test as described in Chapter 5.10 (**Fig. 5-4**). In brief, central to the anastomosis (toward the femoral vein), one forceps occludes upstream the vessel and a second empties the lumen moving 'half-closed' downstream (towards the femoral vein), and closes completely at some point. The first forceps is removed and the lumen is immediately filled up to the second forceps if there is patency.
15. Withdrawal of the yellow plastic background.

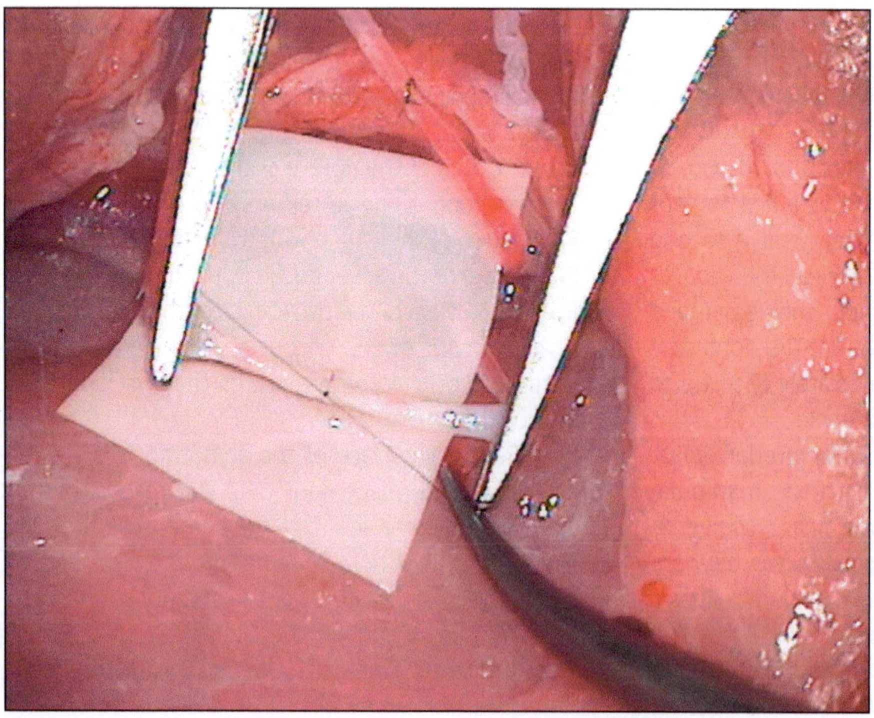

Figure 21-5

Placement of the second corner suture in the anastomosis of the superficial inferior epigastric vein stumps. (From author's photo library)

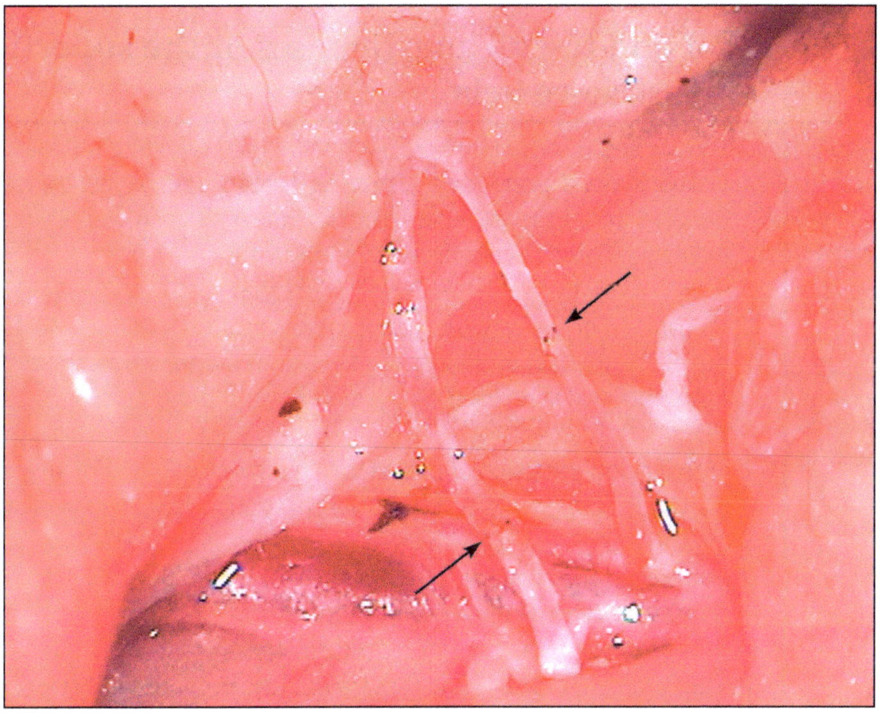

Figure 21-6

Completed anastomoses of the superficial inferior epigastric vessels. (From author's photo library)

The completed anastomoses of the two superficial inferior epigastric vessels can be seen in **Figure 21-6**.

E. Closure of the surgical trauma

The skin and the superficial fascia are closed in one layer with interrupted, non-absorbable 2/0 sutures.

... of end-to-end anastomoses of the superficial inferior epigastric vessels

Synopsis...

A. Positioning of the rat: Dorsal decubitus (supine) position, head away of the surgeon (the longitudinal axis of the rat is perpendicular to the surgeon's frontal plane). The limbs are immobilized on the working surface with adhesive tape.

B. Preparation of the surgical field: A 2-cm incision is made parallel to and 1 cm below the inguinal crease. After opening the fatty layer of the superficial fascia, the superficial inferior epigastric vessels are revealed on the membranous layer.

C. Microsurgical dissection of the vessels: The superficial inferior epigatsric vessels are dissected, starting from the femoral vessels. The artery and the vein are separated and cleaned fully.

D. End-to-end anastomoses

Superficial inferior epigatsric artery: **4 sutures 11/0**

Superficial inferior epigatsric vein: **6 sutures 11/0**

The anastomoses are performed separately, following the same steps:

1. Placement of a yellow plastic background under the vessel.
2. Application of the double clamp.
3. Transection of the vessel.
4. Irrigation of the lumen with warm normal saline.
5. Removal of the adventitia.
6. Approximation of the two clamps of the double clamp.
7. Anastomosis of the vessel. First two are placed as corner sutures.
8. The anterior surface of the anastomosis is completed
   Artery: 1 suture in the middle of the semicircle.
   Vein: 2 sutures placed equidistance from each other and from the corner sutures.
9. Rotation of the double clamp.
10. Checking of the suture(s) of the anterior surface.
11. The posterior surface is completed in similar fashion to the anterior.
12. Release of the vessel from the double clamp.
13. Placement of wet gauze on the anastomosis for 3 minutes.
14. Patency test.
15. Withdrawal of the yellow background.

E. Closure of surgical trauma: The skin and superficial fascia are sutured together with interrupted, non-absorbable 2/0 sutures.

PART IV

TRANSPLANTATIONS

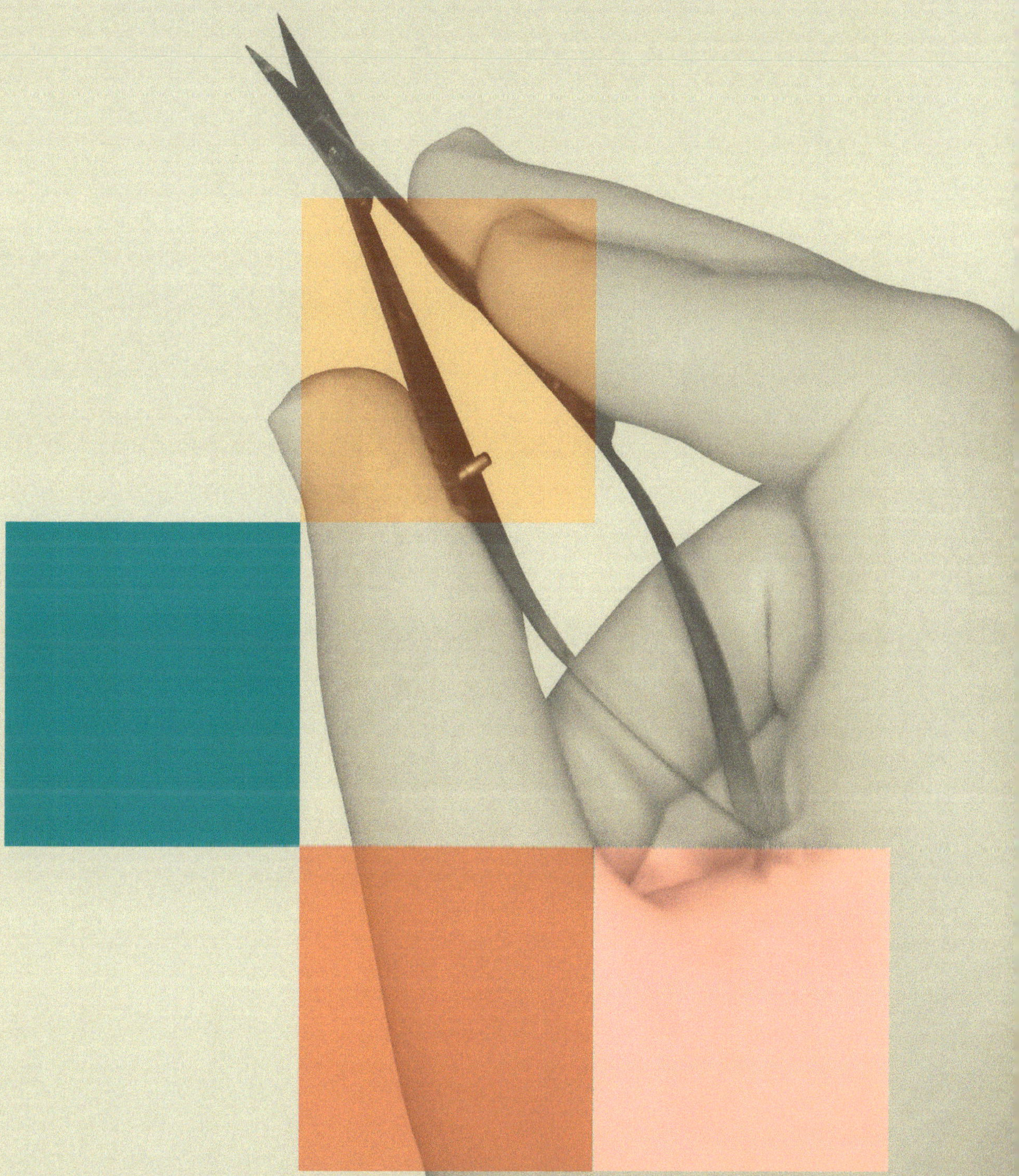

22 Orthotopic autotransplantation of pedicled inguinal skin flap

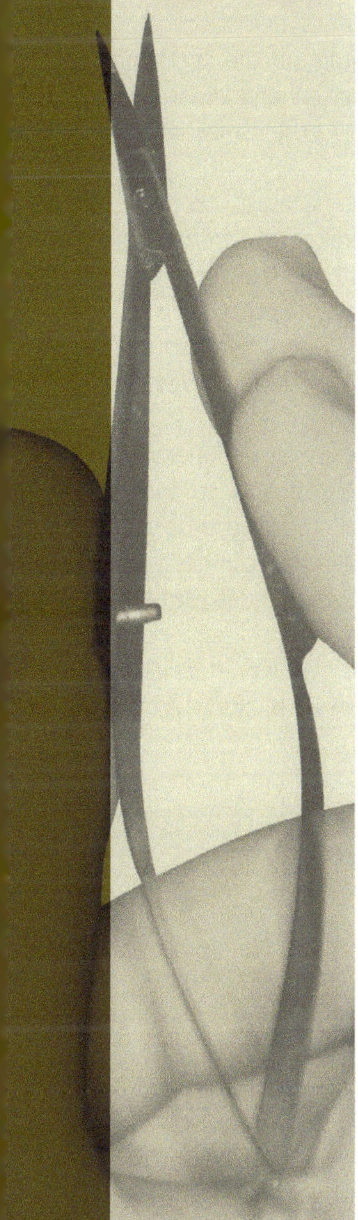

The inguinal skin flap is supplied by the superficial inferior epigastric vessels, which are branches of the femoral vessels. The orthotopic autotransplantation of the inguinal flap will be based on in situ, end-to-end anastomoses of the femoral vessels.

A. Positioning the rat

The rat is placed in dorsal decubitus (supine) position on the working surface. The long axis of the body of the rat is perpendicular to the frontal plane of the surgeon's body, with the head of the rat away from the surgeon. The limbs of the rat are immobilized on the working surface with adhesive tape (**Fig. 22-1**).

B. Preparation of the surgical field

The reader is invited to review Chapter 18.B, where the surgical anatomy and the access to the femoral vessels are described in detail, as well as Chapter 21.B concerning the superficial inferior epigastric vessels. Important elements of surgical anatomy for definition of surgical planes are not repeated here.

A 2 cm incision is made 1 cm below the inguinal crease running parallel to it. (No. 1, **Fig. 22-1**). After opening the superficial fascia, the femoral vessels and the superficial inferior epigastric vessels are exposed, and the rest of the branches/tributaries of the femoral vessels are visualized. The deep fascia is opened with two gauze pads moistened in warm normal saline, providing greater exposure of the femoral vessels along with their branches/tributaries (the full cleaning of the vessels, however, requires microsurgical dissection, see below).

- ➢ During all surgical and microsurgical dissection, preserving the surgical plane of the superficial inferior epigastric vessels is imperative for proper flap harvest (**Fig. 22-2**). These vessels are adhered to the membranous layer of the superficial fascia, which can be separated from the deep fascia investing the lower abdominal wall muscles.

C. Microsurgical dissection of the vessels

The reader is asked to read Chapter 18.C, where the microsurgical dissection of the

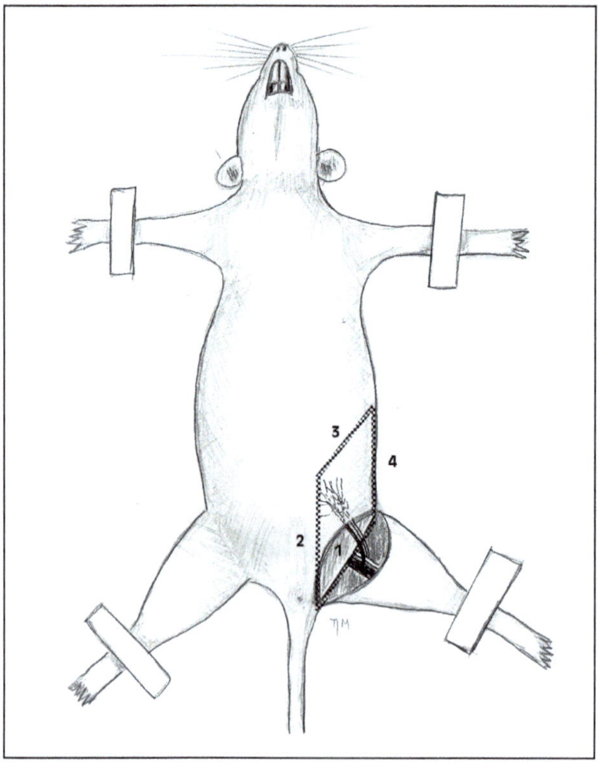

Figure 22-1

The rat in dorsal decubitus (supine) position with the head the away from surgeon and extremities taped to the working surface. The delineation of the flap (skin and superficial fascia) supplied by the superficial inferior epigastric vessels is shown. **1.** subinguinal incision, 2 cm in length, located 1 cm under the inguinal crease, **2.** paramedian incision, 4 cm in length, located 0.5 cm from midline, **3.** incision parallel to the inguinal incision, 2 cm in length, **4.** incision parallel to the paramedian incision, of same length. (Drawing by the author)

surgical field of the femoral vessels is described in detail.

In Chapter 18.C, the microsurgical dissection of the femoral vessels extends from the inguinal ligament to the junction of the superficial inferior epigastric vessels. This includes double-ligation and transection, or selective cauterization and transection of all branches/tributaries of the femoral vessels with the exception of the superficial inferior epigastric vessels. The vessels transected during this dissection include the superficial circumflex vein, the deep branch/tributary on the posterior surface of the vessels, the small artery and larger vein of the adductor muscle, and any other small lateral branches/tributaries encountered.

In the current operation, it is necessary to continue the dissection of the femoral vessels peripheral to the superficial inferior epigastric vessels until reaching the saphenous vein. This ensures that each femoral vessel can be easily ligated peripheral to the junction of the superficial inferior epigastric vessels (see below in E).

The dissection of the femoral vessels peripheral to the junction of the superficial inferior epigastric vessels continues along the femoral artery because the robust arterial wall of the femoral artery can easily be handled (**Fig. 22-3**). The dissection continues with the femoral vein, including the final part of the saphenous vein (peripheral to the saphenous opening). If smaller, lateral tributary veins are encountered, they can be

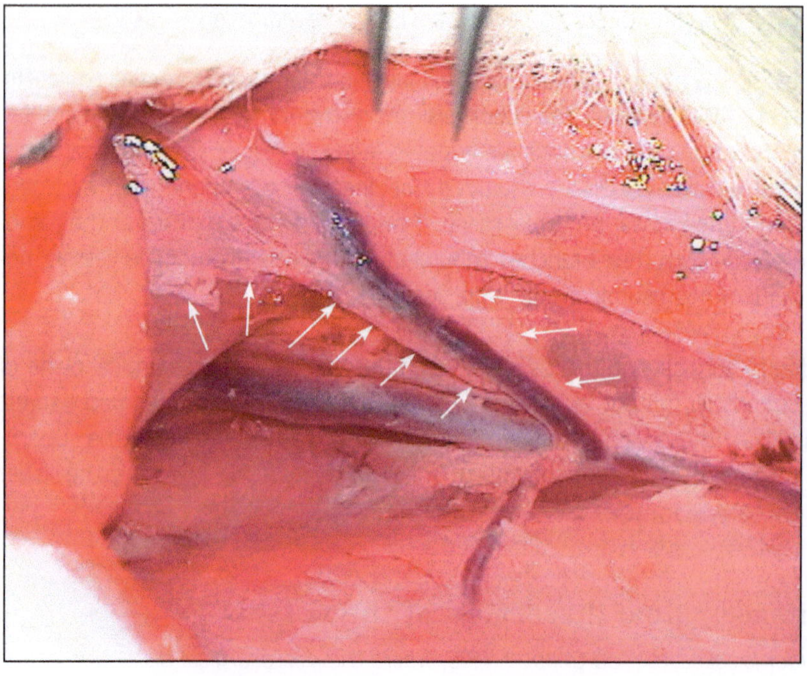

Figure 22-2

Surgical plane of the superficial inferior epigastric vessels. These vessels are found within the superficial fascia, adhered to the membranous layer (white arrows) of this fascia. This layer lies superficial to the deep investing fascia of the anterior abdominal wall musculature. (From author's photo library)

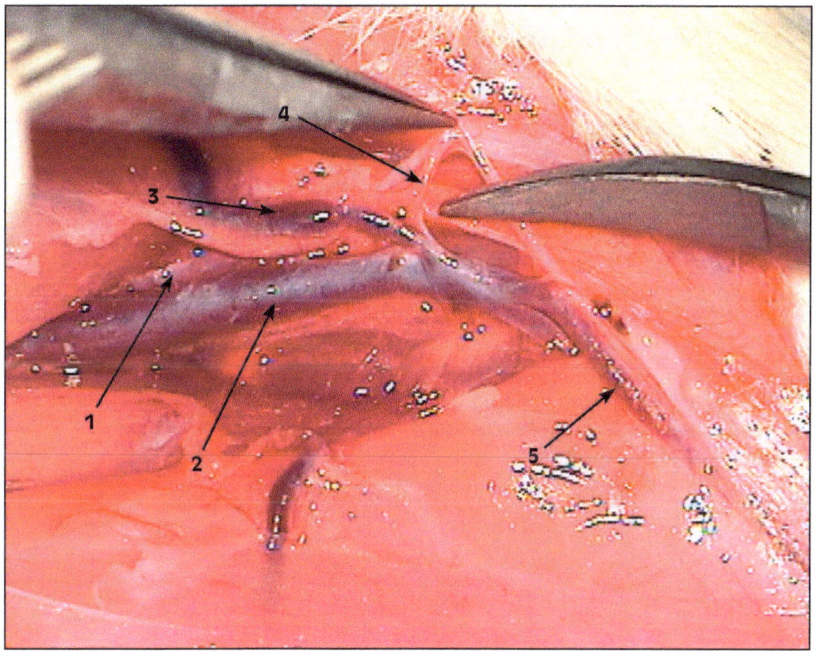

Figure 22-3

Dissection of the femoral vessels peripheral to the junction of the superficial inferior epigastric vessels. Dumont No. 3 forceps lifts the femoral artery at the origin of the superficial inferior epigastric artery, while the scissors develop a plane of separation between femoral artery and femoral vein. **1.** femoral artery, **2.** femoral vein, **3.** superficial inferior epigastric vein, **4.** superficial inferior epigastric artery, **5.** saphenous vein. (From author's photo library)

cauterized (**Fig. 22-4**). The superficial inferior epigastric vessels are also dissected, but only proximal to the femoral vessels in order to preserve the surgical plane when harvesting the flap. This plane is defined between the membranous layer of the superficial fascia, to which the superficial inferior epigastric vessels adhere, and the deep fascia investing the muscles (see below in D).

D. Dissection and mobilization of the flap

The flap is shaped like a rectangle and delineated by: a paramedian incision 4 cm in length located 0.5 cm from the midline and joining the medial end of the subinguinal incision (No. 2, **Fig. 22-1**), an incision parallel to the inguinal incision beginning at the superior apex of the

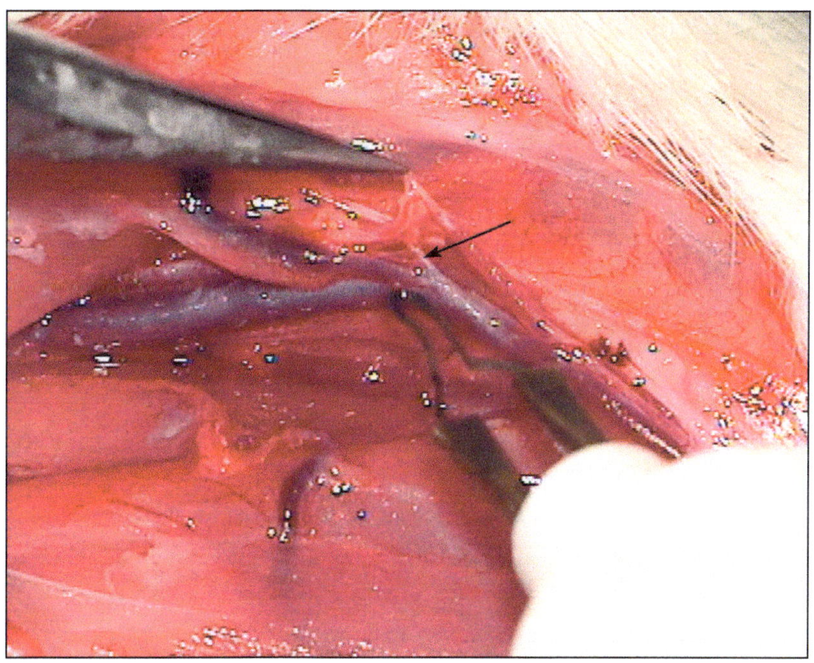

Figure 22-4

Cauterization of a lateral tributary of the femoral vein. The femoral artery has been previously separated from the femoral vein. Using Dumont No. 3 forceps, traction is provided by grasping a residue of the fascia surrounding the superficial inferior epigastric artery. A small lateral tributary vein is revealed (arrow) and will be cauterized with the monopolar diathermy brought in the field. (From author's photo library)

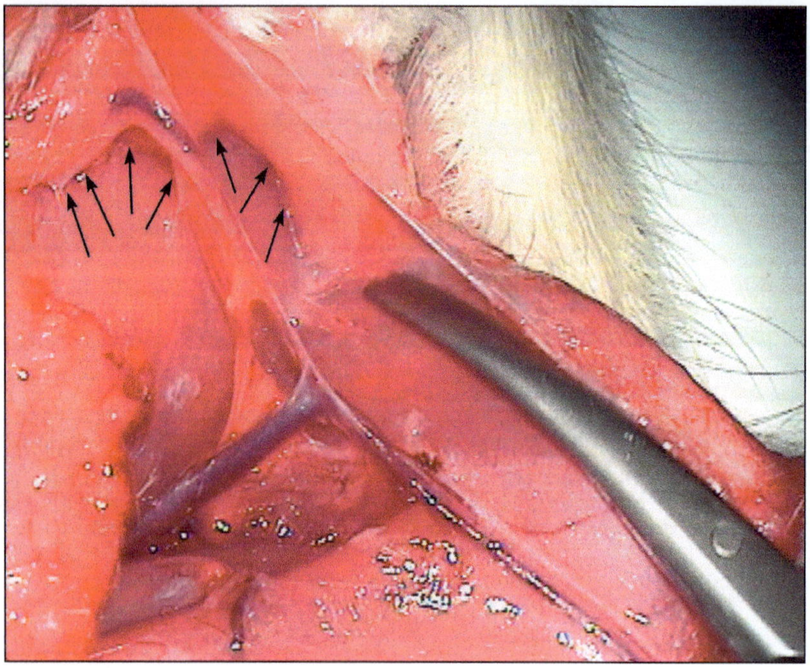

Figure 22-5

Surgical plane of the superficial inferior epigastric vessels after microsurgical dissection of the femoral vessels. The flap is pulled cranially from the edge of the subinguinal incision and the stem of the superficial inferior epigastric vessels is revealed. The plane of separation (arrows) is between the superficial fascia containing the vessels and the deep fascia investing the external oblique muscle. (From author's photo library)

paramedian incision and running the same length as the inguinal (No. 3, **Fig. 22-1**), and a final incision that will be performed after the dissection of the clockwise-rotated 'U', delineated by the three incisions so far.

Traction on the edge of the subinguinal incision assists exposure of the surgical plane of the superficial inferior epigastric vessels (**Fig. 22-5**). Fibro-fatty tissue removed during dissection of the femoral vessels may reduce the thickness of the superficial fascia packing these vessels (compare with **Figure 22-2**). The plane of separation between the deep fascia investing the muscles and the membranous layer of the superficial fascia will be the surgical plane of dissection of the flap. Dissection is performed from medial to lateral using Baby-Metzenbaum scissors. The superficial inferior epigastric vessels are carefully mobilized together with the superficial fascia and skin by precise dissection, staying directly on the investing fascia of the external abdominal muscle (**Fig. 22-6**). Maintaining direct visualization of the superficial inferior epigastric vessels during dissec-

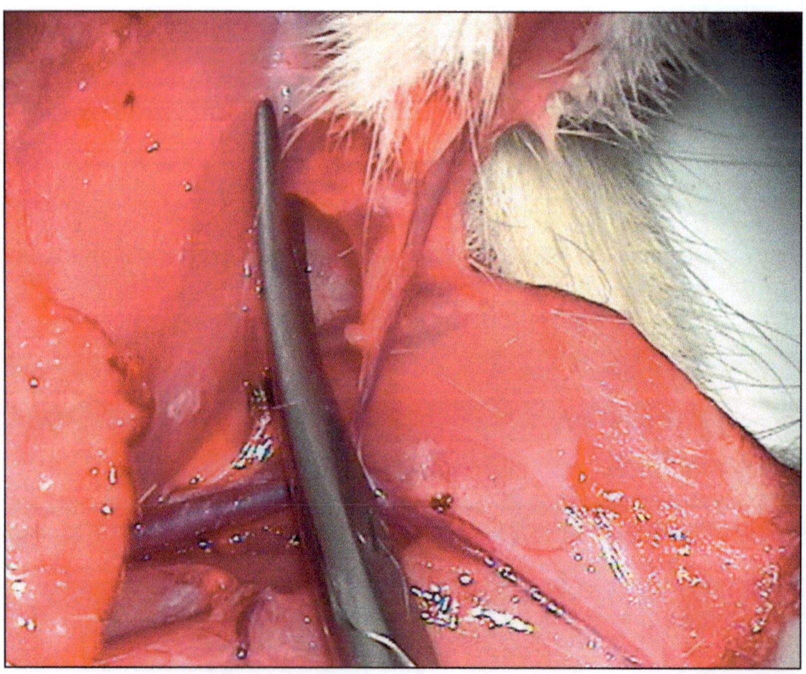

Figure 22-6

Mobilization of the flap from medially to laterally. The flap is lifted and the baby-Metzenbaum scissors sever the attachments between the superficial fascia and the deep fascia investing the external oblique muscle. Attachments are cut as close to the investing fascia of the muscle as possible to allow mobilization of vessels together with the superficial fascia and skin. (From author's photo library) tion will minimize trauma to the vessels. The superficial inferior epigastric vessels should remain in the center of the flap throughout dissection and tension must never be placed on the vasculature of the flap.

Once the flap and its vessels are mobilized, the 4th incision is performed parallel to the paramedian incision (No. 4, **Fig. 22-1**). The flap is now free on all sides attached only by the pedicle of superficial inferior epigastric vessels. The flap is moved laterally with care to avoid torsion, and is placed on either the abdominal wall or on the working surface depending on which location applies the least tension to the vascular pedicle. The internal surface of the flap should be placed on a gauze pad moistened with warm normal saline. A second moistened gauze pad is placed on the hair-side of the flap.

E. Transection of the femoral vessels between two ligations distal to the junction of the superficial inferior epigastric vessels

Peripheral to the junction of the superficial inferior epigastric vessels, each of the femoral vessels is ligated with two 9/0 sutures and transected. The distance between the suture ligations should be sufficient to allow for a comfortable transection of the vessel. The first suture is placed as close as possible to the junction of each of the superficial inferior epigastric vessels.

Vessel ligation and transection should begin with the femoral vein, located superficial to the femoral artery on the surgical field (**Fig. 22-7**). Alternatively, proximal ligation sutures may be placed on both vessels, starting with

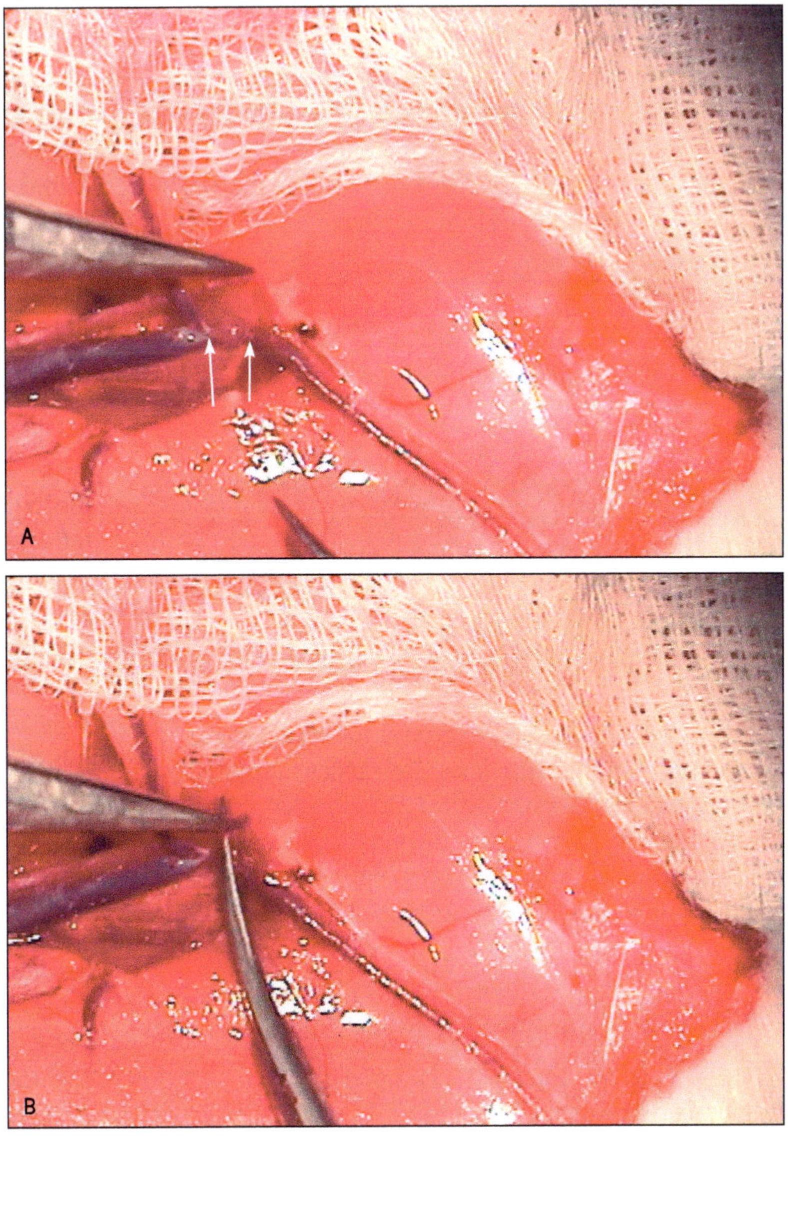

Figure 22-7

Ligation and transection of the femoral vein peripheral to the junction of the superficial inferior epigastric vessels. **A.** Two ligations with 9/0 suture (white arrows) have been placed on the femoral vein. The forceps elevates the femoral artery to reveal them. **B.** The femoral vein is transected between ligations. The forceps lifts the femoral artery to provide sufficient space for scissors to transect the vein. (From author's photo library)

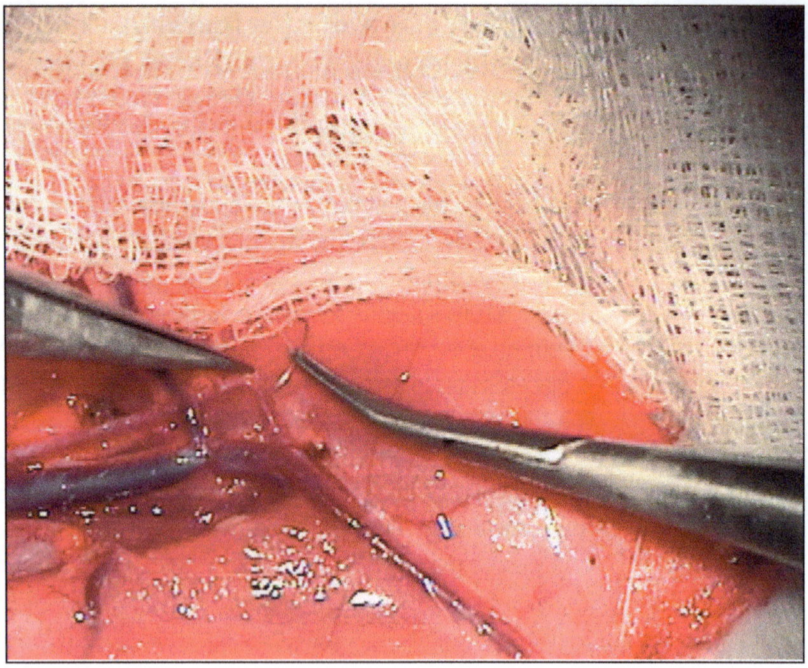

Figure 22-8

Proximal ligation of the femoral artery, placed peripheral to the junction of the superficial inferior epigastric vessels. The proximal ligation of the femoral vein was placed previously. The forceps elevates the femoral artery while the needle-holder grasps the 9/0 suture needle used to place the ligation stitch. (From author's photo library)

the vein, followed by peripheral ligation sutures and transection of both vessels between ligations (**Fig. 22-8**).

F. Placement of the double clamp - Transection of the femoral vessels central to the junction of the superficial inferior epigastric vessels - Irrigation - Removal of the adventitia

A yellow plastic background is placed under the stumps of femoral vessels. The stumps of the femoral vessels are placed together in the clamps of the double clamp. One clamp is placed near the inguinal ligament and the second clamp is placed immediately proximal to the junction of the superficial inferior epigastric vessels. (**Fig. 22-9**).

Using a single cut, the vessels are transected in the middle between the two clamps. Each lumen is irrigated with warm normal saline through a 27G angiocatheter attached to a syringe. The adventitia of the artery is folded in each stump. The adventitia of the vein stump is removed circumferentially around the edges of the vessel.

G. End-to-end anastomoses

The reader will find a detailed description of end-to-end vascular anastomosis in Chapter 5.

- **6 sutures 11/0 are placed in the anastomosis of femoral arteries**
- **6 or 8 sutures 11/0 are placed in the anastomoses of femoral veins**

The anterior surfaces of both vessels are sutured first, the double clamp is rotated together with the flap, and the posterior surfaces are sutured.

The steps of the anastomoses are as follows:

1. Suturing the artery is typically performed first, but is not strictly necessary. Here, the vein is sutured first. In our experience, 8 sutures are usually necessary for the vein: 2 sutures at the corners, 3 sutures on the anterior surface [one in the middle of the semicircle and one in the middle of each quadrant (**Fig. 22-10**), and 3 on the posterior surface placed similarly. If 6 sutures are placed (similar to the artery): 2 sutures at the corners, and 2 sutures on both the anterior and posterior surfaces, placed at equal distances from the corner sutures and between themselves. The completed anastomosis of the anterior surface of the vessels is shown in **Figure 22-11**.
2. The double clamp is rotated to check the sutures of the anterior surface.
3. Suturing of the posterior surfaces of the femoral vein (**Fig. 22-12**) and femoral artery (**Fig. 22-13**) is completed in the same manner as the anterior surfaces.
4. The double clamp and the flap are returned to their initial position and the vessels are released

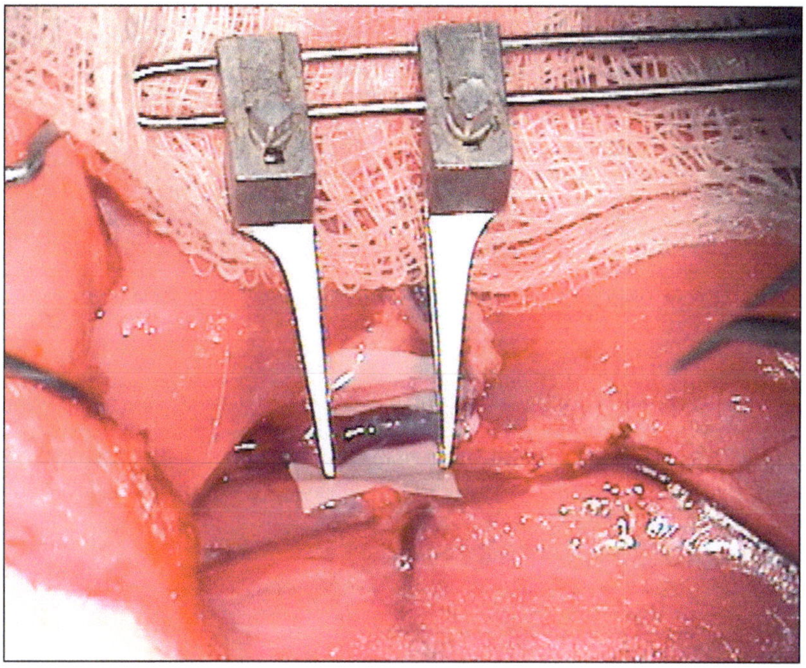

Figure 22-9

Placement of the stumps of the femoral vessels in the double clamp. The central clamp is applied on the vessels near the inguinal ligament, and the peripheral clamp is placed before the junction of the superficial inferior epigastric vessels. A yellow plastic background has been previously placed under the vessels. (From author's photo library)

from the clamps. The peripheral clamp is opened first, followed by the central clamp. Since the double clamp is opened, the patient artery will immediately fill. The venous return from the flap is slow, causing some delay in the filling of the vein (**Fig. 22-14**).

5. A wet gauze pad is placed over the anastomoses for 3 minutes.
6. Patency test, separately for each vessel, as described in detail in Chapter 5.10 (**Fig. 5-4**), described below in brief. Testing occurs following the flow of blood: The arterial anastomosis is tested distal to

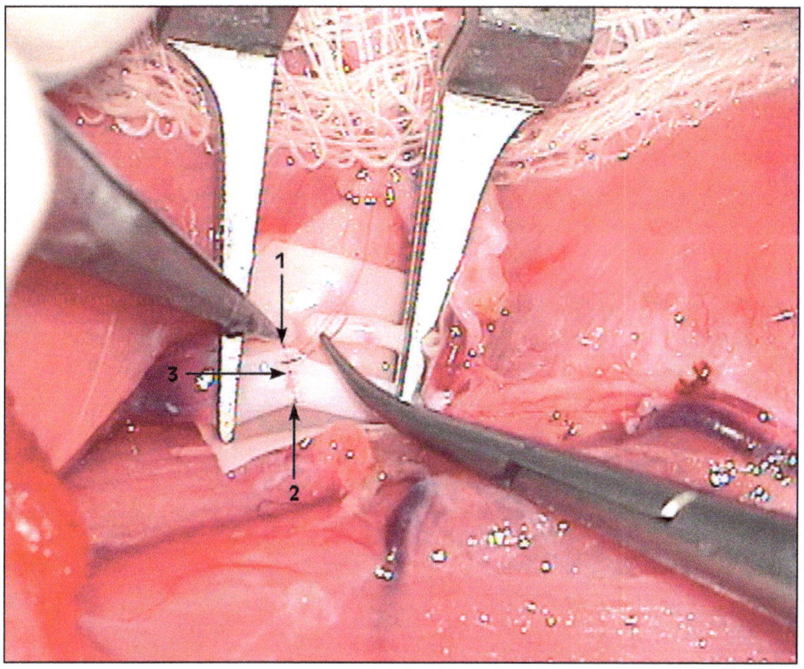

Figure 22-10

Suturing the anterior surface of the femoral vein. Here, the 4th suture is being placed in the middle of one quadrant. The numbers represent the order and the location of the previous sutures. **1** and **2** are the corner sutures, **3** is the suture in the middle of the semicircle. (From author's photo library)

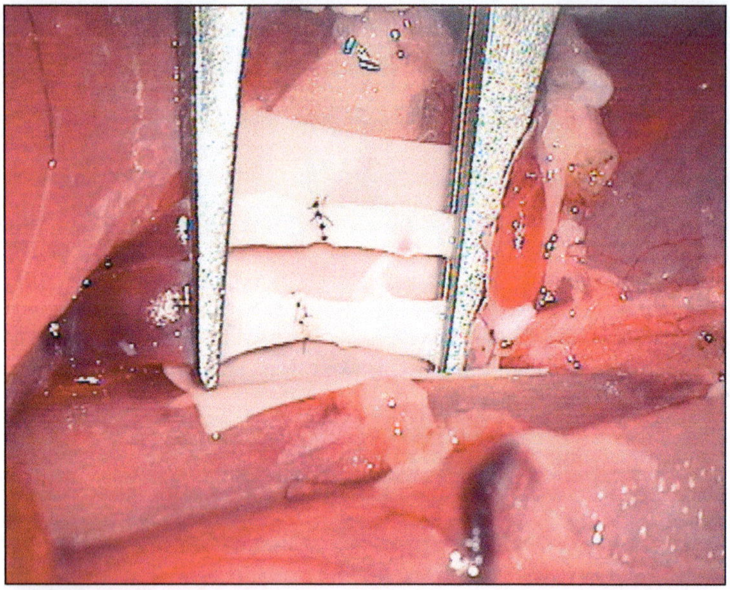

Figure 22-11

Completed suture of the anterior surfaces of the femoral vessels. (From author's photo library)

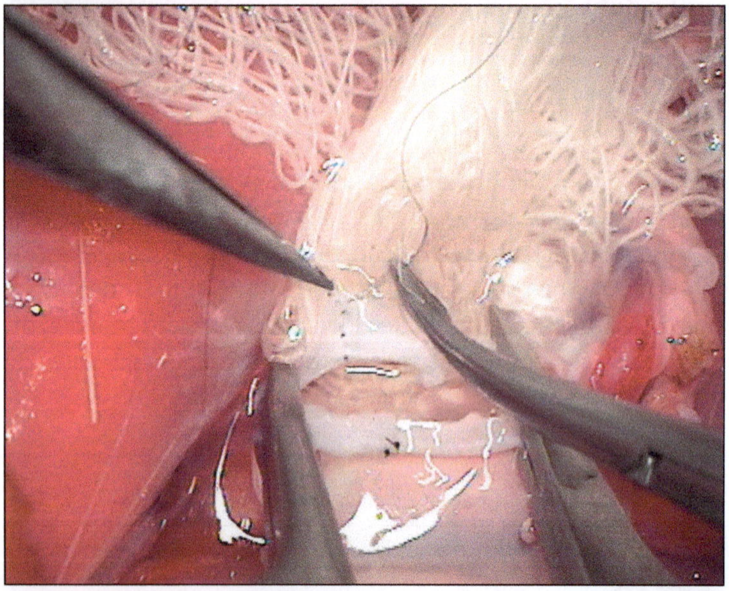

Figure 22-12

Suturing the posterior surface of the femoral vein. The double clamp has been reversed together with the inguinal flap (wrapped in gauze). Rotating the clamp brings the femoral vein laterally. Notice the vessels float in normal saline, keeping the lumen of the vein open. The forceps holds the vein from the corner suture, while the last (8th) suture is placed in the middle of the quadrant (here the suture in the middle of the posterior semicircle has been placed prior to the sutures in the middle of quadrants). (From author's photo library)

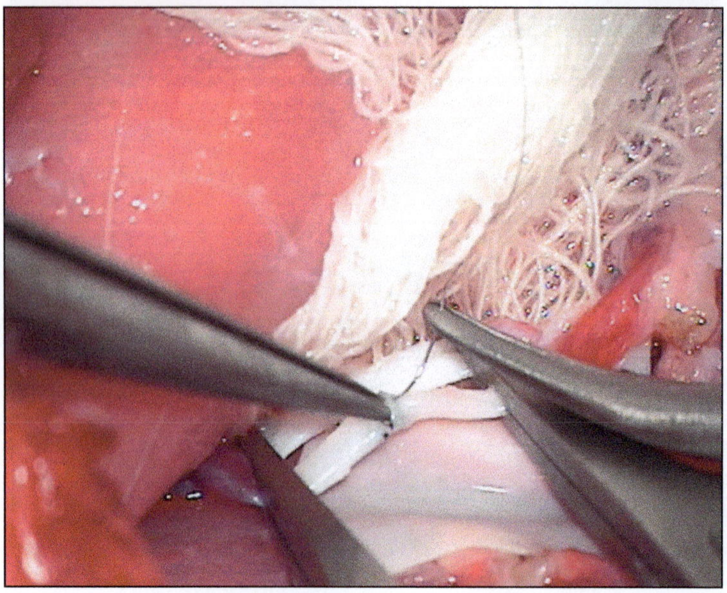

Figure 22-13

Suturing the posterior surface of the femoral artery. The forceps, with its tips slightly open, enters the lumen for support, while the 11/0 suture is now ready to pass through the vessel wall. (From author's photo library)

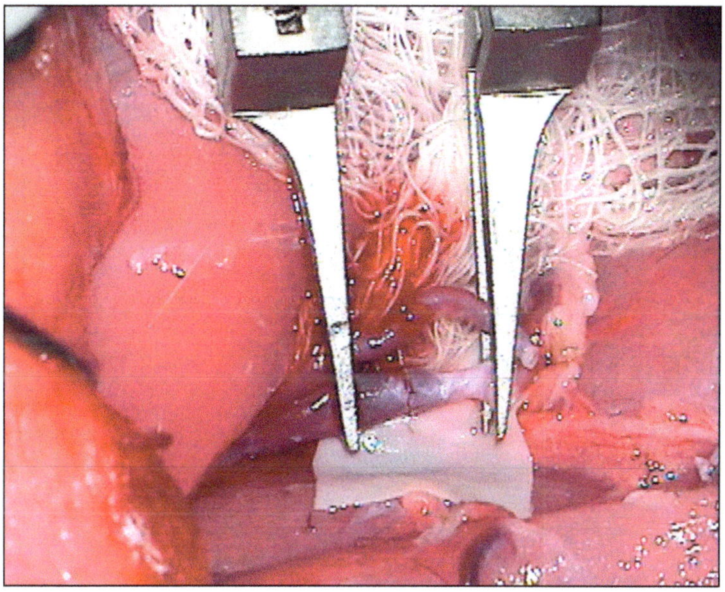

Figure 22-14

Opening of the double clamp. The anastomosed femoral artery fills with blood immediately after removing the clamp. Venous drainage from the flap (wrapped in gauze) is slower to fill the femoral vein. The superficial inferior epigastric vein that serves the flap is the only tributary of the femoral vein. Between the two clamps, retrograde filling of the vein can be seen. (From author's photo library)

the anastomosis and the venous anastomosis is tested proximal to the anastomosis. To test for patency, one upstream forceps is used to occlude the blood flow, while a second downstream forceps is placed initially next to the first forceps and then moves distally while half-closed, thereby 'milking' the vessel, and finally remains closed. The upstream forceps is removed, and if there is patency, the vessel is immediately filled up to the downstream forceps.

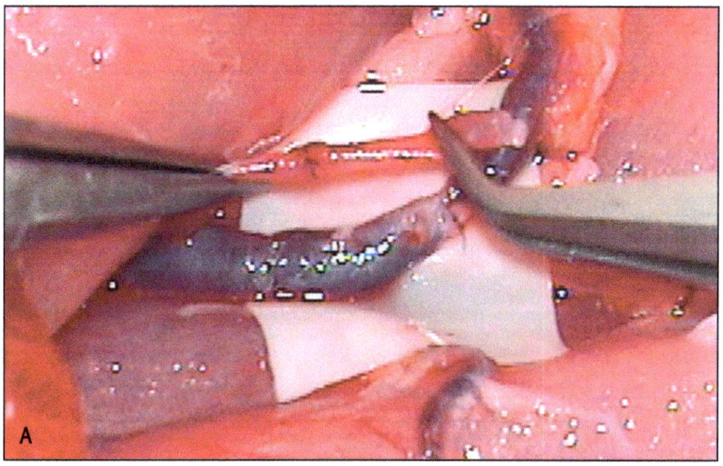

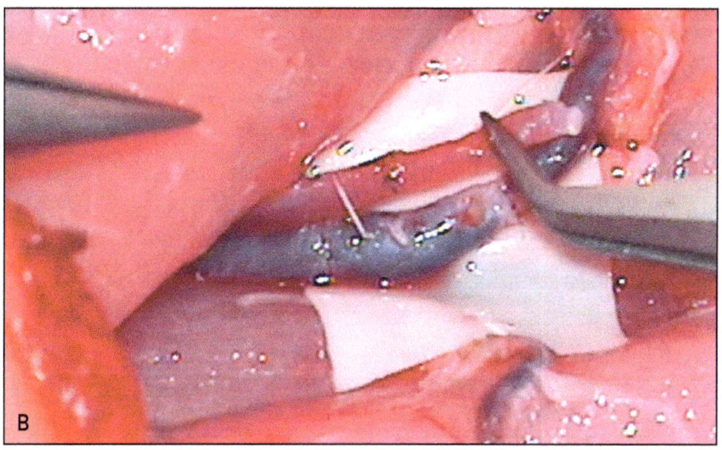

Figure 22-15

Alternative testing the patency of the femoral artery anastomosis. **A.** An upstream forceps stops the blood flow while a downstream forceps empties the lumen and is clamped. **B.** The upstream forceps is removed, while keeping the downstream forceps in place. The lumen of the vessel is filled with blood up to the downstream forceps, demonstrating a patent anastomosis. (From author's photo library)

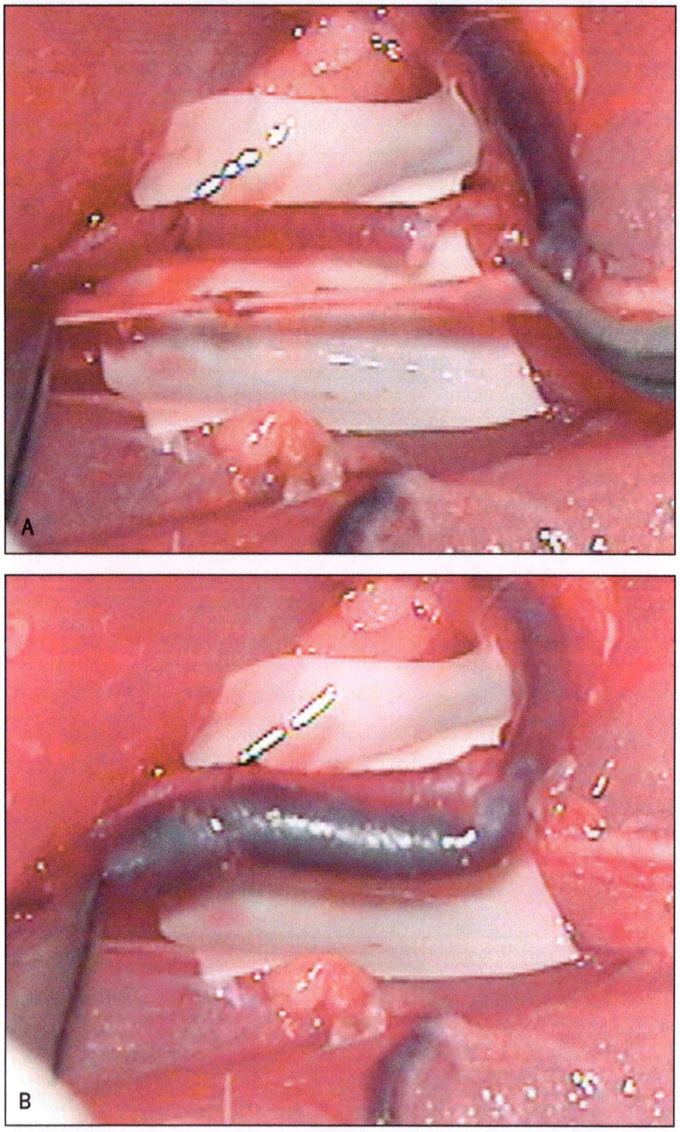

Figure 22-16

Alternative testing the patency of the femoral vein anastomosis. **A.** The (upstream) forceps is placed on the flap-side of the anastomosis, interrupting venous return. The downstream forceps moves half-closed cranially over the anastomosis, emptying the lumen of the vein. **B.** The upstream forceps is removed, keeping the downstream forceps in place. If the anastomosis was successful, the lumen will fill with blood up to the downstream forceps. (From author's photo library)

Here an alternative technique is presented, addressed to more expert surgeons. In the artery, an upstream forceps is placed cranial to the anastomosis to occlude blood flow. A downstream forceps is applied initially next to the first forceps, moved peripherally to 'milk' the vessel, passing over the anastomosis, and eventually closed (**Fig. 22-15A**). The upstream forceps is removed, and causes the arterial lumen to fill with blood up to the downstream forceps if the anastomosis is patent (**Fig. 22-15B**).

Since the blood flow in the vein is opposite, the upstream forceps is placed peripheral to the anastomosis near the flap, while the downstream forceps is run cranially half-open to empty the vein (**Fig. 22-16**).

In both vessels, artery and vein, this alternative technique requires specific attention because the downstream forceps moves of the suture line and may jeopardize it.

7. The yellow plastic background is withdrawn.

H. Closure of surgical trauma

The skin and the superficial fascia are closed in a single layer around the inguinal dermal flap (including the subinguinal incision) with interrupted, non-absorbable 2/0 sutures.

Alternative Technique Using the Superficial Inferior Epigastric Vessels

The operation may performed with end-to-side anastomoses of the superficial inferior epigastric vessels to the femoral vessels, but is far more demanding technically. If this method is chosen, the anastomosis of the artery is performed with **4 sutures 11/0** and that of the vein with **4 or 6 sutures 11/0**.

Synopsis...

... of orthotopic autotransplantation of pedicled inguinal skin flap

A. Positioning of the rat: Dorsal decubitus (supine) with the longitudinal axis of the rat perpendicular to the surgeon's frontal plane and the head facing away from the surgeon. The limbs are immobilized on the working surface with adhesive tape.

B. Preparation of the surgical field: A 2 cm incision is performed parallel and 1 cm inferior to the inguinal crease. After opening the superficial fascia, the deep fascia is torn with two gauze pads moistened with warm normal saline, revealing the femoral vessels and the superficial inferior epigatsric vessels. The membranous layer of the superficial fascia and the fatty layer around the superficial inferior epigastric vessels is preserved.

C. Microsurgical dissection of the vessels: The femoral vessels are dissected from the inguinal ligament to the saphenous vein. All branches/tributaries of the femoral vessels, with the exception of the superficial inferior epigastric vessels, are transected between two ligations (9/0). These include the superficial circumflex vein, the deep branch/tributary of the artery/vein found on the posterior surface of the vessels, the artery and vein of the adductor muscle, and any other small lateral branches/tributaries that can be cut with the diathermy.

D. Dissection and mobilization of the flap: The flap is delineated as a rectangular with the addition of three more incisions: 1) a paramedian incision 4 cm in length located 0.5 cm from the midline, starting at the medial end of the subinguinal incision. 2) a horizontal, 2 cm long incision parallel to the inguinal incision beginning at the superior apex of the paramedian incision. 3) a final incision parallel to the paramedian, after mobilization of the flap based on the superficial inferior epigastric vessels. The plane of dissection of the flap lies between the deep investing fascia of the abdominal wall musculature and the superficial fascia containing the superficial inferior epigastric vessels. Applying traction laterally to the flap, the attachments between the membranous layer and investing fascia are cut with scissors, in close proximity to the muscle.

E. Transection of the femoral vessels between two ligations (9/0 suture, each vessel, separately) distal to the junction of the superficial inferior epigastric vessels.

F. Transection of the femoral vessels central to the junction of the superficial inferior epigastric vessels: After positioning a yellow background, the double clamp is placed along the femoral vessels, and the vessels are transected at the midpoint between the two clamps. The vessel lumens are irrigated and their adventitia is removed.

G. End-to-end anastomoses:

- **6 sutures 11/0 in the anastomosis of femoral arteries**
- **6 or 8 sutures 11/0 in the anastomosis of femoral veins**

1. Placement of the corner sutures followed by suturing the anterior surface of each vessel.
2. Rotation of the clamp and check of the sutures of the anterior surface.
3. Suture of the posterior surface of the vessels is completed.
4. Release of the vessels from the double clamp.
5. Placement of a wet gauze on the anastomoses for 3 minutes.

... of orthotopic autotransplantation of pedicled inguinal skin flap

Synopsis...

6. Patency test, separately for each vessel.
7. Withdrawal of the yellow plastic background.

H. Closure of surgical trauma: The skin and superficial fascia are sutured in a single layer around the flap using 2/0 interrupted, non-absorbable sutures.

23

Contralateral autotransplantation of pedicled inguinal skin flap

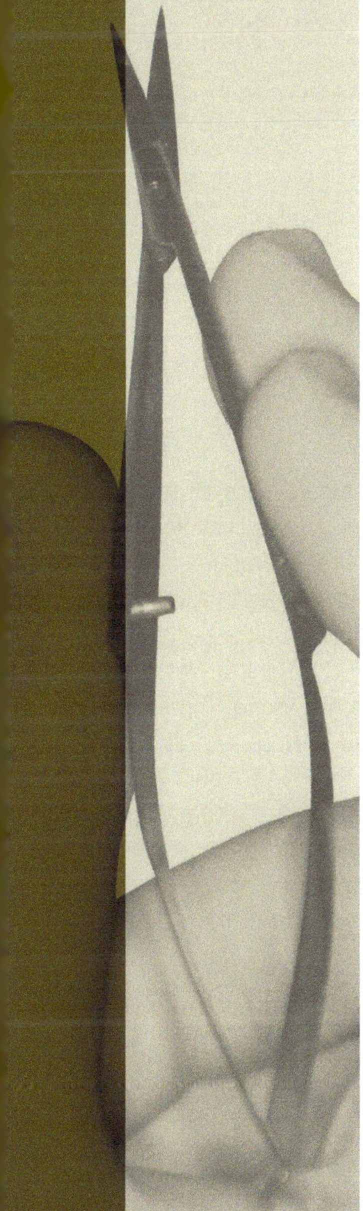

The inguinal skin flap is supplied by the superficial inferior epigastric vessels, which are branches of the femoral vessels. Transplantation is based on end-to-side anastomoses between the femoral vessels of the inguinal skin flap and the femoral vessels of the contralateral side, after the femoral vessels at the donor site are ligated and transected distal to the origin/confluence of the superficial inferior epigastric vessels.

A. Positioning the rat

The rat is placed in a dorsal decubitus (supine) position on the working surface. The long axis of the body of the rat is perpendicular to the frontal plane of the surgeon, with the head of the rat away from the surgeon. The limbs of the rat are immobilized on the working surface with adhesive tape (**Fig. 22-1**).

Left Inguinal Area (Donor Site)

Paragraphs B-E are identical to the corresponding paragraphs in Chapter 22

B. Preparation of the surgical field
C. Microsurgical dissection of the vessels (femoral and superficial inferior epigastric)
D. Dissection and mobilization of the flap
E. Transection of femoral vessels between two ligations (9/0) distal to the junction of the superficial inferior epigastric vessels

Right Inguinal Area (Recipent Site)

F. Preparation of the surgical field

Identical to donor site (see Chapter 22.B).

G. Microsurgical dissection of the femoral vessels

Microsurgical dissection of the femoral vessels is performed from the inguinal ligament to the origin/confluence of the superficial inferior epigastric vessels, as described in detail in Chapter 18.C.

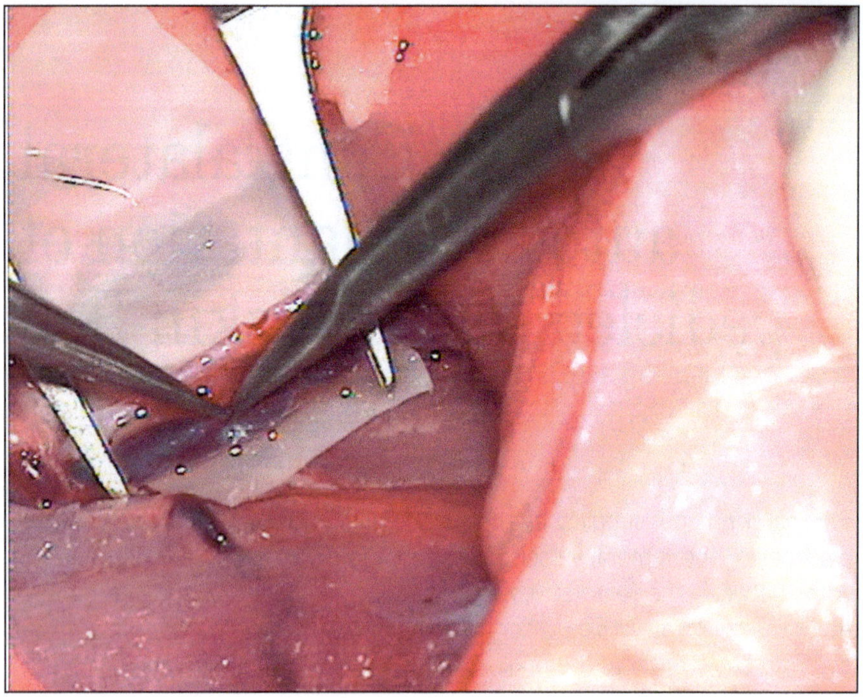

Figure 23-1

Arteriotomy and venotomy of the femoral vessels at the recipient site. The femoral artery and vein were placed in the double clamp and the arteriotomy was performed. Dumont No. 3 forceps elevates the vein while microsurgical scissors are placed perpendicular to make the transverse venotomy using a single motion. Observe that the venotomy is made at a small distance from the arteriotomy. (From author's photo library)

H. Arteriotomy–Venotomy–Irrigation

Once dissection of the femoral vessels is complete, a yellow plastic background is placed under the femoral vessels. The double vascular clamp is then placed on the femoral vessels.

The transverse arteriotomy is performed first, followed by the transverse venotomy (see Chapter 6 for details). Leaving a small distance between them ensures the anastomosis of the artery does not overlap with the anastomosis of the vein (**Fig. 23-1**). The lumens are irrigated with warm normal saline using a syringe attached to a 27G angiocatheter. The adventitia is removed circumferentially around the transverse incision of the femoral artery and the femoral vein.

Left Inguinal Area (Donor Site)

I. Flap harvest

- **Proximal ligation of the femoral vessels, close to the inguinal ligament**
- **Placement of the single vascular clamp distally on the femoral vessels, just before the origin/confluence of the superficial inferior epigastric vessels**
- **Transection of the femoral vessels close to their point of ligation and irrigation of the vessel lumens**

The flap will be supplied by the 'femoral vessels stumps-superficial inferior epigastric vessels' axis. To ensure the anastomoses can be comfortably done at the recipient site, the stumps of the femoral vessels must have adequate length when harvesting. Therefore, both femoral vessels are ligated as close as possible to the inguinal ligament. The femoral artery and vein are ligated simultaneously using a single 9/0 suture (**Fig. 23-2**). Alternatively, it is acceptable to ligate and transect each of the femoral vessels separately.

Prior to transection, a single vascular clamp is applied to both the femoral artery and vein for better handling of the femoral vessels in the suite. The single clamp is placed as close as possible to the origin/confluence of the femoral vessels, in order to maximize the length available for anastomoses during implantation of the flap. The single clamp should not be placed on the superficial inferior epigatsric vessels.

The femoral vessels are transected immediately distal to the proximal ligation suture. The vessel lumens are irrigated with warm normal saline using a 27G angiocatheter (**Fig. 23-3**). During irrigation, the single vascular clamp can be temporarily removed to clear as much blood as possible from the superficial inferior epigastric vessels.

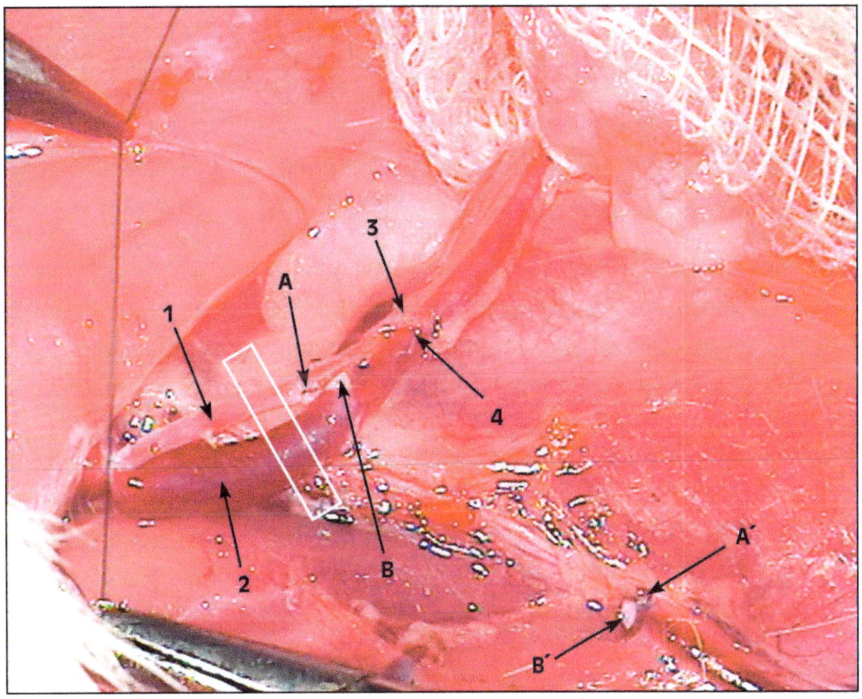

Figure 23-2

Proximal ligation of the femoral vessels before flap harvest. The artery and vein are ligated simultaneously using a single 9/0 suture, placed close to the inguinal ligament. Here, Dumont No. 3 forceps (upper instrument) and a needle holder (lower instrument) make the first simple knot of this ligation. The interrupted-white-line rectangle represents the site where the single vascular clamp will be applied, placed cephalad to the origin/confluence of the superficial inferior epigastric vessels. **A, A′.** sites of ligation and transection of the femoral artery peripheral to the origin/confluence of the superficial inferior epigastric vessels (transection previously performed). **B, B′.** similar for the femoral vein. **1.** femoral artery, **2.** femoral vein, **3.** superficial inferior epigastric artery, **4.** superficial inferior epigastric vein. (From author's photo library)

Right Inguinal Area (Recipent Site)

J. Transfer and placement of the flap, preparation of the vessels

The flap remains covered in a gauze pad, moistened with warm normal saline throughout harvesting. Upon completion of flap harvest, it is transferred wrapped in the gauze to the contralateral side of the rat without removing the single vascular clamp attached to the stumps of the femoral vessels. Transport of the free flap should be performed with great care taken to avoid torsion of the vessels.

At the recipient site, a piece of skin (and superfi-

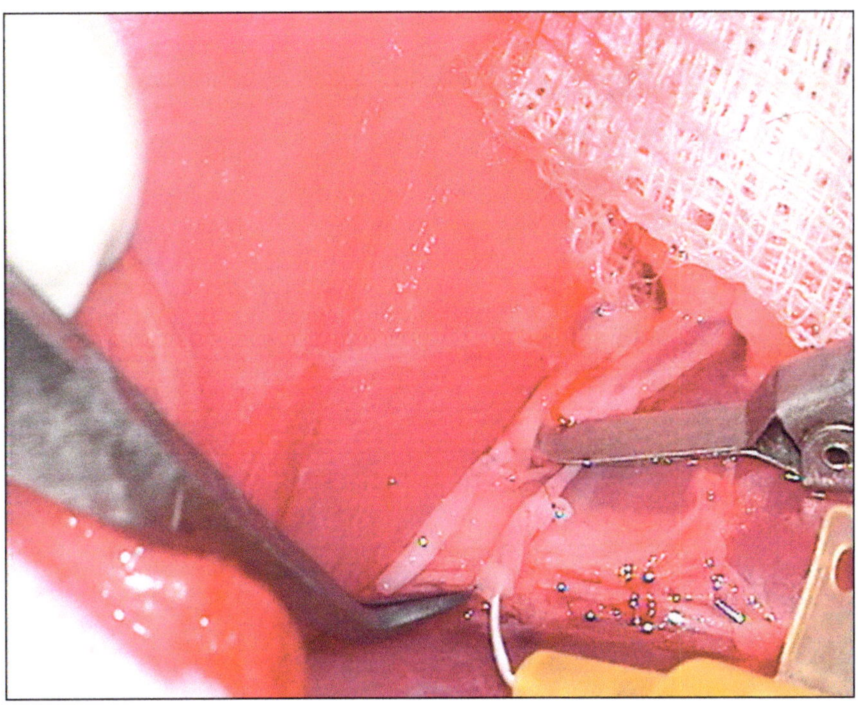

Figure 23-3

Irrigation of the stumps of the femoral vessels after transection. Curved forceps holds the femoral vein by the ligation suture of the tributary vein from the adductor muscle, while the angiocatheter irrigates the lumen with normal saline. The single clamp is temporarily removed from the vessels and used to occlude the superficial inferior epigastric vein, which is then washed up to this point. Note the lumen that has been washed from the cut edge to the clamp, while distal to the clamp (toward the flap) the lumen still contains blood. This stepwise irrigation of the vein can be extended toward the flap (enveloped in gauze). (From author's photo library) cial fascia) must be removed to place the flap. A rectangle of skin and subcutaneous tissue the same dimensions as the flap is cut, and can be removed after cauterization and transection of the superficial inferior epigastric vessels. The area created by the removal of this tissue becomes the recipient site for the flap.

The flap is placed in this area so the interior surface lies on the external oblique muscle and the vessels of the pedicle reach the site of arteriotomy/venotomy of the recipient femoral vessels without tension. Alternatively, the flap may be positioned laterally with the vessels' pedicle in a straight-line, perpendicular to the recipient femoral vessels. The skin flap then rests on gauze pads moistened with warm normal saline. Attention is needed when positioning the single clamp so that the flap vessels do not undergo torsion or kinking (angulation). Supporting the clamp with a small gauze pad may be required.

To prepare for the anastomosis, the adventitia is removed from the perimeter of the edges of the flap vessels. In the femoral artery, the adventitia can be folded (**Fig. 23-4**). In the femoral vein, folding of the adventitia is difficult. The preferred method of removal of the adventitia is to remove it in pieces by pulling with forceps and cutting with scissors.

Before starting the anastomoses, the flap vessels are placed near the transverse incisions of the recipient femoral vessels. If the arteriotomy was made larger than the width of the flap artery, dilation of the artery may be accomplished using microsurgical forceps (**Fig. 23-5**). Given the more distensible venous lumen, this maneuver will likely be unnecessary for the vein.

K. End-to-side anastomoses

The reader will find a detailed description of end-to-side anastomoses technique with rotation of the double clamp in Chapter 6.1.

- **6 sutures 11/0 are placed in the anastomosis of femoral arteries**
- **6 or 8 sutures 11/0 are placed in the anastomosis of femoral veins**

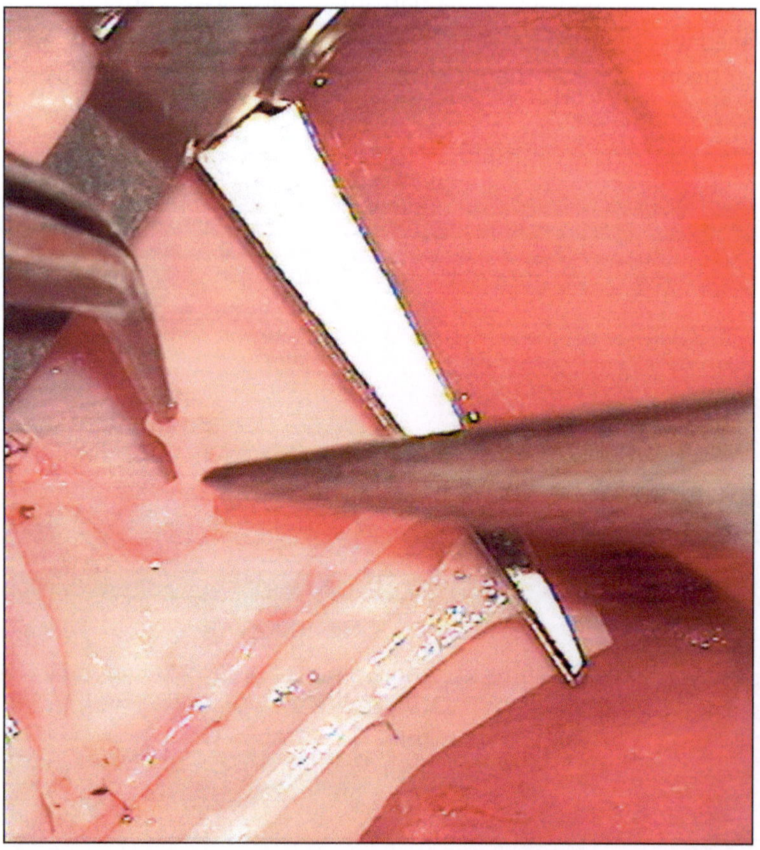

Figure 23-4

Folding the adventitia at the edge of the stump of the flap femoral artery. Curved forceps holds the outer surface of the arterial wall, while Dumont No. 3 forceps refolds the adventitia. The femoral vessels at the recipient site were placed in the double clamp, and an arteriotomy and venotomy have been performed. The opening of the arteriotomy is seen on the femoral artery (upper vessel). Note the femoral vein of the flap lies on the recipient femoral artery (by coincidence). (From author's photo library)

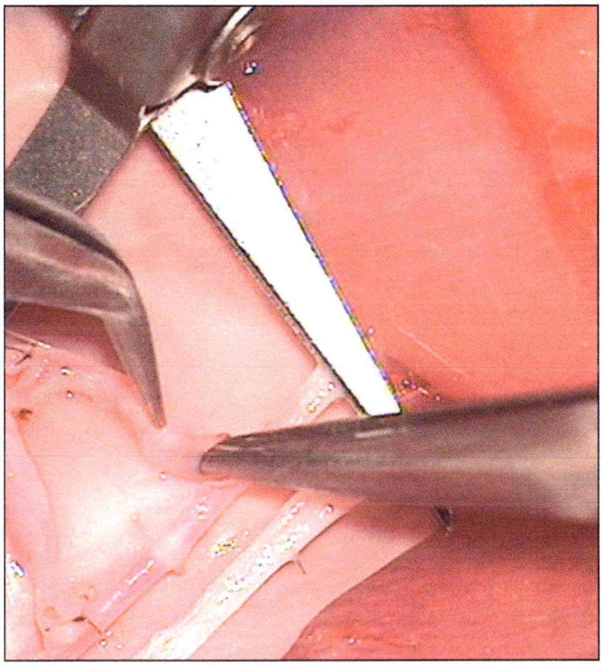

Figure 23-5

Dilatation of the flap's femoral artery lumen. The vessel preparation is continued from Figure 23-4, where is evident that the arteriotomy has been made larger than the width of the artery of the flap. Here, curved forceps holds the artery, while Dumont No. 3 forceps gradually opens within the lumen, causing dilatation. (From author's photo library)

The steps of end-to-side anastomoses are as follows:

1. The anastomosis begins with suturing of the anterior surface of the artery. The 2 corner sutures are placed first, followed by 2 additional sutures positioned at equal distances between themselves and from the corner sutures (**Fig. 23-6A**).
   In the vein, again, 2 corner sutures are placed first (**Fig. 23-6A**). If placing 8 sutures on the vein, the middle suture is placed next, followed by 1 suture in the middle of each quadrant (**Fig. 23-6B**). If placing 6 sutures, they are placed in the same manner as the artery.
2. The flap and the single clamp are rotated, and the correct placement of the sutures of the anterior surfaces is checked.
3. Suturing of the posterior surfaces of the artery and the vein is completed in the same manner as the anterior surfaces (**Fig. 23-7**).
4. All clamps are removed. First, the single clamp is rele-

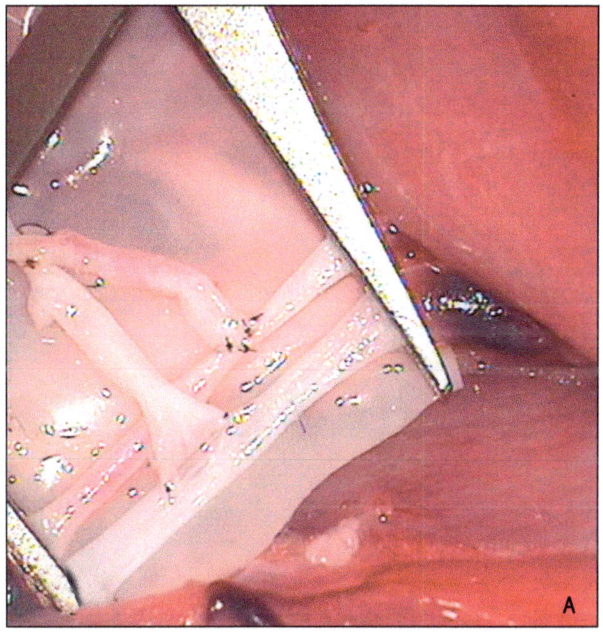

A

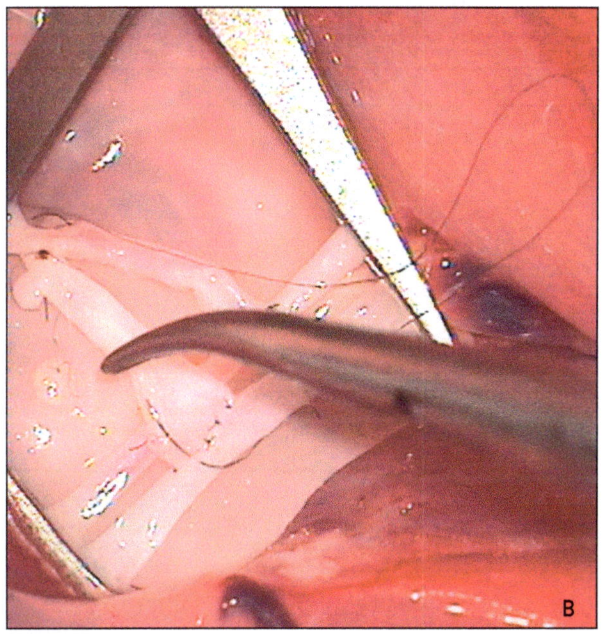

B

Figure 23-6

End-to-side anastomoses of the femoral vessels of the flap to the femoral vessels of the recipient side, anterior surfaces. **A.** Suturing the anterior surface of the artery has been completed. The corner sutures have also been placed on the vein. **B.** Suturing of the vein. The 5th suture is placed in the middle of the remaining quadrant (the needle has only passed through the wall of the recipient femoral vein and is released from the needle-holder). Note: Mistakes in technique are shown in this photo. In order to acquire adequate space, the single clamp has been placed on the superficial inferior epigastric vessels, which, in addition, cross each other. These mistakes should be avoided. The single clamp should only be placed on the femoral vessels of the flap as there is ample space to perform the anastomosis without clamping the superficial inferior epigastric vessels, and the vessels should not cross each other in order to minimize the risk of torsion (From author's photo library)

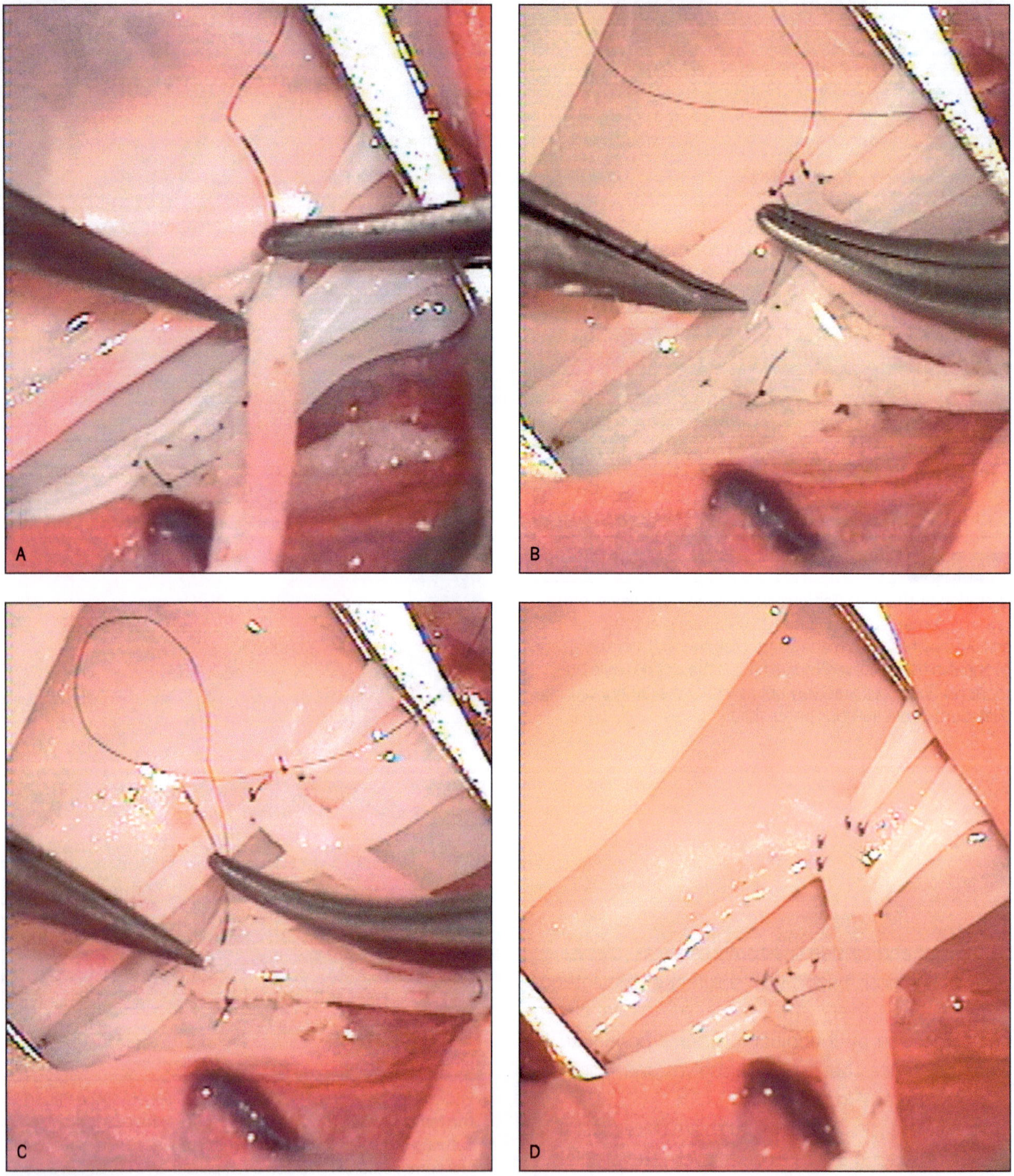

Figure 23-7

Suture of the posterior surfaces of the artery and vein. The flap and the single clamp have been rotated. **A.** The 5th suture of the anastomosis is placed through the walls of the arteries in one step, while the forceps holds the wall of the artery of the flap. **B, C.** Vein anastomoses. The 6th suture is placed in two steps in the middle of the posterior surface. **D.** Completed anastomoses. (From author's photo library)

ased followed by the double clamp. The immediate filling of the vessels of the flap is very encouraging for the eventual patency of the anastomoses (**Fig. 23-8**).

5. A wet gauze pad is placed over the anastomoses for 3 minutes.
6. Patency test, separately for each vessel. The patency

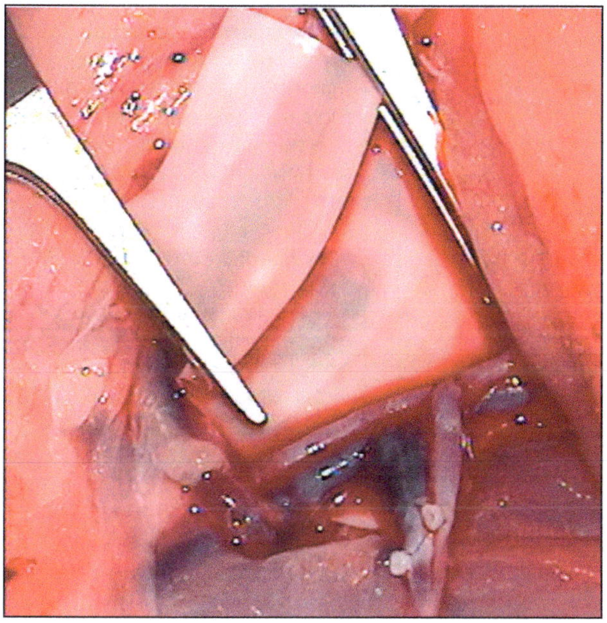

Figure 23-8

Release of the double clamp. The single clamp has been previously removed. The hemorrhage seen is expected and due to temporary leakage of blood between sutures. The immediate filling of the vessels is an encouraging sign for the ultimate patency of the vessels. (From author's photo library)

away from the anastomosis and empty the recipient femoral vein. Then, when they re-approach quickly, if the anastomosis is patent, the lumen between the forceps gets immediately filled.

7. The yellow plastic background is withdrawn.

test is performed as usually, applying the technique described in Chapter 6.9.

The patency testing for the artery is shown in **Figure 23-9** (also see **Figure 6-9**). In brief, an upstream forceps is placed in the artery of the flap, just after the anastomosis (toward the flap), and occludes the blood flow. A second forceps is placed just next to the first, empties the lumen by moving 'half-closed' downstream and is closed in a final position. The upstream forceps is removed, and if the anastomosis is patent, the lumen is immediately filled up to downstream forceps.

The patency test for the vein is shown in **Figure 23-10** (also see **Figure 6-10**). Two forceps move half-closed in opposite directions

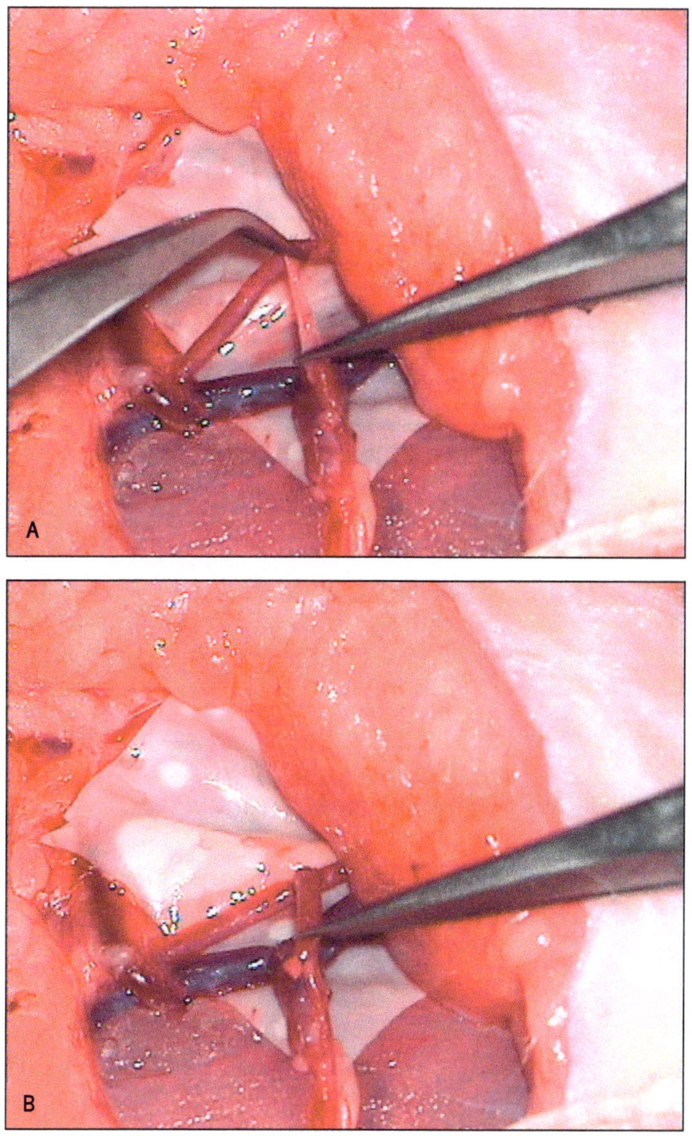

Figure 23-9

Patency test of the end-to-side anastomosis of the femoral arteries. **A.** The curved forceps occludes the blood flow downstream to the artery of the flap. Dumont No. 3 forceps moves half-closed emptying the lumen downstream towards the flap, emptying the lumen (here, the flap is temporarily placed medially) and finally stays closed. **B.** The upstream forceps is removed while the downstream forceps stays closed in its position. Immediate filling of the lumen is noted, demonstrating a successful anastomosis. (From author's photo library)

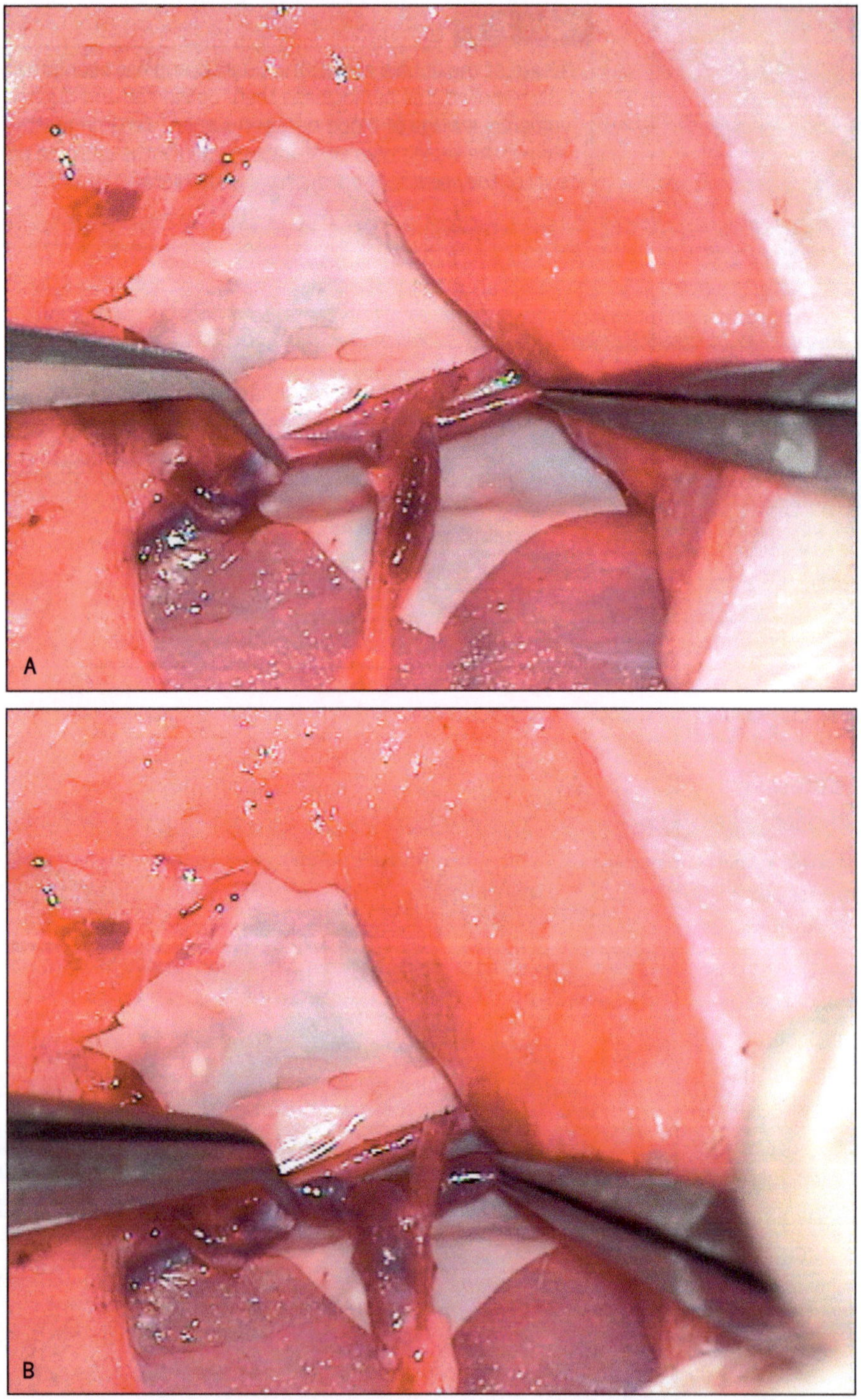

Figure 23-10

Patency test of the end-to-side anastomosis of the femoral veins. **A.** Two forceps are applied on the recipient femoral vein, move half-closed upstream and downstream on either side of the anastomosis, thus emptying the vein (and close at a final position). **B.** In a quick motion, the two forceps reapproach each other. Immediate filling of the lumen in the space between the forceps demonstrates a successful anastomosis. (From author's photo library)

L. Closure of the surgical traumas

On the recipient side, the perimeter of the skin flap is sutured with the skin of the inguinal area using interrupted, non-absorbable 2/0 sutures. The skin gap on the donor side is closed in a similar fashion.

Alternative Technique with Anastomosis of the Superficial Inferior Epigastric Vessels

The flap may be positioned using end-to side anastomosis of the superficial inferior epigastric vessels of the flap onto the femoral vessels of the recipient side. This technique, however, is much more difficult than the technique described above. If this method is chosen, the anastomoses will be performed with **4 sutures 11/0** on the artery and **6 sutures 11/0** sutures on the vein.

... of contralateral autotransplantation of pedicled inguinal skin flap

Synopsis...

A. **Positioning the rat:** Dorsal decubitus (supine) with the head away from the surgeon. The limbs are immobilized on the working surface with adhesive tape.

LEFT INGUINAL AREA (DONOR SITE)

B. **Preparation of the surgical field:** A 2 cm incision is performed parallel and 1cm inferior to the inguinal crease. After opening the superficial fascia, the deep fascia is torn with two gauze pads moistened with warm normal saline, revealing the femoral vessels and the superficial inferior epigatsric vessels. The membranous layer of the superficial fascia and the fatty layer around the superficial inferior epigastric vessels is preserved, making the vascular pedicle of the flap.

C. **Microsurgical dissection of the vessels:** The femoral vessels are dissected inferiorly from the inguinal ligament to the saphenous vein. All branches/tributaries of the femoral vessels, with the exception of the superficial inferior epigastric vessels, are transected between two ligations (9/0). These include the superficial circumflex vein, the deep branch/tributary of the artery/vein found on the posterior surface of the vessels, the small artery and large vein of the adductor muscle, and all other small lateral branches/tributaries that can be cut with the diathermy.

D. **Dissection and mobilization of the flap:** The flap is designed as a rectangle with 3 more incisions: 1) a paramedian incision 4 cm in length, 0.5 cm from the midline, starting at the medial end of the subinguinal incision. 2) a horizontal incision, 2 cm long, parallel to the inguinal incision, begining at the superior apex of the paramedian incision. 3) a final incision parallel to the paramedian, performed after mobilization of the flap based on the superficial inferior epigastric vessels. The plane of dissection of the flap lies between the deep investing fascia of the abdominal wall musculature and the superficial fascia containing the superficial inferior epigastric vessels. Applying traction laterally to the flap, the attachments between the membranous layer and investing fascia are cut with scissors, in close proximity to the muscle.

E. **Transection of the femoral vessels between two ligations (9/0 suture, each vessel, separately) distal to the junction of the superficial inferior epigastric vessels.**

RIGHT INGUINAL AREA (RECIEPENT SITE)

F. **Preparation of the surgical field:** Identical to donor site (see B).

G. **Microsurgical dissection of the femoral vessels** from the inguinal ligament to the origin/confluence of the superficial inferior epigastric vessels.

H. **Placement of the double clamp** proximal to the superficial inferior epigastric vessels. **Arteriotomy-Venotomy** of the femoral vessels is performed, leaving a small distance in between. **Irrigation, Removal of the adventitia** is performed circumferentially at the perimeter of the vessel edges.

... of contralateral autotransplantation of pedicled inguinal skin flap

Synopsis...

LEFT INGUINAL AREA (DONOR SITE)

I. **Flap harvest:** The femoral vessels are ligated using 9/0 suture close to the inguinal ligament. A single vascular clamp is placed on both vessels, near the origin/confluence of the superficial inferior epigastric vessels. The femoral vessels are transected and their lumens are irrigated.

RIGHT INGUINAL AREA (RECIEPENT SITE)

J. **Transfer and placement of the flap,** removal of the adventitia.

K. **End-to-side anastomoses**

6 sutures 11/0 in the anastomosis of femoral arteries

6 or 8 sutures 11/0 in the anastomosis of femoral veins

1. The anterior surface of the artery is sutured first: 2 corner sutures and 2 additional sutures at equal distances from the corner sutures and from each other. The vein follows: 2 corner sutures, 1 in the middle of the semicircle, and 1 in the middle of either quadrant.
2. Rotation of the clamp and check of the sutures of the anterior surface.
3. Suture the posterior surface of the vessels is completed in the same manner as the anterior surface.
4. Release of the vessels from the single (first) and double clamp.
5. Placement of a wet gauze pad on the anastomoses for 3 minutes.
6. Patency test, separately for each vessel.
7. Withdrawal of the yellow plastic background.

L. **Closure of the surgical traumas:** the flap on the recipient side and the incision gap on the donor side are sutured with 2/0 interrupted, non-absorbable sutures.

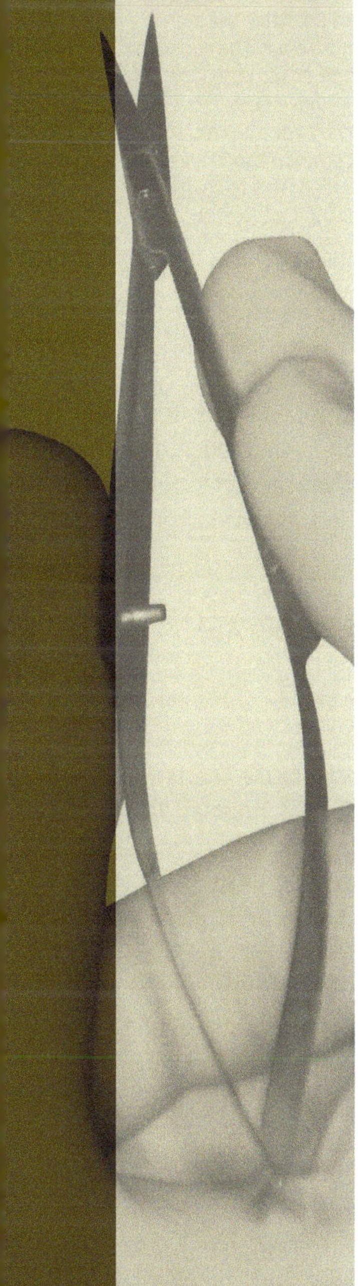

24 Autotransplantation of free inguinal skin flap to the neck

The inguinal skin flap is supplied by the superficial inferior epigastric vessels. Autotransplantation of the inguinal flap to the neck is achieved through end-to-side anastomoses between the femoral vessels (from which the superficial inferior epigastric vessels originate) with the common carotid artery and the external jugular vein.

A. Positioning the rat

The rat is placed in dorsal decubitus (supine) position on the working surface. The long axis of the body of the rat is parallel to the frontal (coronal) plane of the surgeon with the head of the rat on the surgeon's left. The limbs of the rat are immobilized on the working surface with adhesive tape (**Fig. 24-1**).

RIGHT INGUINAL AREA (DONOR SITE)

Paragraphs B-E are identical to the corresponding paragraphs in Chapter 22.

B. Preparation of the surgical field
C. Microsurgical dissection of the vessels (femoral and superficial inferior epigastric)
D. Dissection and mobilization of the flap
E. Transection of the femoral vessels between two ligations (9/0) distal to the junction of the superficial inferior epigastric vessels

NECK (RECIEPENT SITE)

The reader is invited to study Chapter 9, where he/she will find a detailed description and depiction of the preparation of the surgical field and microsurgical dissection of the neck vessels. In the following paragraphs F and G, only a summary is given.

F. Preparation of the surgical field in the neck

A horizontal incision is performed from shoulder to shoulder at the base of the neck. A retractor is used to reflect the superficial fascia and the submandibular salivary glands cranially. On the right side, another retractor is used to laterally displace the superficial fascia containing the external jugular vein. The sternohyoid and sternothyroid muscles

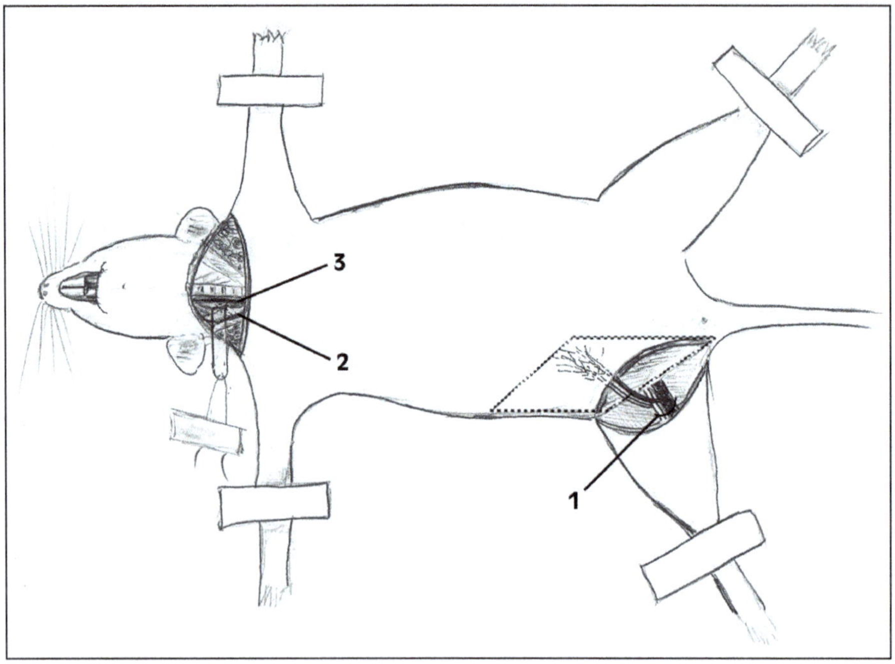

Figure 24-1

Positioning the rat and incisions. First the subinguinal incision is performed, revealing the femoral and superficial inferior epigastric vessels. The inguinal flap is represented by a dot-line rectangular. Its vascular pedicle is comprised of the superficial inguinal vessels originating at the femoral vessels **(1)**. The incision at the base of the neck reveals the right external jugular vein **(2)**. After the sternohyoid muscle and the superficial fascia (together with the external jugular vein) have been moved laterally using a paper-clip retractor, the right common carotid artery **(3)** can be seen next to the trachea. (Drawing by the author)

are also displaced en bloc with this retractor (**Fig. 24-1**). Alternatively, a separate retractor may be used to displace these muscles. The dissection then focuses on the common carotid artery.

Access to the common carotid artery is obtained through the midline between the sternohyoid muscles (see Chapter 9.II.B.1). For beginners, and operations where more space is needed, the sternal portion of the sternocleidomastoid muscle can be transected (this process is described in detail in Chapter 9.II.B.2). For the current procedure, the recommended approach is to follow the atraumatic midline access with displacement of the sternohyoid and sternothyroid muscles. Nevertheless, if the trainee feels that he/she needs more comfort and space, it is acceptable to proceed with transection of the sternocleidomastoid muscle; however, mastery of the midline access must be achieved.

G. Microsurgical dissection of the vessels in the neck

I. Dissection of the right carotid artery

For details see Chapter 9.II.B.1.b

The carotid sheath is opened. The carotid artery is mobilized and separated from the internal jugular vein and the vagus nerve. This dissection should be performed carefully to avoid traumatizing the vagus nerve (found behind and between the carotid artery and the internal jugular vein) and the recurrent laryngeal nerve (found in the groove between trachea and esophagus or on the trachea).

II. Dissection of the right external jugular vein

For details see Chapter 9.I.C

The retractor holding the superficial fascia and the right external jugular vein (and the strap muscles) laterally, is removed. Dissection of the vein starts from the superior margin of the pectoralis major muscle and is continued until the trifurcation of the vein. The external jugular vein is meticulously cleaned of fatty tissue and the outer covering of its wall is removed. The small lateral tributary veins are cauterized or ligated, and transected.

III. Preparation of the right common carotid artery (arteriotomy-irrigation)

After completion of its dissection, the external jugular vein is pulled laterally en bloc with the strap muscles, allowing access to the dissected carotid artery. Since the superficial fascia has been dissected from the external jugular vein, a single retractor holding the vein and strap muscles is now sufficient to expose the surgical

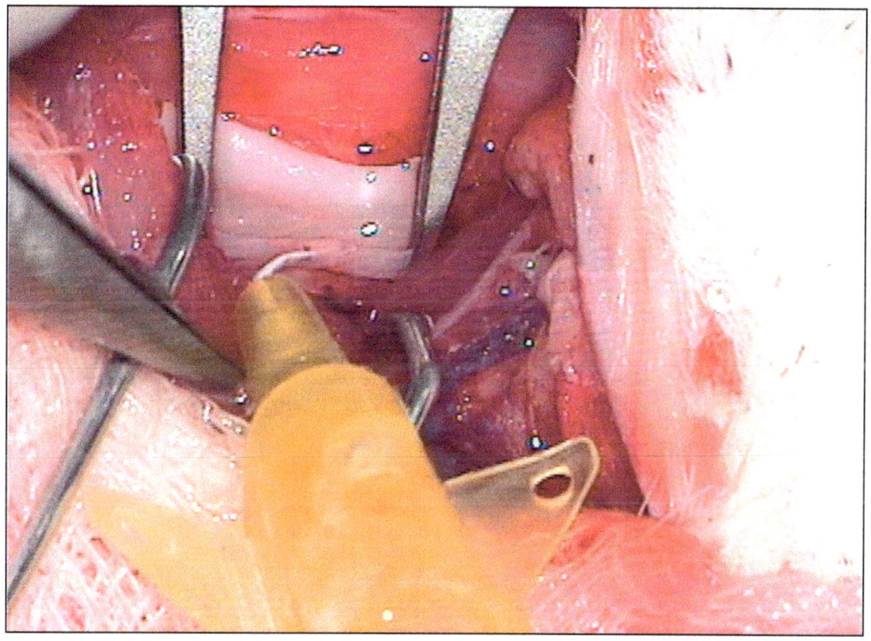

Figure 24-2

Irrigation of the lumen of the carotid artery following arteriotomy. The central part of the artery is irrigated with warm normal saline through a bent angiocatheter. The catheter is then removed and reinserted in the opposite direction to wash the peripheral portion. (From author's photo library)

field of the carotid artery. Ensure the retractor does not press or traumatize the dissected external jugular vein when positioned.

Then, a yellow plastic background is placed under the common carotid artery and the double clamp is applied. A transverse arteriotomy is performed, and the lumen is irrigated with warm normal saline through a 27G angiocatheter (**Fig. 24-2**). The adventitia is removed around the perimeter of the incision (**Fig. 24-3**).

➢ The transverse venotomy of the external jugular vein will be performed just prior to vein anastomosis

The reason is that prolonged occlusion of the external jugular vein while carrying out the arterial anastomosis (performed first, see below), greatly increases risk of vein thrombosis.

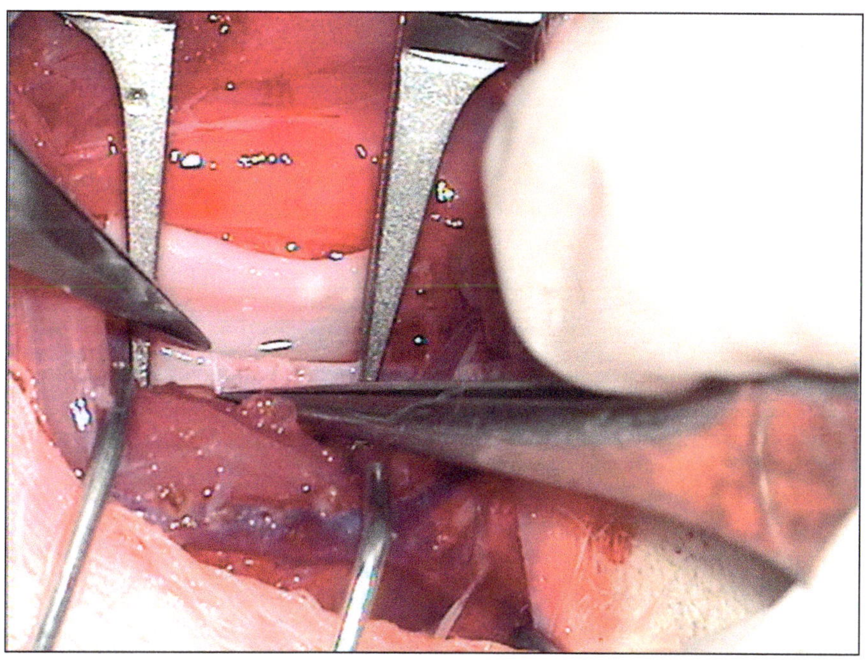

Figure 24-3

Removal of the adventitia. Dumont No. 3 and No. 5 forceps pull the adventitia cranially, easily detaching it from the rest of the coverings of the vessel wall. The same maneuver is performed in the opposite direction. (From author's photo library)

Right Inguinal Area (Donor Site)

H. Flap harvest

The reader is referred to Chapter 23.I for a detailed description of flap harvest on the left. Below, harvesting of the flap is performed on the right with ligation and transection of the femoral vessels presented again in brief. The relationship between femoral artery and vein on the right is a mirror image of the contralateral side.

- **Proximal ligation of the femoral vessels, close to the inguinal ligament**
- **Placement of the single vascular clamp distally on the femoral vessels, just before the origin/confluence of the superficial inferior epigastric vessels**
- **Transection of the femoral vessels close to their point of ligation and irrigation of the vessel lumens**

As mentioned in paragraph E, the femoral vessels have already been transected between two ligations placed peripheral to the origin/confluence of the superficial inferior epigastric vessels (see **Figures 22-7** and **22-8**). The femoral vessels are then ligated as close as possible to the inguinal ligament using a 9/0 suture. This suture can comprise both vessels—as described in Chapter 23 (see **Figure 23-2**) – or, as presented here, each vessel can be ligated separately (**Fig. 24-4**). The

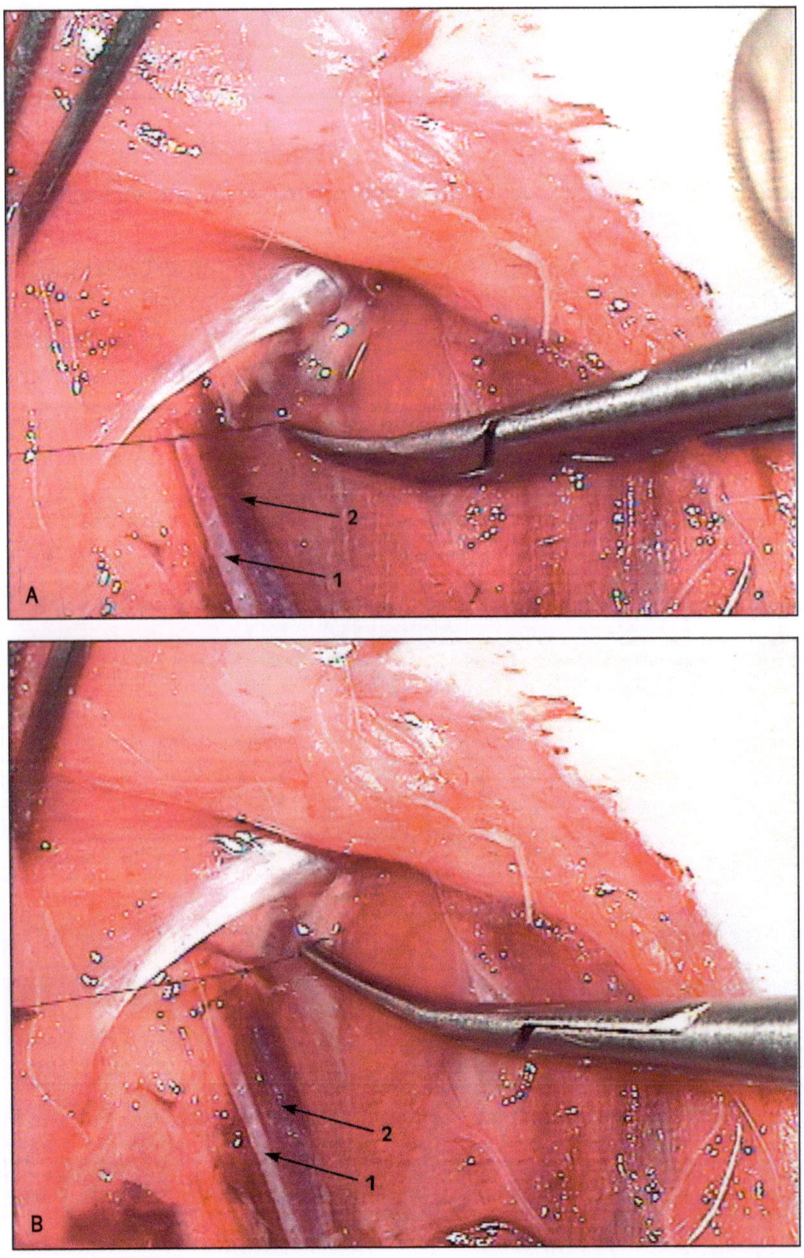

Figure 24-4

Ligation of the right femoral vessels close to the inguinal ligament with 9/0 suture. Each vessel is ligated separately. **A.** Ligation of the femoral artery. **B.** Ligation of the femoral vein. Anatomical forceps (upper left) bends the lowest part of the external oblique muscle, revealing the fibrous inguinal ligament seen as a whitish transverse band over the vessels. **1.** femoral artery, **2.** femoral vein. (From author's photo library)

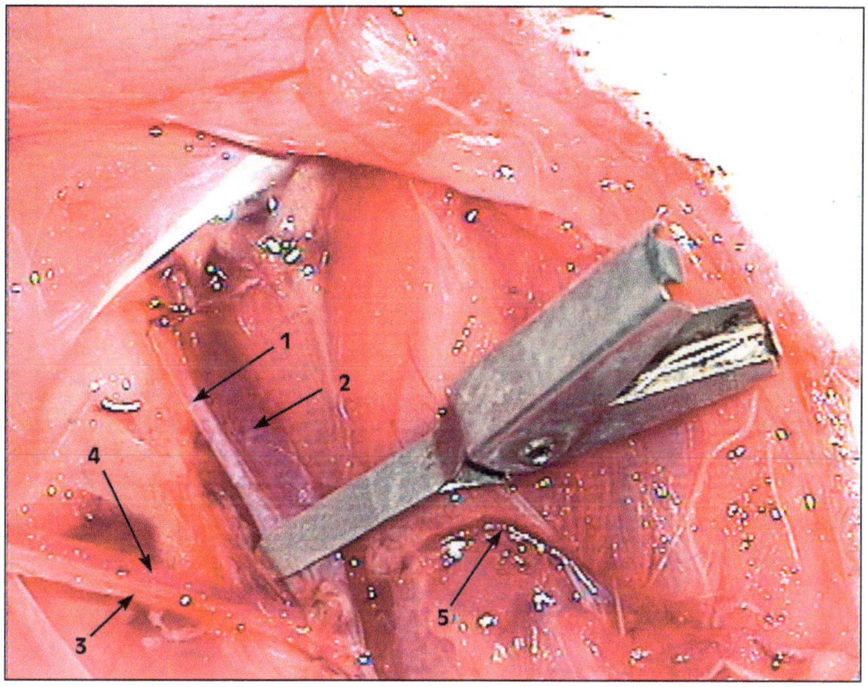

Figure 24-5

Placement of the single clamp on the femoral vessels, right side. The clamp is applied to both vessels, placed close to the origin/confluence of the superficial inferior epigastric vessels. **1.** femoral artery, **2.** femoral vein, **3.** superficial inferior epigastric artery, **4.** superficial inferior epigastric vein, **5.** muscular tributary vein (from the adductor muscle). (From author's photo library)

single clamp is applied to both vessels together, as close as possible to the origin/confluence of the superficial inferior epigastric vessels (**Fig. 24-5**). The femoral vessels are transected as close as possible to their ligation at the inguinal ligament, so that the vessel stumps have the maximal length toward the flap (**Fig 24-6**). Then, the stumps of the vessels of the flap are irrigated with warm normal saline through a 27G angiocatheter. The artery is irrigated under light pressure (**Fig. 24-7A**), while, in the vein, a few drops open the lumen (**Fig. 24-7B**), followed by gentle continuous irrigation.

Folding of the adventitia in the arterial stump and removal of the adventitia in the vein stump preferably performed after transfer of the flap into the surgical field of the neck (see below, J.1.1. for the artery and J.2.a for the vein, respectively).

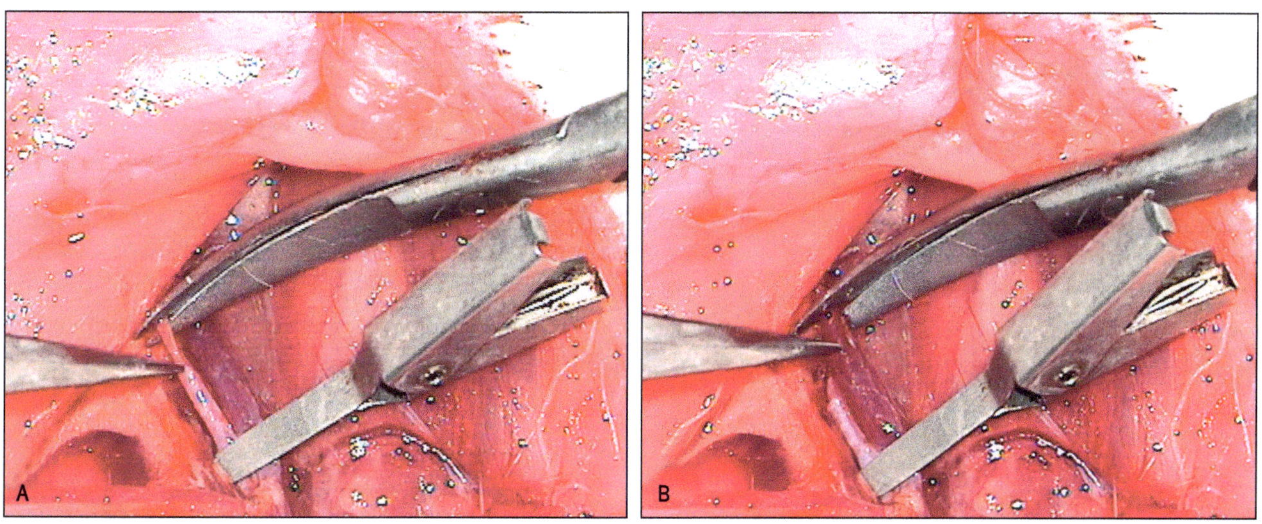

Figure 24-6

Transection of the right femoral vessels. The single clamp has previously been applied on both vessels. **A.** Transection of the femoral artery. Dumont No. 3 forceps lifts the artery from the adventitia and pulls it laterally, away from the adjacent vein, while microsurgical scissors are brought perpendicular to the vessel and cut it. **B.** Transection of the femoral vein is performed in a similar fashion. Observe the shortening of the stump of the femoral artery. (From author's photo library)

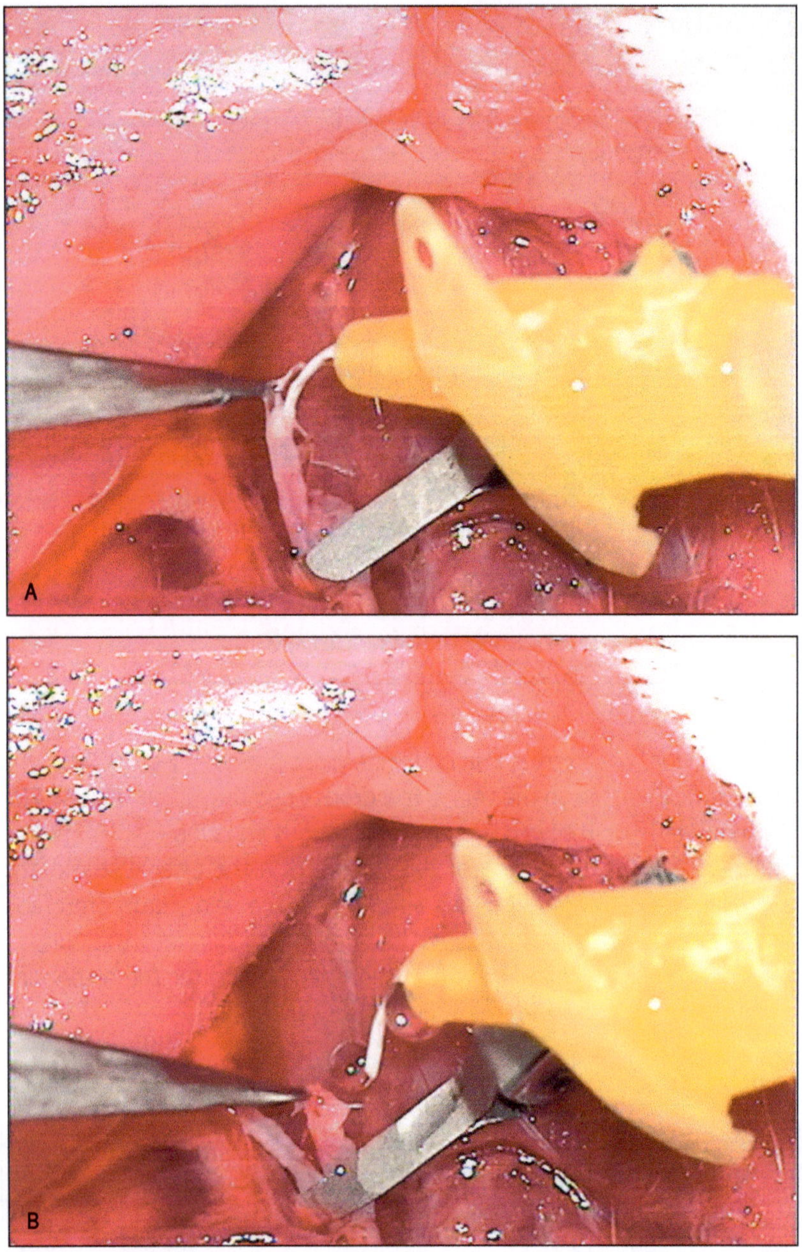

Figure 24-7

Irrigation of the lumen of the transected right femoral vessels. **A.** Dumont No. 3 forceps holds the artery from the adventitia, while the 27G angiocatheter is placed a short distance into the lumen without traumatizing the endothelium. Normal saline is injected into the lumen under light pressure. **B.** A few drops of normal saline from the catheter are used to separate the edges of the transected vein. A continuous current of irrigation under pressure would make the vein walls collapse further. When the opening of the lumen becomes obvious, the vessel can be irrigated similarly to the artery. (From author's photo library)

Neck (Reciepent Site)

I. Transfer and placement of the flap

The flap is transferred to the neck enveloped in a gauze pad moistened in warm normal saline. Attention must be paid to the single vascular clamp during the transfer to avoid torsion of the vessels. The flap is positioned on the left neck so that the flap vessels stumps are brought perpendicular to the dissected right common carotid artery and external jugular vein (recipient vessels). The vessel stumps of the flap should comfortably reach the site where the arteriotomy has already been performed (see above, G.III) and the site where the venotomy is going to be performed (see below J.1.2).

J. End-to-side anastomoses

A detailed description of the arterial and venous end-to-side anastomoses can be found in Chapter 6. The steps are summarized here.

The arterial anastomosis is performed first, followed by the vein anastomosis.

Figure 24-8

Folding the adventitia of the femoral artery stump of the flap. Dumont No. 3 forceps holds the wall of the artery, while Dumont No. 5 forceps folds the adventitia. **1.** femoral artery (stump), **2.** femoral vein (stump), **3.** common carotid artery; the arrow points at the arteriotomy, **4.** external jugular vein, **5.** superficial inferior epigastric artery, **6.** superficial inferior epigastric vein. (From author's photo library)

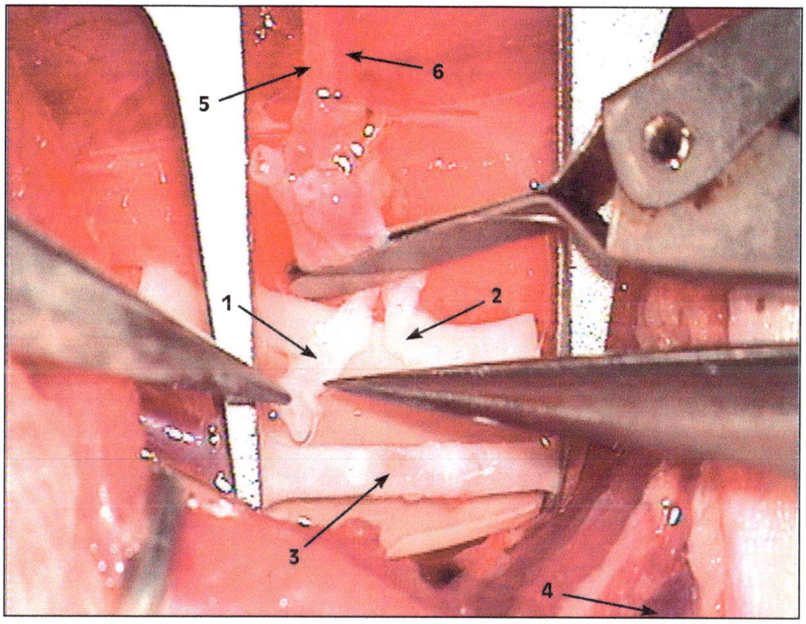

1. Anastomosis of the stump of the femoral artery with the common carotid artery

- The end-to-side arterial anastomosis is performed using **6 sutures 11/0**.

Before starting the anastomosis, the adventitia of the femoral artery of the flap is folded (**Fig. 24-8**).

The steps of the process of the end-to-side arterial anastomosis are as follows:

1. The 2 corner sutures (at 3 and 9 o'clock) are placed first (**Fig. 24-9**). The anterior surface is completed by 2 sutures placed at equal distances between themselves and from the corner sutures.
2. The flap rotates, i.e. is brought laterally (to the ri-

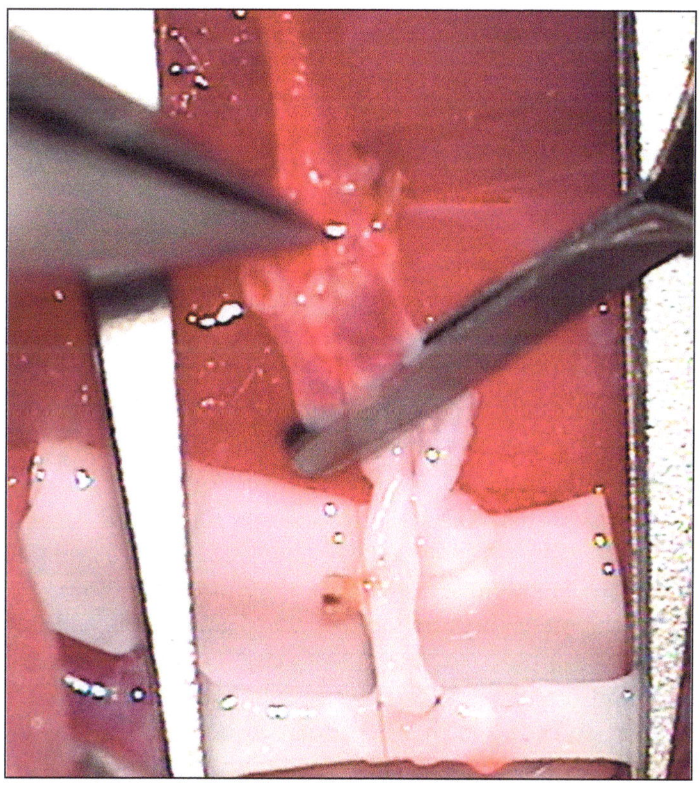

Figure 24-9

Placement of the 9 o'clock suture (2nd corner suture) at the anastomosis between the stump of the femoral artery of the flap and the common carotid artery. (From author's photo library)

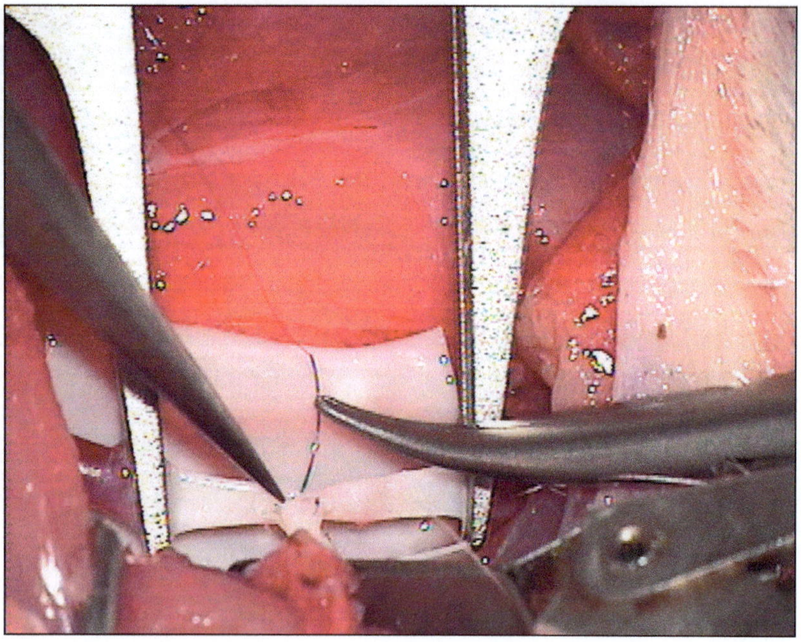

Figure 24-10

Placement of the 6th (last) suture on the posterior surface of the anastomosis between the stump of the femoral artery of the flap and the common carotid artery. The needle is seen passing through the wall of carotid artery, while the forceps lifts the wall of the femoral artery so the needle is passed through both walls in a single step. (From author's photo library)

ght), so the hair on the flap lies on the working surface, supported by gauze pads moistened in warm normal saline. The sutures of the anterior surface are checked.

3. In the posterior surface, 2 sutures are placed at equal distances, as in the anterior surface (**Fig. 24-10**).
4. The flap is returned to its initial position at the left side of the neck, still enveloped in gauzes moistened with warm normal saline.
5. The double clamp is removed from the common carotid artery, followed by the single clamp on the vascular pedicle of the flap.
6. A wet gauze pad is placed over the anastomosis for 3 minutes.
7. Patency test.
   It is necessary to have venous return from the flap into the unsutured femoral vein, denoting that the arterial anastomosis is patent. This sign, however, does not replace the classic test for proving vessel patency, described in Chapter 6.9.1 (**Fig. 6-9**). The classic test for patency starts with central occlusion of the artery of the flap using a forceps placed upstream (just after the anastomosis). A second forceps is applied just peripherally to the first forceps and moves half-closed downstream toward the flap, emptying blood from the lumen and is closed after a short distance (**Fig. 24-11A**). The upstream forceps is removed, and if there is patency, the arterial lumen is immediately filled (**Fig. 24-11B**).
8. The yellow plastic background is redrawn.

2. Anastomosis of the stump of the femoral vein with the external jugular vein

a. Rearrangement of the surgical field, transverse incision of the external jugular vein, and removal of the adventitia

The retractor holding en bloc the sternohyoid and sternothyroid muscles, together with the superficial fascia and the external jugular vein, is withdrawn. The muscles are left to return to their native position. The now anastomosed femoral artery supplying the flap courses through the midline toward the carotid artery, which has also returned to its initial position in the paratracheal groove.

Attention is then focused in the stump of the femoral vein of the flap. A single vascular clap is placed on the vein stump. Without causing tension, the vein stump is positioned near the previously dissected (see above, F. II) external jugular vein at a perpendicular angle. A yellow background is placed under the external

Figure 24-11

Patency test of the end-to side anastomosis between the femoral artery stump of the flap and the common carotid artery. **A.** A first Dumont forceps is placed on the femoral artery upstream, just after the anastomosis. A second Dumont forceps has moved half-closed downstream, toward the flap to empty the lumen. It is then closed after a short distance (as shown). **B.** The upstream forceps has been removed. The immediate filling of the lumen until the downstream forceps demonstrates the patency of the anastomosis. (From author's photo library)

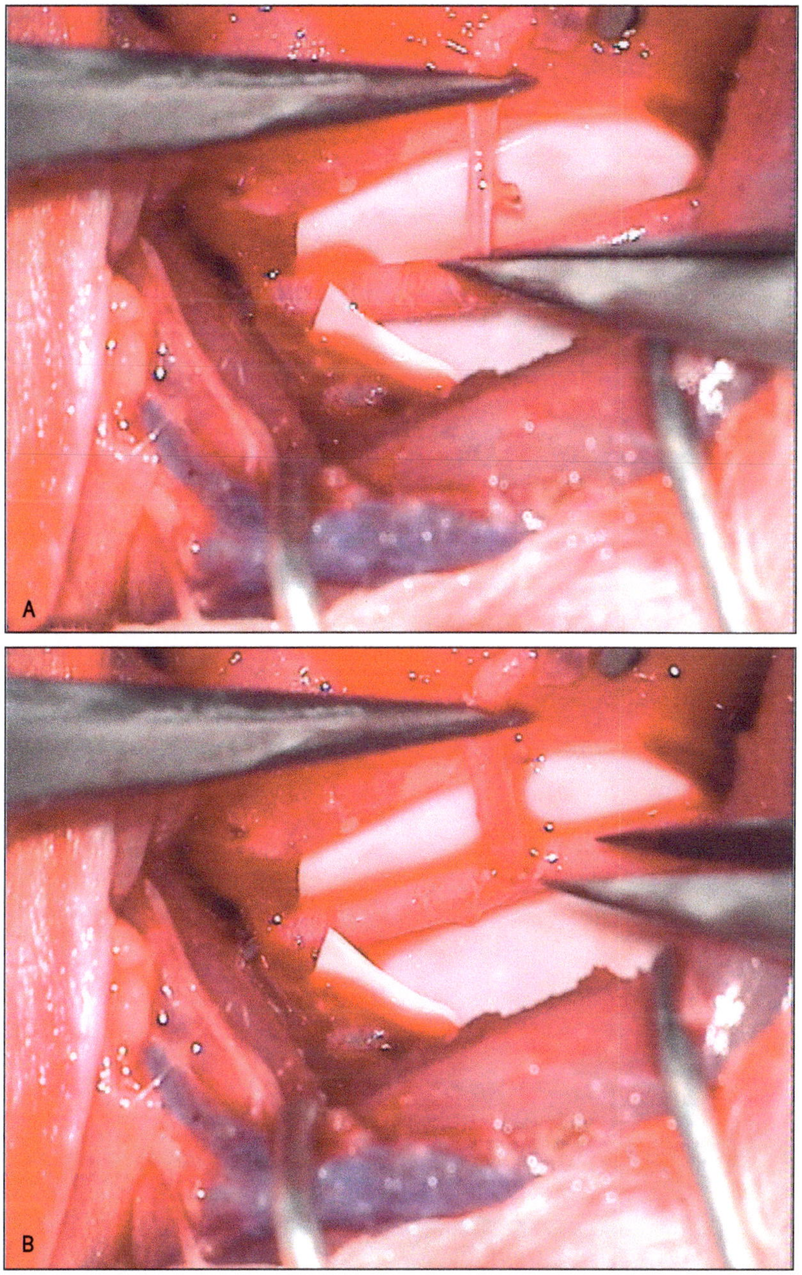

jugular vein, on which the double clamp is applied (**Fig. 24-12**).

Then, a transverse venotomy is performed in the external jugular vein (**Fig. 24-13A**) followed by irrigation of the lumen (**Fig. 24-13B**). If the cleaning of the external jugular vein performed during dissection of the neck (see above F. II) has left the adventitia of vein intact at the site of the venotomy, or removal is incomplete, it must be removed by cutting it into pieces and detaching them from the vein wall to obtain a clean area at the perimeter of the venotomy. Also, in the stump edge of the femoral vein of the flap, the adventitia must be removed. Any remaining adventitia within the completed anastomosis can cause it to fail. If removal of the adventitia proves difficult at the edge of the femoral vein stump of the flap, a small portion of the stump can be transected and removed to make a new, clean edge for removal of the adventitia. Bear in mind, especially for the veins, cleaner vessels edges make easier anastomoses.

b. Anastomosis of the veins

- The end-to-side venous anastomosis is performed using **6 or 8 sutures 11/0**

During anastomosis of the veins, the flap cannot rotate because the completed arterial anastomosis pre-

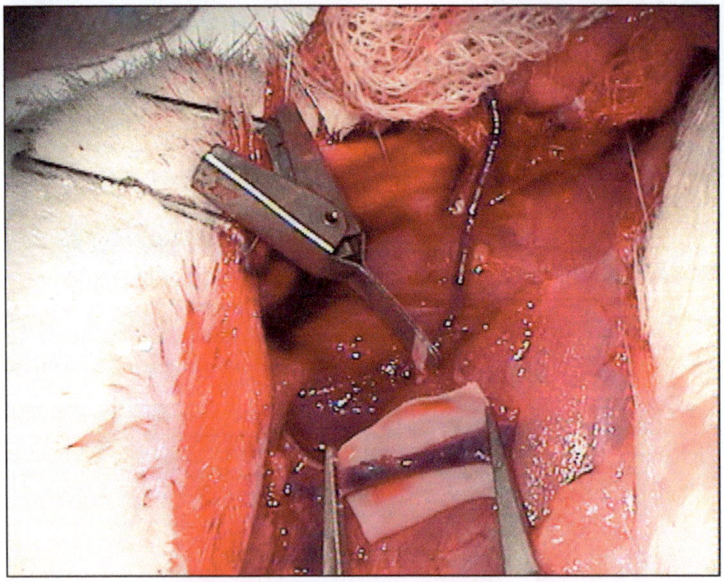

Figure 24-12

Arrangement of the surgical field for the anastomosis between the femoral vein stump of the flap and the external jugular vein. Observe that the vein axis 'superficial inferior epigastric-femoral stump' fills with blood to the level of the single clamp, denoting the success of the preceding arterial anastomosis. Note that the artery of the flap is behind the vein (can be seen in higher magnification in Figure 24-14) (From author's photo library)

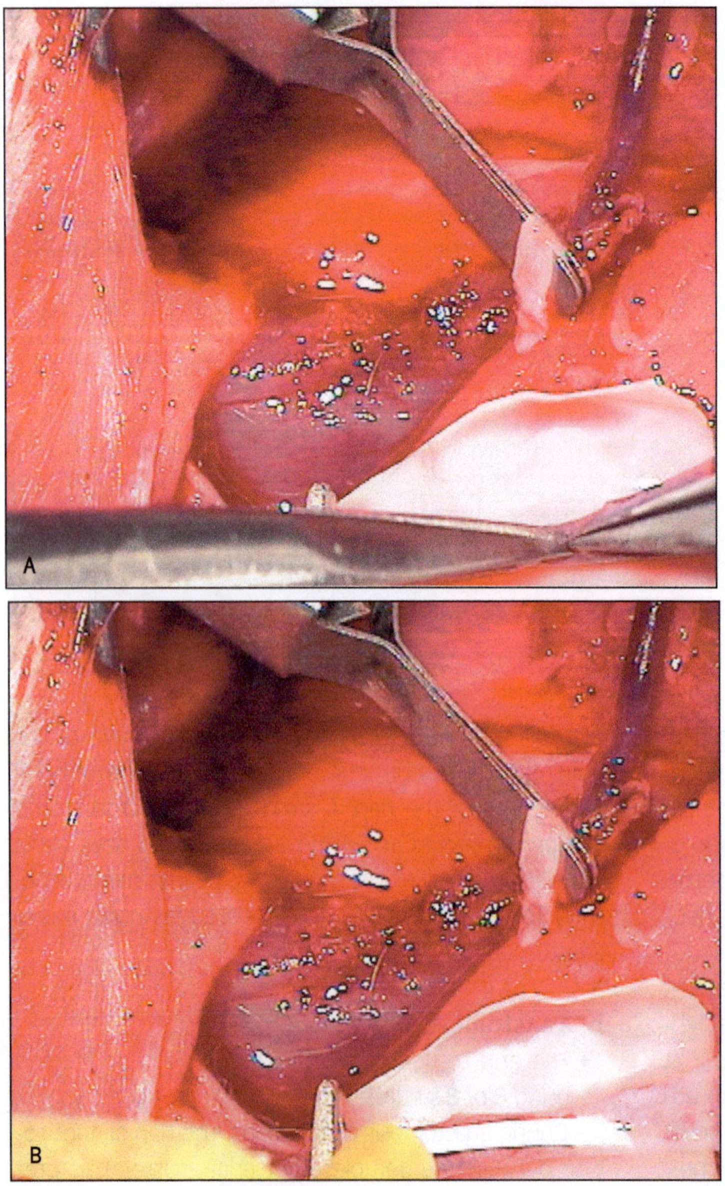

Figure 24-13

A. Transverse incision in the external jugular vein. Dumont No. 3 forceps holds the vein wall while microsurgical scissors are brought at an angle to perform the venotomy. **B.** The edge of a 27G angiocatheter (yellow catheter, partially visible in bottom left corner) carefully enters the vessel lumen (white tube in the transparent lumen, bottom right corner). This step should be performed gently to prevent trauma to the endothelium. The lumen is irrigated under light pressure. (From author's photo library)

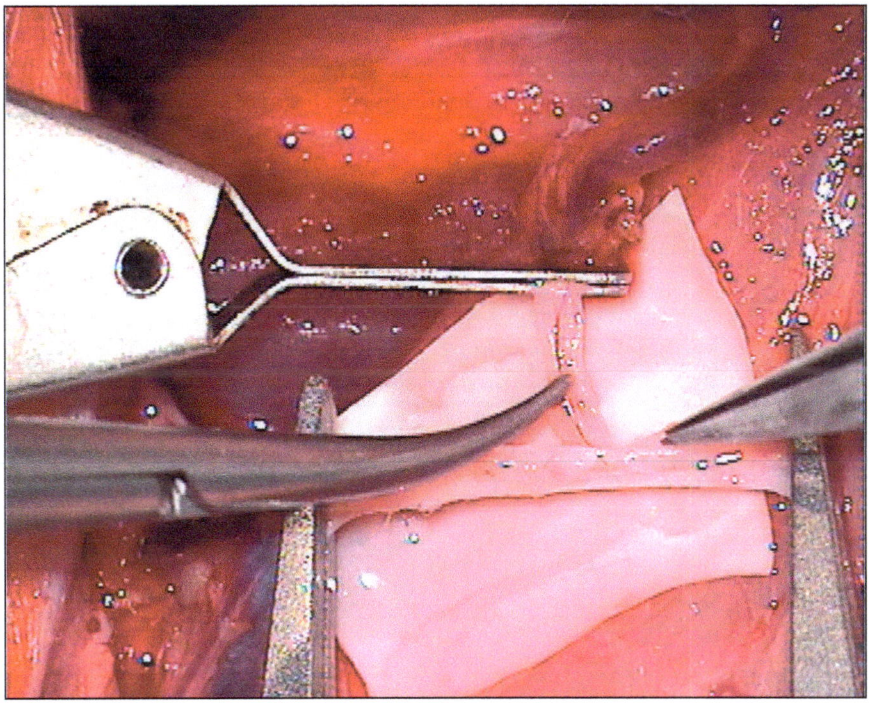

Figure 24-14

Placement of the 1st suture in the middle of the posterior surface of the anastomosis between the femoral vein stump of the flap and the external jugular vein. The needle-holder (shown here in the surgeon's left hand) passes the needle from outside to inside on the wall of the external jugular vein. The needle will then be passed through the wall of the femoral vein stump from inside to outside. The knot will be placed outside of the lumen. (From author's photo library)

vents the flap from rotating. The posterior surface, however, is accessible for suture placement and therefore, the anastomosis is performed as described in Chapter 6.2.I.

The steps of the end-to-side venous anastomosis are as follows:

1. The anastomosis begins by placing the 1st suture in the middle of the posterior surface, with the knot outside of the lumen (**Fig. 24-14**). The 2nd and 3rd sutures will be placed on the posterior surface at equal distances from the first suture on either side. The 4th and 5th sutures are placed on the anterior surface, at equal distances from the 2nd and 3rd (the distant is equal to the distance 1st-2nd and 1st-3rd), while the 6th is put in the middle of the distance 4th-5th sutures. In case that 8 sutures 11/0 are needed, the 1st suture is placed in the middle of the posterior surface, the 2nd and 3rd at equal distances on either side, the 4th and 5th as corner sutures of 3 and 9 o'clock, the 6th and 7th at equal distances on the anterior surface, and the 8th in the middle of the remaining distance in the anterior surface.
   An alternative technique for this case of anastomosis is the following: the 1st suture is placed in the middle of the posterior surface, and the 2nd suture is positioned in the middle of the anterior surface. The remaining sutures are placed in the right and left half-circles. The anterior sutures can be placed easily (**Fig 24-15A**). The posterior sutures can be placed by pulling the femoral vein anteriorly toward the contralateral side (**Fig 24-15B**).
2. Release of the vessels from the clamps, first the single clamp, followed by the double clamp.
3. A wet gauze pad is placed over the anastomoses for 3 minutes.
4. Patency test.
   A very promising sign for patency is the filling of the external jugular vein after removing the single clamp from the femoral vein [before releasing the double clamp from the external jugular vein] (**Fig 24-16**). While helpful, this sign is not a substitute for the classic test of patency described in Chapter 6.9.2 (**Fig. 6-10**). In brief, two forceps are applied on the external jugular vein and move half-closed in opposite directions, away from the anastomosis, and close; this maneuver empties the lumen. Then, they are brought closer to each other with a quick movement and if there is patency, the lumen between the forceps fills immediately.
5. The yellow plastic background is redrawn.

K. Closure of surgical traumas

The surgical traumas in the inguinal and neck regions are closed using interrupted, non-absorbable 2/0 sutures.

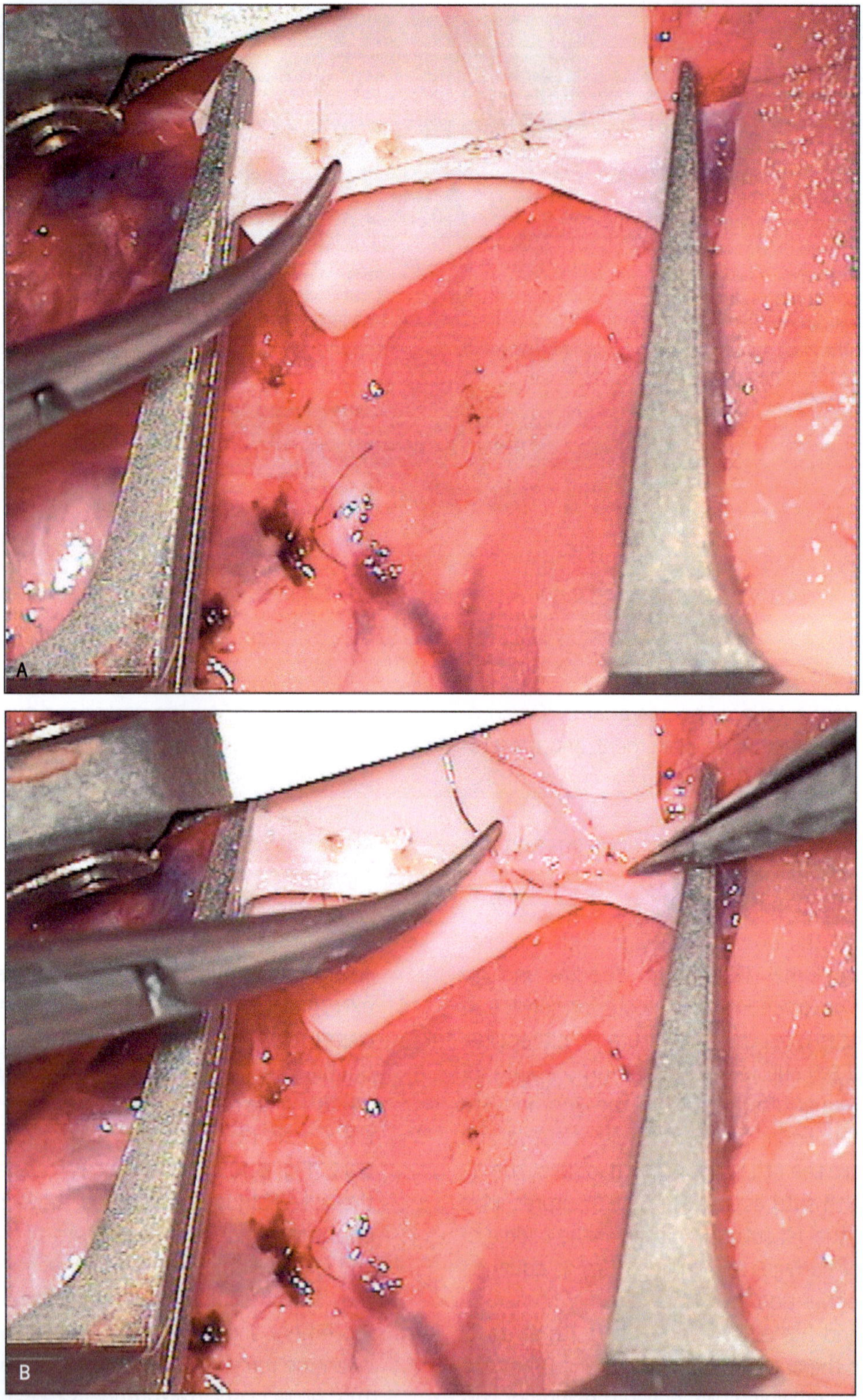

Figure 24-15

Alternative way of suture the end-to-side anastomosis between the fermoral vein stump of the flap and the external jugular vein, from the middle of the posterior surface to the middle of the anterior surface. **A.** Placement of the 5th suture, anteriorly, in the left half-circle. Here, the 1st suture has been placed in the middle of the posterior surface, and cannot be seen. The 2nd suture has been placed in the middle of the anterior surface, the 3rd and 4th can be seen placed on the right half-circle. **B.** Placement of the 8th suture, posteriorly, in the left half-circle. The femoral vein is pulled in the opposite direction with Dumont No. 3 forceps, while the needle holder guides the needle to pass, in a single step, the external jugular vein from outside-inside, and the fermoral vein from inside-outside. The 6th and 7th sutures have been placed previously in the same way (From author's photo library)

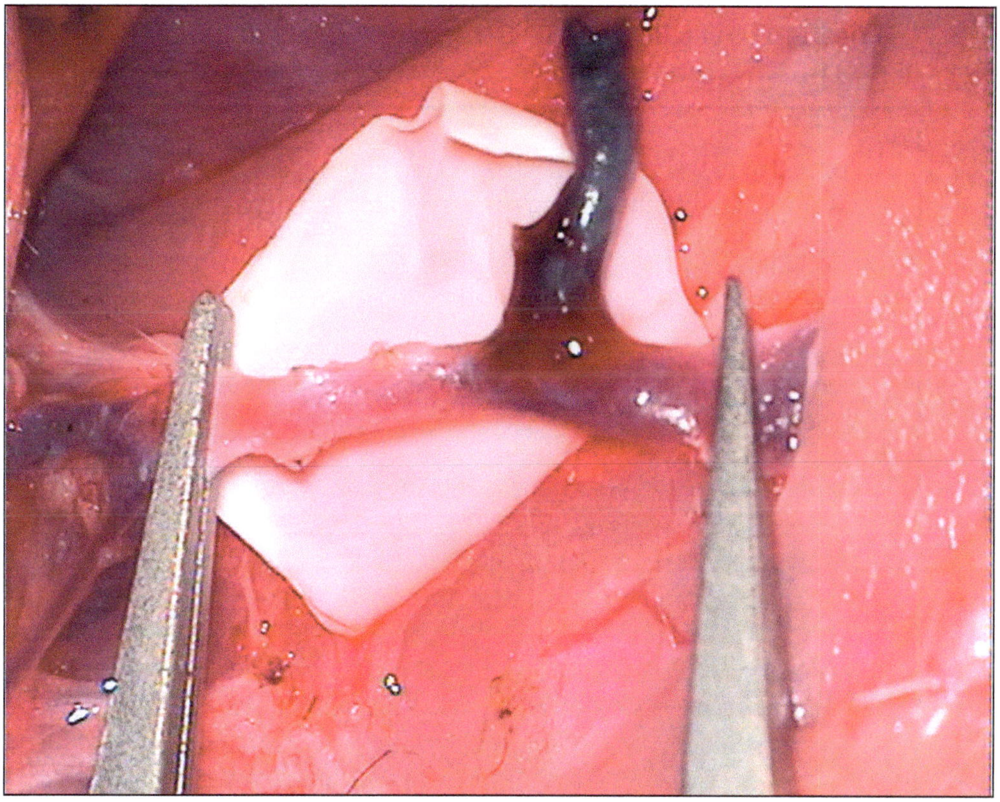

Figure 24-16

Sign indicating patency of the anastomosis between vein of the flap and external jugular vein. After removal of the single clamp from the femoral vein of the flap, the lumen of the external jugular vein fills. The standard patency test will follow (From author's photo library).

Synopsis...

... of autotransplantation of free inguinal skin flap to the neck

A. **Positioning the rat:** Dorsal decubitus (supine) with the head on the surgeon's left. The limbs are immobilized on the working surface with adhesive tape.

RIGHT INGUINAL AREA (DONOR SITE)

B. **Preparation of the surgical field:** A 2 cm incision is performed parallel and 1 cm inferior to the inguinal crease. The deep fascia is torn using two gauze pads moistened with warm normal saline, revealing the femoral vessels and the superficial inferior epigastric vessels.

C. **Microsurgical dissection of the vessels:** The femoral vessels are dissected inferiorly from the inguinal ligament to the saphenous vein. All branches/tributaries of the femoral vessels, with the exception of the superficial inferior epigastric vessels (dissected only in the initial part), are transected between two ligations (9/0).

D. **Dissection and mobilization of the flap:** The flap is designed as a rectangle with 3 more incisions: 1) a paramedian incision 4 cm in length, 0.5 cm from the midline. 2) a horizontal incision parallel and equal to the inguinal incision beginning at the superior apex of the paramedian incision 3) a final incision parallel to the paramedian performed after mobilization of the flap based on the superficial inferior epigastric vessels. The plane of dissection of the flap lies between the deep investing fascia of the abdominal wall musculature and the superficial fascia containing the superficial inferior epigastric vessels. Applying traction laterally to the flap, the attachments between the membranous layer and investing fascia are cut with scissors, in close proximity to the muscle.

E. **Transection of the femoral vessels between two ligations (9/0 suture, each vessel, separately) distal to the junction of the superficial inferior epigastric vessels.**

NECK (RECIEPENT SITE, RIGHT SIDE)

F. **Preparation of the surgical field in the neck:** A horizontal incision is made at the base of the neck, from shoulder to shoulder. A retractor is placed, reflecting the submandibular glands toward the mandible. The superficial fascia containing the external jugular vein is moved laterally (to the right) using a second retractor. The surgical plane is opened in the midline and a retractor is used to move the right sternohyoid and sternothyroid muscles laterally.

G. **Microsurgical dissection**

I. **Common carotid artery:** The carotid sheath is opened. The common carotid artery is mobilized and separated from the internal jugular vein and the vagus nerve.
II. **External jugular vein:** The retractor holing the vein is withdrawn. The vein is dissected from the superior margin of the pectoralis major up to its trifurcation. Any small, lateral tributary veins are transected between two ligations or after cauterization.
III. **Common carotid artery preparation (arteriotomy-irrigation):** The retractor displacing the external jugular vein and the strap muscles is put back, allowing access to the common carotid artery. A yellow plastic background is placed under the carotid artery. The double clamp is applied, a transverse arteriotomy is performed, the lumen is irrigated and the adventitia is removed from the perimetry of the incision.

Synopsis...

... of autotransplantation of free inguinal skin flap to the neck

RIGHT INGUINAL AREA (DONOR SITE)

H. Flap harvest: The femoral vessels are ligated close to the inguinal ligament using 9/0 suture. A single vascular clamp is placed on both vessels simultaneously, near the origin/confluence of the superficial inferior epigastric vessels. The vessels are transected near the ligation and the lumens are irrigated.

NECK (RECIEPENT SITE, RIGHT SIDE)

I. Transfer and placement of the flap towards the left side, so that the femoral vessel stumps are brought perpendicular to the dissected recipients vessels of the neck.

J. End-to-side anastomoses

1. Femoral artery stump-common carotid artery

Prior to anastomosis, the adventitia in the femoral artery stump is folded.

1. Placement of **6 sutures 11/0**. The anterior surface of the artery is sutured first: 2 corner sutures and 2 additional sutures at equal distances from the corner sutures and from each other.
2. Rotation of the flap, and check of the sutures of the anterior surface.
3. Placement of 2 equidistant sutures on the posterior surface.
4. Return of the flap to its initial position.
5. Release of the clamps.
6. Placement of a wet gauze pad on the anastomosis for 3 minutes.
7. Patency test.
8. Withdrawal of the yellow plastic background.

2. Femoral vein stump-external jugular vein

a. **Rearrangement of the surgical field and preparation for veins anastomosis:** The retractor holding the muscles, superficial fascia, and external jugular vein is withdrawn. A yellow plastic background is placed under the external jugular vein and a double clamp is applied. A transverse venotomy is performed, followed by irrigation of the lumen. A single clamp is placed on the femoral vein of the flap.

b. **Vein anastomosis:** Placement of **6 or 8 sutures 11/0**. The flap cannot rotate, but the posterior surface is accessible.

1. The 1st suture is placed in the middle of the posterior surface, with the knot outside. The remaining sutures are placed on alternating sides equidistant from the middle suture, advancing toward the middle of the anterior surface. Alternatively, the 1st suture is placed in the middle of the posterior surface and the 2nd is placed in the middle of the anterior surface. Two or three sutures are placed on the right and left half-circles. The anterior surface is directly visible; the posterior surface is visualized by pulling the vein in opposite direction.
2. Release of the clamps.
3. Placement of a wet gauze pad on the anastomosis for 3 minutes.
4. Patency test.
5. Withdrawal of the yellow plastic background.

K. Closure of surgical traumas: (inguinal, neck) using interrupted, non-absorbable 2/0 suture.

25

Autotransplantation of the posterior limb

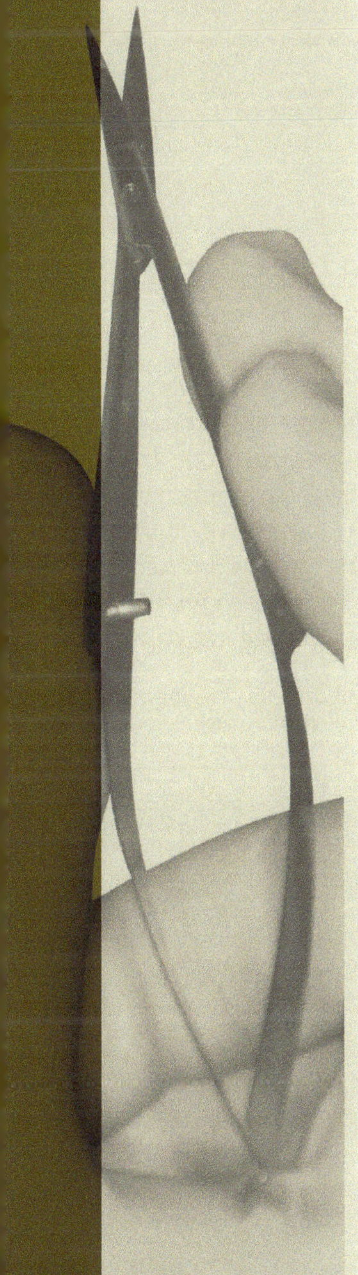

The operation is described for the left posterior limb. Paragraphs in which the surgical microscope is used are annotated "(microsurgically)" in the title.

A. Positioning the rat

The rat is placed in dorsal decubitus (supine) position on the working surface. The long axis of the body of the rat is perpendicular to the frontal plane of the surgeon, with the head of the rat away from the surgeon. The limbs of the rat are immobilized on the working surface with adhesive tape (**Fig. 18-1**).

B. Transection of the limb

The transection of the limb is performed starting antero-medial and proceeding postero-lateral. On the anterior surface, the incision is placed 1 cm below the inguinal crease and runs parallel to it.

1. Dissection of the femoral vessels (microsurgically)

A brief overview of the dissection of the femoral vessels is presented here. The reader is referred to Chapter 18\.B and C for a more detailed description.

After the incision is made, the superficial fascia containing the superficial inferior epigastric vessels is dissected. Under the transparent deep fascia, the femoral vessels and the rest of their branches/tributaries (superficial circumflex vein, tributary vein from the adductor muscle) can be visualized (**Fig. 18-3**). The deep fascia is torn using two gauze pads moistened in warm normal saline. This maneuver fully reveals the femoral vessels and their branches/tributaries (**Fig. 18-4**). The femoral artery and vein are dissected separately from the origin/confluence of the superficial inferior epigastric vessels to the inguinal ligament using the surgical microscope. Any branches/tributaries identified during dissection are transected between two ligations (9/0) or after cauterization.

2. Extension of skin incision and transection of anterior muscles

The dissection continues with minimal magnification under the microscope, or without the microscope. While not strictly necessary, it is advised to continue using

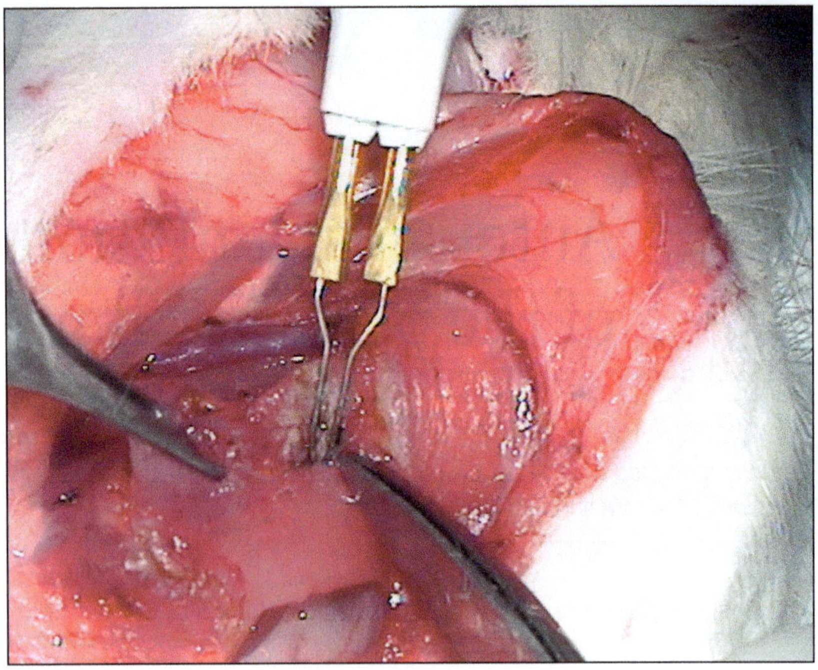

Figure 25-1

Transection of the anterior muscles of the thigh using electrocautery. (From author's photo library)

the microscope in order to economize time. The incision on the anterior surface of the limb is largely extended medially and laterally. The anterior muscles are then transected antero-posteriorly in the middle of the thigh using the monopolar cautery (**Fig. 25-1**).

3. Dissection and transection of the sciatic nerve (microsurgically)

After transection of the muscles, the sciatic nerve is easily visualized (**Fig. 25-2**). Dissection of the nerve requires high magnification using the surgical microscope (it is reinserted if moved during the previous step). The dissection starts cephalad, and begins by creating a 'window' in the deep fascia attaching the nerve on the underlying muscles (**Fig. 25-3A**). The 'window' is extended until the nerve is mobilized in its whole length available in the field (**Fig. 25-3B**). Once complete, the nerve is transected.

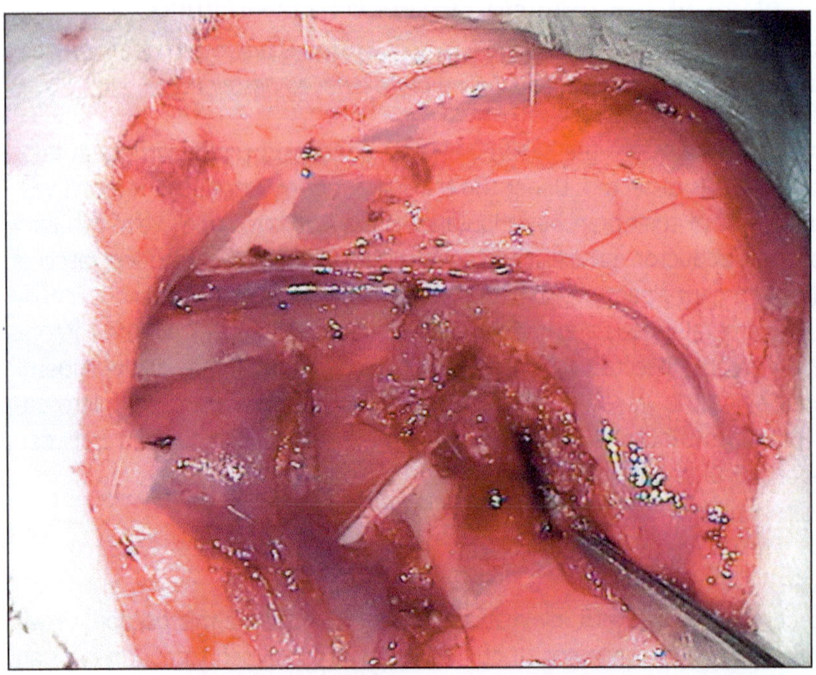

Figure 25-2

The sciatic nerve easily visualized after transection of the anterior muscles of the thigh. (From author's photo library)

Figure 25-3

Dissection of the sciatic nerve. **A.** Using the tip of microsurgical scissors, and by opening slightly the legs, a "window" is created in the deep fascia attaching the nerve on the underlying muscles. **B.** Completed dissection of the nerve. (From author's photo library)

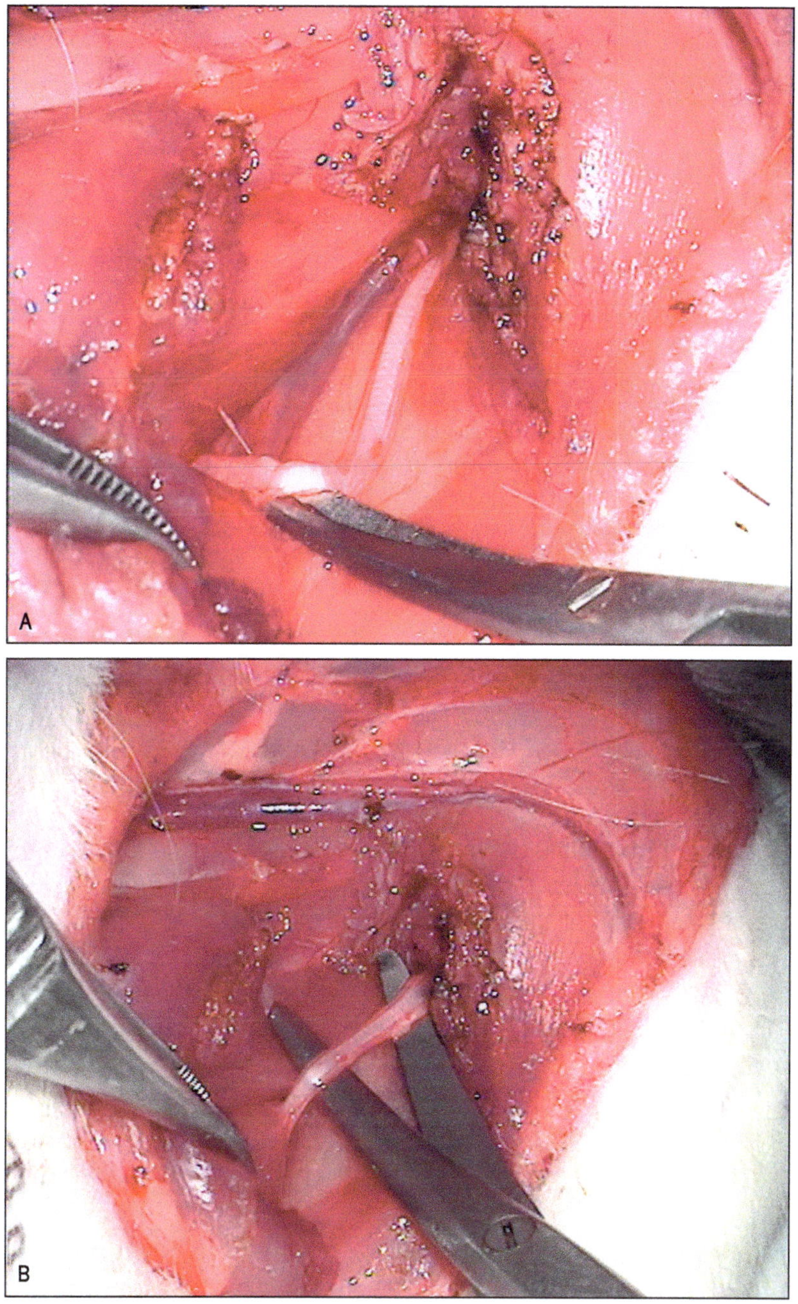

4. Transection of the posterior muscles and skin

Dissection continues without the microscope or, preferably, with the microscope set to minimal magnification. The posterior muscles are transected using electrocautery until the only attachments between the limb and trunk are the femur, femoral vessels and nerve, and the sciatic nerve (**Fig. 25-4**). The skin is cut circumferentially by continuing the skin incision onto the posterior surface of the thigh.

5. Occlusion and transection of the femoral vessels (microsurgically)

Two single vascular clamps are applied close to each other, occluding both the femoral artery and vein simultaneously. The midpoint between the clamps should be found at the plane of transection of the limb.

If autotransplantation of the limb is immediately performed, a double vascular clamp with a small distance between the two clamps can be placed on the femoral vessels instead of two single clamps. Given that

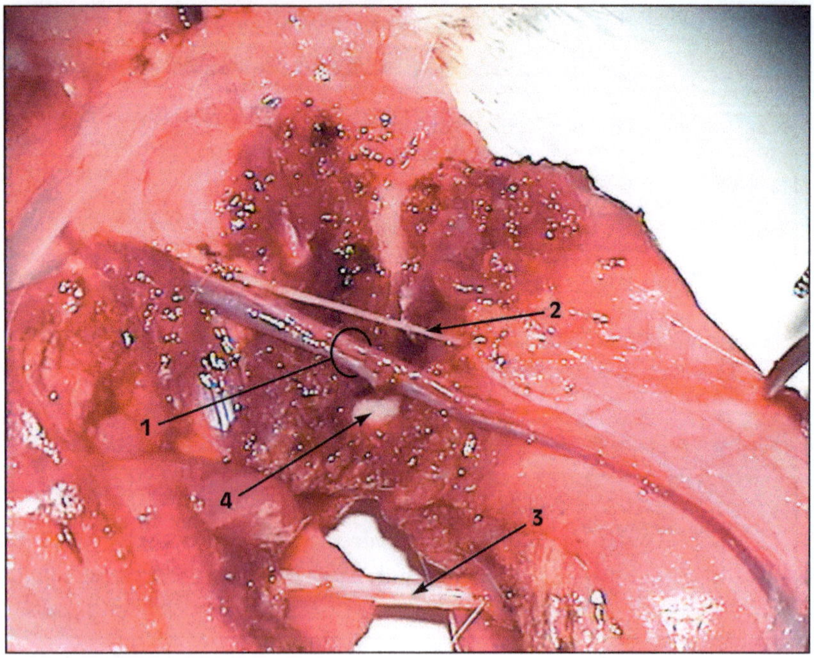

Figure 25-4

In this limb, the posterior muscles have been transected [the sciatic nerve has not been transected in this photo to show its position]. **1.** femoral vessels, **2.** femoral nerve (shown displaced), **3.** sciatic nerve, **4.** femur. (From author's photo library)

transection of the femur will follow, the double clamp must rest on gauze pads placed in proper position to support the weight of the limb and prevent damage of the double clamp. If this cannot be achieved, it may be preferable to place two single clamps initially, then replacing them with a double clamp before rejoining the limb.

The femoral vessels are transected and their lumens irrigated with warm normal saline through a 27G angiocatheter.

6. Transection of the femur

After creating an incision through the periosteum, the femur is transected using a file. When complete, a 0.5 mm piece of bone is removed from the edge of the peripheral stump. This creates a clean surface of bone that will easily join with the counterpart after rejoining the limb.

The limb, now fully transected, is removed.

C. Rejoining of the limb

1. Rejoining of the femur

The stumps of the femur are joined and aligned through internal fixation using a pin, wire nail, or clip of 1 mm diameter.

2. Suturing of the posterior muscles

Suturing begins on the posterior surface and continues internally toward the bone. Each muscle layer is sutured separately using interrupted 3/0 absorbable suture.

3. Suturing of the sciatic nerve (microsurgically)

The reader is referred to Chapter 17.E for a detailed description. A summary is provided below.

A yellow plastic background is placed under the nerve. The sciatic nerve suture starts with 2 sutures 9/0 placed diametrically on the epi-perineurium (perineurium and epineurium overlap in the sciatic nerve of the rat) (**Fig. 25-5**). Correct orientation and direction of neurons is critical to successful anastomosis of the nerve. Carefully observe the outer covering of the nerve during dissection and use a landmark for realignment, such as a vessel on the epi-perineurium or residue of the deep fascia. As stressed in Chapter 17, we recommend placing a total of 4 sutures in the nerve to prevent 'overflow' of the neurons from the edges of the nerve stumps (**Fig. 17-7B** and **Fig. 25-5C**).

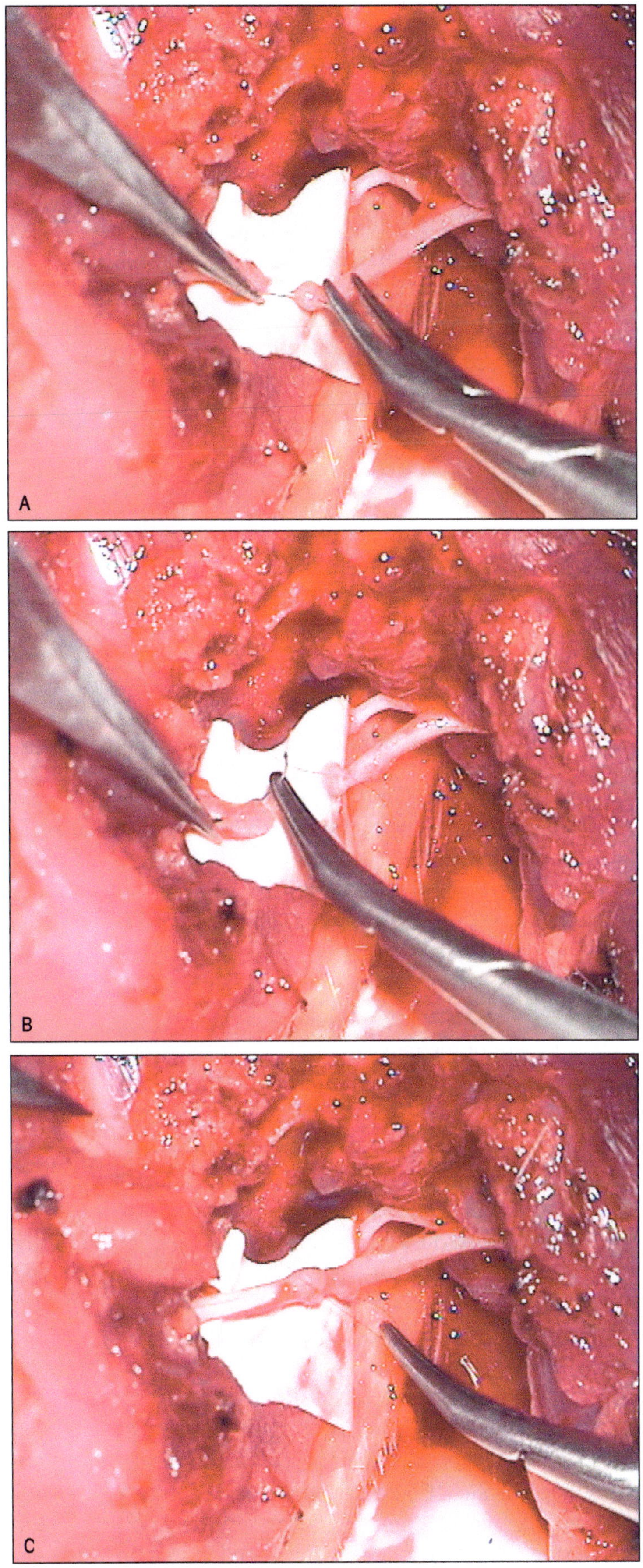

Figure 25-5

Suturing the sciatic nerve. **A.** The first 9/0 suture passes through the epi-perineurium of the peripheral stump of the nerve. Here, the needle has been released from the needle-holder and is held by Dumont No. 3 forceps **B.** In the central stump, the needle-holder pushes the needle through the epi-perineurim while the stump is supported by Dumont No. 3 forceps. **C.** The second knot is tied in the second (diametric to the first) suture. Notice the projection of nerve fibers from the edges of the anastomosed stumps. To prevent this, placement of 4 sutures is recommended. (From author's photo library)

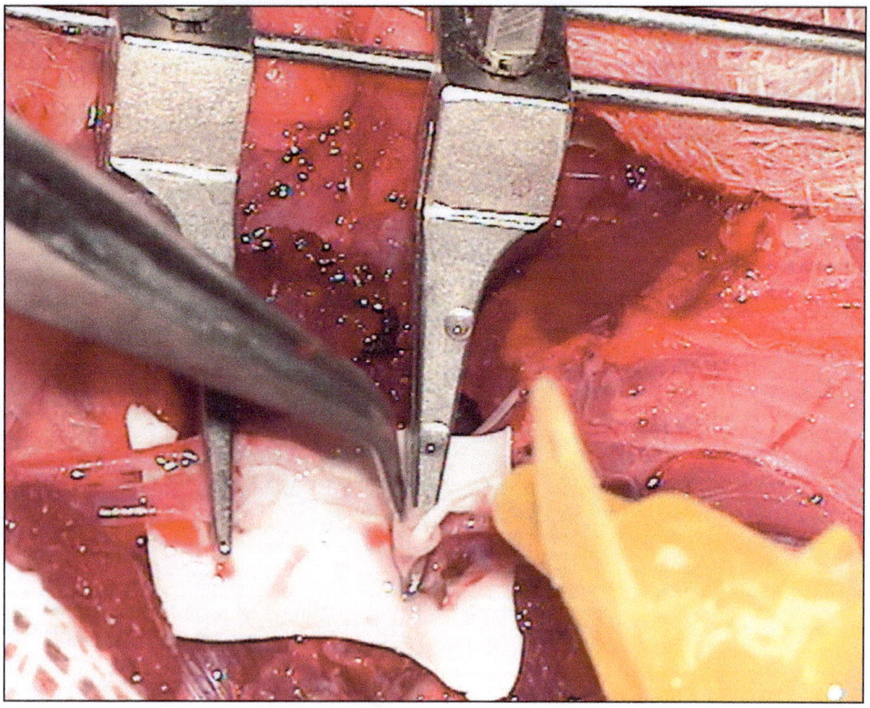

Figure 25-6

Irrigation of the femoral vein before anastomosis. Curved forceps grasp the outer covering of the vein while warm normal saline is injected in the lumen through a 27G angiocatheter. The catheter is inserted for a small distance in the lumen, but does not touch the vein wall to prevent trauma to the endothelium. (From author's photo library)

4. Anastomoses of the femoral vessels

A yellow plastic background is placed under the femoral vessels, and a double vascular clamp is applied on both vessels. If single vascular clamps were applied before transection of the vessels, they are removed before placement of the double clamp. Attention is needed in supporting the double clamp using gauze pads placed in the gap between the two stumps of the posterior limb.

The lumens of the femoral vessels are irrigated with warm normal saline through a 27G angiocatheter (**Fig. 25-6**). The adventitia is folded at the edges of the arterial stumps, while it is removed in the vein stumps.

End-to-end anastomoses

- **Artery: 6 sutures 11/0**
- **Vein: 6 or 8 sutures 11/0**

The anterior surfaces of the vessels are sutured first. The anterior surface of each vessel, artery or vein, can be completed individually before advancing to the other. Given the difficulty of working in this surgical field–compared with the simple anastomosis described in Chapter 18–, an alternative technique may be used when creating these anastomoses: The 4 corner sutures, 2 on each vessel, are placed in first to hold the stumps together, followed by suturing of the anterior surfaces.

The steps of the anastomoses are numbered below:

1. Regarding the arterial anastomosis, after placement of the 2 corner sutures, 2 more are required in the anterior surface placed at equal distances between themselves and from the corner sutures. In the vein, we suggest placement of 8 sutures, i.e. after the 2 corner sutures, 3 more are required on the anterior surface starting with the 1st, which is placed in the middle of the semicircle, and then 1 in the middle of each quadrant on either side. Completed suturing of the anterior surfaces is shown in **Figure 25-7**.
2. The clamp is rotated, and the sutures on the anterior surfaces are checked.
3. Suturing of the posterior surface is completed, identical to the anterior sutures. Sometimes, this may prove difficult given the small distance between the clamps and the problematic support of the vessels (there is gap under the yellow background). In such cases, when performing the vein anastomosis, the two sutures in the middle of the quadrants on either side are placed before the middle suture (**Fig. 25-8**). This variant in technique allows for a better view of the lumen during the passage of the

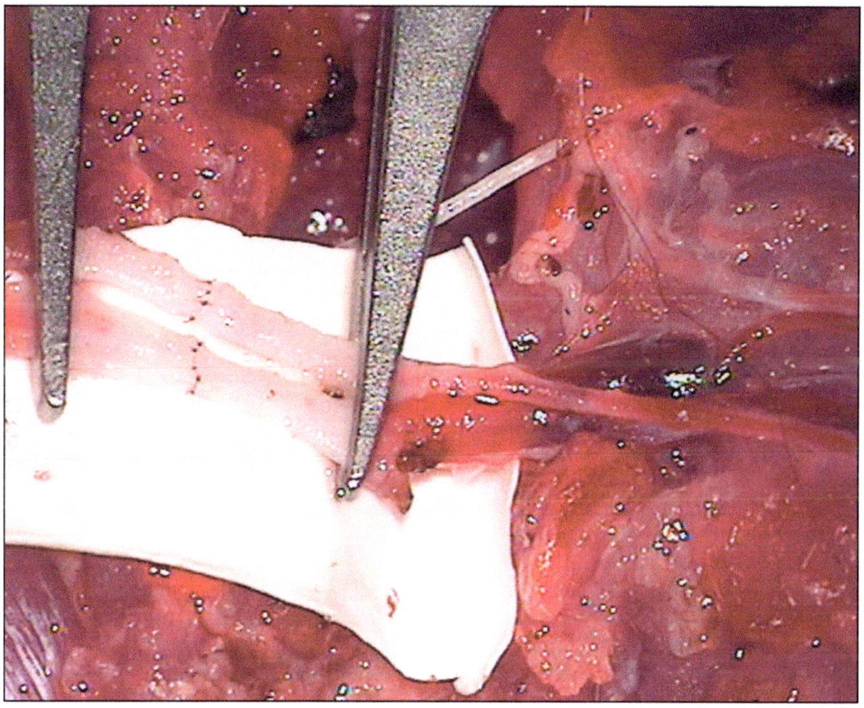

Figure 25-7

Completed suturing of the anterior surfaces of the femoral vessels during rejoining of the posterior left limb. (From author's photo library)

mid-quadrant sutures and helps to avoid catching the anterior wall, which will inevitably lead to failure of the anastomosis.

4. The double clamp is released.
5. A wet gauze is placed on the anastomoses for 3 minutes.
6. Patency test, separately for each vessel as decribed in Chapter 5.10 (**Fig. 5-4**). In brief, distal to the anastomosis (following the blood flow), an upstream forceps occludes the vessel, and a second forcpes moves half-closed downstream and closes. The upstream forceps is withdrwan, and, if there is patency, the vessel fills in immediately up to the downstream forceps. The patency test for the artery is shown in **Figure 25-9** and for the vein in **Figure 25-10**.

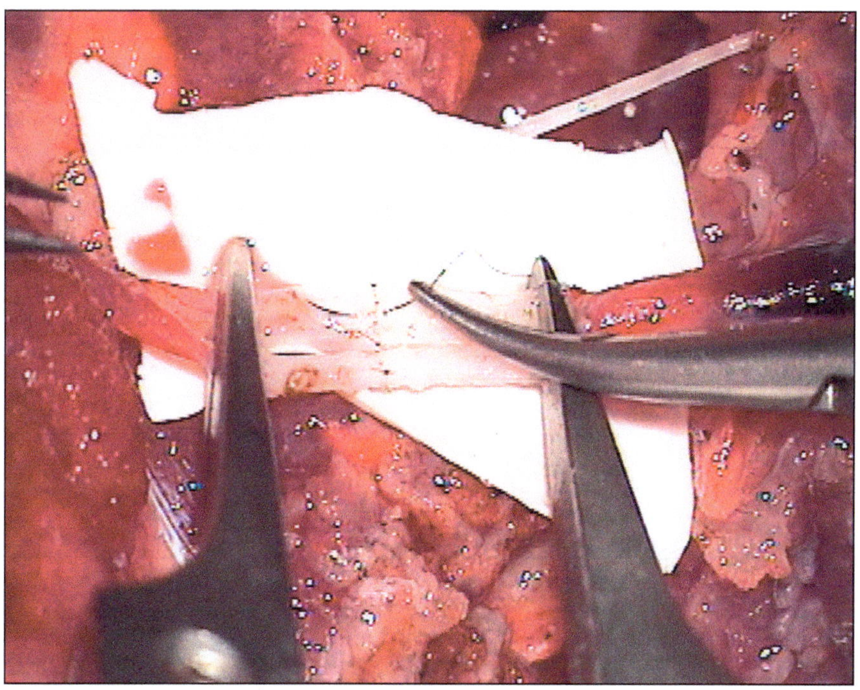

Figure 25-8

Anastomosis of the posterior surface of the femoral vein, rejoining the posterior left limb. One suture has been placed in the middle of each quadrant on either side first. The middle suture on the posterior surface here is placed last, allowing a better view of the lumen during placement of the previous two sutures. (From author's photo library)

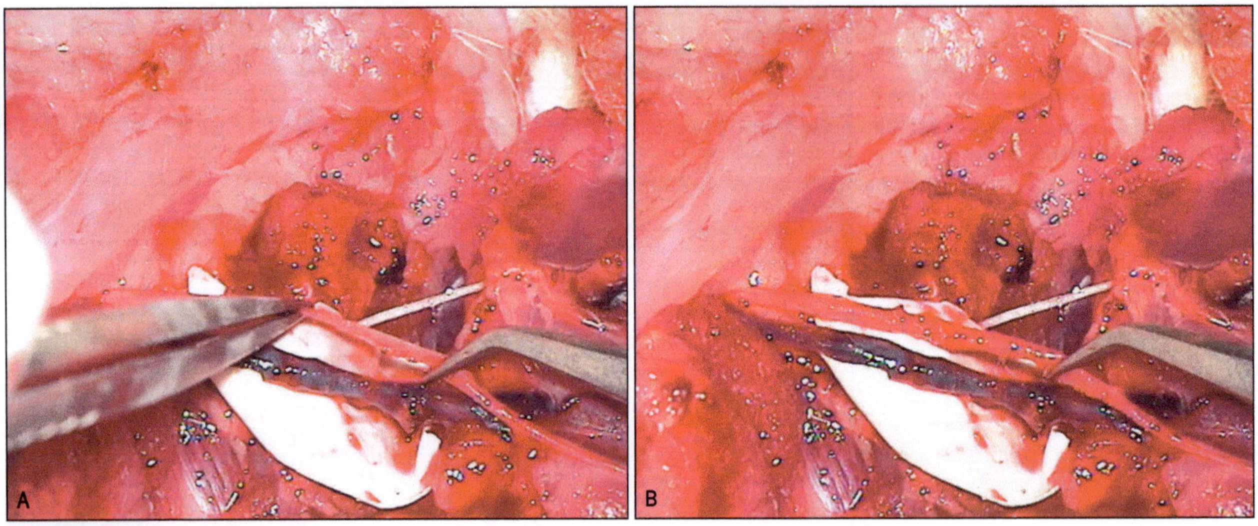

Figure 25-9

Patency test of the anastomosis of the femoral artery. Rejoining of posterior left limb. **A.** The upstream Dumont No. 3 forceps occludes blood flow just after the anastomosis, while the curved forceps, starting next to the No. 3 forceps, moves half-closed downstream to empty the lumen, eventually closing after a short distance. **B.** The upstream forceps is removed. Filling of the lumen up to the curved forceps proves patency of the anastomosis. (From author's photo library)

7. The yellow plastic background is withdrawn.

5. Suturing of the anterior muscles and skin

Each anterior muscle is sutured separately using interrupted 3/0 absorbable suture. Finally, the skin is sutured circumferentially using interrupted 2/0 non-absorbable suture.

Follow up: The leg must be pinkish in color. Postoperative edema is normal and will resolve within three days.

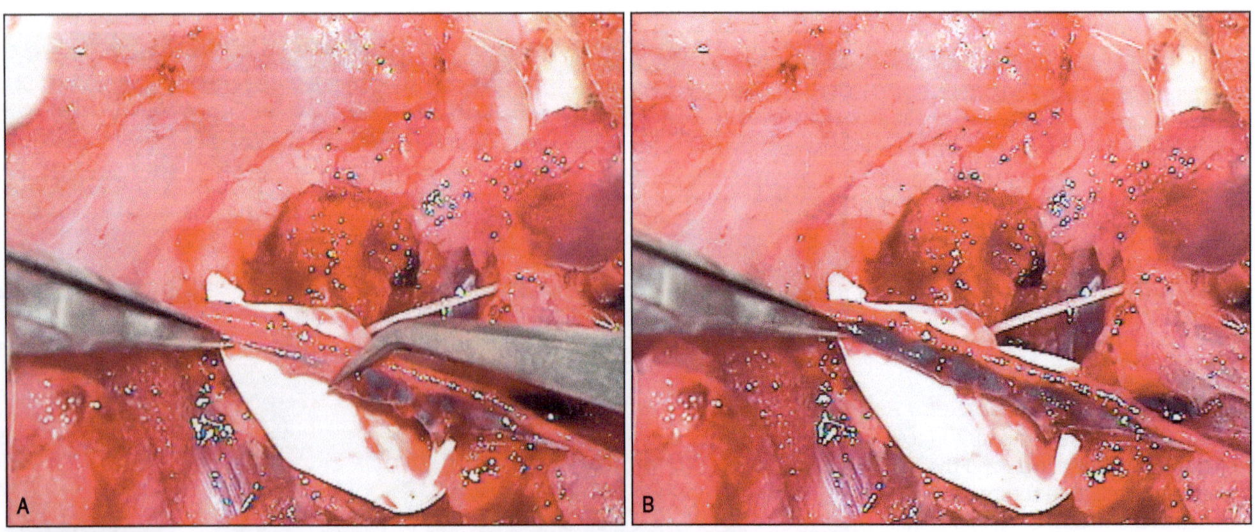

Figure 25-10

Patency test of the anastomosis of the femoral vein. Rejoining of posterior left limb. **A.** The curved forceps is applied just cranial to the anastomosis, occluding the vein. The straight forceps is initially placed cephalad, next to the curved forceps, then moves 'half-closed' downstream to empty the lumen, eventually closing after a short distance. **B.** The curved forceps is removed. Filling of the vessel up to the straight forceps proves patency of the anastomosis. (From author's photo library)

Synopsis...

... of autotransplantation of the posterior limb

A. **Positioning the rat:** Dorsal decubitus (supine) with the head away from the surgeon. The limbs are immobilized on the working surface with adhesive tape.

B. **Transection of the limb:** Incision is parallel to and 1 cm below the inguinal crease.

1. **Dissection of the femoral vessels (microsurgically):** The superficial fascia containing the superficial inferior epigastric vessels is dissected. The deep fascia is opened using two wet gauze pads, revealing the femoral vessels and their branches/tributaries. Each of the femoral vessels is microsurgically dissected from the origin/confluence of the superficial inferior epigastric vessels up to the inguinal ligament. All branches/tributaries found are transected between two ligations (9/0) or after cauterization.
2. **Transection of the skin and anterior muscles** using electrocautery, until the sciatic nerve is visualized.
3. **Dissection and transection of the sciatic nerve (microsurgically).**
4. **Transection of the posterior muscles and skin.**
5. **Occlusion and transection of the femoral vessels (microsurgically):** Two single vascular clamps or the double clamp can be used. The vessels are transected between the clamps.
6. **Transection of the femur** using a file, after opening the periosteum. A 0.5 mm piece is removed from the peripheral stump of the bone.

The limb is now fully transected and can be removed.

C. **Rejoining of the limb**

1. **Rejoining of the femur with internal fixation,** using a paper clip 1 mm in diameter
2. **Suturing of the posterior muscles** using absorbable 3/0 interrupted sutures.
3. **Suturing of the sciatic nerve (microsurgically)** using 2 or 4 (recommended) 9/0 sutures on the epi-perineurium.
4. **Anastomoses of the femoral vessels**
   - A yellow plastic background is placed under the femoral vessels.
   - The femoral vessels are placed together in the double vascular clamp. If single vascular clamps were applied before transection of the vessels, they are removed. The double clamp is supported with gauze pads in the gap between the stumps.
   - The lumens are irrigated and the adventitia is removed.

End-to-end anastomoses
Artery: 6 sutures 11/0
Vein: 6 or 8 sutures 11/0

1. The corner sutures are placed and the anterior surfaces of the vessels are sutured.
2. The clamp is rotated and the sutures on the anterior surfaces are checked.
3. The posterior surfaces are sutured, similar to the anterior.
4. The douple clamp is released.
5. A wet gauze is placed on the anastomoses for three minutes.
6. Patency test, separately for each vessel.
7. The yellow plastic background is withdrawn.

5. **Suturing of the anterior muscles** (3/0 absorbable sutures) **and skin** (2/0 non-absorbable, circumferentially).

Follow up: The leg must be pinkish in color. Postoperative edema is normal and will resolve within three days.

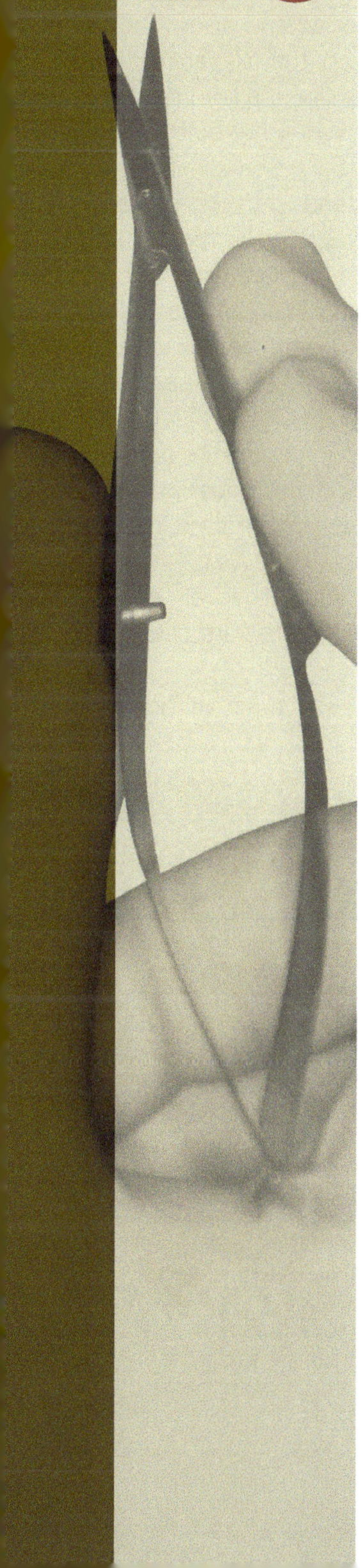

26 Orthotopic autotransplantation of the left kidney

The technique is described here for the left kidney because its vascular stalk is longer. The procedure on the right kidney is much more difficult due to its shorter vascular stalk.

A. Positioning of the rat

The rat is placed in dorsal decubitus (supine) position with the head on the surgeon's left. The limbs are immobilized on the working surface with adhesive tape.

B. Preparation of the surgical field

For a detailed presentation and imaging, the reader is invited to read the section on preparation in Chapter 8.B and C.1.

A median incision is performed, starting 5 mm caudal to the end of the cartilage of the xiphoid process (the xiphoid process ends in cartilage in the rat) and ending 5 mm cranial to the pubic symphysis. The skin and superficial fascia are detached from the investing fascia of the muscles with blunt dissection, using baby-Metzenbaum scissors.

The recti abdomini muscles are separated at the linea alba. Using fine, toothed forceps, the abdominal wall is elevated in the midline and a small transverse incision is made on the midline with baby-Metzenbaum scissors. Then, one leg of the scissors enters the abdominal cavity, and the incision is extended cranially and caudally. When extending the incision cranially, the border of the liver is met. This must be protected and preserved. Once fully extended, retractors are placed on either side of the incision.

Next, a piece of gauze moistened with warm normal saline is placed on the table, to the right side of the rat. The intestines are displaced from the abdominal cavity and enveloped in the gauze. Manipulation of the intestine must be performed with two wide atraumatic forceps. Since this procedure is being performed on the left kidney, *the small and large intestines are displaced to the right side.* The rectum is also moved to the right.

Finally, the posterior peritoneum is opened with two moistened gauzes that are drawn laterally, on either side, moving away from the midline, thus tearing the posterior peritoneum. This technique serves to bluntly dissect the retroperitoneal space and expose the inferior vena cava, aorta, left renal vein, and possibly the gonadal vein (**Fig. 26-1**).

The beginner should terminate macroscopic dissection of the surgical field at this point. Any effort to further dissect with gauze may tear the renal vein or inferior vena cava, leading to hemorrhage. However, with experience, it is possible to continue blunt dissection of the renal vessels until the renal artery becomes visible.

C. Microsurgical dissection of the renal fascia, renal vessels and ureter

In order to improve clarity, the microsurgical dissection of the renal fascia and its contents is presented in discrete sections. However, during an actual dissection, it is important that the surgeon perceive the wholeness of the surgical field, the continuation of the process, and realize that he or she will be required to revisit previous stages of the dissection.

I. Elements of surgical anatomy

The opening of the posterior peritoneum and retroperitoneal space with the two gauzes does not help with understanding surgical layers, which are torn blindly. Behind the posterior peritoneum and until the investing fascia of the muscles (transversalis fascia), there is the retroperitoneal space, which contains—among others—the kidney and its vessels. The renal fascia (Gerota's) envelops the kidney and the perirenal fat. It is continued toward the midline, surrounding the renal vessels and their perivascular fat and finally attaches to the adventitia of the aorta and the inferior vena cava (**Fig. 26-2**). In fact, the perivascular fat is the continuation of the perirenal fat.

Cranially, the renal fascia extends to envelop the adrenal glands. Since the branches of the renal vessels addressed to the adrenal (inferior adrenal artery and vein) are contents of the renal fascia, they also are packed by the perirenal fat. As a reminder, the left inferior adrenal vein empties in the renal vein, while on the right it exits in the inferior vena cava.

Caudally, the renal fascia extends into the pelvis and contains the ureter and its vasculature. The renal fascia envelops the ureter and the periureteral fat in the same way it does for the kidney and perirenal fat. The renal fascia also contains the gonadal vessels. These vessels course in front of the ureter because the gonad develops in front of the kidney, and this embryogenetic relation is maintained in the mature organism. On the left side, the gonadal vein empties in the left renal vein, as opposed to emptying into the inferior vena cava like the right gonadal vein. Also, as said above, on the left side the inferior adrenal vein empties in the renal vein. These asymmetries are due to

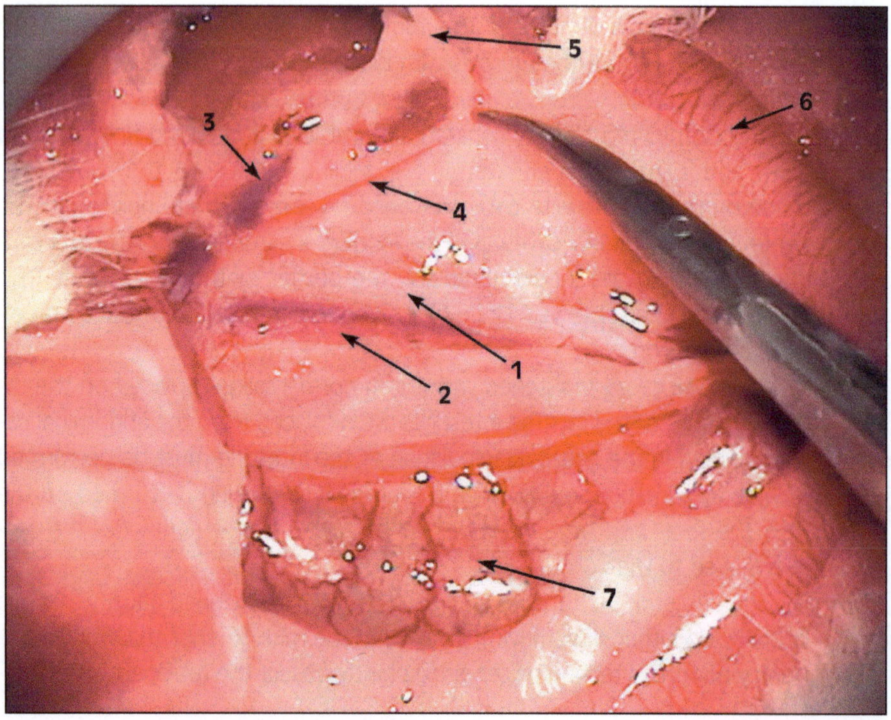

Figure 26-1

View of the surgical field after opening of the posterior peritoneum and retroperitoneal space with two gauzes. This maneuver reveals the aorta, the inferior vena cava, the renal vein, and, here, the gonadal vein. Here, the renal fascia is removed, together with the perirenal fat, with Dumont No. 3 forceps and baby Metzenbaum scissors. Observe that the perirenal fat is in continuation with the perivascular fat on the renal vessels. **1.** aorta, **2.** inferior vena cava, **3.** left renal vein, **4.** left gonadal (ovarian) vein, **5.** perirenal fat, **6.** left horn of the uterus, **7.** rectum, moved to the right. (From author's photo library)

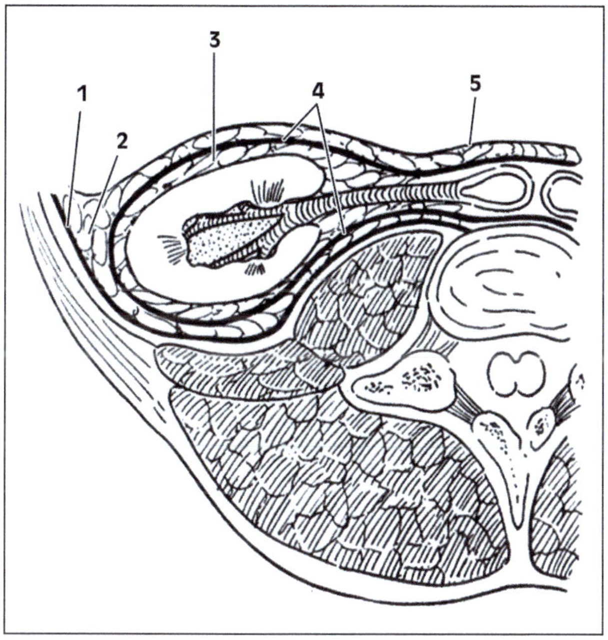

Figure 26-2

Diagram of the renal fascia and its relations, axial cross section in human. **1.** transversalis fascia, **2.** pararenal fat, **3.** perirenal fat, **4.** renal fascia, **5.** peritoneum. (Modified from W. H. Hollinshead. Anatomy for Surgeons, Vol 2, The Thorax, Abdomen, and Pelvis. New York: Horber-Happer Inc, 1956: p. 537, Fig. 392)

the fact that, during development, there existed a left inferior vena cava—comprised of the left gonadal, left adrenal, and a portion of the left renal vein where the former two vessels empty—which regresses during maturation.

Since the opening of the retroperitoneum is performed bluntly with the gauzes, it is probable to encounter the origins of vessels addressed to the intestine (e.g. superior mesenteric artery). We clear that these vessels are not related with the renal fascia. They arise retroperitoneally, at the same anatomical level where the renal fascia—enveloping the renal vessels—is attached to the adventitia of the aorta (and inferior vena cava); soon afterward, however, the intestine vessels are packed in the mesentery addressed to the respective intraperitoneal splanchna. The splanchnic veins mostly empty in the portal vein, and also are not related with the renal fascia.

The parietal vessels, such as the lumbar vessels, which are branches/tributaries of the aorta/inferior vena cava, are addressed to the muscles of the posterior abdominal wall; therefore they are found behind the posterior leaf of the renal fascia. The retroperitoneal nerves are found on top of the muscles, consequently also behind the posterior leaf of the renal fascia.

The renal fascia constitutes the border of the surgical layer delineating the kidney, renal vessels and ureter. The renal fascia is avascular, and external to its boundaries there are no vessels that communicate with the vessels internal to the fascia. The only possible exclusion is the space where the renal fascia surrounds the renal vessels, specifically close to the great vessels (aorta and inferior vena cava). There, deep tributary veins may be encountered, thought to originate from the muscles of the posterior abdominal wall.

If the surgeon is aware of the above few key points, then he/she is able to perceive the surgical layer undertaken for dissection of the kidney, renal vessels and ureter. The renal fascia per se is a thin transparent layer, which is usually opened unconsciously. Characteristic is the confusion between renal fascia and perirenal fat, terms inappropriately considered synonymous. While the latter mistake is not serious, ignoring surgical layers and their importance certainly is.

II. Microsurgical dissection

1. Renal fascia and perirenal fat

During the rough dissection of the surgical field using gauzes as described above, the renal fascia is detached from the adventitia of the aorta and inferior vena cava, and the perivascular fat from the renal vessels. This exposes the renal artery, renal vein, and some of their branches/tributaries.

Dissection and removal of the renal fascia and perirenal fat starts at the perivascular fat of the renal vessels. By advancing toward the kidney, a portion of the perirenal fat is also removed together with the surrounding renal fascia. The surgeon should have in mind that the perivascular fat is continued with the perirenal fat, and both are enveloped by the renal fascia.

The dissection of the renal fascia and perirenal fat is performed using two forceps or forceps and scissors. The anterior surface of the kidney is cleaned off first (**Fig. 26-1**). After rotating the kidney medially, renal fascia and perirenal fat have to be removed from the posterior surface (**Fig. 26-3**).

While the perirenal fat is easily detached from the renal capsule around the kidney, specific attention is needed at the hilum of the kidney. There, perirenal fat occupies the space between segmental branches of the renal vessels (branching of renal vessels takes place in the hilum before their entrance in the kidney) and adheres to the adventitia of the vessels. Therefore, this dissection of the perirenal fat near the hilum of the

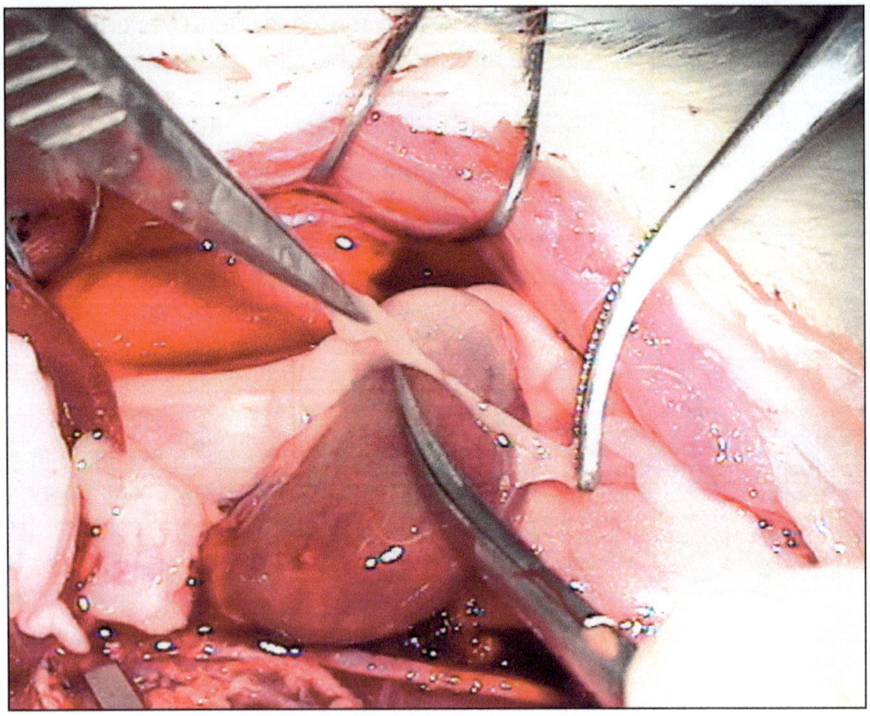

Figure 26-3

Dissection of the renal fascia and perirenal fat in the posterior surface of the kidney. The kidney has been rotated medially and downward. The curved mosquitos holds caudally the leaf of the opened renal fascia and perirenal fat, the Dumont No. 3 forceps lifts the cranial leaf, while the scissors are placed closed between the capsule of the kidney and the perirenal fat. (From author's photo library)

kidney is combined with the dissection of the renal vessels. According to our experience, it is best to stop the lateral to medial dissection of the perirenal fat at some point within the hilum and complete it later by meticulously dissecting the renal vessels from medial to lateral (from the aorta and inferior vena cava toward the hilum as described below). In any case, at some point it will be necessary to combine the dissection of the renal fascia and perirenal fat with the dissection of the perivascular fat of the renal vessels and their branches/tributaries.

During removal of the renal fascia and perirenal fat, specific attention is needed at the medial surface of the upper and lower poles of the kidney, as there are often accessory renal vessels that must be preserved. If such an accessory renal artery gets traumatized, blood supply to the respective segment of the kidney is jeopardized. Remember that accessory arteries are often segmental, i.e., responsible for the sole blood supply of a renal segment.

2. Renal vein and artery

It is very useful to have dissected first the great vessels, the inferior vena cava and the aorta, at the area of confluence of the renal vein and origin of the renal artery. **Microsurgical dissection starts with the renal vein,** since it is superficial to the artery. Dissection starts from the confluence of the renal vein with the inferior vena cava and advances toward the hilum of the kidney.

Technically, the renal vein is stripped of the perivascular fat and connective tissue attaching it to the renal artery (as opposed to stripping the fat off of the vein). This is performed with blunt dissection using two Dumont forceps (using one to hold the vein and the other to dissect) or with a combination of blunt and sharp dissection (where microsurgical scissors are used for dissection and cutting away perivascular tissues).

After dissecting the anterior surface of the renal vein, tributary veins become visible. The renal vein accepts the inferior adrenal vein cranially, the gonadal vein caudally, and the deep tributary veins posterolaterally (**Fig. 26-4**).

In detail:

- The *inferior adrenal vein* courses parallel and superficial to the inferior adrenal artery and, therefore, is dissected first (**Fig. 26-5**). Note that the inferior adrenal artery can be fully dissected at this point, but it is better to wait before ligating and transecting this artery. Early transection of the adrenal branch will detach the renal artery cranially. If this occurs, the artery is free to move caudally, and cause trouble during the dissection between renal artery and vein.
- Caudally, the greatest vein is the *gonadal vein.* Dis-

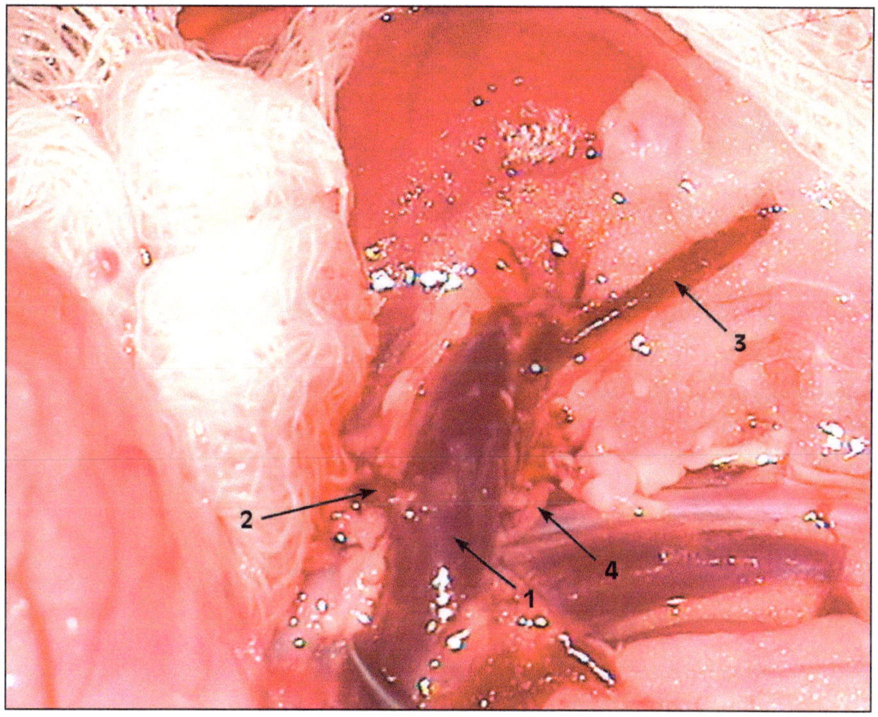

Figure 26-4

Tributaries of the renal vein. Partially dissected (frontal surface only) are seen the aorta, the inferior vena cava, the renal vein and its tributaries: the inferior adrenal vein is seen cranially, the gonadal vein caudally, and one deep tributary vein posterolaterally (crossing over the aorta). **1.** renal vein, **2.** inferior adrenal vein, **3.** gonadal vein, **4.** deep tributary veins. (From author's photo library)

section of this vein has to be start at its confluence with the renal vein (**Fig. 26-6**). Then the vein is stripped caudally off the perivascular fat (continuation of the perirenal fat) for some length to allow double ligation. As for all veins, the caudal ligature is placed first (**Fig. 26-7**) and the cranial ligature follows, placed close to the renal vein wall. The gonadal vein is then transected between the two ligations.

- *The deep tributary veins* arise from deeper muscle layers. These veins vary and may empty in the corner of the confluence of the renal vein with the inferior vena cava (No. 4, **Fig. 26-4**) or near the confluence of the gonadal vein with the renal

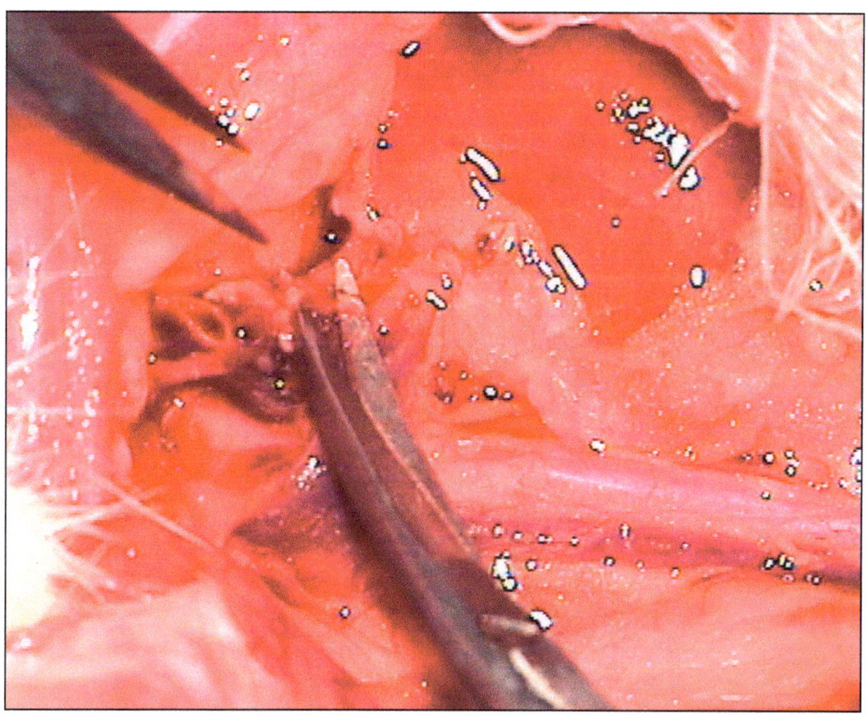

Figure 26-5

Dissection of the inferior adrenal vein. The Dumont No. 3 forceps, seen open here, has just left the translucent inferior adrenal vein that overlies the parted tips of the microsurgical scissors. The vein is now ready to be ligated. (From author's photo library)

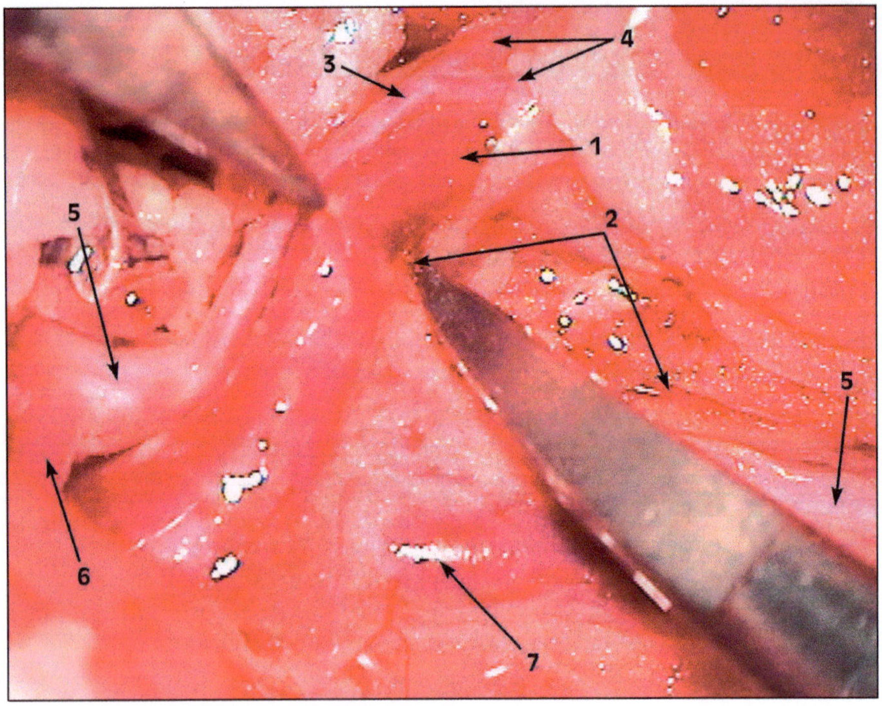

Figure 26-6

Dissection of the gonadal vein. The renal vein is held with Dumont No. 3 forceps from a residue of fat, while the blunt microsurgical scissors (closed) dissect the confluence of the gonadal vein with the renal vein. Observe the course of the gonadal vein. Cranial to the renal vein, the renal artery can be seen, partially dissected past its "bifurcation"; further dissection may reveal that there are more than two branches in the renal hilum. **1.** renal vein, **2.** gonadal vein, **3.** left renal artery, **4.** branches of the renal artery, **5.** aorta, **6.** right renal artery, **7.** inferior vena cava. (From author's photo library)

vein. Others are found to empty in the posterior surface of the renal vein. The ligation and transection of the deep tributary veins must be done with attention and fine movements, since the available space for suture placement is very limited. It is strongly advised to avoid cauterization of these veins. Transection of the deep tributary vein is required for the rotation of the renal vein so that the posterior surface can be approached. Avoid grasping the stumps of transected deep tributaries for handling the renal vein.

Attention is needed in the case of anatomic varia-

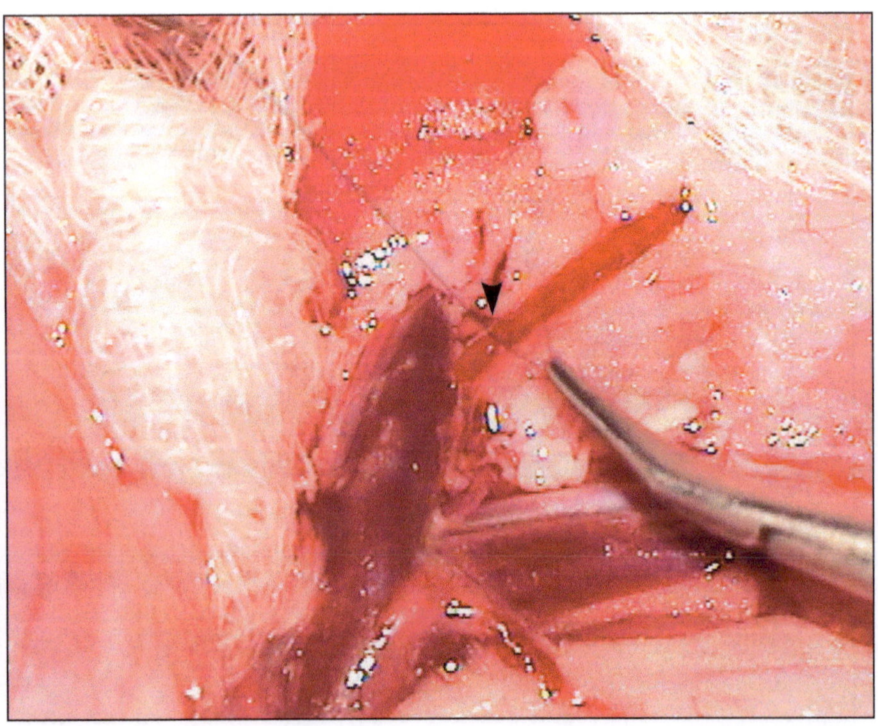

Figure 26-7

Ligation of the gonadal vein. This dissection continues from that shown in Figure 26-4. Here, the caudal ligation is placed, at a distance from the renal vein to allow space for transection after placement of the cranial ligation. An arrowhead denotes the knot with 9/0 suture. (From author's photo library) tions which, as known, are not rare phenomena for veins. Beyond the expected configuration of the renal vein, see if you can recognize the following in your surgical field:

- An additional vein for the lower pole (most common) or upper pole of the kidney
- A vein coming from a renal segment that empties into the renal vein away from the hilum of the kidney

Such veins should not be perceived as inferior adrenal, gonadal or deep tributary veins and be ligated by mistake. For this reason all the tributary veins of the renal vein should be identified before ligation.

After all tributary veins have been transected, the renal vein is dissected and separated from the renal artery. As a rule, the artery is found deep to the vein and is strikingly smaller in caliber. The walls of the vessels are attached to each other by loose connective tissue. To separate them, the vein is grasped from a residue of fat or from the adventitia (not from the wall per se), and, with blunt microsurgical scissors, a 'window' is created between the two vessels (**Fig. 26-8**). The scissors are held closed and gently enter the loose connective tissue between the two vessels with slow and repeated movements. When the window becomes transparent, the scissors can fully enter the space between the vessels and the legs can open. The renal vein, now detached from the artery, can be lifted or partially rotated in order to gain access and fully dissect the posterior surface. To achieve this, a residue of adventitia is left near the cranial or caudal edge of the anterior surface of the vessel in order to grasp the vein and this residue is removed latter.

Dissection of the renal artery is performed starting from its origin at the aorta until the hilum of the kidney. We repeat that it is necessary to dissect the aorta at the origin of the renal artery. Then, the renal artery is followed to the hilum and all branches are dissected, ligated or cauterized, and transected. The expected branches of the renal artery are the *inferior adrenal artery* and a *ureteral branch*. The ureteral branch, supplying blood to the cranial portion of ureter, is preserved if its origin is close to the hilum of the kidney. However, if it arises quite far from the hilum, it can be sacrificed without compromising ureteral blood supply, since lower arteries supplying the ureter will compensate (see below).

Because dissection of the renal vein includes the separation of the vein form the renal artery, it is evident that at many instances of the dissection, the surgeon may interchangeably dissect along either vessel. It is also evident that the surgeon will prefer to grasp the ad-

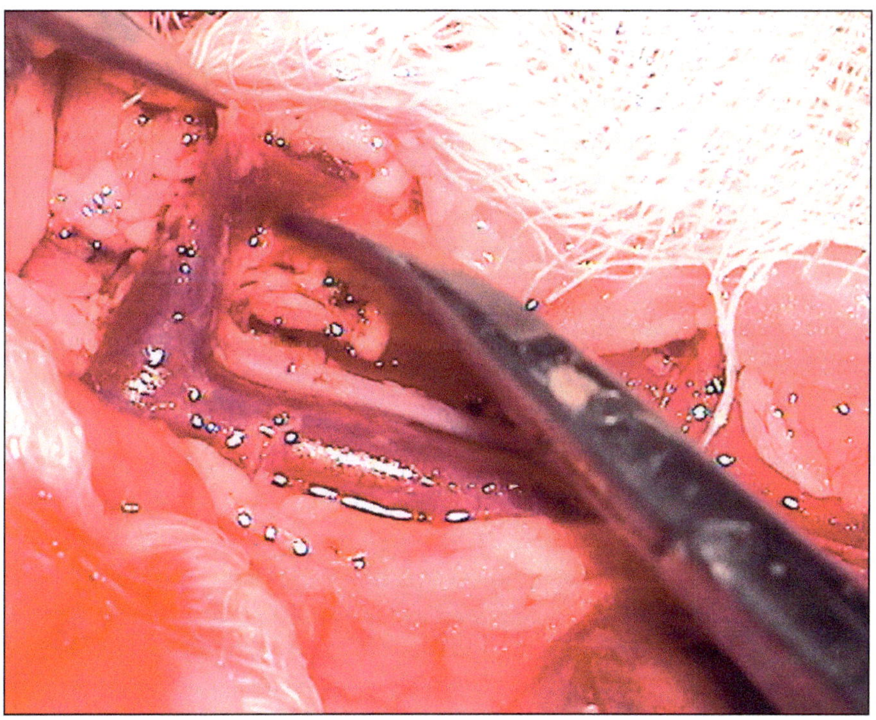

Figure 26-8

Detachment of the renal vein from the renal artery. Observe that previous to this, the inferior vena cava and the aorta have been meticulously cleaned at the origin/confluence of the renal vessels and that all the tributaries of the renal vein have been ligated and transected. The vein is elevated with Dumont No. 3 forceps from a piece of fat left on the anterior surface during dissection, while the blunt scissors open a window between the renal vein and the artery found beneath it. (From author's photo library) ventitia of the artery, as opposed to that of the vein (which is prone to rupture). Dissection of the artery must precede that of the vein in rare cases where it is almost anterior to the vein (**Fig. 26-9**). Handling the artery must be done with care, as it is prone to spasm. In general, it is recommended to grasp the wall of the renal vessels as little as possible.

➢ It is of extreme importance to perform a meticulous dissection of the renal vessels and avoid leaving tissue residues on the walls. The cleaner the vessels, the healthier the anastomoses will be. This is especially valid for the renal vein.

3. Ureter

Dissection of the ureter consists of stripping the ureter of periureteral fat and renal fascia. It is reminded that the renal fascia packs the ureter and periureteral fat, and also contains the gonadal vessels (found in front of the ureter). Dissection of the ureter sounds simple. However, one major issue is that "defatting" the ureter carries a high risk of ischemia. The explanation for this is found in the blood supply of the ureter. As in the human, the ureter has no specific supply from the aorta, i.e. there is no official ureteral artery. Instead, blood supply comes from arteries that vary throughout the course of the ureter according to the height. For example, at the level of kidney, the ureter is supplied by a branch of the renal artery, further on from a branch of the gonadal artery, and in the pelvis [in the rat] from the umbilical artery (branch of the internal iliac artery). All of these branches are contained in the periureteral fat. Through the surgical microscope, one or more small branches can be seen coursing longitudinally in the periureteral fat as well as on top of the ureter (**Fig. 26-10**). In order to preserve blood supply from the vessels of the periureteral fat, it is suggested to open a 'window' between the fat and the ureter only in the area where the ureter is going to be transected and anastomosed (**Fig. 26-10**). Pay attention not to unintentionally advance to total removal of the periureteral fat from the ureter at its whole length as a continuation of the dissection of the kidney, because this is obviously endowed with ischemia risk.

Other authors suggest not to dissect any of the 'periureteral fascia' (meaning the periureteral fat) in order to preserve the blood supply of the ureter. We disagree about not dissecting the periureteral fat from the part of ureter that will be anastomosed, because, with the ureter carrying fat and with no clear edges, the anastomosis is at risk. According to our experience, it is safe to separate a small area of periureteral fat (No 3, **Fig. 26-10**) from the ureter. In fact, by doing so, it is evident that there are one or more arterial branches in the ad-

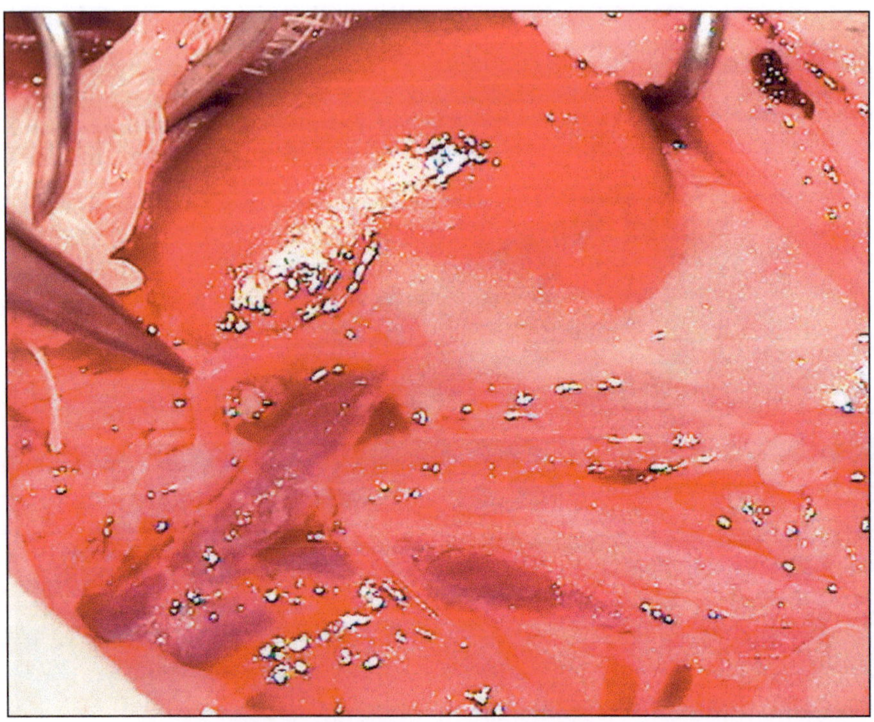

Figure 26-9

Dissection of the renal artery prior to the renal vein, since the artery was found in front of the vein. Observe the difference in caliber between the two vessels. The artery wall is grasped only from the adventitia in order to avoid spasm of the vessel. (From author's photo library)

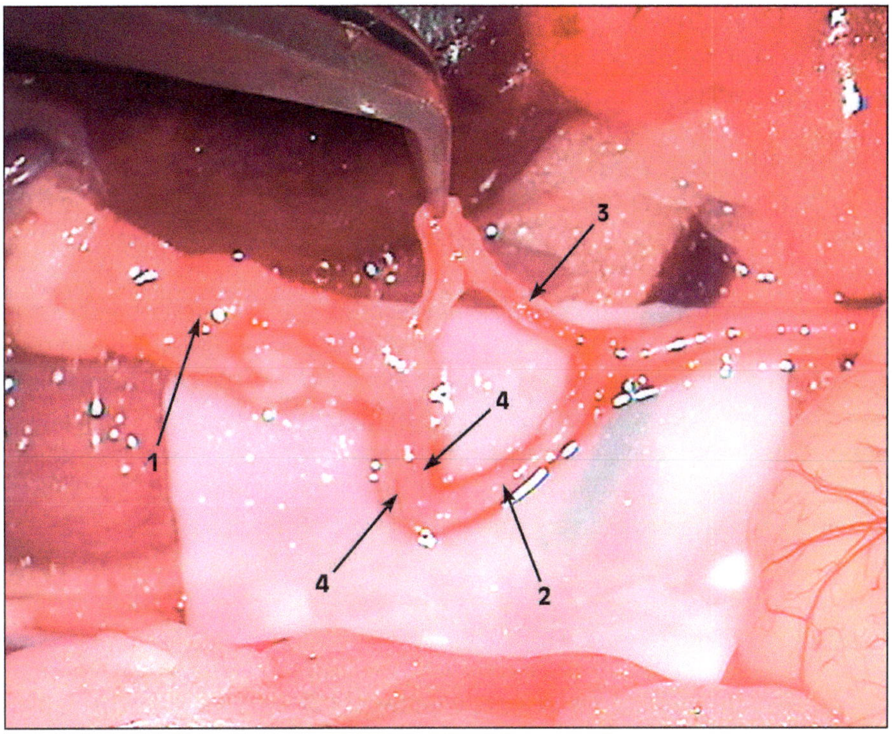

Figure 26-10

Dissection of the ureter. The renal fascia and part of the periureteral fat have been removed. Cranially, the ureter is surrounded by residual periureteral fat. More caudally, the periureteral fat has been detached from the ureter (a "window" has been created) and can be seen lifted by the curved microsurgical forceps. Observe the vessel contained in the periureteral fat. On the adventitia of the ureter, two small arterial branches are also visible. **1.** ureter and periureteral fat, non-separated, **2.** ureter, dissected, **3.** periureteral fat, dissected, **4.** longitudinal small arterial branches on the ureter. (From author's photo library)

ventitia of the ureter (No. 4, **Fig. 26-10**) which are adequate to supply the ureter after the anastomosis.

From a surgical anatomy point of view, opening a 'window' between the periureteral fat and the ureter is justified as follows: The vessels carried by the periureteral fat (No 1, **Fig. 26-11**), arise from local arteries supplying the ureter at each level of its descent toward the bladder (renal, gonadal, and umbilical arteries). From vessels of the periureteral fat, longitudinal vessels are

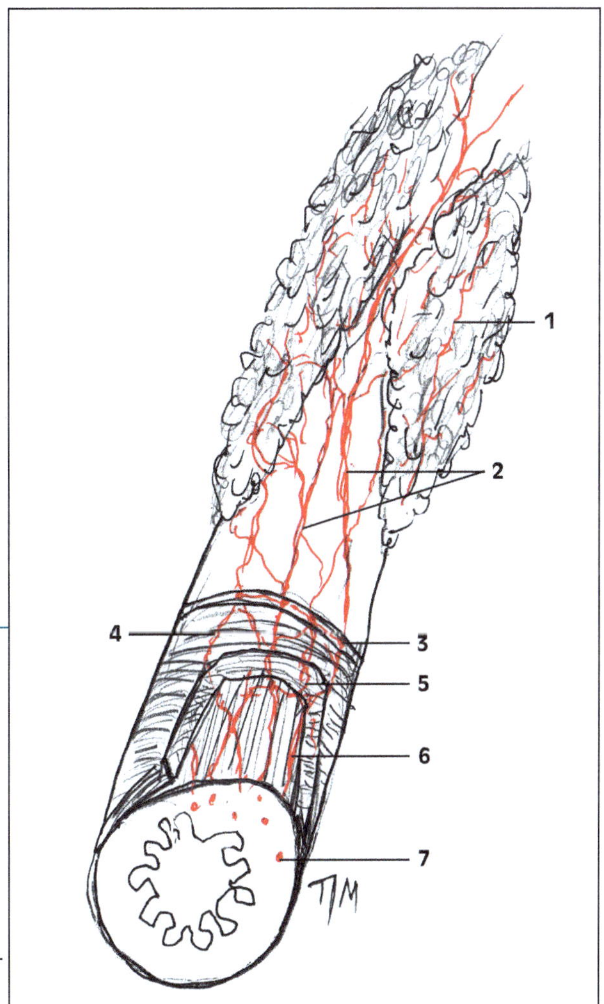

Figure 26-11

Blood supply of the ureter. Originating from arteries of the periureteral fat are long longitudinal branches that course along the adventitia (superficial network). The longitudinal branches communicate already from the point they emerge and along their entire length with the deep vascular network through penetrating branches. Similarly, the deep network comprises longitudinal vessels and penetrating branches at every stratum of the ureteral wall, from muscular layers to the endothelium. **1.** arteries in the periureteral fat, **2.** longitudinal branches on the adventitia, **3.** penetrating branches of the adventitia, **4.** longitudinal branches of the circular muscle layer, **5.** penetrating branches of the circular muscle layer, **6.** longitudinal branches of the longitudinal muscle layer, **7.** small arterial branches in the lamina propria. (Drawing by the author) supplied to the adventitia (No 2, **Fig. 26-11**). These vessels may course cranially or caudally and have a long course from where they first meet the adventitia. Therefore, detachment of the periureteral fat does not disturb the longitudinal vessels given higher or lower than the ends of the 'window'. The vessels of the adventitia communicate throughout their entire length with the deep vascular plexus through penetrating branches (which also communicate between themselves) (No 3, **Fig. 26-11**). The deep vascular network includes vessels in all strata of the ureter: longitudinal vessels of the circular muscular layer, which in turn give penetrating branches to the longitudinal vessels of the longitudinal muscular layer found internally, which give arterioles deeper to the lamina propria and the endothelium of the ureter (**Fig. 26-11**). The fact that there are longitudinal vessels on the adventitia after the detachment of the periureteral fat (**Fig. 26-10**) and that these vessels communicate more cranially or caudally with the deep vascular network, reassure that the blood supply of the ureter in the 'window' between periureteral fat and ureter is preserved.

In the *in situ* autotransplantation of the kidney (without removal of the kidney) described here, the periureteral fat is separated from the ureter without transection. It is moved aside to provide space for the anastomosis of the ureter. Thus, vessels contained in the fat are preserved. In the orthotopic autotransplantation with removal and repositioning of the kidney (as well as in the orthotopic or heterotopic transplantation described in the next chapters), the periureteral fat is transected along with the ureter. At the edges of the ureteral stumps of donor and recipient, the periureteral fat is dissected in order to obtain a 'clean' anastomosis. In these cases, transection and removal of the terminal periureteral fat does not disturb nearby longitudinal vessels on the adventitia. The communication of these vessels with the deep network reassures the blood supply of the anastomosed stumps of the ureter.

D. Placement of the double clamp – Transection of vessels – Irrigation – Removal of the adventitia

⇨ ***ATTENTION: The duration of occlusion of vessels in the kidney cannot surpass the limit of 30 minutes***

After placing a background under the prepared vessels, the double vascular clamp is brought in the field. The base of the double clamp rests on the left hypohondrium. The renal artery and vein are placed together near the tips of the clamps, at a small distance from each other.

➢ After the double clamp is closed, start a chronometer: you have only 30 minutes to complete the anastomoses

The vessels are transected with a clear cut. Although the classic instruction is to perform both transections midway between the two clamps, we suggest offsetting the arterial and venous transection of the first sutured vessel. This will prevent the tied sutures of the anastomosis of the first sutured vessel from interfering with the anastomosis of the other. However, it is not a mistake at all to cut the vessels in the same line, as it is a matter of preference for the surgeon.

The lumens of the stumps of the renal vessels are irrigated with normal saline using an angiocatheter 27G without entering the lumen. The adventitia on each end of the transected artery is then folded back. For vein stumps, the adventitia is carefully cut away. The clamps are approximated, to avoid tension while performing the anastomoses.

E. End-to-end anastomoses of the vessels

The end-to-end anastomoses are performed according to the principles described in Chapter 5.

The following number of sutures are placed:

- **Renal artery anastomosis: 8 sutures 11/0**
- **Renal vein anastomoses: 10 or 12 sutures 10/0**

From the arrangement of the vessels in the clamp, it is obvious that the anterior surfaces of both vessels will be sutured first, the clamp will be rotated, and suturing of the posterior surfaces will be completed.

The exact steps of the process of the anastomoses are numbered below:

1. First is sutured the anterior surface of the artery. The corner sutures are placed first, at 12 o'clock and 6 o'clock (**Fig. 26-12**). The 3rd suture is placed in the middle of the anterior surface. The 4th and the 5th sutures are placed midway between the middle suture and the corner sutures.
2. Suturing of the vein starts also with placement of corner sutures (**Fig. 26-13**). The suite is dictated by

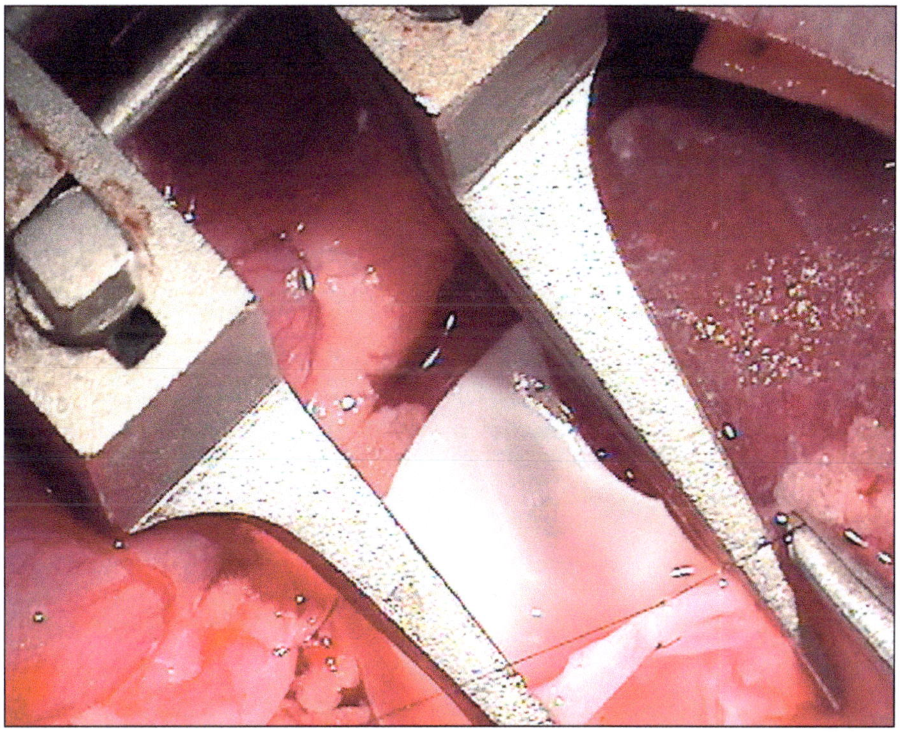

Figure 26-12

Anastomosis of the renal artery with 11/0 sutures. Here the 6 o'-clock corner suture has already been placed and the 12 o'clock suture is being tied. (From author's photo library)

the number of sutures needed on the vein. If a total of 10 sutures are required, there are 4 left for the anterior surface, which will be placed at estimated equal distances from the corner sutures and between themselves, first the lateral (toward the corner sutures), then the more central (see **Figure 5-2D**). If 12 sutures are needed, there are 5 left for the anterior surface. The 1st suture will be placed in the middle of each semicircle and then 2 at equal distances in each quadrant, starting laterally and approach-

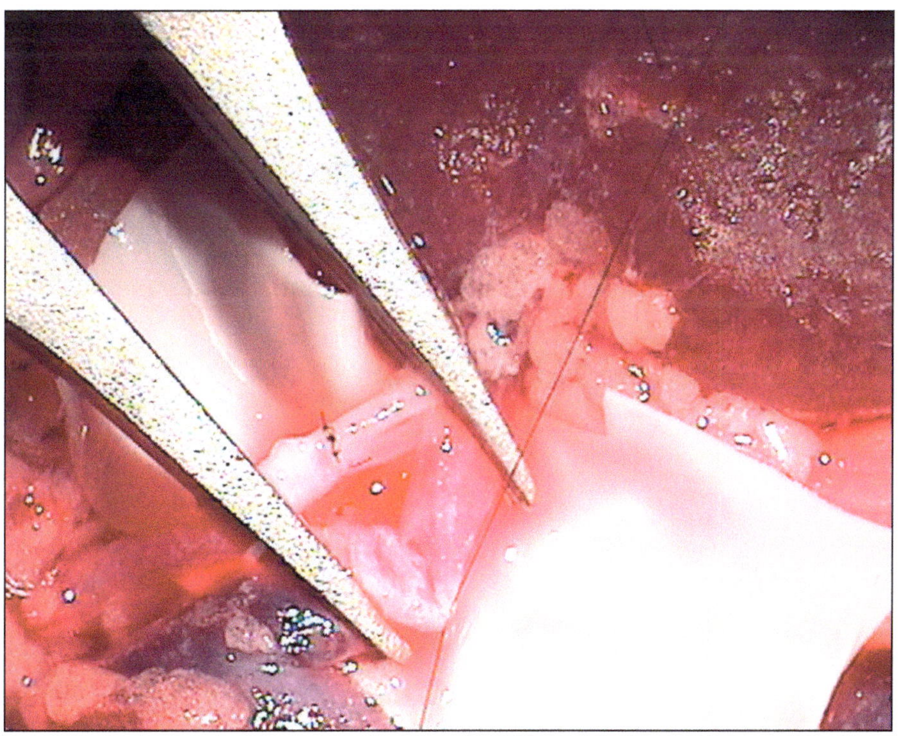

Figure 26-13

Anastomosis of the renal vein with 10/0 sutures. Here the knot of the 6 o'clock suture is placed. (From author's photo library)

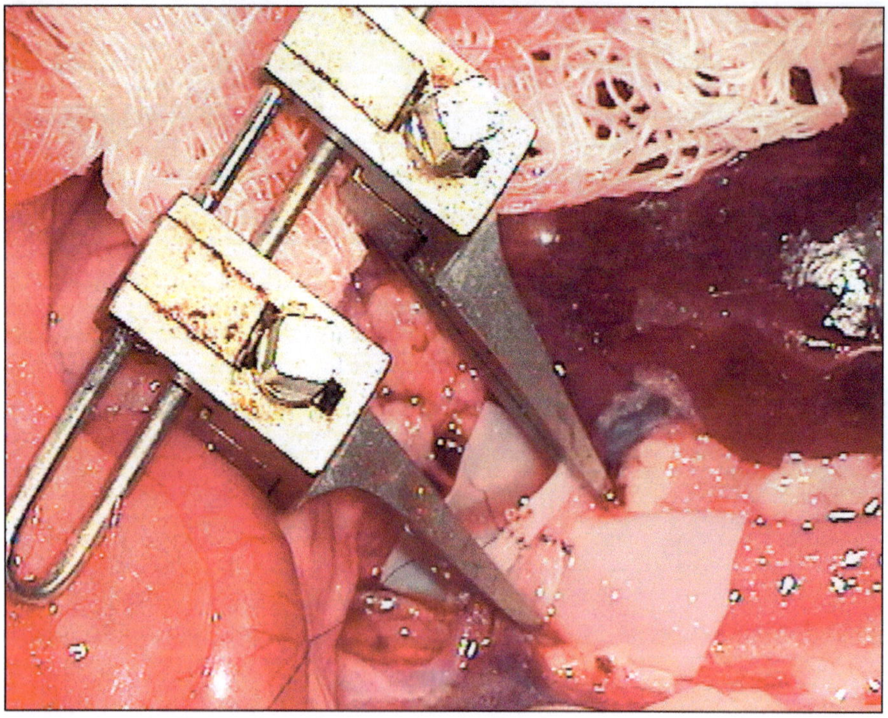

Figure 26-14

Completely sutured anterior surfaces of the renal artery and renal vein. (From author's photo library)

ing the middle of the anterior surface (see **Figure 5-2E**). Completed suturing of the anterior surfaces of both artery and vein is shown in **Figure 26-14**.

3. The double clamp is rotated and the sutures of the anterior surface are checked.
4. Suturing of the posterior surface of the artery and vein is completed in the same way as the anterior surfaces (**Fig. 26-15**).
5. The vessels are released from the double clamp (**Fig. 26-16**).

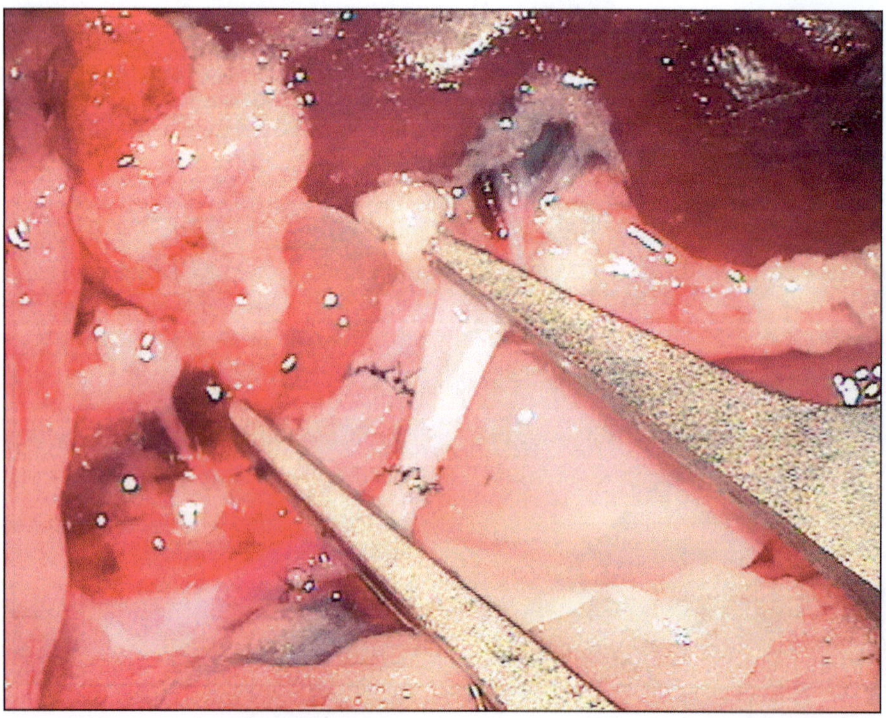

Figure 26-15

Completely sutured posterior surfaces of the renal artery and renal vein. (From author's photo library)

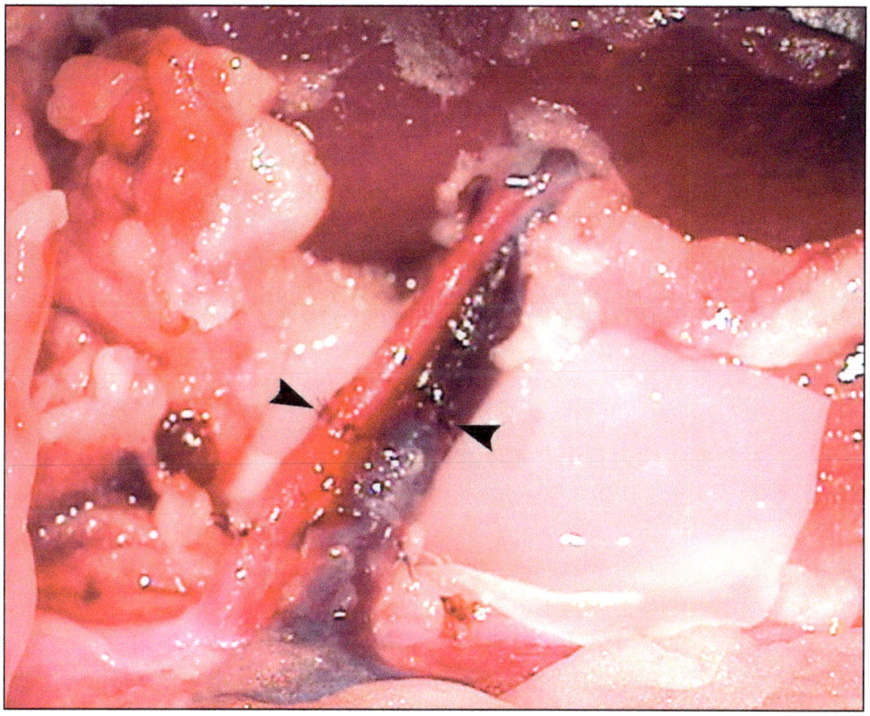

Figure 26-16

Sutured renal vessels after removal of the double clamp, with suture lines marked by arrowheads. (From author's photo library)

6. Wet gauze is placed on the vessels over the anastomosis for 3 minutes.
7. The patency test is performed separately for each vessel. The test is described in detail in Chapter 5.10 (**Fig. 5-4**). In short, peripheral to the anastomosis (according to blood flow), a 1st forceps occludes the vessel and a 2nd forceps empties the lumen by moving half-closed and remains closed at a final point. The 1st forceps is removed, and, if the vessel is patent, it is immediately filled up to 2nd forceps.
8. The yellow plastic background is removed.

F. Transection and anastomosis of the ureter

Following the above dissection, the ureter has been detached from the periureteral fat (**Fig. 26-10**). This detachment takes place for a length of ureter that will make the anastomosis comfortable. We repeat that transection for the in situ autotransplantation should comprise only the ureter and not the periureteral fat.

- Ureteral anastomosis: **4 sutures 11/0** are placed

The steps of the process of the anastomosis are the following:

1. The transection of the ureter is performed **without placement of double vascular clamp,** only the yellow plastic background is put under the ureter.
2. The anastomosis of the ureter is done with 4 sutures 11/0 following the technique for end-to-end-terminal anastomosis of vessels.
3. The patency test of the ureter is performed with injection of methylene blue in the renal parenchyma. If the ureter is patent, the methylene blue will be seen to flow peripheral to the anastomosis (**Fig. 26-17**). In addition, the tightness of the anastomosis is judged on whether there is a leak of methylene blue from the suture line. The patency test should not be done immediately after the anastomosis of the ureter; as for vessels, we wait a few minutes.
4. The yellow plastic background is withdrawn from behind the ureter.

G. Closure of the surgical trauma

The splanchna are positioned back in the abdomen and

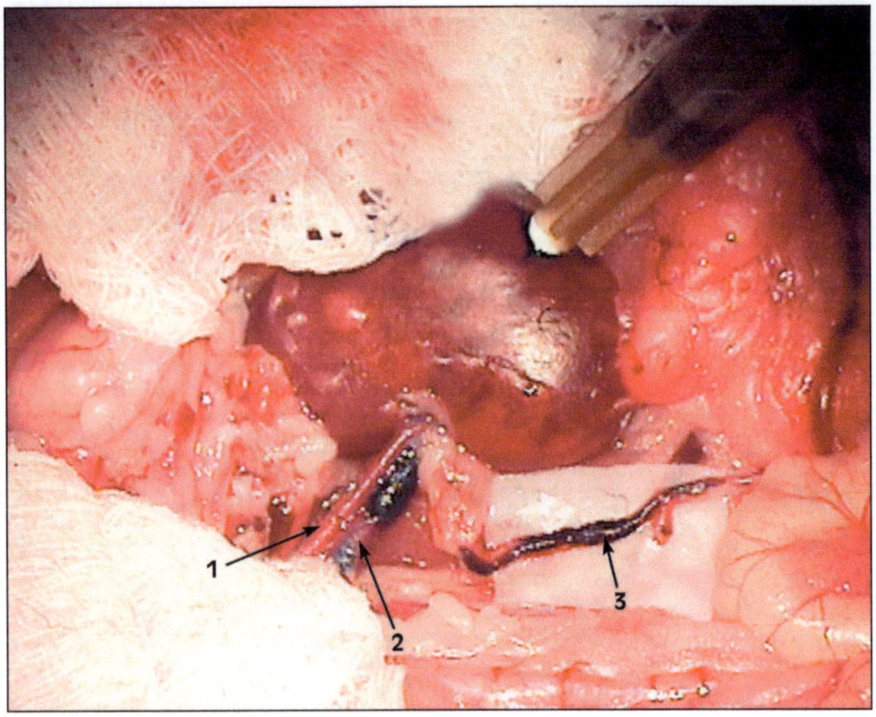

Figure 26-17

Patency test of the ureter. Injection of methylene blue in the renal parenchyma is followed by observing for the flow of color in the ureter distal to the anastomosis. If seen, this confirms patency of the ureter. Check to be sure that there is no leak of dye on the yellow plastic background, which shows the tightness of the anastomosis. **1.** renal artery, **2.** renal vein, **3.** ureter full of methylene blue. (From author's photo library)

the abdominal wall is closed in two layers with non-absorbable 2/0 sutures. The muscles are closed in a continuous suturing fashion, while the subcutaneous and skin are approximated with interrupted sutures.

Synopsis... of orthotopic autotransplantation of the left kidney

A. **Positioning of the rat:** Laid on its back, head to the surgeon's left. The limbs are immobilized on the working surface with adhesive tape.

B. **Preparation of the surgical field:** A median incision is performed, from xiphoid process to the pubic symphysis, and the linea alba is opened. The small intestine is mobilized and placed as a whole to the right of the rat. The posterior peritoneum and retroperitoneum is opened with two gauzes moistened in warm normal saline.

C. **Microsurgical preparation of the renal fascia and perirenal fat, renal vessels and ureter:** The renal fascia is opened (envelops the perirenal fat, kidney, the renal vessels and perivascular fat, the ureter and periureteral fat, and the gonadal vessels). The perirenal fat is dissected around the kidney and removed; similar for the perivesacular fat (continuation of the perirenal fat) on the renal vessels. The renal vein is dissected, starting from its confluence with the inferior vena cava. Then the renal artery is dissected, from the aorta to the hilum of the kidney. The branches/tributaries of the renal vessels are transected between two ligations (9/0): inferior adrenal vein and artery, gonadal vein, and deep tributary veins of the renal vein. The kidney is rotated and the posterior surfaces of the renal vessels are dissected. Finally, the ureter is dissected by opening a "window" between the ureter and the periureteral fat, (which carries blood supply to the ureter), where the transection and anastomosis of the ureter will be performed. A yellow plastic background is placed under the renal vessels.

D. **Placement of the double clamp –Transection of vessels – Irrigation – Removal of adventitia**

⇨ ***ATTENTION: The duration of occlusion of renal vessels cannot surpass 30 minutes***

1. Placement of the renal artery and vein together in the clamps of the double clamp, so that the base of the clamp rests on the left hypohondrium and the tips of the clamps point to the pelvis.
2. Transection of the vessels.
3. Irrigation of the lumens with warm normal saline.
4. Approximation of the clamps.
5. Folding of the adventitia from the cut ends of the artery and removal from the cut ends of the vein.

E. **End-to-end anastomoses of the vessels**

- **Renal artery: 8 sutures 11/0**
- **Renal vein: 10 or 12 sutures 10/0**

1. The anterior surfaces of the anastomoses are sutured first, starting from with the artery with placement of 4 sutures (first the corner sutures, then 2 at equal distances). Then the vein is sutured with 5 sutures (first the corner sutures, 1 in the middle, 1 in the middle of each quadrant) or 6 sutures (first the corner sutures, then 4 at equal distances).
2. The double clamp is reversed and the anterior sutures are checked.
3. Suturing of the posterior surfaces is completed.
4. Release of the double clamp.
5. Placement of wet gauze on the anastomosis for 3 minutes.
6. Patency test.
7. Withdrawal of the yellow plastic background.

... of orthotopic autotransplantation of the left kidney

Synopsis...

F. Transection and anastomosis of the ureter

1. Placement of yellow plastic background under the ureter.
2. Transection of the ureter **without placement of vascular clamp.**
3. Anastomosis of the ureter with **4 sutures 11/0**, following the same technique as in vascular anastomosis.
4. Patency test of the ureter with injection of methylene blue into the renal parenchyma. If the ureter is patent, the blue will flow peripheral to the anastomosis. The patency test is performed a few minutes after the anastomosis is completed.
5. The yellow background is withdrawn.

G. Closure of the surgical trauma: Repositioning the intestines in the abdomen and suturing of the abdominal wall in 2 layers with non-absorbable 2/0 suture. A continuous stitch is used in the muscles and an interrupted stitch is used in the subcutaneous and skin.

27

Orthotopic transplantation of the left kidney

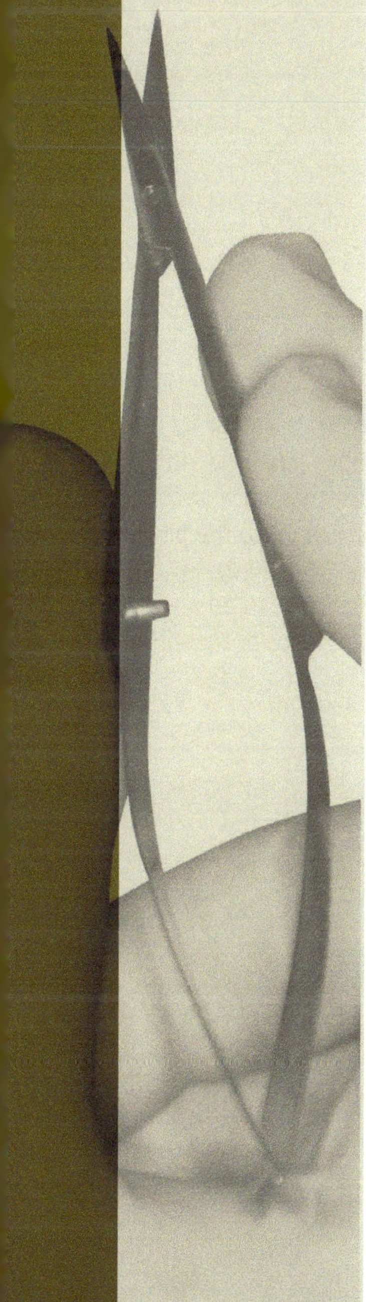

I. Preparation of the Donor

The reader is refered to Chapter 26 for sections A and B.

A. Positioning

B. Preparation of the surgical field

C. Microsurgical dissection of the renal fascia, renal vessels and ureter – Dissection of the aorta for flushing of the graft

The reader is referred to Chapter 26 for a detailed presentation of the dissection of the renal fascia, renal vessels and ureter. Here we focus on specific differences and the additional maneuvers during the steps of this particular dissection.

1. Renal fascia and perirenal fat

As in Chapter 26.C.II.1.

2. Dissection of vessels

a. Renal vein and artery

➢ **In transplantation of the kidney, dissection of the renal vessels must be meticulous throughout their entire length.** The steps are repeated here in brief:

- Dissection of the aorta cranially and caudally to the origin of the renal artery (here of the left kidney). The origin of the renal artery is meticulously dissected.
- Dissection of the anterior surface of the inferior vena and the confluence of the left renal vein.
- Dissection of renal vessels toward the renal hilum.

The dissection of the renal fascia and perirenal fat (in the anterior and posterior surface of the kidney) may be combined with the dissection of the renal vessels, as described in Chapter 26 C.II.2. However, in kidney transplantation it is best to prepare the renal vessels first throughout their entire length, from the aorta and inferior vena cava to the renal hilum. During rotation of the kidney for dissection of the renal fascia and perirenal fat at the posterior surface, it must be verified that the renal vessels do not suffer compression or torsion.

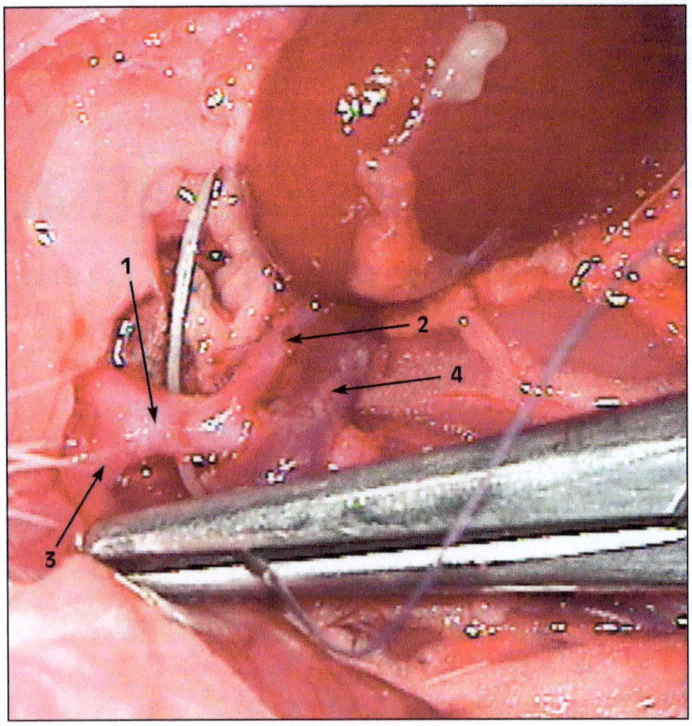

Figure 27-1

Preparation for ligation of the aorta cranial to the origin of the left renal artery. After a 'window' has been opened between the aorta and the inferior vena cava, a 5/0 suture needle passes behind the aorta. This suture will not be tied, but wait until harvesting the kidney **1.** aorta, **2.** left renal artery, **3.** right renal artery, **4.** left renal vein. (From author's photo library)

b. Dissection of the aorta for flushing of the graft

- **In transplantation of the kidney, the donor kidney must be flushed with heparin solution** administrated via injection into the aorta at the level of the renal artery, after the aorta is occluded cranially and caudally to the renal artery origin. Microsurgical dissection starts with **making a 'window' posterior to the aorta, cranial to the origin of the left renal artery (Fig. 27-1), and proceeds with making a second 'window' posterior to the aorta, cranial to the bifurcation into common iliac arteries (Fig. 27-2).** In these sites, the aorta is dissected from the inferior vena cava so it can be occluded (with clamps or ligations).

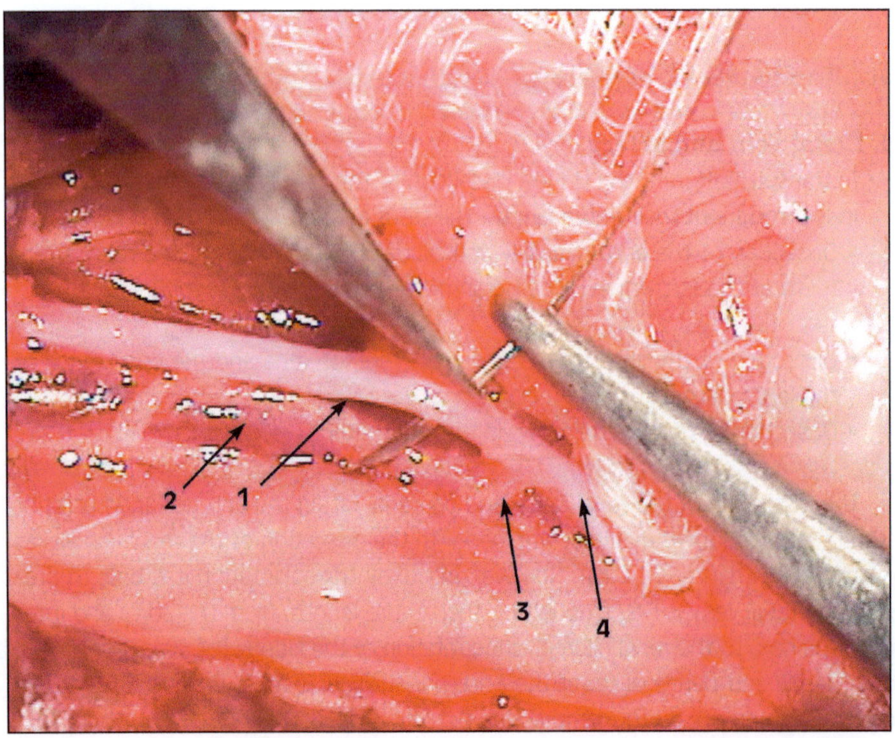

Figure 27-2

Preparation for ligation of the aorta cranial to its bifurcation. After a 'window' has been opened between the aorta and the inferior vena cava, a 5/0 suture needle passes behind the aorta. The width of the 'window' is restricted caudally by a lumbar artery. The suture will not be tied, but wait until harvesting the kidney. **1.** cranial end of the 'window' between aorta and inferior vena cava, **2.** inferior vena cava, **3.** right lumbar artery, **4.** bifurcation of the aorta into common iliac arteries. (From author's photo library)

As presented in **Figures 27-1** and **27-2** the sutures can be placed in the 'windows' created between the aorta and inferior vena cava and stay untied. The occlusion of the aorta for flushing the kidney will be performed later, at the stage of taking the graft (section III.A)

3. Ureter

➢ **In transplantation of the kidney, the ureter and the periureteral fat have to be transected.**

The periureteral fat is dissected and separated from the ureter only at the site where the ureter is going to be transected. However, the separated periuriteral fat cannot remain intact, as in in situ autotransplantation of the kidney, but has to be transected during harvesting of the graft (see below, section III.B). Verify that vessels can be seen along the adventitia of the ureter.

The periureteral fat transfers blood supply to the ureter, part of which is given from the renal artery (or sometimes also from the gonadal artery). Therefore, in order to preserve this blood supply to the ureter, it is wise to keep as short as possible the cranial separation of the periureteral fat from the ureter (**Fig. 27-3**). However, the terminal portion the periureteral fat, near the site of transection, has to be removed in order to obtain a 'clean' ureteral edge for anastomosis in the recipient.

The donor animal stays on the working surface during the next step and must be kept warm. The kidney is periodically irrigated with warm normal saline.

II. Preparation of the Recipient

A. Position of the rat

As in the donor.

B. Preparation of the surgical field

As in the donor.

C. Microsurgical dissection of the renal fascia, renal vessels and ureter

As in the donor, except that there is no need to dissect behind the aorta to open 'windows'. No flushing of the kidney with heparin solution is done.

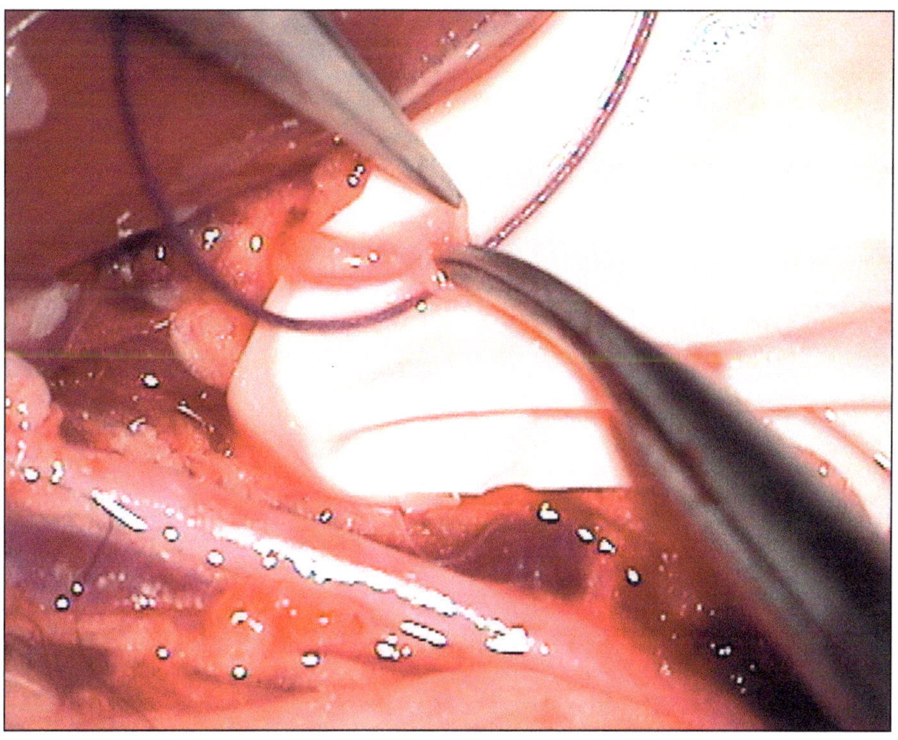

Figure 27-3

Dissection of the donor ureter. Cranial to the site where the ureter is going to be transected, only a small part of periureteral fat is dissected away in order to preserve the vascular supply to the ureter. Dumont No. 3 forceps lifts the periureteral fat and scissors separate it from the ureter. On the yellow plastic background behind the ureter, a 5/0 Vicryl suture has been placed, waiting to ligate the peripheral part of the ureter that will stay in the donor. (From author's photo library)

III. Graft Harvestig (Donor)

A. Flushing of the kidney

The aim of flushing the donor kidney with heparin solution is to remove all blood from the intrarenal vasular network. Otherwise, this blood will clot and render the kidney useless for transplantation.

To properly flush the kidney, heparin solution should enter the renal artery and exit from the renal vein. In order to direct the solution to the kideny only and avoid diffusion of heparin throughout the general circulation, the aorta is occluded above and below the renal artery. In addition, to avoid enrtrance of the solution into the inferior vena cava, the renal vein is transected before its confluence. This way, as the solution is injected into the *cranially and caudaly occluded aorta,* heparin will flow to the kidney via *the untouched renal artery* and exit from *the cut renal vein.*

The technical steps of the process are the following:

- In the 'window' that has been created cranial to the origin of the renal artery, a ligation is performed with 5/0 Vicryl suture, or, as said above, the suture placed during dissection of the aorta (**Fig. 27-1**) is ligated at this point. Of course, a single clamp can be used instead of ligation.
- In the caudal 'window', before the bifurcation of the aorta, another ligation is performed with 5/0 Vicryl suture or, as presented above, the suture which as been placed in this window during aorta dissection (**Fig. 27-2**) is ligated at this moment. Evidently, a single clamp can be used instead.
- The renal vein is ligated adjacent to its confluence with the inferior vena cava (**Fig. 27-4**) and transected just distal to the ligature, so that a maximal length of the stump of renal vein is retained.
- Flushing of the kidney by **injecting cold heparin solution in normal saline (25.000 IU/ml)** until the kidney obtains a whitish color. A 5 ml syringe is used, in which a fine needle has been attached. The needle is bent so that the stream of the injected fluid will follow the direction of the lumen (**Fig. 27-5**). The volume of injected solution is 1-3 ml. This is done with a gentle and controlled pressure, so that there will be no back-flow and leak from the needle's entrance point.

B. Technique of graft harvesting

- The renal vessels are placed in the jaws of the lateral arm of the double vascular clamp. The base of the double clamp, on which the arms move, rests on the left hypochondrium. The dissected and preserved renal artery is placed in the clamp first, followed by the stump of the cut renal vein. The clamp should grasp the vessels close to the hilum of the kidney, leaving enough vessels length toward the midli-

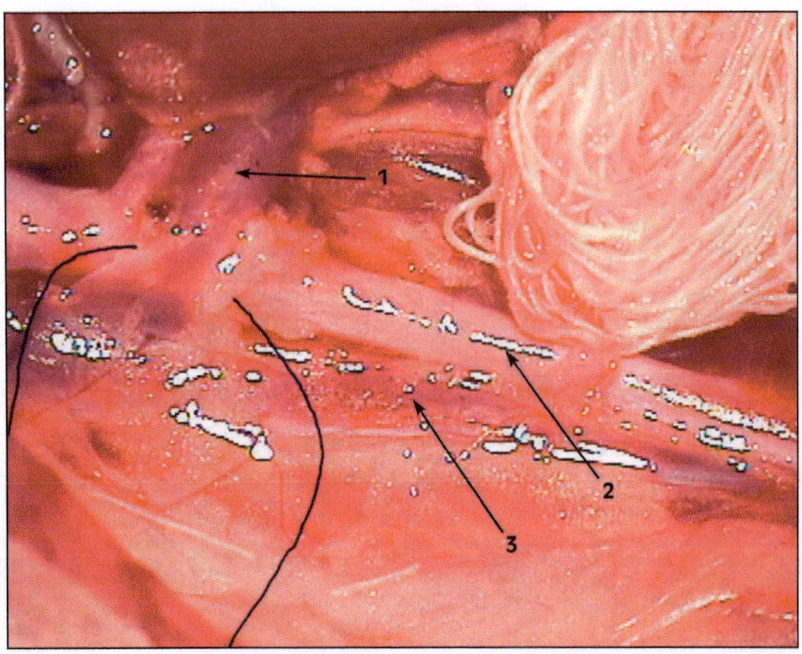

Figure 27-4

Ligation of the renal vein. A 9/0 Nylon suture passes under the renal vein and is about to be tied (the line of the suture has been artificially enhanced in this photo for emphasis). **1.** left renal vein, **2.** aorta, **3.** inferior vena cava. (From author's photo library)

Figure 27-5

Flushing of the donor kidney with injection of cold heparin solution in the aorta, which has been ligated cranially to the renal artery and before the bifurcation. Observe the site of injection into the distal aorta and the curved needle in the aorta lumen. The heparin solution rinses the kidney and exits from the renal vein, seen here as 'venous blood' filling the opened retroperitoneun to the left of the aorta. **1.** ligation of the aorta, cranial to the renal artery, **2.** ligation of the aorta cranial to its bifurcation, **3.** renal artery, **4.** transected renal vein, **5.** ureter. Observe the Vicryl suture passing under the ureter and lying on the kidney. It will be used later to ligate the peripheral stump of the ureter that will remain in the donor. (From author's photo library)

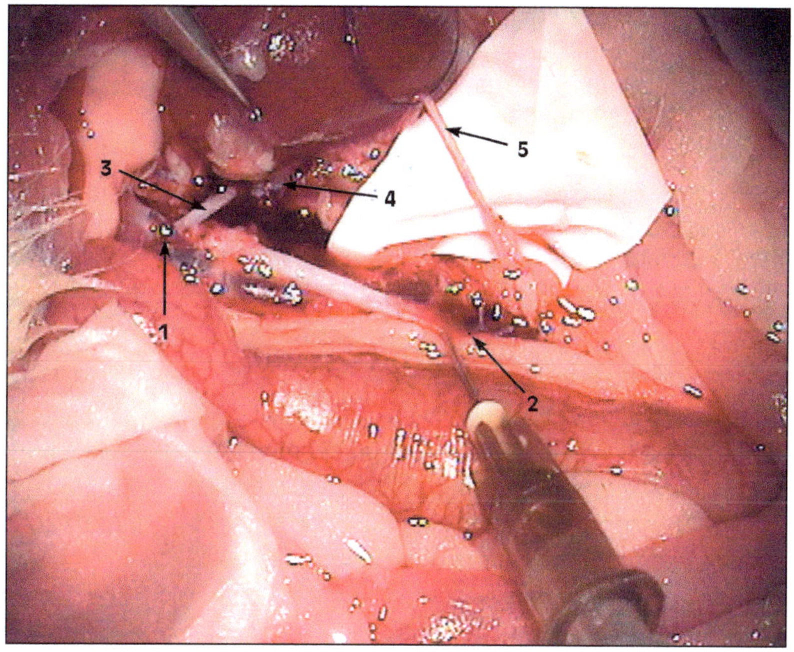

ne for comfortable anastomoses in the recipient. The site of placement of the clamp is usually indicated by the bifurcation of the renal artery, which should be left peripheral to the point of occlusion, so that we ultimately have one main artery for anastomosis.

- The renal artery is ligated with 9/0 suture at its origin from the aorta and transected just distal to the ligation.
- The ureter is ligated with 5/0 Vicryl suture at the caudal end of the 'window' opened between the ureter and the periruteral fat, and cut proximal to the ligation. Transection is performed with the microsurgical scissors perpendicular to the long axis of the ureter with one clean cut. The separated periureteral fat is also transected at the same place.

The free graft is then taken and enveloped in a gauze moistened with cold heparin solution (same as used in flushing of the kidney).

After harvest of the graft, the aorta ligations (or clamps) are removed so that the rat-donor does not suffer any ischemic damage to abdominal viscera or posterior limbs.

IV. Graft Implantation (Recipient)

The graft, together with the double clamp whose lateral arm occludes the renal vessels, is placed in the surgical field adjacent to the kidney of the recipient that will be replaced by the graft.

A. Removal of the recipient's kidney – Placement of the stumps of its vessels in the free clamp

- The renal vessels of the recipient are placed in the free medial arm of the double clamp. The double clamp is placed as in the donor, i.e., with the base resting on the left hypochondrium. This placement has to be accompanied by proper positioning of the donor kidney. Attention is needed in the arrangement of the surgical field with the two kidneys present.

  The renal artery and vein of the recipient are occluded as proximally as possible to the origin of the renal artery from the aorta with the free arm of the double clamp.
- The renal vessels of the recipient should be transected far enough from the site of occlusion, i.e. just before the bifurcation of the renal artery, because of the contraction they will undergo after transection (especially the artery). This length will also be useful in making modifications (e.g. lumen dilatation) that may be required to the recipient vessels.
- The ureter of the recipient is transected together

with the periureteral fat. The remaining peripheral ureteral stump is cleaned of periureteral fat at its end, in preparation for the anastomosis.

The kidney of the recipient is then ready to be removed from the field and the graft is placed in its bed.

B. Preparation of the donor and recipient renal vessel stumps

First, the diameters of the renal vessels are checked for any disproportion in lumen size. If a disproportion is found, it can be corrected with dilatation of the smaller vessel. This is accomplished by inserting a Dumont No. 3 forceps into the smaller lumen and allowing the tips to gradually open. This maneuver can be repeated in order to achieve the desired amount of dilation. In rare cases, more advanced correction techniques are needed; such as oblique section or 'fish mouth' cuts of the smaller lumen. These techniques are described in Chapter 5.

Then, the length of the donor and recipient vessels are checked. Donor vessels that are left too long can kink, which will disturb blood flow, placing vessel patency and donor kidney survival at risk. If the vessels have been left too long, they should be transected at a site obviating their ability to kink.

Next, the vessels of recipient and donor are prepared in the same way as for any anastomosis. The lumens are irrigated with warm normal saline using a fine angiocatheter 27G. The adventitia is folded in the arteries, and removed in the veins in order to provide clean vessel ends.

The clamps are approximated to bring the vessels of the donor exactly opposite to the corresponding vessels of the recipient, so that the anastomoses will be performed correctly and comfortably.

C. End-to-end anastomoses of vessels and ureter

End-to-end anastomoses of renal vessels and ureter have been described in detail in Chapter 26.

1. Renal Vessels

The following number of sutures is placed

- **Renal artery anastomosis: 8 sutures 11/0**
- **Renal vein anastomoses: 10 or 12 sutures 10/0**

The anterior surfaces of the two vessels will be sutured first, the double clamp will be rotated together with the graft, and suturing of the posterior surfaces will be completed.

➢ **There is always the time restriction that the anastomoses of the renal vessels must be completed within 30 minutes from the obstruction of the donor's vessels**

The steps of the end-to-end anastomoses are the following:

1. First the anterior surface of the arterial anasto-

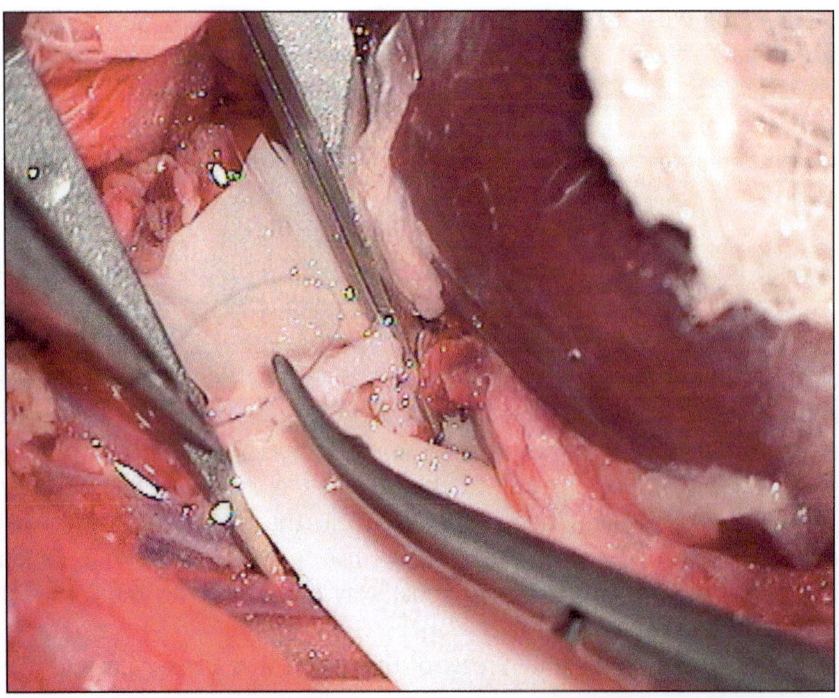

Figure 27-6

Suturing of the anterior surface of the renal artery, performed prior to the vein. Here, after placement of the two corner sutures, is put the suture in the middle of the anterior surface, in one step. The needle can be seen through the wall of the artery. (From author's photo library)

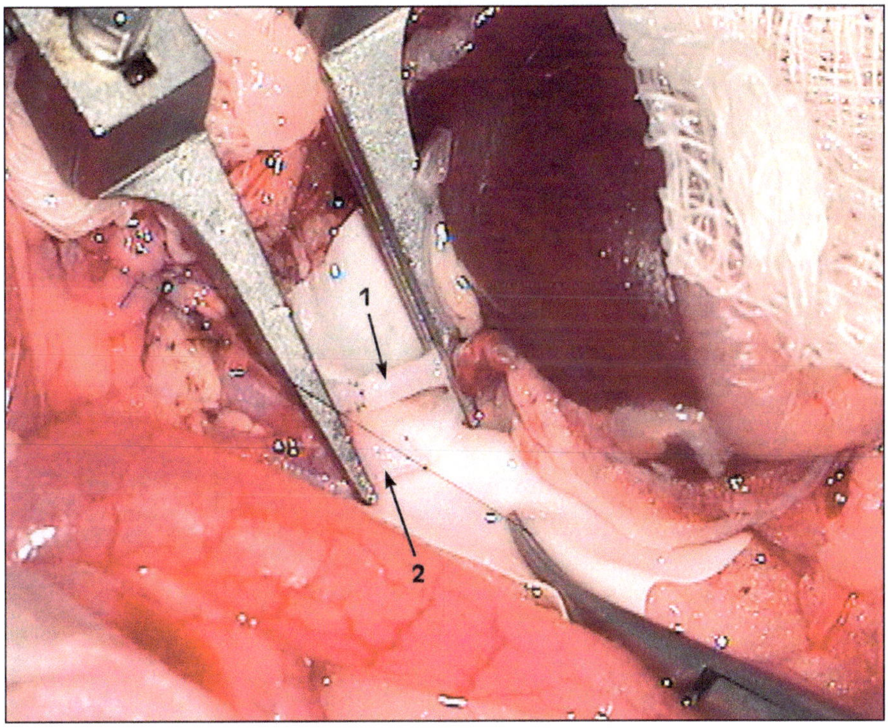

Figure 27-7

Suturing of the anterior surface of the renal vein. The 2nd corner suture is placed in the 6 o'clock position. The anterior surface of the artery has been completed previously. **1.** renal artery, **2.** renal vein. (From author's photo library)

mosis is sutured (**Fig. 27-6**), followed by the anterior surface of the vein (**Fig. 27-7**).

2. The double clamp is rotated and correct placement of anterior sutures is checked.
3. Posterior surfaces of the anastomoses are completed (**Fig. 27-8**).
4. Release of the vessels from the double clamp.
5. Placement of wet gauze on the anastomoses for 3 minutes.
6. Patency test (separate test for each vessel) (**Fig. 27-9**).
7. Withdrawal of the yellow plastic background.

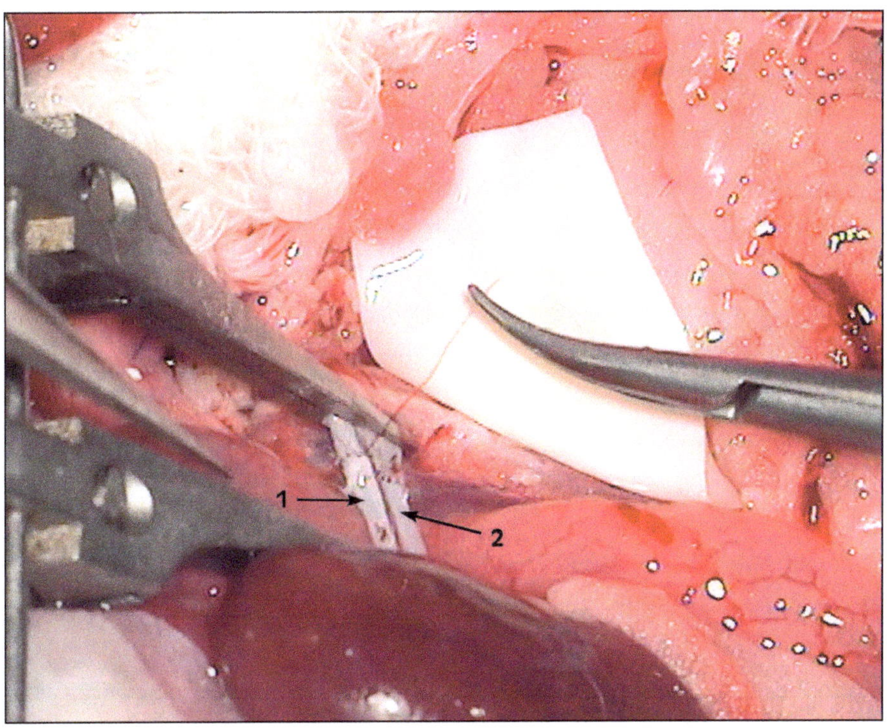

Figure 27-8

Suturing of the posterior surfaces of the renal vessels. The kidney and the double clamp have been rotated medially. Here, suturing of the posterior surface of the renal artery is performed. The needle holder and the Dumont No. 3 forceps hold the 11/0 suture. Suturing of the posterior surface of the vein will follow (the sutures seen in the vein belong to the anterior surface). **1.** renal artery, **2.** renal vein. (From author's photo library)

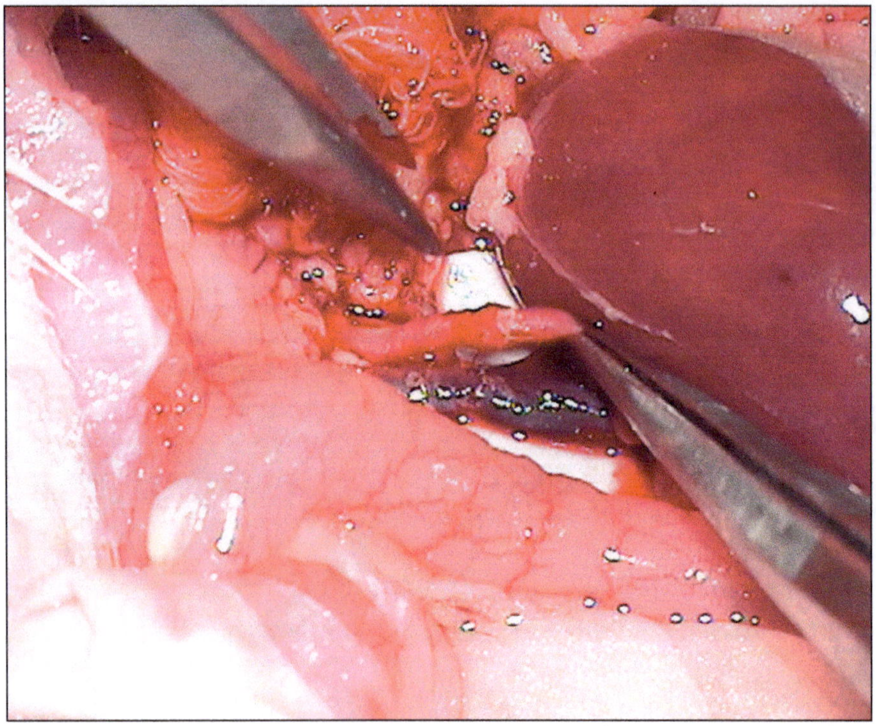

Figure 27-9

Patency test of the renal artery anastomosis. Peripheral to the anastomosis (following the blood flow), the closed forceps occludes the blood flow. The other forceps, seen open here, was initially closing the lumen distal to the anastomosis, while the 2nd forceps was emptying the lumen moving downstream, until the final position, where it was closed. The fact that the vessel is filled up until the closed forceps proves the patency of the anastomosis. (From author's photo library)

2. Ureter

- **Ureteral anastomosis: 4 sutures 11/0 are placed**

The steps of the anastomosis are the following:

1. Placement of the yellow plastic background under the ureter with no vascular clamp placed on the ureter.
2. Anastomosis of the ureter with 4 sutures 11/0, following the same technique as in end-to-end anastomosis of vessels (**Fig. 27-10**).
3. Patency test of the ureter, with injecting methylene blue in the renal parenchyma (**Fig. 27-11**).
4. Withdrawal of the yellow plastic background.

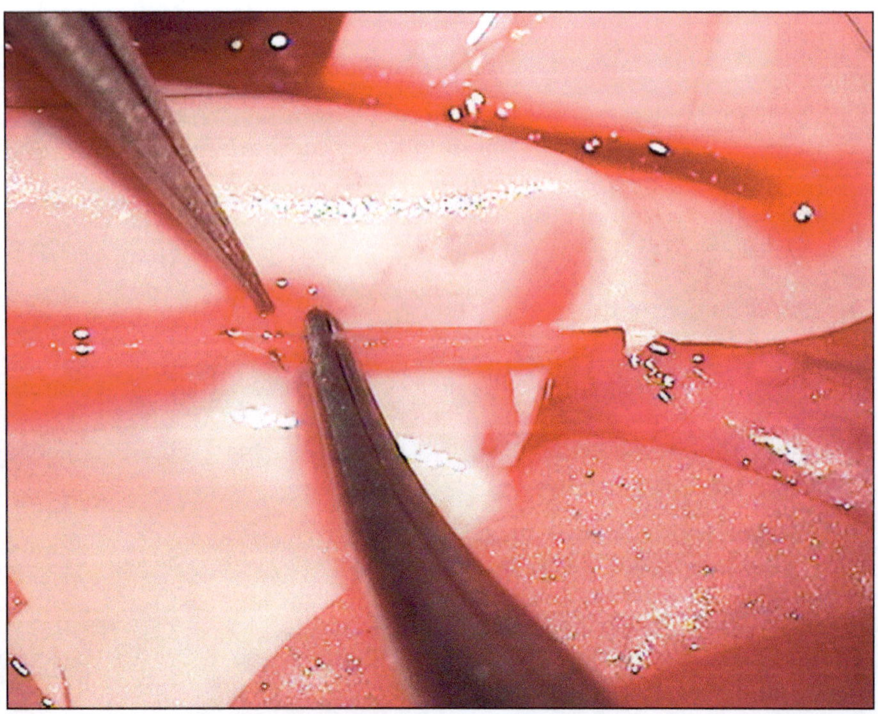

Figure 27-10

Suturing of the ureter with 11/0 suture. Here, the medial suture of the anterior surface is placed and the corner sutures have been placed previously (the 6' o'clock suture can be seen). (From author's photo library)

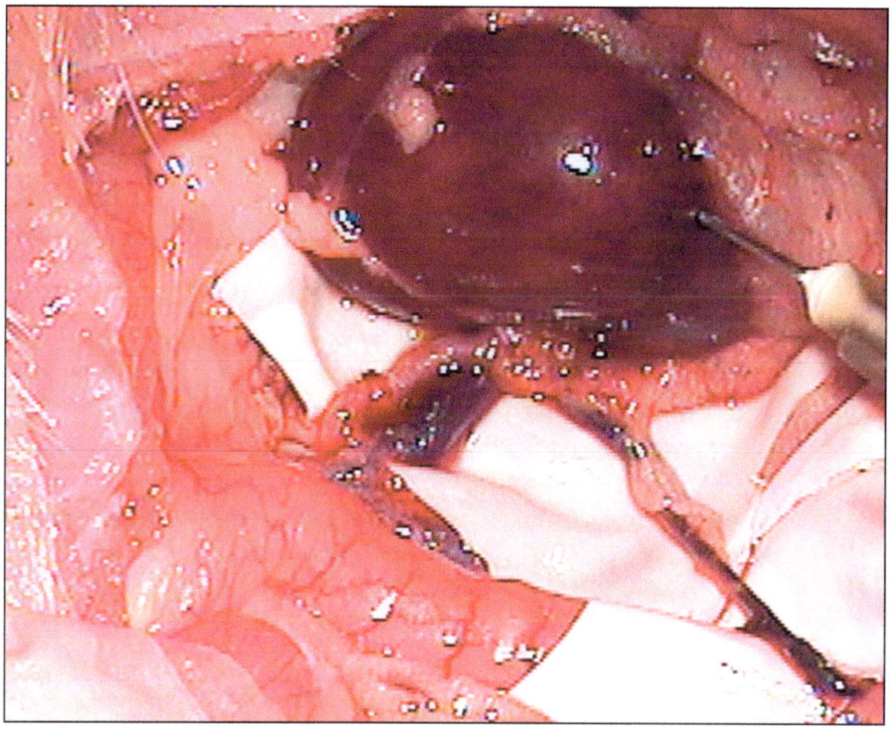

Figure 27-11

Patency test of the ureter. Methylene blue is injected in the renal parenchyma. The fact that color passes in the ureter distal to the anastomosis proves that the anastomosis is patent. Observe the absence of leak. (From author's photo library)

5. Closure of Surgical Traumas

First in the recipient and then in the donor, the splanchna return to the abdominal cavity and the abdominal wall is closed in two layers with non-absorbable 2/0 sutures. (muscles with continue suturing and subcutaneous and skin with interrupted sutures).

... of orthotopic transplantation of the left kidney

Synopsis...

I. PREPARATION OF THE DONOR

A. Positioning: Dorsal decubitus (supine) position, head to the left of the surgeon, with limbs immobilized on the working surface with adhesive tape.

B. Preparation of the surgical field: A median incision is performed from the xiphoid process to the pubic symphysis and the linea alba is opened. The small intestine is mobilized and placed as a whole to the right of the rat. The posterior peritoneum and retroperitoneum are opened with two gauzes moistened in warm normal saline.

C. Microsurgical preparation of the renal fascia and vessels, and dissection of the aorta for flushing the graft

- The renal fascia is opened, and the perirenal fat is dissected and removed around the kidney.
- The renal vein and artery are dissected, from the inferior vena cava and aorta to the hilum of the kidney. All branches and tributaries are transected between two ligations: inferior adrenal vein and artery, gonadal vein, and deep tributary veins of the renal vein. The kidney is mobilized from its bed, rotated and the posterior surfaces of the vessels are dissected.
- The aorta is dissected by creating a 'window' between it and the inferior vena cava in two locations; cranially to the left renal artery and caudally just proximal to the aortic bifurcation.
- The ureter is dissected off the periureteral fat in the site of planned transection.

The rat is kept warm and the kidney is periodically irrigated with warm normal saline.

II. PREPARATION OF THE RECIPIENT

A. Positioning

B. Preparation of the surgical field

C. Microsurgical dissection of the renal fascia, renal vessels, and ureter

A, B, C as in the donor, except for dissection of the aorta.

III. GRAFT HARVERSTIG (DONOR)

A. Flushing of the kidney

- Ligation of the aorta cranial to the origin of the left renal artery (5/0 suture).
- Ligation of the aorta cranial to its bifurcation (5/0 suture).
- Ligation of the renal vein (9/0 suture) close to its exit into the inferior vena cava and transection just distal to the ligation.
- **Cold solution** of **heparin in normal saline (25.000 IU/ml) is injected into the aorta, below the origin of the left renal artery,** until the kidney obtains a whitish color.

B. Graft harvesting

- Placement of the renal vessels in the lateral arm of the double clamp, close to the renal hilum.

Synopsis... of orthotopic transplantation of the left kidney

- Ligation (9/0 suture) and transection of the renal artery near its origin from the aorta.
- Ligation (5/0 suture) and transection of the ureter.
- The graft is removed and kept in gauze soaked in cold heparin solution.
- After harvest of the graft, the aorta ligations (or clamps) are removed.

IV. GRAFT IMPLANTATION (RECIPIENT)

Placement of the graft adjacent to the left kidney of the recipient

A. Removal of the recipient's kidney – Placement of the stumps of its vessels in the free clamp

- Placement of the recipient's renal vessels in the free arm of the double clamp, close to the origin of the renal artery.
- Transection of the recipient's renal vessels just proximal to the artery bifurcation.
- Transection of the recipient's ureter and cleaning of periureteral fat from the end of the s-tump.
- Removal of the recipient's kidney and placement of the graft in its bed.

B. Preparation of the vessels

- Irrigation of recipient and donor the vessel lumens and removal of the adventitia. Approximation of the clamps.

C. End-to-end anastomoses

1. Renal vessels

ATTENTION: **Duration of occlusion of the graft vessels should not surpass 30 minutes**

Anastomoses with placement of **8 sutures 11/0** in the artery and **10 to 12 sutures 10/0** in the vein.

1. The anterior surfaces of both vessels are sutured first.
2. The double clamp is rotated and correct placement of anterior sutures is checked.
3. The posterior surfaces of the anastomoses are completed.
4. Vessels are released from the double clamp.
5. A wet gauze is placed over the anstomoses for 3 minutes.
6. Patency test (separate tests for each vessel).
7. Withdrawal of the yellow plastic background.

2. Ureter

1. Placement of a yellow plastic background under the ureter.
2. Anastomosis of the ureter with **4 sutures 11/0, without using double vascular clamp.**
3. Patency (and leak) test with injection of methylene blue into the renal parenchyma.
4. Withdrawal of the yellow plastic background.

5. CLOSURE OF THE SURGICAL TRAUMAS

In recipient and donor, repositioning the splanchna into the abdomen and suturing of the abdominal wall in 2 layers with 2/0 sutures, continuous in the muscles, interrupted in the skin.

28

Heterotopic (Auto)transplantation of the left kidney

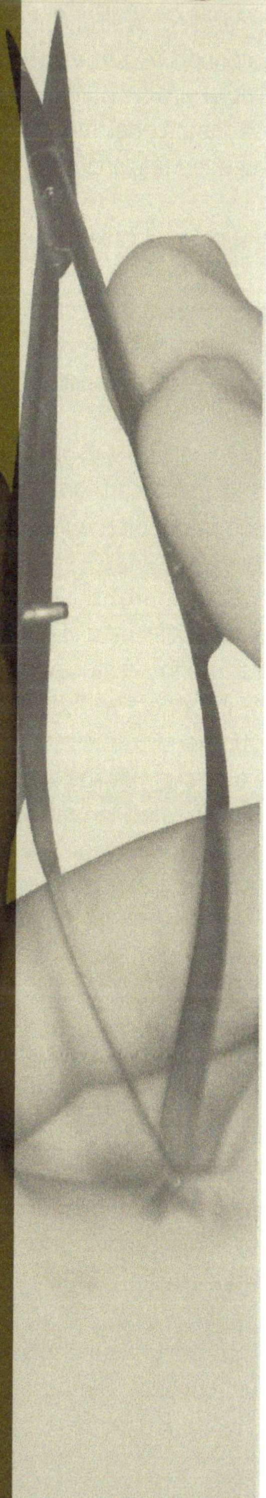

Prior to attempting the heterotopic kidney transplantation the reader must have performed the orthotopic in situ autotranspalation (Chapter 26) and the orthotopic transplantation (Chapter 27)

Heterotopic transplantation of the kidney described in this Chapter relies on anastomoses of the renal vessels to the aorta and inferior vena cava or to the common iliac vessels, which are performed end-to-side. Therefore, the reader is referred to Chapter 6 for details of the technique.

The heterotopic kidney transplantation with anastomoses to the aorta/inferior vena cava or to the common iliac vessels may be an auto-transplantation or transplantation from a donor. For your practice, start with auto-transplantation, which is more simple with regard to dissection and shorter in duration (there is no transfer of graft from the donor), taking into consideration that **there is always the time restriction of 30 minutes from the moment of vessel occlusion of the donor kidney up to completion of anastomoses.**

In the heterotopic auto-transplantations described in this Chapter, preparation of the surgical field and microsurgical dissection of the renal fascia, renal vessels and ureter are similar to those described in Chapter 26. Then, microsurgical dissection is extended in the areas of the aorta/inferior vena cava or in the common iliac vessels, where the anastomoses with graft vessels will be performed. In the heterotopic transplantation from a donor, the kidney will be received from another rat as described in Chapter 27.

The heterotopic transplantations described hereafter are performed as autotransplantations; therefore, dissection and anastomosis of the ureter is not performed. In case that these operations are heterotopic transplantations from a donor, it is evident that the ureter has to be dissected and anastomosed as described in Chapter 27.

I. Transplantation with anastomoses in the aorta - Inferior vena cava

For the sections A-C that follow, the reader is referred to the respective sections of Chapter 26. Here, to avoid repetition, only a short summary is given.

A. Positioning of the rat

The rat is placed in dorsal decubitus (supine) position with the head on the surgeon's left. The limbs of the rat are immobilized on the working surface with adhesive tape.

B. Preparation of the surgical field

A median incision is performed from the xiphoid process to the pubic symphysis. The intestines are enveloped in a gauze moistened with warm normal saline and placed outside of the abdomen contralateral to the side of transplantation. The retroperitoneal space is entered via blunt dissection with two gauzes moistened in warm normal saline. The so-created surgical field is wide, extending from the kidney to the aortic bifurcation. Placement of retractors must be designed to offer a spacious view of the surgical field. It is recommended to place at least two retractors on the left border of the incised abdominal wall and one or two retractors on the right border.

C. Microsurgical dissection of the renal fascia, renal vessels and ureter

The kidney is cleaned off the renal fascia and perirenal fat up to the hilum, where dissection of the renal fascia is combined with dissection of the renal vessels. The latter have to be cleaned from the perirenal fat through their entire length, the artery from its origin from the aorta, the vein up to its confluence with the inferior vena cava. The ureter, as said above, is not dissected off the periureiteral fat in the heterotopic autotransplantation of the kidney; however, it is necessary to mobilize the ureter from the retroperitoneum, so that it can follow the kidney in its new position. In the heterotopic transplantation from a donor, the edge of the ureter stamp of the donor must be cleaned of the periureteral fat to be prepared for a clean anastomosis with the recipient ureteral stamp.

D. Microsurgical dissection of the aorta and inferior vena cava

The aorta and the inferior vena cava must be meticulously dissected. Time 'lost' here will lead to enormous gain of time during anastomoses.

a. Microsurgical dissection of the aorta

The reader is referred to Chapter 8.C.

b. Microsurgical dissection of the inferior vena cava

Microsurgical dissection of the inferior vena cava has been presented in Chapter 16.D, but only for the region between renal veins. In the heterotopic kidney transplantation, a wide dissection of the inferior vena cava is required.

After the aorta is fully dissected, the inferior vena cava will be dissected in the area between the left renal vein and the confluence of common iliac veins.

The dissection of the inferior vena cava is extremely dangerous and needs much attention:

- The inferior vena cava can be handled by lifting it from a residue of adventitia or connective tissue that will be left attached on the vessel wall on purpose (this will be removed latter). Use the broader microsurgical forceps Dumont No. 3 or even fine anatomical forceps.
- Avoid in any case lifting the inferior vena cava from the wall per se.
- For lateral movement, push the inferior vena cava with the closed tip of blunt microsurgical scissors or curved forceps; the convex surface of the instrument should touch the vein wall.
- The lumbar veins are better off ligated (9/0) and transected rather than cauterized, because there is the risk of thermal transport and injury of the vein wall (the diathermy is monopolar).

After this general advice, the dissection of the inferior vena cava will be presented in detail. The dissection comprises mobilization of the inferior vena cava, meticulous dissection of the areolar connective tissue and fat off the vein wall, and ligation and transection of the lumbar tributary veins. The dissection of the anterior surface of the vena cava is performed in continuation of the dissection of the aorta, after opening a window in the areolar connective tissue between the two vessels. Take care to leave a residue of adventitia on the anterior wall of the inferior vena cava for handling it. Mobilization of the lateral and posterior surfaces of the inferior vena cava requires the transection between two ligations of the lumbar veins, which join posterolaterally with the inferior vena cava. The dissection of the lumbar veins is not simple and differs between sides (left and right). In both sides, remember that–as for all veins–the peripheral (distal) ligation is placed before the central (proximal) ligation in order to avoid entrapment of blood between the two ligations.

On the left side, ligation of the cranial (superior) left lumbar veins is more difficult because they are covered by the aorta, which, below the left renal vein

Figure 28-1

Dissection of the inferior vena cava, ligation and transection of a superior (cramial) left lumbar vein. **A.** The needle holder has just released the 9/0 suture, and now is used to push with the convex surface of its tip the aorta and inferior vena cava to the right, simultaneously rotating medially the inferior vena cava. The microsurgical forceps Dumont No. 3 has grasped the needle of the suture. **B.** Descending of the knot of the peripheral suture on the lumbar vein, while the assistant moves the aorta medially, and also the inferior vena (with medial rotation), using the convex surface of a curved microsurgical forceps. **C.** After the central ligation has been placed, the lumbar vein is pulled by the peripheral (distal) suture, which has been left long, and is transected with microsurgical scissors. (From author's photo library)

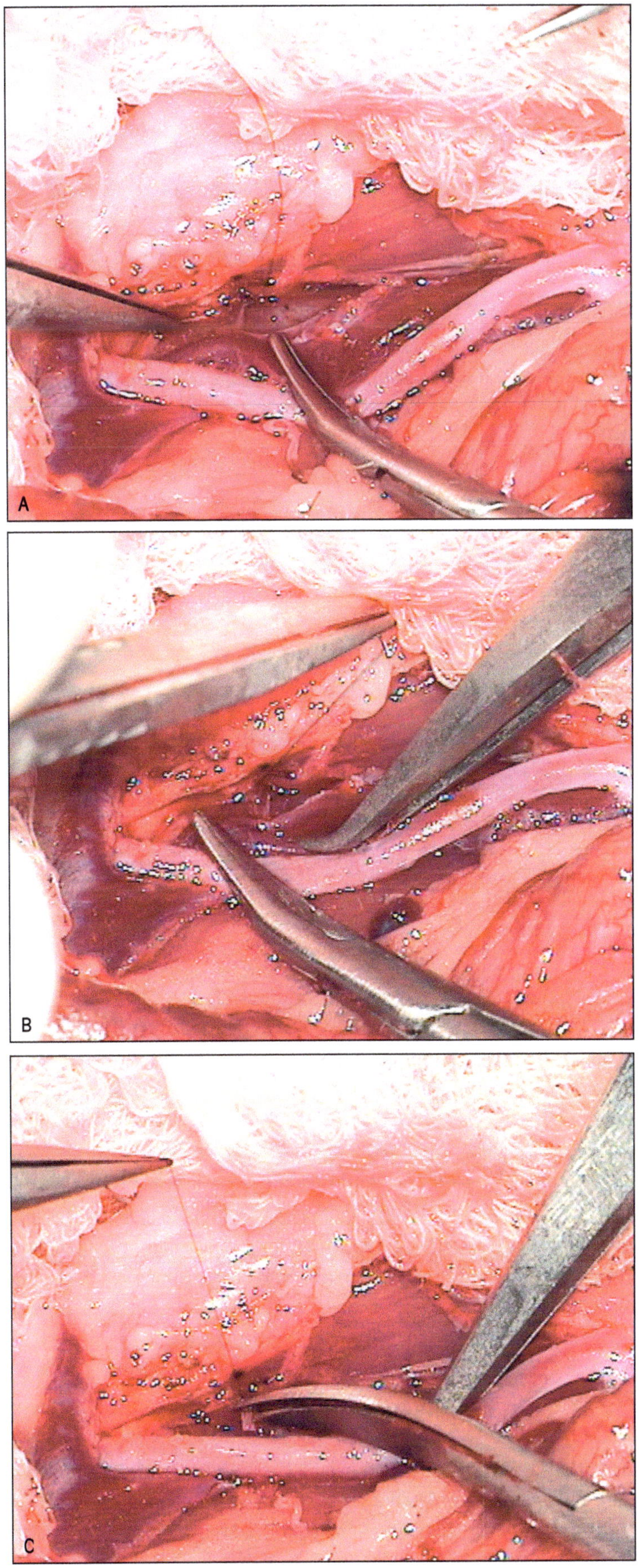

is in front and mostly on the left of the inferior vena cava. In order to expose and dissect the superior left lumbar tributaries, it is necessary to move the aorta to the right side, and to push the inferior vena cava also to the right while rotating it medially (**Fig. 28-1A**). While to lift the inferior vena cava from a residue of the adventitia has a relatively low risk for rupture, to rotate the inferior vena cava by pulling it from the adventitia is more hazardous. It is advised to push and slightly ro-

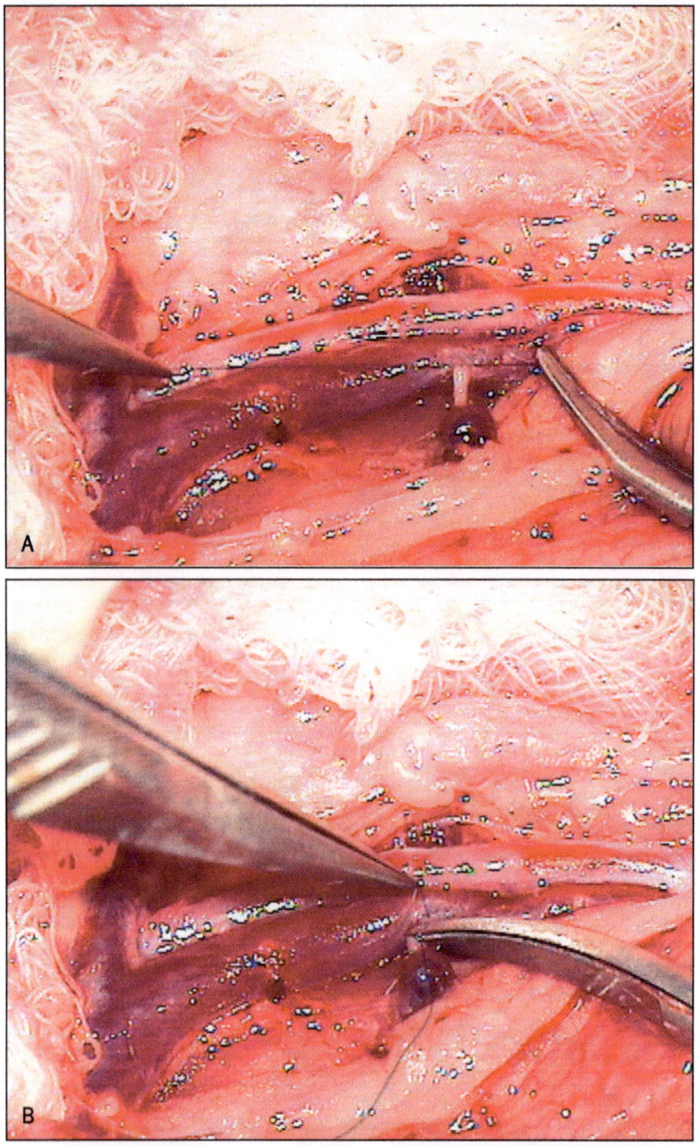

Figure 28-2

Dissection of the inferior vena cava: double ligation and transection of a right lumbar tributary vein. **A.** Placement of the 2nd simple knot in the central (proximal) ligation of the lumbar vein. Observe the distension of the vein lateral to the distal ligation of the vein (which has been placed prior to the central ligation). **B.** Transection of the lumbar vein. The vein is lifted with Dumont No. 3 forceps from the suture of the central ligation that has been left on purpose long, and is transected with the microsurgical scissors brought perpendicular to the vein. (From author's photo library)

tate the inferior vena cava with the convex surface of the tip of the needle holder or curved forceps in order to adequately expose a superior left lumbar vein and obtain enough space to place the two ligations (**Fig. 28-1A, B**). Then, by leaving long the suture of the lateral ligation, and using it as a stay-suture to lift the vein, the latter can be easily transected between the ligations (**Fig. 28-1C**).

On the right side, the lumbar veins are directly visible and can be dissected, ligated and transected without much difficulty (**Fig. 28-2**).

The complete dissection and ligation of the right lumbar veins allows the mobilization of the posterior surface of the inferior vena cava, which permits a different exposure of the remaining lower left lumbar veins: the freed inferior vena cava can be transferred to the left of the aorta pulled from a residue of the adventitia or from the suture of the peripheral ligation of a lower left lumbar vein; this maneuver makes comfortable the placement of the central ligation and transection of the left lower lumbar vein between the ligations (**Fig. 28-3**).

After transection of the right lumbar veins, the inferior vena cava is freed from the right side; thus an alternative access to a superior left lumbar vein is offered from the right side, posterior to the inferior vena

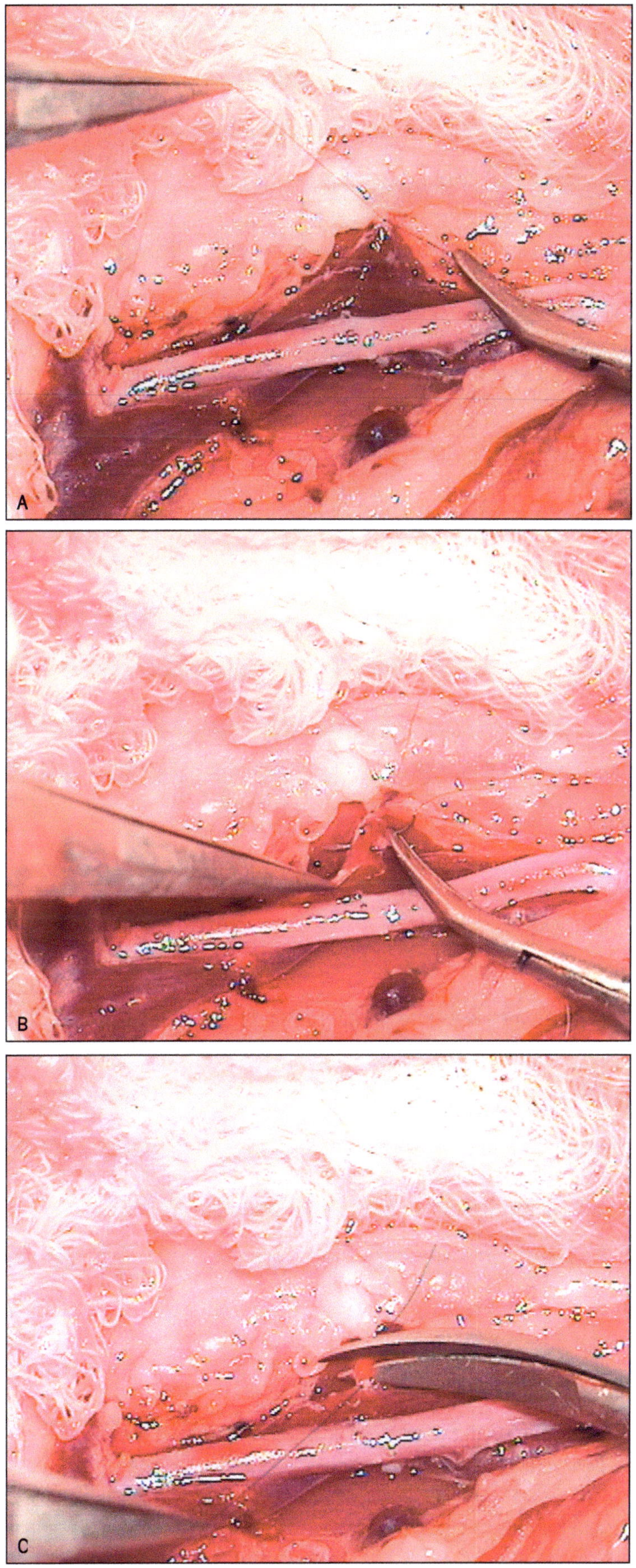

Figure 28-3

Double ligation and transection of a lower left lumbar vein. After transection of the right lumbar veins and mobilization of the posterior surface, the freed inferior vena cava is pulled to the left by the peripheral ligation placed on the lower left lumbar vein. **A.** Placement of the peripheral suture in the left lumbar vein. **B.** Placement of the central suture: the needle guided by the needle holder passes under the vein, while the vein is lifted with Dumont No. 5 forceps from a residue of the adventitia. **C.** The vein is lifted from the central suture, left long, while the scissors are brought perpendicular to the vein, ready to transect it. (From author's photo library)

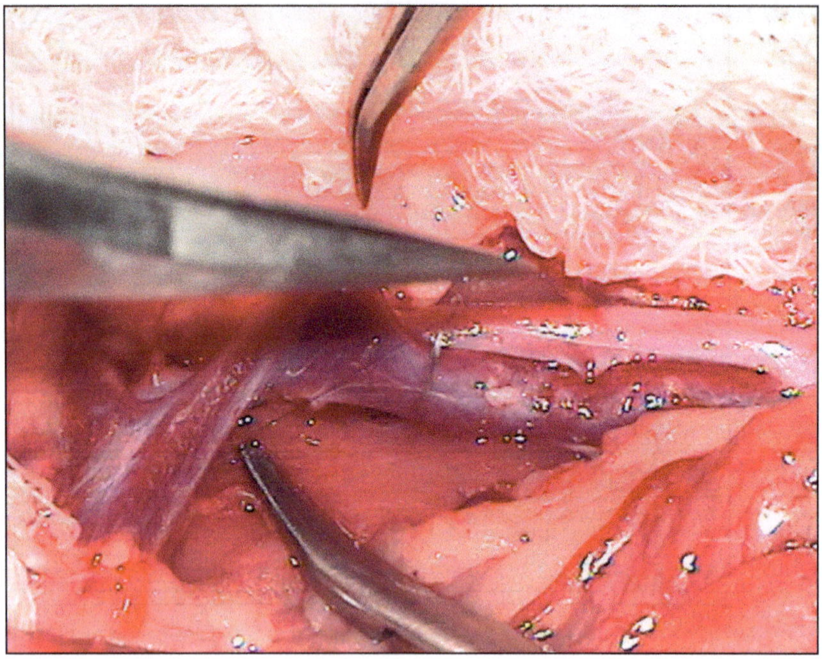

Figure 28-4

Ligation of a superior left lumbar vein with access from the right side, posterior to the inferior vena cava. Previously, the right lumbar veins have been transected and the posterior surface of the inferior vena cava has been mobilized. The curved microsurgical forceps lifts the inferior vena cava (from a residue of the adventitia, not seen here because is hidden behind the straight microsurgical forceps), while the Dumont No. 3 forceps and the needle holder place the 1st simple knot. (From author's photo library)

cava (**Fig. 28-4**). This access may be chosen if you encounter difficulties in moving the aorta to the right and rotating the inferior vena cava medially as in **Figure 28-1**. However, as can be seen in **Figure 28-4**, the access from the right side is endowed with a much greater risk of rupture of the inferior vena cava as the vessel is lifted and rotated to a greater degree than in the access from the left side

➢ All the above directions aim to avoid trauma of the inferior vena resulting in massive—and probably fatal—hemorrhage. If this happens: occlude IMMEDIATELY the blood flow with two single vascular clamps, wash and aspirate the surgical field, and suture the vein (10/0, continuous suturing). The sutured area is not suitable for the end-to-side anastomoses that will follow, therefore extend the dissection of the inferior vena cava.

E. Preparation of the recipient vessels

- **Occlusion of the aorta & inferior vena cava with the double clamp**

The vessels are placed together in the jaws of the double clamp. The aorta, located in front and to the left of the inferior vena cava, is moved to the left (of the rat), while the inferior vena cava remains to the right. A yellow plastic background is placed under the vessels (**Fig. 28-5**).

- **Arteriotomy – Venotomy – Irrigation**

A small transverse incision is made in the aorta and the inferior vena cava. Each vessel is lifted with Dumont No. 3 forceps and microsurgical scissors are used (the technique is described in detail in Chapter 6).

➢ It is advised to make the venotomy a bit more caudal to the arteriotomy. The small distance between them will allow the subsequent end-to-side anastomoses to be performed comfortably.

Then, the vessel lumens are irrigated with warm normal saline (**Fig. 28-6**). The adventitia is removed from the perimeter of the transverse openings.

F. Graft harvesting

- Ligation of the renal artery (9/0 suture) at its origin from the aorta.
- Ligation of the renal vein (9/0 suture) at its exit into the inferior vena cava.

These ligations are placed very close to the great vessels.

- Placement of the renal vessels in a single vascular clamp.

The single clamp is placed as peripherally as possible,

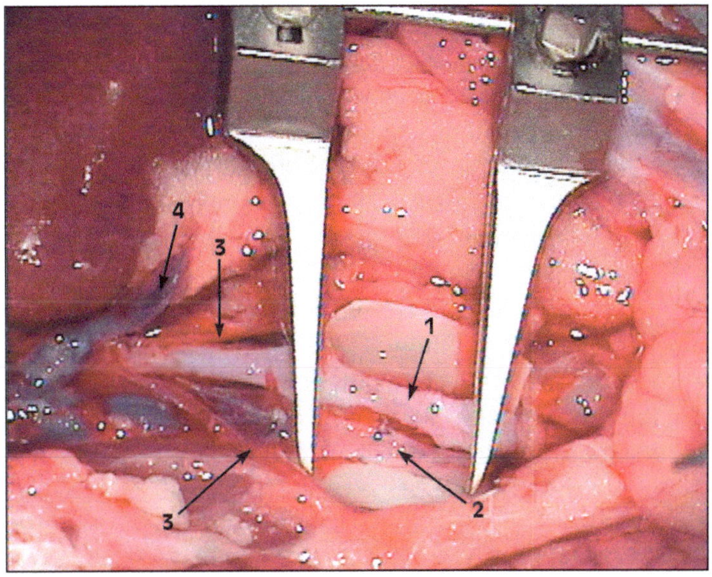

Figure 28-5

The aorta and the inferior vena cava are placed in the double clamp. The aorta is positioned on the left. **1.** aorta, **2.** inferior vena cava, **3.** gonadal arteries, **4.** left renal vein. (From author's photo library)

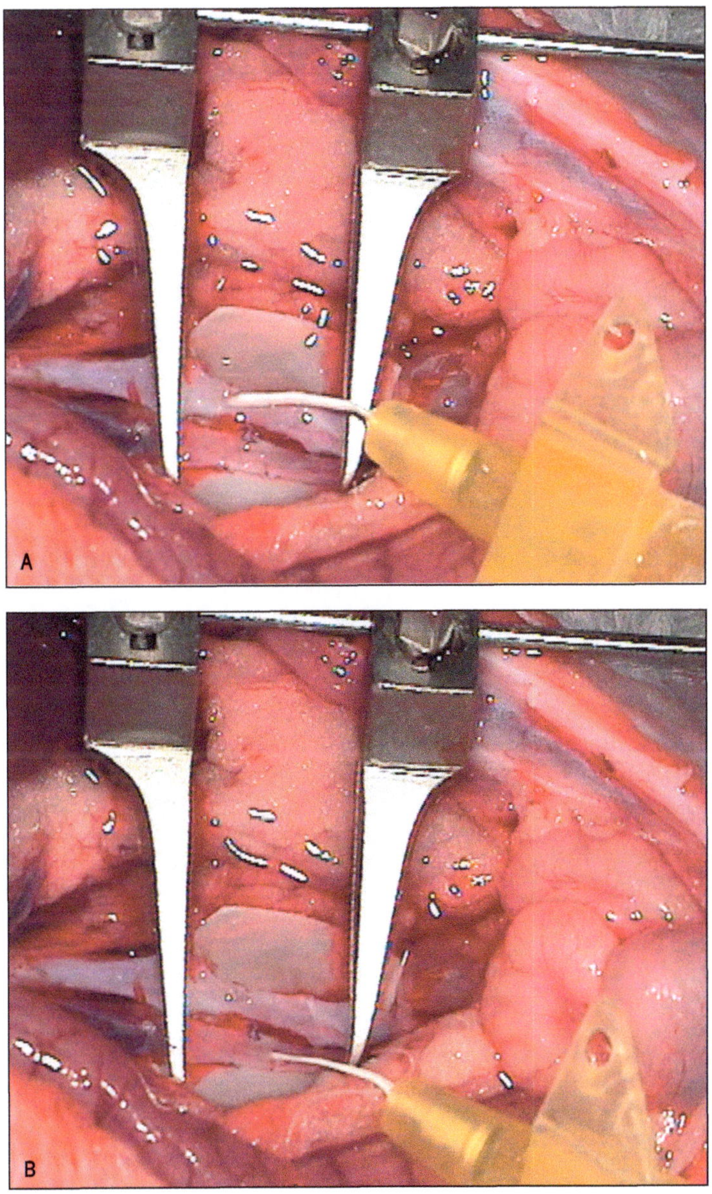

Figure 28-6

Irrigation of the lumen by injecting warm normal saline through a 27G angiocath in the aorta **(A)** and inferior vena cava **(B)**. (From author's photo library) toward the hilum of the kidney. The site of placement of the clamp is usually indicated by the bifurcation of the renal artery, which should be left peripheral to the point of occlusion, so that finally we should have one artery for anastomosis and not two. The aim is to have enough length of renal artery and vein that will allow rotation of the clamp in the subsequent end-to-side anastomoses.

- Transection of the renal vessels, each close to the ligation (**Fig. 28-7**).
- Irrigation of the stumps of the renal vessels with warm normal saline.
- Folding back of the adventitia (in the artery) or removal of the adventitia (in the vein).

G. Graft implantation

The graft is transferred caudally—together with the single clamp—parallel to its initial position, and is placed in the surgical field so that the stumps of the renal vessels will be brought perpendicular to the aorta and the inferior vena cava, at the height of the transverse incisions. The ends of the stumps of the renal vessels are positioned close to the openings of the aorta and inferior vena cava, so that the anastomoses will be comfortably performed.

End-to-side anastomoses

The reader is referred to Chapter 6.6.1, for a detailed description of the technique of the end-to-side anastomoses with rotation of the clamp.

The following number of sutures are placed in each vessel

- **Anastomosis renal artery-aorta: 8 sutures 11/0**
- **Anastomosis renal vein-inferior vena cava: 10 or 12 sutures 10/0**

In these end-to-side anastomoses the graft and the single clamp can be rotated.

➤ **Effective is the time restriction of 30 minutes from the moment of occlusion of the vessels of the kidney**

It is recommended to place first the corner sutures in both vessels, (first the two corner sutures in one vessel and then in the other) in order to stabilize them in place.

The steps of the end-to-side anastomoses of the renal vessels with the big vessels are the following:

1. The anastomosis of the renal artery stump of the graft with the aorta starts with suturing the anterior surface (**Fig. 28-8**). Since the 2 corner sutures are placed first, for a total of 8 sutures, there are 3 remaining for each surface: the first placed is the one

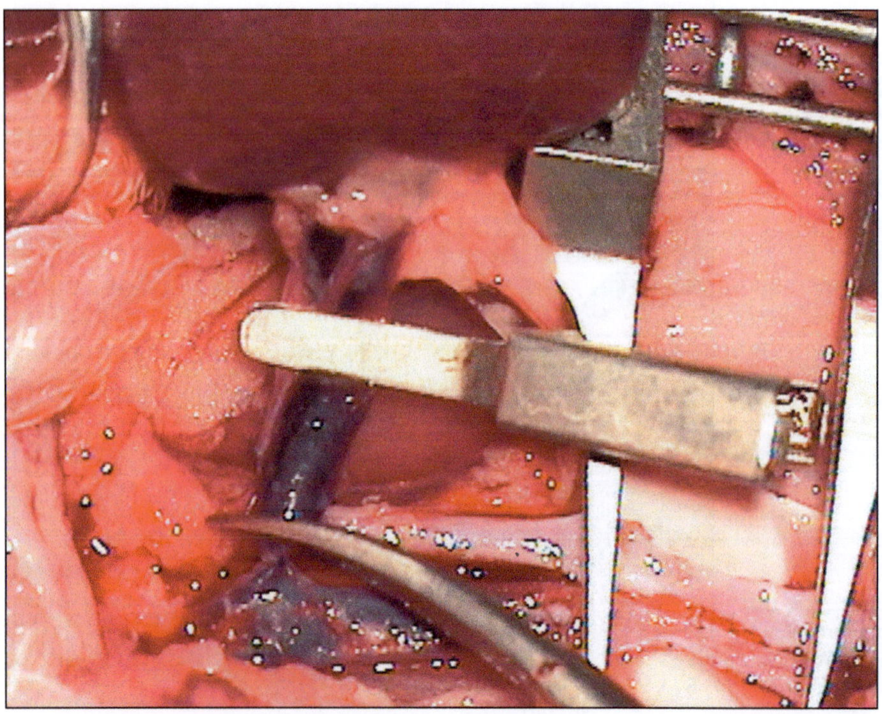

Figure 28-7

Harvesting the graft – Transection of the renal vein. The renal artery and the renal vein have been ligated very close to the aorta and the inferior vena cava respectively. The single clamp occludes the renal vessels peripherally, leaving enough length for each until the point of transection. Observe that here the bifurcation of the renal artery is placed in the single clamp in order to obtain length for the artery. The scissors are ready to transect the renal vein. More caudally, the aorta and inferior vena cava have been placed in the double clamp and have been prepared to be anastomosed end-to-side with the renal vessels. (From author's photo library)

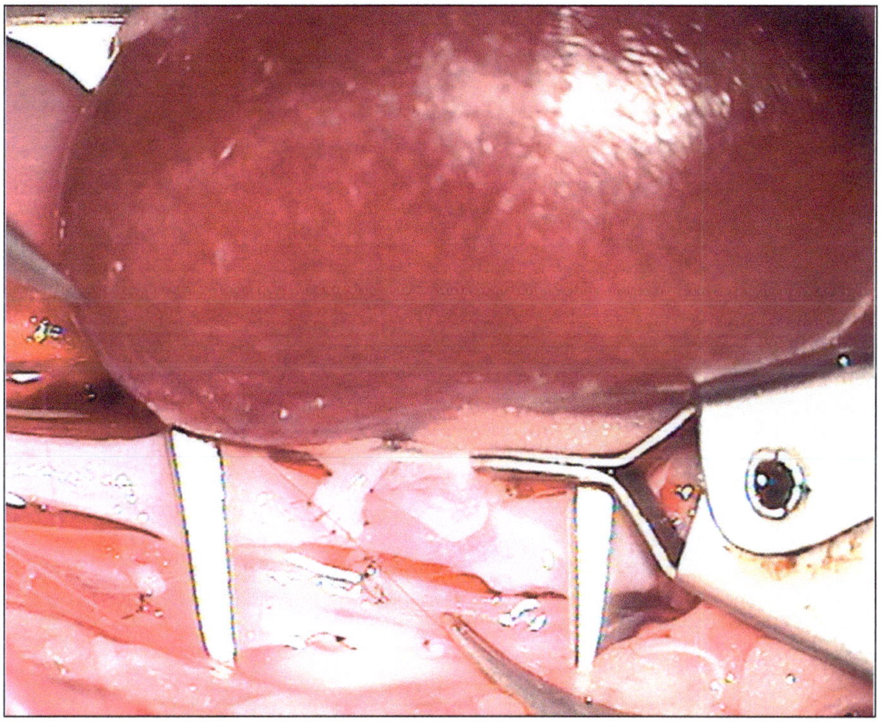

Figure 28-8

Placement of the 5th and last suture (11/0) in the middle of the 2nd cranial quadrant of the anterior surface of the anastomosis of the renal artery with the aorta. (From author's photo library)

in the middle of the semicircle, and then one in the middle of each quadrant on either side.

Similarly, in the anastomosis of the renal vein stump with the inferior vena cava, the anterior surface is sutured first. Again, the two corner sutures are placed first. Then, for a total of 10 or 12 sutures, there are 4 or 5 remaining sutures left for each surface, respectively. If 4, they are placed in symmetrical pairs, at equal distances, from lateral toward the middle of the semicircle. For 5 sutures: first the middle one is placed and then 2 in each quadrant, at equal distances from the middle and corner sutures.

In **Figure 28-9**, the completed sutures of the ante-

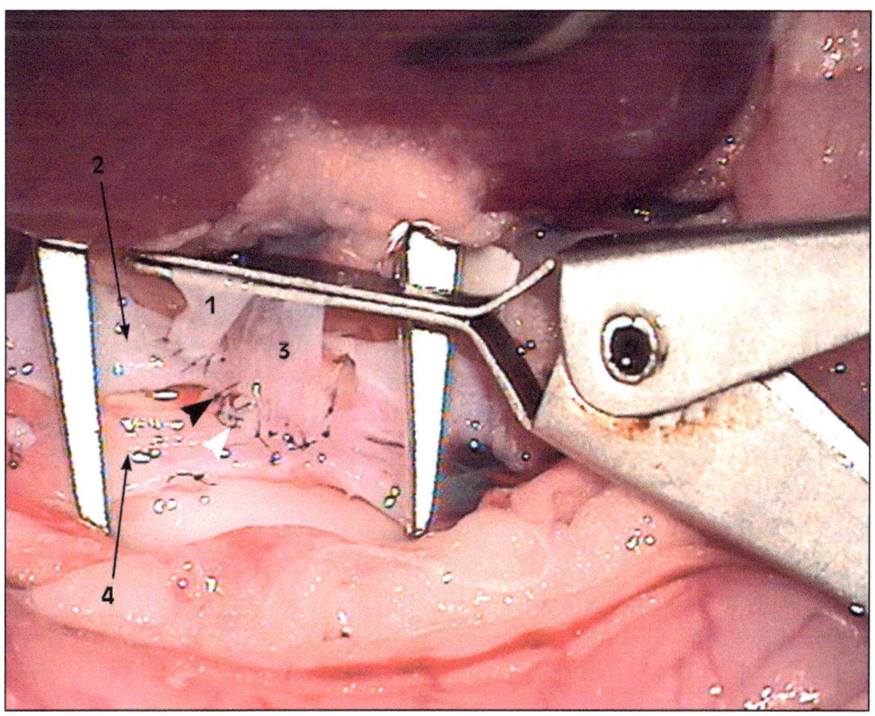

Figure 28-9

Completed sutures of the anterior surfaces of the anastomoses of the renal vessels. In the anterior surface of the renal vein, 6 sutures have been placed (12 in total, see also Figure 28-10). Because a greater than expected number of sutures is seen in the vein anastomosis, it is clarified that the suture annotated with black arrowhead belongs to ligation of a lumbar tributary vein, while the two sutures pointed by the white arrowhead belong to double ligation of the inferior adrenal vein, the stump of which lies on the anastomosis. **1.** renal artery, **2.** aorta, **3.** renal vein, **4.** inferior vena cava. (From author's photo library)

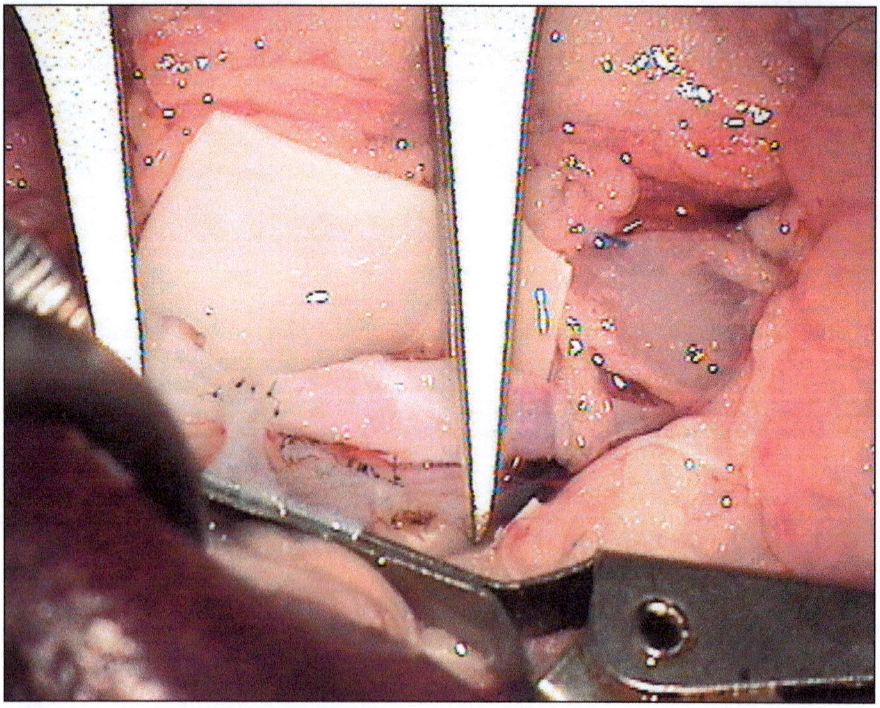

Figure 28-10

The kidney and the single clamp holding the renal vessels have been rotated medially and suturing of the posterior surfaces of the anastomoses has been completed. In this figure, the arterial anastomosis is found above and the venous anastomosis is below. (From author's photo library)

rior surfaces of the renal artery and vein can be seen.

2. The graft is rotated together with the single clamp and the correct placement of the sutures of the anterior surfaces is checked.
3. The posterior surfaces of the anastomoses are completed (**Fig. 28-10**).
4. The single and the double clamps are released and removed (first the single and then the double clamp).
5. Placement of a wet gauze on the anastomoses for 3 minutes.
6. Patency test, separately for each vessel. The patency test is performed as described in Chapter 6.9.1 (**Fig. 6-9A**) for the renal artery, and 6.9.2 (**Fig. 6-9B**) for the renal vein..

   A simple test is shown in **Figure 28-11**: after occlusion of the inferior vena cava with a single clamp caudal to the anastomosis, the inferior vena cava is filled cranial to the clamp, indicating patency of the anastomosis with the renal vein. This testing is not reliable, because the inferior vena cava may be filled retrogradely (from cranial), resulting in a false positive result. Therefore, this test is just an indication of patency of the vein anastomosis and cannot replace the classic patency test.
7. Withdrawal of the yellow plastic background.

H. Closure of the surgical trauma

The splanchna are returned to the abdomen and the abdominal wall is closed in two layers with non-absorbable sutures 2/0, the muscles with continuous suturing, and then the subcutaneous and skin with interrupted sutures.

II. Transplantation with Anastomoses in the Common Iliac Vessels

For the following sections A,B,C, the reader is referred to the respective sections of part I.

A. **Position of the rat**

B. **Preparation of the surgical field**

C. **Microsurgical dissection of the renal fascia, renal vessels and ureter**

D. Microsurgical preparation of the common iliac vessels

Surgical anatomy of the common iliac vessels is presented first in Chapter 15.D and in detail in Chapter 29.C.1.

The microsurgical dissection of the common iliac vessels can either be the caudal continuation of the dissection

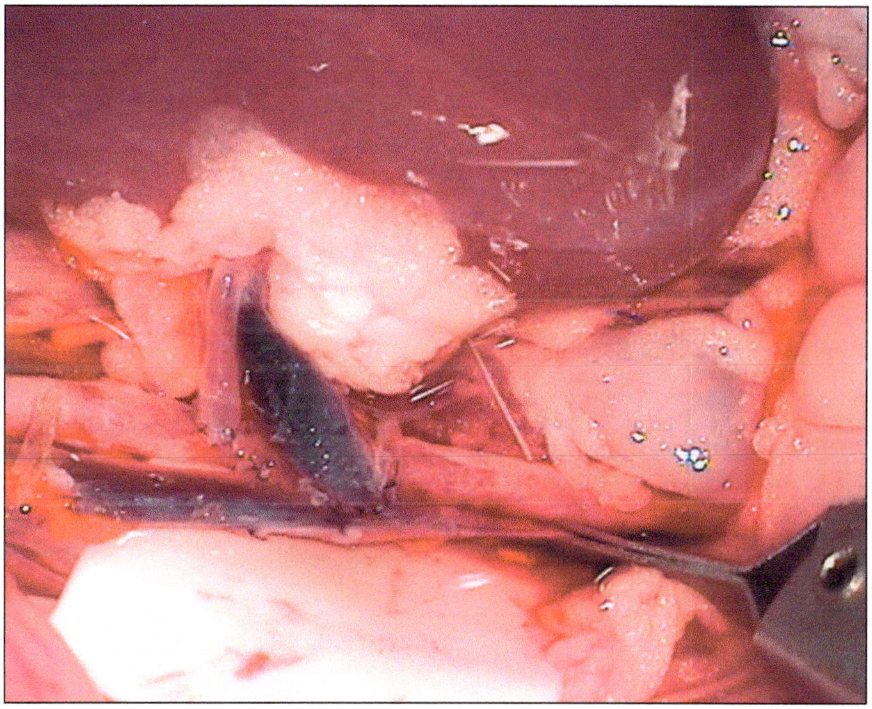

Figure 28-11

A simple test, indicative of patency of the renal vein anastomosis. The inferior vena cava is occluded with a single clamp caudal to the anastomosis, and seems to fill in cranial to the occlusion, supplied by the renal vein. This test does not replace the classic patency test for end-to-side anastomoses (see Chapter 6.9.1). (From author's photo library)

of the aorta and inferior vena cava, or the dissection may start and be restricted to the common iliac vessels. Hereafter, both techniques are presented and discussed so that the surgeon makes his/her choice, but we strongly advise the trainee to start the dissection from the aorta and inferior vena.

1. Dissection of the common iliac vessels in continuation of the dissection of the aorta and inferior vena cava

Dissection of the common iliac vessels starts as a dissection of the caudal part of the aorta and inferior vena cava (**Fig. 28-12**) and is continued caudally to the com-

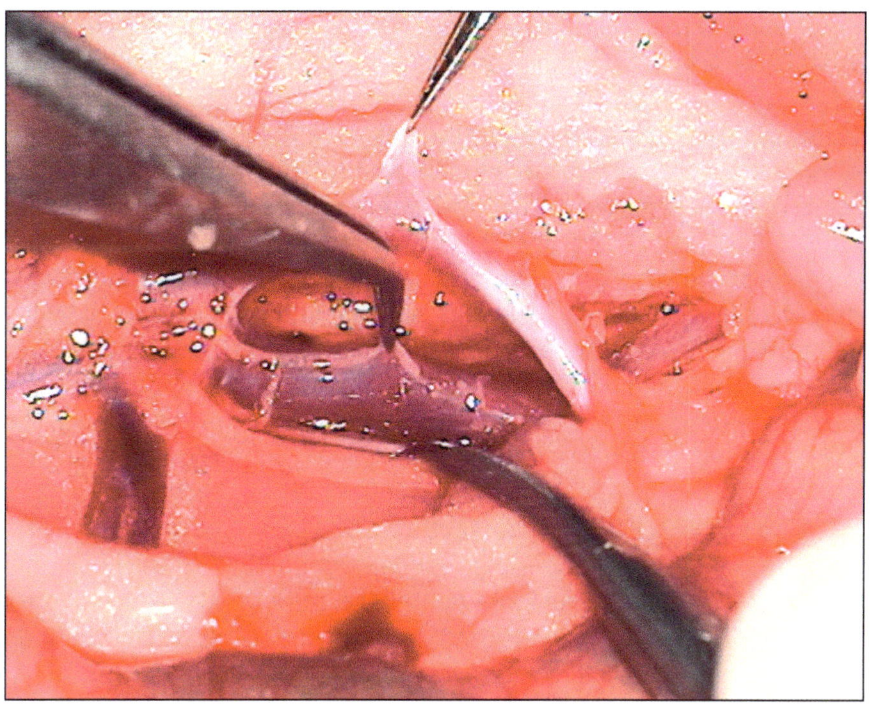

Figure 28-12

Dissection of the common iliac vessels starts as dissection of the aorta cranial to the bifurcation, and of the inferior vena cava cranial to the confluence of common iliac veins. The aorta is lifted from the adventitia with straight forceps and the inferior vena cava with curved forceps, while the microsurgical scissors dissect the posterior surface of the inferior vena cava. (From author's photo library)

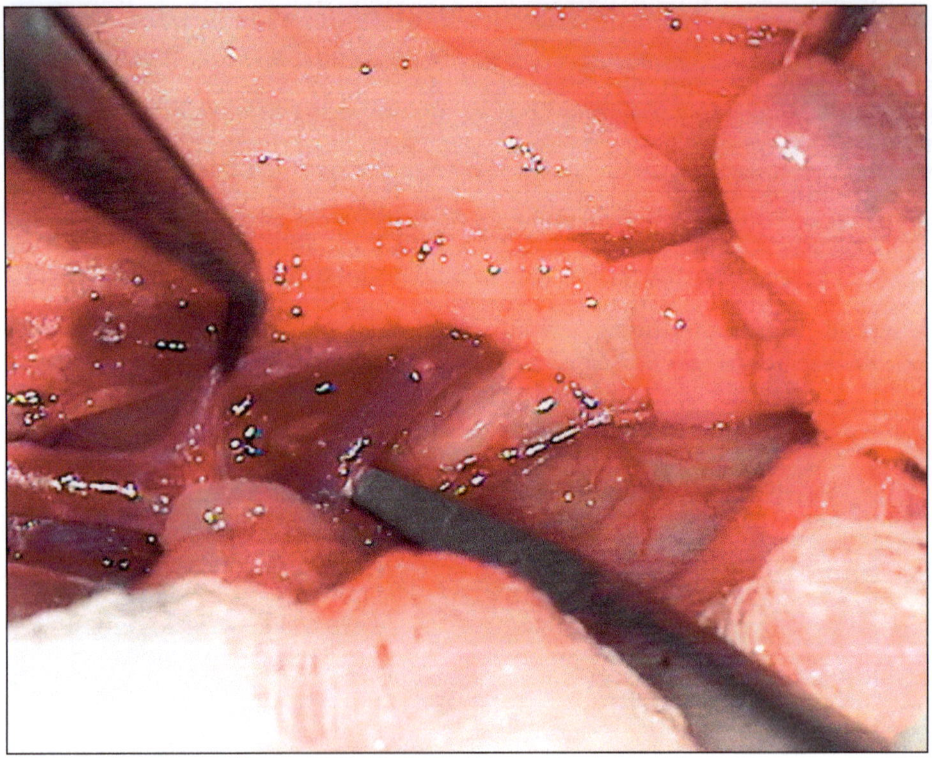

Figure 28-13

Dissection of the left common iliac vessels. The forceps lifts the common iliac artery, which has been fully dissected and mobilized. The common iliac vein has been dissected in the anterior surface. The blunt microsurgical scissors enter closed behind the common iliac vein in order to detach it so that the vein will be able to be lifted and the posterior surface dissected. (From author's photo library)

mon iliac artery and vein of the chosen side, here on the left (**Fig. 28-13**).

For dissection of the caudal part of the aorta, the lower lumbar arteries are cauterized or ligated and transected, and a window is opened between the aorta and inferior vena cava. During dissection of the aortic bifurcation the *middle sacral artery* will be met (discussed in Chapter 15.D see **Figure 15-1**). By lifting up the aorta bifurcation, the middle sacral artery is exposed and can be transected after cauterization, or more securely, as it goes deep, after double ligation. The dissection will continue peripherally in the left common iliac artery. Dissection of the latter comprises mobilization of the artery, detachment from the homonymous vein found deep to the artery, and transection after cauterization of the small posterior parietal branches. *The first big division of the common iliac artery is the origin of the internal iliac artery.*

The dissection of the inferior vena cava will be performed as described above (see above, section I.D.b), and will continue with dissection of the confluence of the common iliac veins and then with the left common iliac vein. In the posterior surface of the confluence of the common iliac veins, when lifting up the inferior vena cava, the middle sacral vein will be found. This vein has to be double ligated before transection.

- Do not even think to use diathermy on the middle sacral vein, because it is connected with the sacral vein plexus, and if the plexus bleeds it is difficult to stop the hemorrhage. In microsurgery of the rat there are no wax and pins (for the old school) or hemostatic gauzes (for the new school) as in human surgery!

The dissection of the common iliac vein comprises ligation and transection of the small posterior parietal tributaries, if encountered. Note that the small arterial posterior parietal branches are not necessarily accompanied by venous counterparts. The first 'big division' of the common iliac vein is the confluence of the internal iliac vein. This confluence is found deep and more caudal to the 'big division' of the common iliac artery, i.e. the internal iliac artery.

Remember

- The end of the dissection for the common iliac artery and vein is dictated by the first big division of the artery.

The dissection of the common iliac vessels in continuation of the dissection of the aorta and inferior vena cava offers a wide surgical field in which are adequately exposed and comfortably transected (after ligation or cauterization, accordingly) the middle sacral artery and vein and the small posterior parietal arterial branches (sometimes accompanied by respective tributary veins).

2. Dissection of the common iliac vessels only

Another strategy often described is to dissect only the common iliac vessels, from the aorta bifurcation and the confluence of the common iliac vessels until the first big division of the common iliac artery. Without implicating the middle sacral vessels, the common iliac artery will be freed from the homonymous vein, the posterior parietal branches will be dissected and cauterized, and similarly for the common iliac vein (if posterior tributaries are found).

The above tactic surely requires more experience, has risks and, to our opinion, has disadvantages for the beginner:

- The space yielded from dissection solely of the common iliac vessels should be adequate to have the clamps of the double clamp at a proper distance, otherwise you will have to work with end-to-side anastomoses found too close to each other and you will have restricted freedom in your movements.
- During access to the posterior branches/tributaries, internal and external rotation of the common iliac vessels is not allowed because their movements are restricted centrally by the middle sacral vessels and peripherally (downstream) by other branches of the common iliac vessels (see Chapter 29.C.I).
- Most importantly, the middle sacral vessels are jeopardized because of the manipulation of the common iliac vessels. The tension created by lifting the common iliac vessels and dissecting their branches/ tributaries is transferred to the middle sacral artery and vein. The vein can easily rupture with an abrupt accidental movement (the consequences were mentioned above).

After the dissection of the iliac vessels has been completed, a yellow plastic background is placed under the vessels (**Fig. 28-14**).

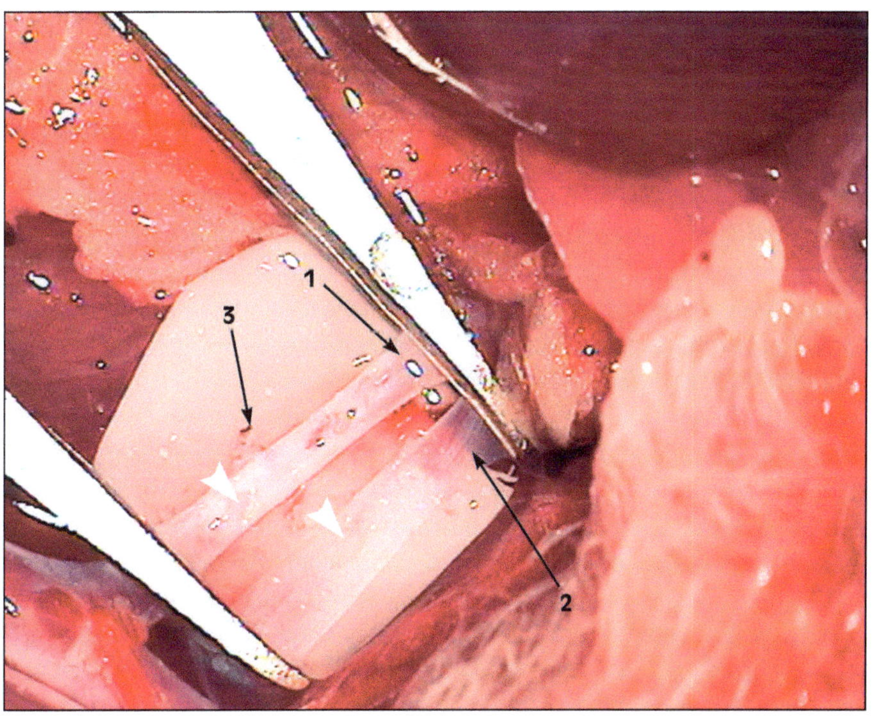

Figure 28-14

Dissected left common iliac vessels, placed in the double clamp. The artery has been placed laterally, the vein is left medially. Observe the distance between the transverse incisions of the arteriotomy and venotomy (white arrowheads), so that the end-to-side anastomoses that follow will not overlap (see Figure 28-15). **1.** left common iliac artery, **2.** left common iliac vein, **3.** cauterized parietal branch of the artery. (From author's photo library)

E. Preparation of the recipient vessels

- **Occlusion of the common iliac vessels with the double clamp**

The common iliac vessels are placed together in the jaws of the clamps. The artery, found superficial to the vein in normal position, is moved laterally, while the vein stays in place and is placed medially in the clamp (**Fig. 28-14**).

- **Arteriotomy – Venotomy – Irrigation**

A transverse incision is opened in both the common iliac artery and vein, leaving a small distance between the two that will facilitate the subsequent end-to-side anastomoses (**Fig. 28-14**). If this distance is not allowed and the two transverse incisions are aligned, evidently the hole on one vessel will be under cover of the other sutured vessel, and this will happen during suturing of the anterior and posterior surfaces.

To perform the transverse incision, each vessel is lifted with Dumont No. 3 forceps and the hole is opened with microsurgical scissors (the technique is described in detail in Chapter 6). The vessel lumens are irrigated with warm normal saline. The adventitia is removed from the perimeter of the openings.

F. Graft harvesting

- As described above, in part I, section F. For a more detailed description see Chapter 7.III.B,

G. Graft implantation

The graft is transferred caudally—together with the single clamp—and is placed in the surgical field. The stumps of the renal vessels are brought perpendicular to the common iliac vessels so that the edge of each stump lies on the respective transverse incision of the common iliac artery/vein.

End-to-side anastomoses

- **Renal Artery-Common Iliac artery: 8 sutures 11/0**
- **Renal Vein-Common Iliac vein: 10 or 12 sutures 10/0**

Here, as in all heterotopic kidney tranplantations, we deal with end-to-side anastomoses, in which the graft and the single clamp can be rotated.

➢ **Effective is the time restriction of 30 minutes from the moment of occlusion of the vessels of the kidney**

The technique is described above, in part I. section G. **Figure 28-15** shows the completed suturing of the anterior surfaces of the anastomoses between the renal and common iliac vessels.

H. Closure of the surgical trauma

The splanchna are returned to the abdomen and the abdominal wall is closed in two layers with not absorbable sutures 2/0, the muscles with continuous suturing, and then the subcutaneous and skin with interrupted sutures.

III. Remarks on all Kidney Transplantations

1. Transplantation of kidney with vessel variation

What are you going to do if you come across an anatomical variation in the renal vessels?

In the first description of dissection of the kidney in Chapter 26, we have already discussed the attention needed in the case of accessory renal vessels. We have not, however, discussed the technique to be followed in such a case.

A. Anomalies (variations) of the renal arteries

The embryologic development of the kidney predisposes it to vascular variations. Because the definitive kidney of the embryo (metanephros) ascends from the pelvis to the lumbar area, its vascular supply changes continuously. As it moves cranially, different renal arteries originating from the aorta appear, while the caudal arteries disappear. The end result is the lone renal artery and involution of the embryonic vascular supply. Sometimes these embryonic vessels do not involute. Therefore, it is relatively common (20-40% in humans) to have a remaining embryonic artery that originates from the aorta and coexists with the main renal artery. Such an artery is defined as accessory artery. In rare cases (<5% in humans) there are two accessory arteries.

Figure 28-15

Completed suturing between the anterior surfaces of the anastomoses of the renal artery to the common iliac artery **(1)** and renal vein to the common iliac vein **(2)**. (From author's photo library)

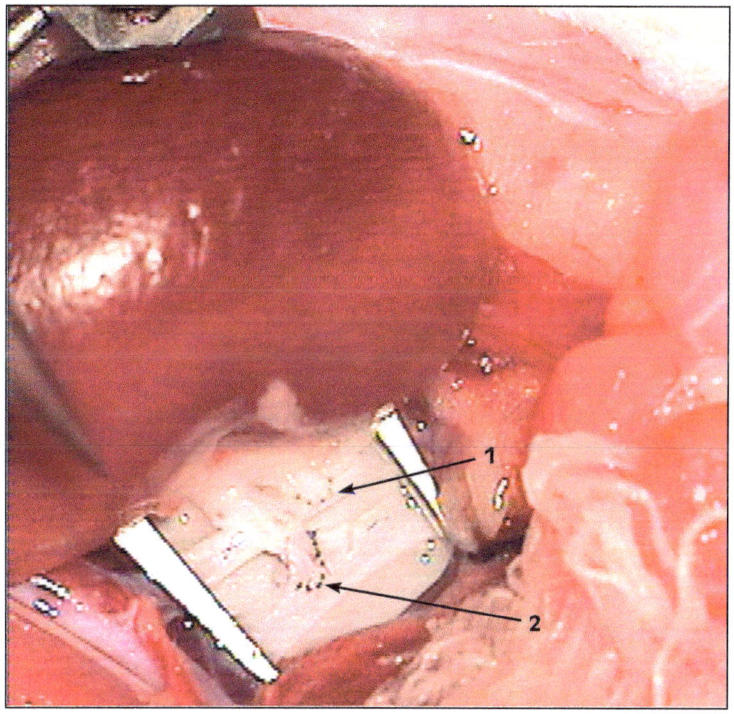

Accessory renal arteries usually originate from the part of the abdominal aorta facing the kidney. In very rare cases an accessory artery may arise form the thoracic aorta or the common iliac arteries. In such cases it is defined as ectopic accessory renal artery.

An accessory renal artery is usually addressed to a renal pole, most often to the lower pole. If there is such a polar artery, the respective segmental arteries to this pole given from the renal artery are usually absent. The accessory artery is 'segmental', i.e., addressed to a single renal segment. Although the term 'accessory' implies that this artery has an auxiliary role, this is a misnomer. The accessory artery is the only artery responsible for a segment's blood supply, because that there is no vascular communication between segments of the kidney and consequently no indirect contribution of the main renal artery via an adjacent segment.

In very rare cases a double renal artery is encountered. The differences from the variation of accessory artery are the following: The main renal artery is present in the case of accessory artery, addressed to the hilum of the kidney, and gives its usual branches. In the case of double renal artery, there are two arteries entering the hilum, and they can give branches corresponding to those of the lone main artery (e.g. inferior adrenal) or other unexpected ones (e.g. the lower artery has been reported to give an additional gonadal branch in human). Sometimes, an artery originating from the renal artery at a distance from the hilum of the kidney is incorrectly considered as 'accessory'. Evidently, it is a branch of the renal artery and not an accessory artery, and its branches may be addressed to more than one renal segment.

Finally, for reasons of completeness, and because the terminology of arterial variations is often erroneous, we refer to the 'replacing' artery. The term signifies an ectopic artery–coming from a source other than the aorta facing the kidney–that replaces the main artery of the viscerum (the main artery is absent). This nomenclature is usually used in the liver, e.g. an ectopic left hepatic artery originating from the superior mesenteric artery, while the normal left hepatic artery is absent. In the kidney, due to the specific pattern of development of the arteries, the 'replacing-ectopic' renal artery is unlikely, since there is usually a renal artery from the aorta. The most profound variation encountered in the kidney is rather the 'accessory-ectopic' artery, as the one given from the iliac artery mentioned above.

Management of renal arterial variation in kidney transplantation

In order to avoid missing an 'additional' renal artery (accessory artery or double renal artery or long branch (early bifurcation) of the renal artery], the aorta must be meticulously dissected, and the renal artery identified and fully dissected.

- ➢ In any case, it is forbidden to ligate the 'additional' artery, because of the risk to harm the blood supply of one or more renal segments.
- ➢ The existence of a 'double' renal artery in the donor transforms the transplantation into heterotopic, because the two arteries of the graft cannot be anastomosed with the single renal artery of the recipient. Thus, the only solution is the heterotopic end-to-side anastomosis with the aorta or the common iliac artery of the recipient.

Management of a 'long branch' of the renal artery varies:

- If the branch is given far from the renal hilum, there will be two arteries to anastomose. Therefore the solution is heterotopic transplantation and anastomoses of the two arteries to the aorta or the common iliac artery of the recipient.
- If the branch arises from the renal artery close to the hilum of the kidney (i.e. the configuration of the 'classic bifurcation' of the renal artery) an orthotopic transplantation is feasible, taking care, however, to place the single clamp away enough from the hilum, so that you will have to deal with one artery to anastomose and not two.

A case with double renal artery

If you managed to read the Chapters on renal transplantation up to here, and have practiced the described techniques, you may look forward to finding a case with double renal artery. Here we present the technique with a double renal artery:

In the donor, the left kidney was dissected as usual. Dissection revealed 2 renal arteries of equal size, directed to the hilum and 1 renal vein. The two renal arteries were both giving an inferior adrenal branch. The renal vein was accepting the inferior adrenal vein and the gonadal vein (**Fig. 28-16**).

The implantation of the graft in the recipient was performed heterotopically, in the common iliac vessels. The technique applied was that of end-to-side anastomoses with clamp rotation. The anastomoses of the smaller caliber renal arteries required a lesser number of 11/0 sutures. The vein anastomosis was performed as usual.

The anterior surfaces of the 3 vessels were sutured first (**Fig. 28-16**). The graft was rotated and suturing of the posterior surfaces of the vessels was completed (**Fig. 28-17**). The patency test for the venous anastomosis was performed in the usual way (see Chapter

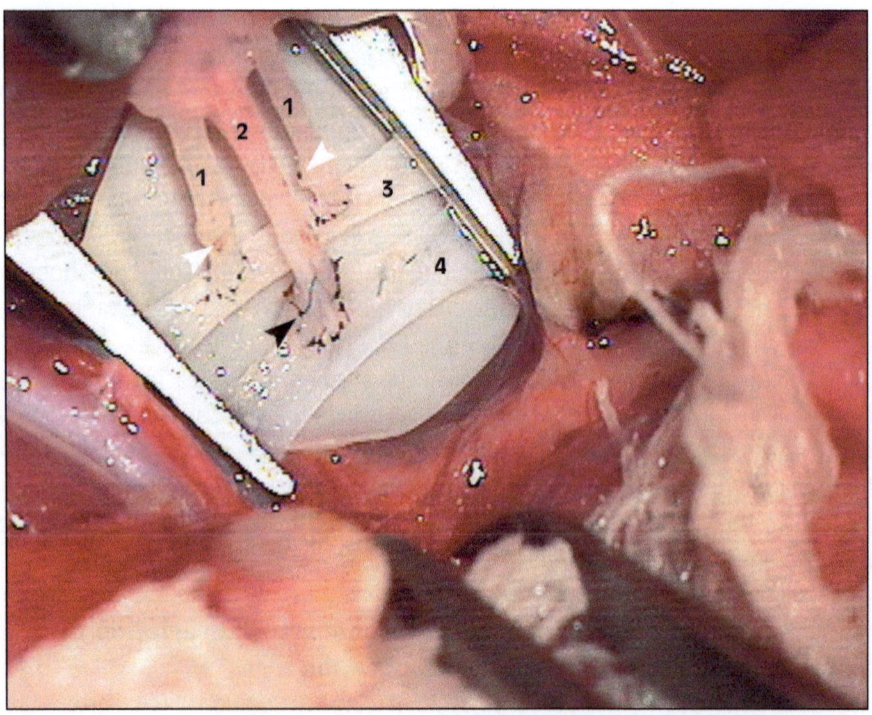

Figure 28-16

A case of kidney transplantation with double renal artery. Suturing of the anterior surfaces of the anastomoses of two renal arteries and renal vein has been completed. Observe that the renal arteries were each giving an inferior adrenal branch (white arrowheads). The ligation and the stump of the inferior adrenal vein can also be seen on the renal vein (black arrowhead). **1.** renal arteries, **2.** renal vein, **3.** left common iliac artery, **4.** left common iliac vein. (From author's photo library)

Figure 28-17

Suturing of the posterior surfaces of the two renal arteries and single renal vein. The graft has been rotated towards the pelvis with the Metzenbaum scissors. Here, the posterior surface of the vein has been completed. Now is placed the last suture in one of the renal arteries. Suturing of the other artery will follow (on which the two already placed corner sutures can be seen). (From author's photo library)

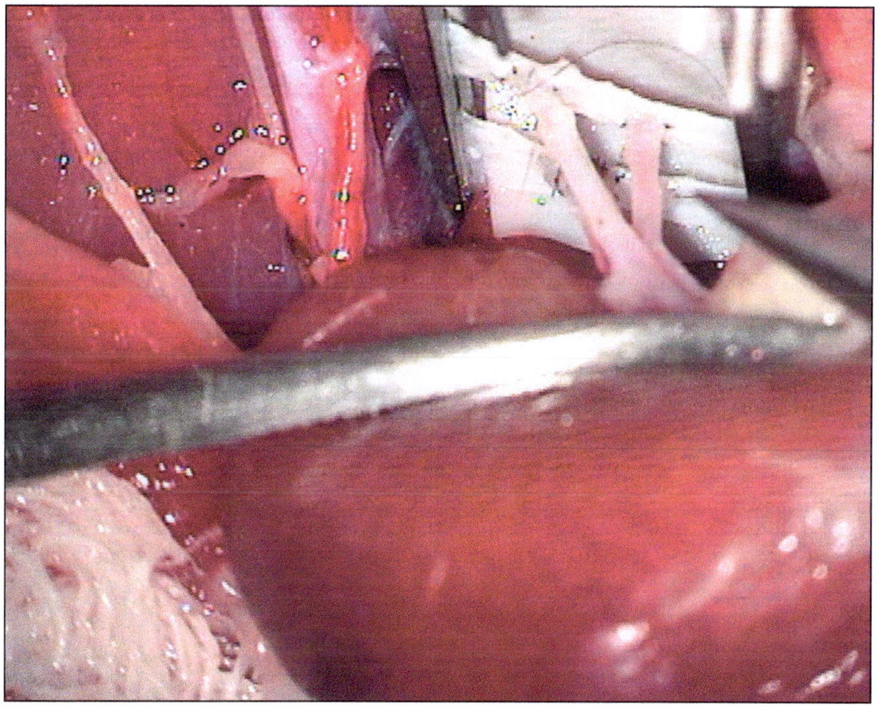

6.9.2) (**Fig. 28-18**). As for the renal arteries, a first indication of patency is the presence of pulsation in the central renal artery, which can be amplified by occluding the common iliac artery between the two arterial anastomoses (**Fig. 28-19**). The same can be done for the peripheral renal artery with occlusion of the common iliac artery peripheral to its anastomosis. Then, necessarily, the classic patency test for each renal artery must be tested separately—with the common iliac free—first the central and then the peripheral, following the known technique. First, a forceps occludes the lumen of the renal artery after the anastomosis. A

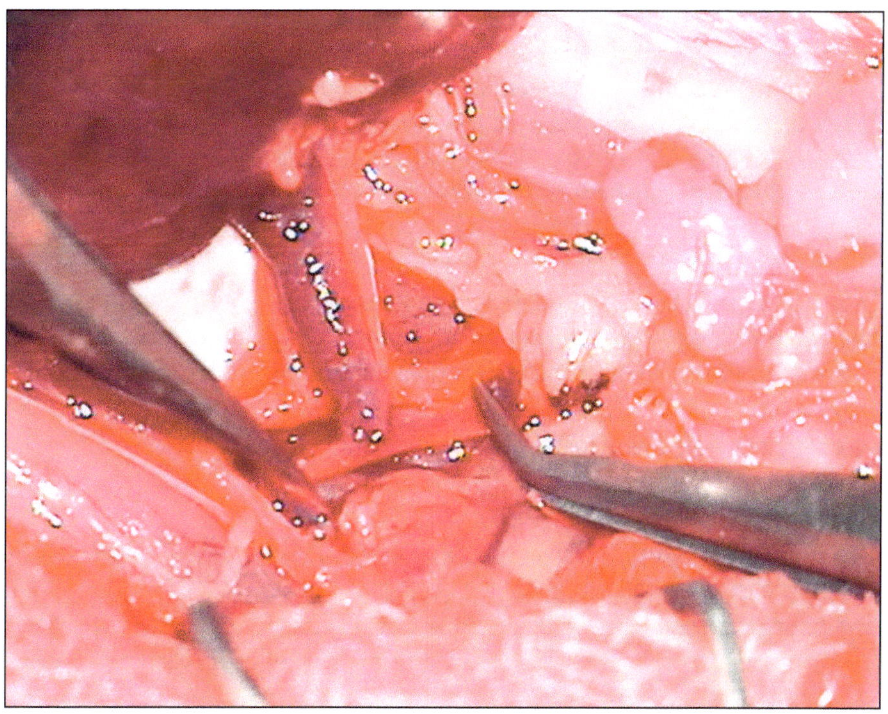

Figure 28-18

Patency test of the anastomosis of the renal vein with the common iliac vein. The two forceps move away from each other and empty the lumen of the common iliac vein. If the anastomosis is patent, when the two forceps re-approach, the part of the common iliac vein between them will be filled immediately. (From author's photo library)

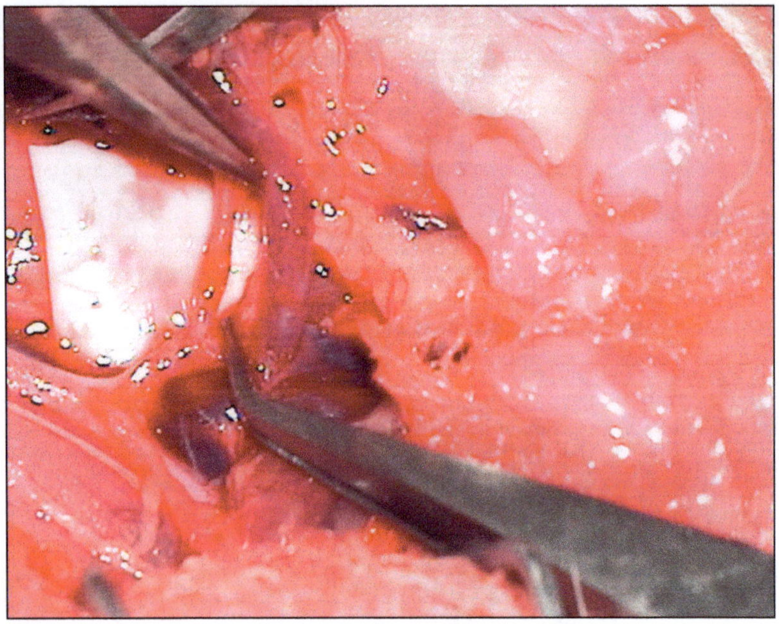

Figure 28-19

Amplification of the blood flow through the 1st arterial anastomosis when looking for pulsation of the central renal artery as an index of patency. The curved forceps occludes the common iliac artery between the anastomoses of the renal arteries, and the flow is directed from the common iliac artery of the recipient in the central renal artery of the graft. (From author's photo library).

second forceps is placed on the renal artery adjacent to the first forceps, moves away 'half-closed', thus milking the lumen, and stays closed after a short distance. The first forceps is removed, and if there is patency in the anastomosis, the lumen of the renal artery will be filled in immediately up to the second forceps (see **Figure 6-9**).

B. Anomalies of the renal veins

In Chapter 26.C, where we first described the renal vein dissection, it was mentioned that variations of the veins are common. It was underlined that attention must be paid not to perceive an accessory vein or a tributary emptying far from the hilum as inferior adrenal vein or deep tributary or gonadal vein and erroneously ligate it.

The embryologic pattern of renal arterial development discussed above is also valid for the veins. As the permanent kidney of the embryo (metanephros) ascends from the pelvis to the lumbar area, new veins appear cranially while caudal veins regress. However, veins do not have a firm pattern of development compared with the arteries (for instance, in many organs veins are more numerous than arteries, and in the pelvis they form plexuses such as prostatic, uteral, etc). Therefore, more variation is expected in renal veins than in renal arteries.

Thus, an accessory vein, especially at the lower pole of the kidney, is a relatively common finding. Sometimes, the veins are subject to greater malformation, such as forming a vein ring around the aorta in the left side (before emptying as single vein in the inferior vena cava). And these malformations may coexist with a typical accessory renal vein.

The matter in kidney transplantation is if one or more than one renal veins are recognized. Similar to the variations of the renal arteries, the following are valid in case that an 'additional' vein is found:

- It is not permitted to ligate any 'additional' renal vein.
- An 'additional' vein is in opposition to an orthotopic transplantation with end-to-end anastomoses of the renal vessels (two vessels in the graft versus one vessel in the recipient) and dictates heterotopic implantation of the kidney with end-to-side anastomoses of the two (or more) veins to the inferior vena cava or common iliac vein.

As seen above in arteries, if more than one veins are encountered, they are expected to be of lesser caliber, and fewer sutures will be placed in each anastomosis.

2. Flushing of the graft in autotransplantation

In this book, there is no mention of irrigating the kidney

graft in othotopic autotransplantation (Chapter 26) and heterotopic autotransplantaion (Chapter 28). Our experience has shown that in both orthotopic and heterotopic autotransplantations the kidney worked immediatelly without flushing. However, no long term follow-up was undertaken.

For security, and if your experimental needs demand so, you can proceed with flushing of the graft in renal autotransplantations. The solution must be injected in the renal artery, wash the kidney, and exit from the renal vein. Therefore the renal vessles must be freed from clamps and some rearrangemnt will be needed in the surgical field:

- In **orthotopic autotransplantaion,** at the step of occlusion of the renal vessels centrally (toward the aorta) and peripherally (toward the kindney) with the double clamp, the peripheral clamp should open to release the vessels. Before opening the peripheral clamp, the renal vein should be transected in the middle of the distance of the two clamps; if the transection is performed after opening the clamp, the vein will shrink, and most likely the cut will not be in the middle and the following anastomoses will not be aligned. Then the stumps of the vein are irrigated as usual with warm normal saline.

  For flushing the graft, a small syringe (2 or 5 ml) will be used with its needle bent into right angle. The needle enters the lumen of the renal artery, headed toward the kidney. The entrance point is beyond the mid-length of the artery, near the hilum of the kidney (in order to minimize the length of the vessel to be washed, and consequently the resistance).

  Flushing can be done either with injection of cold heparin solution without transection of the artery, as described here, or as others suggest, with entrance of the needle (or angiocath) in the lumen after transection of the artery mid-way between the clamps. If transection of the artery is chosen, the central stump should be washed now with warm normal saline to avoid clot formation. The peripheral stump of the artery should be temporarily ligated—while containing the needle or angiocath—in order to avoid leak during injection due to difference of caliber between the needle or catheter and the artery. Take care, this ligation should not be placed very close to the edge of the lumen, neither be too tight, in order to avoid harm to the artery wall or endothelium, which are pressed against the needle or catheter. For this reason it is here suggested to inject the renal artery; this has no need of a ligation, because, even if a small amount of heparin solution flows back, the artery is intact and occluded centrally by the clamp, that is there no way for leak. Some others, however, suggest injecting with the needle as we do, but then to surround and ligate the artery containing the needle in order to avoid back flow. We disagree and consider this ligation useless (and dangerous for the endothelium), because even if back blow occurs, it will simply wash the artery centrally, which is of no harm.

  After flushing the graft, the intact renal artery (if punctured) or the peripheral stump of the artery (if 'transection-needle in lumen-ligation' is chosen), and the stump of the renal vein are repositioned in the peripheral clamp. Following the method shown here, transection of the renal artery follows, in the middle of the distance of the clamps. The peripheral stump has already been washed with the heparin solution; the central stump should be irrigated with warm normal saline through a fine angiocath, as usually.

- In **heterotopic autotransplantation,** after the renal vessels have been ligated centrally (toward the aorta), the renal vein should be transected just after its ligation close to the inferior vena cava, as in **Figure 28-7**, but with no placement of single clamp occluding the renal artery and vein.

  Flushing of the kidney with cold heparin solution will be performed by puncturing the renal artery, as described above in orthotopic transplantation. It can also be done with 'transection of the artery-needle in lumen-ligation', as described by others (see above in orthotopic transplantation).

  After flushing the kidney, the renal vein is placed in the single clamp together with the artery. Transection of the renal artery follows, close to its ligated origin from the aorta. Peripheral to the injection site (toward the kidney), the arterial stump has been washed with the heparin solution. It is advised to irrigate again the artery with warm normal saline through a fine angiocath, in order to clean completely the part of the artery between the transection and puncture points.

Solutions for graft flushing

In this book, flushing of the graft is described to be performed only with cold heparenized saline. However, many other protocols can be found in the literature, varying from Ringer's to specific solutions (e.g. Ros). You should search for the technique that is most suitable for the needs of your research.

Synopsis... of heterotopic (auto)transplantation of the left kidney

I. TRANSPLANTATION WITH ANASTOMOSES IN THE AORTA – INFERIOR VENA CAVA

A. **Position of the rat:** Laid on its back, head on the left of the surgeon. The limbs are immobilized on the working surface with adhesive tape.

B. **Preparation of the surgical field:** Median incision, from the xiphoid process to the pubic symphysis. Mobilization of the small intestine and placement of the intestines, enveloped in a wet gauze, outside of the abdomen, contralateral to the transplantation side. The retroperitoneum is opened with two gauzes moistened in warm normal saline.

C. **Microsurgical dissection of the renal fascia, renal vessels and ureter:** The renal fascia is opened and the fat enveloping the kidney, renal vessels and ureter is dissected off them. The renal vein and artery are dissected from the inferior vena cava and aorta to the hilum of the kidney transecting between two ligations all branches/tributaries: inferior adrenal vein and artery, gonadal vein (left side), and deep tributary veins of the renal vein. The kidney is mobilized from its bed, rotated medially, and the posterior surface of the vessels is dissected (the ureter is not dissected if only vessels anastomoses are practiced).

D. **Microsurgcial dissection of the aorta and inferior vena cava:** Transection between two ligations of lumbar and branches and tributaries, and meticulous dissection of the aorta and inferior vena cava in the area where anastomoses with the graft vessels will be performed.

E. **Preparation of the recipient vessels:** Occlusion of the aorta and inferior vena cava with the double clamp. Placement of a yellow plastic background under the vessels. Arteriotomy – Venotomy – Irrigation of the vessels lumens.

F. **Graft harvesting:** The renal vessels are ligated (separately) close to the aorta-inferior vena cava with 9/0 suture. A single clamp is placed on both vessels close to the hilum of the kidney. Transection of the vessels close to ligations, irrigation, removal of the adventitia.

G. **Graft implantation:** The graft is transferred in the field so that the renal vessels are brought perpendicular to the aorta and inferior vena cava, with the edges adjacent to the arteriotomy and venotomy.

End-to-side anastomoses

- **Renal Artery: 8 sutures 11/0**
- **Renal Vein: 10 or 12 sutures 10/0**

➢ **Time restriction of 30 minutes from the moment of occlusion of the vessels of the kidney**

1. Corner sutures are placed in both vessels.
2. Suturing of the anterior surface of the artery first, then of the vein.
3. Rotation of the graft and check of the sutures of the anterior surfaces.
4. Suturing of posterior surfaces is completed.
5. Release of the clamps, first the single then the double.
6. Placement of a wet gauze on the anastomoses for 3 minutes.
7. Patency test, separately for each vessel.
8. Withdrawal of the yellow plastic background.

... of heterotopic (auto)transplantation of the left kidney

Synopsis...

H. Closure of the surgical trauma in two layers with non-absorbable 2/0 sutures, muscles with continuous suturing, subcutaneous and skin with interrupted sutures.

II. TRANSPLANTATION WITH ANASTOMOSES IN THE COMMON ILIAC VESSELS

A. Position of the rat

B. Preparation of the surgical field

C. Microsurgical dissection of the renal fascia, renal vessels and ureter
Same as in I.A, B, C (see above).

D. Microsurgical preparation of the common iliac vessels: Dissection of the caudal part and bifurcation of the aorta, and similarly the inferior vena cava and confluence of the common iliac veins. Ligation and transection of the middle sacral artery and vein. Continuation of the dissection in the left common iliac artery and vein, by ligating and transecting branches and tributaries met, until the first large branch of the common iliac artery (internal ileac artery). Placement of a yellow plastic background under the vessels.

E. Preparation of the recipient vessels: Occlusion of the common iliac artery and vein with the double clamp. Arteriotomy –Venotomy – Irrigation of the lumens of the vessels.

F. Graft harvesting: As in I.F (see above).

G. Graft implantation: The graft is transferred in the field so that the renal vessels are brought perpendicular to the iliac vessels, with the edges adjacent to the openings of the arteriotomy and venotomy.
End-to-side anastomoses: as in I.G (see above).

H. Closure of the surgical trauma: as in I.H (see above).

29

Autotransplantation of the uterine horn-fallopian tube-ovary

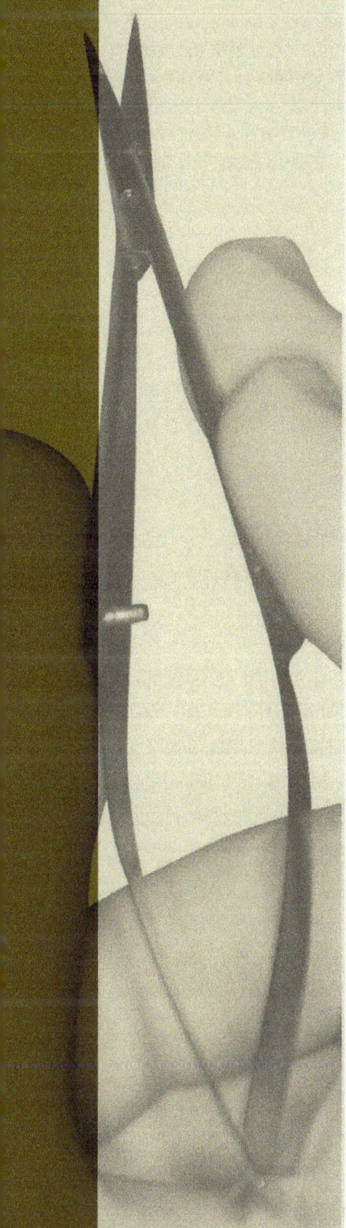

The procedure is described in this Chapter as performed on the right side. It can be identically performed on the left side, with the only change being the placement of the intestines to the right side during preparation of the surgical field.

A. Positioning of the rat

The rat is placed in dorsal decubitus (supine) position on the working surface with the head on the left side of the surgeon. The limbs of the rat are immobilized on the working surface with adhesive tape.

B. Preparation of the surgical field

The reader will find a detailed description and imaging of the preparation of the surgical field of the aorta in Chapter 8.B and C.1. Here only a summary pertaining to this procedure is provided.

A median incision is performed through the skin and superficial fascia 5 mm inferior to the xiphoid process cranially to a position 5 mm superior to the pubic symphysis caudally. The aponeuroses at the linea alba are then opened followed by the peritoneum. Two retractors are placed symmetrically on both sides of the incision.

The lobes of the liver are removed from the field using a retractor wrapped in gauze. Beginning at the cecum, the intestine is mobilized and moved out of the surgical field using broad atraumatic (anatomical) forceps. The autotransplantation will be performed on the right side, thus, the intestine is placed on a moistened gauze on the left side of the rat. It should be covered by another gauze moistened in warm normal saline and periodically irrigated. The rectum is then moved to the left in the peritoneal cavity.

The retroperitoneum is opened widely from the renal vessels to the pelvis with two gauzes moistened in warm normal saline. This maneuver exposes the microsurgical field of the aorta, inferior vena cava, and common iliac vessels along with their branches/tributaries.

The morphology of the uterine horns may look strange to the unaccustomed eye due to differences between the rat and human uterus, and this deserves special mention. The uterus of the rat is 'double', with two long horns that unite low in the pelvis (**Fig. 29-1**). The body of the uterus, formed by the union of the two uterine horns, is short and contains the distal lumens of both horns. These lumens open in the vagina. This V-like configuration justifies the term 'double' uterus used here ('duplex' is also accurate); the term 'bicornuate' (double horn) is not ju-

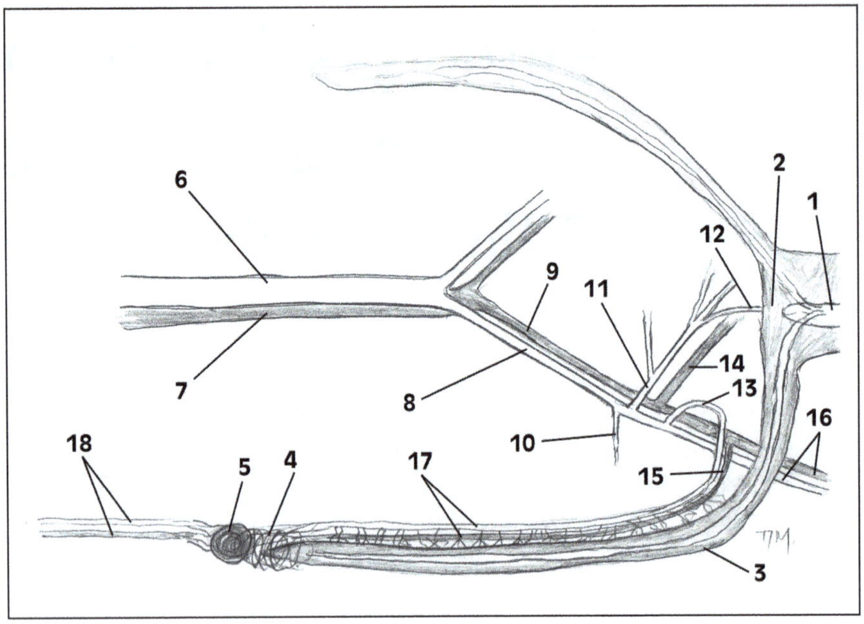

Figure 29-1

Schematic representation of the morphology and vasculature of uterus, fallopian tube, and ovary in the rat (right side). **1.** vagina, **2.** uterine body, **3.** right uterine horn, **4.** fallopian tube (salpinx), **5.** ovary, **6.** aorta, **7.** inferior vena cava, **8.** common iliac artery, **9.** common iliac vein, **10.** posterior parietal branch, **11.** internal iliac artery, **12.** uterine or utero-vaginal branch of the internal iliac artery, **13.** artery of the uterine horn, **14.** internal iliac vein, **15.** vein of the uterine horn, **16.** external iliac vessels, **17.** vessels of the uterine horn and small vertical arterial branches/vein tributaries to/from the horn, **18.** gonadal (ovarian) vessels. (Drawing by the author)

stified, because it refers to a Y-like configuration. The horns of the uterus have a mesentery, the mesometrium, which attaches them to the posterolateral abdomino-pelvic wall. The peritoneum envelops the horns, except from their posterior surface, and its two leaves continue on the wall as parietal peritoneum. The vessels of the horn are comprised of an artery arising from the common iliac artery and a vein emptying into the common iliac vein. These vessels enter the mesometrium after traveling for a short distance retroperitoneally. In the mesometrium, they follow the horn (No. 17, **Fig. 29-1**); small arterial branches and vein tributaries from the vessels of the horn are given to/come from the uterine horn.

The fallopian tube (salpinx) of the rat is also significantly different than from a human's. In the rat, the fallopian tube, sometimes also referred to as the oviduct in books of anatomy, can be described as a long duct. It starts as a funnel-like opening near the ovary, coiling around the ovary and continuing around the cranial part of the horn for 1-2 cm before penetrating the wall of the uterine horn (No. 4, **Fig. 29-1**). The diameter of the duct is very small, about 0.5 mm.

C. Microsurgical dissection

Given the complexity of the procedure, a separate description of the vasculature involved and the design of the operation precedes the presentation of the dissection.

I. Elements of surgical anatomy (vasculature of the uterine horn, fallopian tube, and ovary)

In Chapter 15.D and Chapter 28. II.D.1, the branches of the common iliac artery were mentioned. The autotransplantation of the uterine horn, fallopian tube, and ovary in the rat requires detailed knowledge of their vasculature, thus enabling feasible and comfortable dissection. Unfortunately, given the differences in the anatomy of the rat, just having knowledge of human anatomy will not suffice.

The *middle sacral artery* arises from the posterior surface of bifurcation of the aorta, which is important in the rat because it continues as the caudal artery (see more in Chapter 15.D and **Figure 15-1**). Near the bifurcation of the aorta, a posterior parietal branch is also encountered. In addition, small parietal branches may be found along the course of the common iliac artery, arising from the posterior surface and addressed to muscles of the posterior abdomino-pelvic wall. Similarly, posterior parietal tributary veins enter along the posterior surface of the common iliac vein.

Knowledge of the branches of the common iliac artery is extremely important for understanding the surgical field and the design of the operation. The common iliac artery, in accordance with the pattern encountered in human anatomy, is expected to bifurcate into the external and internal iliac arteries. The external iliac is addressed to the lower limb and lower anterior abdominal wall and the internal iliac artery is addressed to the pelvis and perineum. In the female rat, however, the common iliac artery also gives off a visceral branch, the artery for the uterine horn from its anterior surface (No. 13, **Fig. 29-1**). This artery, as stated above, initially courses retroperitoneally before entering the mesometrium where it follows the horn, giving off several small arterial branches perpendicular to the horn (No. 17, **Fig. 29-1**). The cranial part of the artery of the horn supplies the coiled fallopian tube and helps supply the ovary along with the gonadal artery, which is the main vessel supplying the ovary. The vein of the uterine horn mirrors the course of its respective artery as it passes through the mesometrium and then courses in the retroperitoneum to empty into the common iliac vein (No. 15, **Fig. 29-1**). Note that the origin of the artery of the horn is found cranial to the confluence of the vein. Additionally, the artery of the horn has a greater length and a more curved course compared the vein.

Frequently, the artery and vein of the horn are referred to as the '*uterine artery*' and '*uterine vein*'. These terms incorrectly signify that these vessels are responsible for the vasculature of both the horn and body of the uterus on that respective side. As in the human, however, the ipsilateral internal iliac artery gives a branch for the body of the uterus (No. 12, **Fig. 29-1**) as well as utero-vaginal branches. Consequently, we suggest that the terms *artery of the uterine horn and vein of the uterine horn* should be applied for the vessels that follow the course of the horn of the uterus, and the terms 'uterine artery' and 'uterine vein' should be reserved for the uterine/utero-vaginal branches of the internal iliac artery and the tributaries of the homonymous vein, respectively.

Along its posteromedial surface, the common iliac artery gives off a large pelvic branch (No. 11, **Fig. 29-1**), which is referred to as the '*internal iliac artery*'. This implies that this vessel is responsible for the parietal and visceral supply of the pelvis and perineum. This definition is not justifiably fulfilled, however, as the artery of the uterine horn, a visceral pelvic branch, arises from the common iliac artery. The respective pelvic vein, called the '*internal iliac vein*' (No. 11, **Fig. 29-1**) is of greater caliber than the artery. Similarly to the artery, the vein of the uterine horn enters the common iliac vein. In spite of this, we are going to use here the terms 'internal iliac artery' and 'internal iliac vein' in order to avoid polyphony.

Remember that

- In the rat, the common iliac artery preserves the pattern of division into the external and internal iliac arteries as in humans. Additionally in the rat, however, the common iliac artery gives off the artery of the uterine horn (the same pattern is valid for the common iliac vein, which receives blood flow from the vein of the uterine horn).

After the internal iliac artery and the artery of the uterine horn takeoff from the common iliac artery (Nos. 11 and 13, **Fig. 29-1**), the artery can be named the external iliac artery in correspondence to human anatomy. This artery is responsible for supplying the lower limb and for providing deep branches to the muscles of the lower anterior abdominal wall (e.g. deep inferior epigastric artery, etc.). We remind the reader that the femoral vessels contribute, among others, the respective superficial branches to the lower anterior abdominal wall (e.g. superficial inferior epigastric artery, etc.). The nomenclature and course of the veins of the region follow the arterial pattern (**Fig. 29-1**).

In the area where the internal iliac artery and the artery of the uterine horn takeoff from the common iliac artery, a *posterior parietal arterial branch* is also consistently seen (No. 10, **Fig. 29-1**). This branch arises from the posterior surface of the common iliac artery, slightly cranial to the internal iliac artery and the artery of the uterine horn. In our experience, the posterior parietal arterial branch is not necessarily accompanied by a corresponding vein.

Beyond the accessory supply from the artery of the uterine horn, the ovary receives its blood flow from the *gonadal (ovarian) artery,* which originates from the aorta just caudal to the ipsilateral renal artery. The *gonadal vein,* which for a large distance follows the artery, empties on the right side directly into the inferior vena cava and into the left renal vein on the left side. The gonadal vessels (No. 18, **Fig. 29-1**) are packed in the suspensory ligament of the ovary, which extends from the ovary to the renal area due to the embryologic descent of the ovary following its development in front of the kidney. In the rat, the suspensory ligament of the ovary is short as the ovary is located relatively high outside of the pelvis due to the long uterine horn. The suspensory ligament and the gonadal vessels contained within are superficial to the ureter because the ovary develops on the anterior surface of the kidney in the embryo.

II. Design of the operation

This operation aims to make the vessels (artery and vein) of the uterine horn the only supply to the complex 'uterine horn-fallopian tube-ovary'. Additionally, these vessels will become the only arterial branch and tributary vein of their respective common iliac vessels. This allows for the transplantation of the uterine horn, fallopian tube, and ovary en block by anastomosing only the common iliac vessels.

In order to accomplish these aims, the following steps have to be performed (the numbering of the steps listed below corresponds with **Figure 29-2**):

1. The posterior parietal arterial branch **(1A)**, the internal iliac artery and vein **(1B),** and the external iliac vessels **(1C)** should be ligated and divided to make the artery and vein of the uterine horn the only intact vessels in communication with the common iliac artery and vein.
2. The gonadal vessels should be ligated and divided, thus making the vessels of the uterine horn the only vessels supplying the uterine horn, fallopian tube and ovary.
3. The uterine horn, fallopian tube, and ovary should be mobilized en bloc with the vascular supply from the common iliac vessels. This means that both the common iliac vessels **(3A),** and the uterine horn at its base **(3B)** will have to be ligated and divided.

III. Microsurgical dissection

1. Dissection of the common iliac vessels (and aorta-inferior vena cava, at their bifurcations)

The reader is referred to Chapter 8.C.2 for the detailed dissection of the aorta and to Chapter 28.I.D.b for the inferior vena cava.

Microsurgical dissection starts by developing a plane of separation between the aorta and the inferior vena cava, cranial to the bifurcation of the aorta. Ligation (or cauterization) and division of one or two lumbar arteries will allow for the aorta to be lifted and the middle sacral artery to be exposed. The plane of separation is then extended to the right common iliac artery, which is detached from the right common iliac vein and lifted together with the aorta. One or two posterior parietal branches of the right common iliac artery should be cauterized and divided. Lifting the right common iliac artery will allow further exposure of the middle sacral artery. Although other authors do not deal at all with the middle sacral artery in this operation, we suggest that the middle sacral artery should be divided between two ligations (double-ligated) as opposed to cauterized. This avoids the risk of rupture from the manipulations that will follow, especially for the less experienced surgeon.

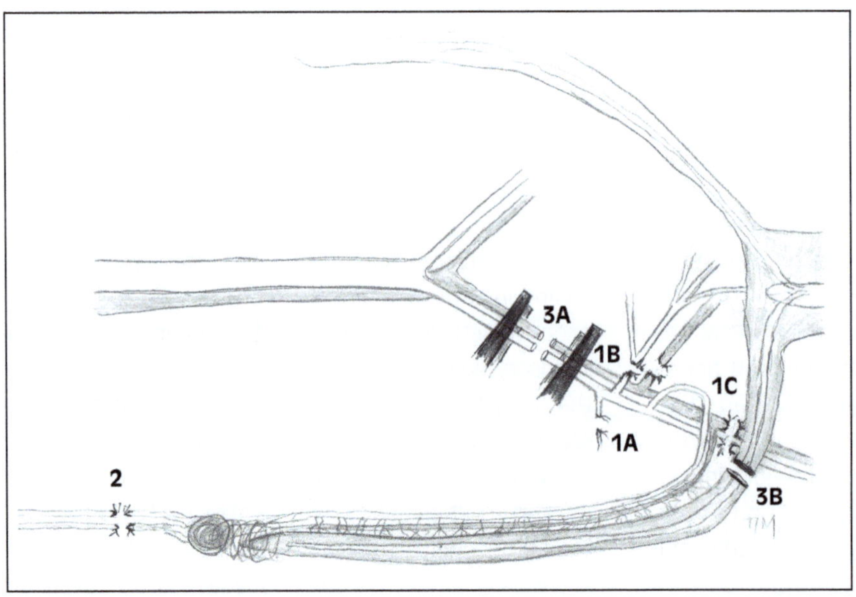

Figure 29-2

Design of the autotransplantation of the 'uterine horn-fallopian tube-ovary' complex. The order of steps taken to mobilize the uterine horn, fallopian tube, and ovary en bloc with the vascular supply from the common iliac vessels, is as follows. **1.** Ligation and division of the: **A.** posterior parietal branch of the common iliac artery, **B.** internal iliac vessels, **C.** external iliac vessels (caudal to the origin/confluence of the vessels of the uterine horn. **2.** Ligation and division of the gonadal vessels. **3.** Transection of the: **A.** common iliac vessels, **B.** horn of the uterus. The stumps of the common iliac vessels have been placed in the jaws of the double clamp (Drawing by the author)

The takeoff of the artery of the right horn of the uterus is evident on the anterior surface of the caudal aspect of the right common iliac artery. The dissection to this point is shown in **Figure 29-3**.

Next, the inferior vena cava is dissected at the area of the confluence of the common iliac veins; the dissection will be extended along the right common iliac vein. For the posterior dissection of the inferior vena cava, the surgeon should double-ligate and divide (or cauterize and divide for the more experienced surgeon) one or, rarely, two lower lumbar veins on either side. On the right side, the lower right lumbar vein can easily be dissected, double-ligated and transected (**Fig. 28-2**). After mobilization of the posterior surface of the inferior vena cava, the lower left lumbar vein can be directly accessed from the left (**Fig. 28-3**). Additionally, the final part of a lower left lumbar vein at its entrance on the posterolateral surface of the inferior vena cava can be accessed from the right, under the inferior vena cava (**Fig. 29-4**). The dissection is continued towards the right common iliac vein, facilitated by elevating the inferior vena cava; then, under direct visualization, the posterior parietal tributary veins are cauterized or double-ligated and divided (the detailed dissection of the common iliac vein will be described below).

In other books of microsurgery, the instruction is often to dissect the common iliac vessels only, sparing the aorta or the inferior vena cava from dissection. In Chapter 28, where the dissection along the common iliac artery was extended up to the 'first big division of the common iliac artery' (meaning the internal iliac artery), we were skeptical that dissection of only the common iliac vessels would be adequate (see Chapter 28. II.D.2). This was done because we felt that there would not be sufficient space for the double clamp, and access to the posterior branches/tributaries of the common iliac vessels would be limited. In the current procedure, the surgeon could dissect the common iliac vessels without further dissection of the aorta and inferior vena cava, but only those with experience should perform this. When dissecting only the common iliac artery without dissection of the aorta, one or two small posterior parietal branches must be cauterized and transected while taking care to preserve the middle sacral artery (**Fig. 29-5**). During the dissection of only the common iliac vein without dissection of the inferior vena cava, dissection and division of the small posterior parietal tributary veins running into the common iliac vein can be quite difficult in the narrower window created posterior to the vein, requiring careful, meticulous, and precise technique. In addition, as discussed in Chapter 28.II.D.2, the middle sacral vein and its connections to the sacral vein plexus are at risk for rupture during

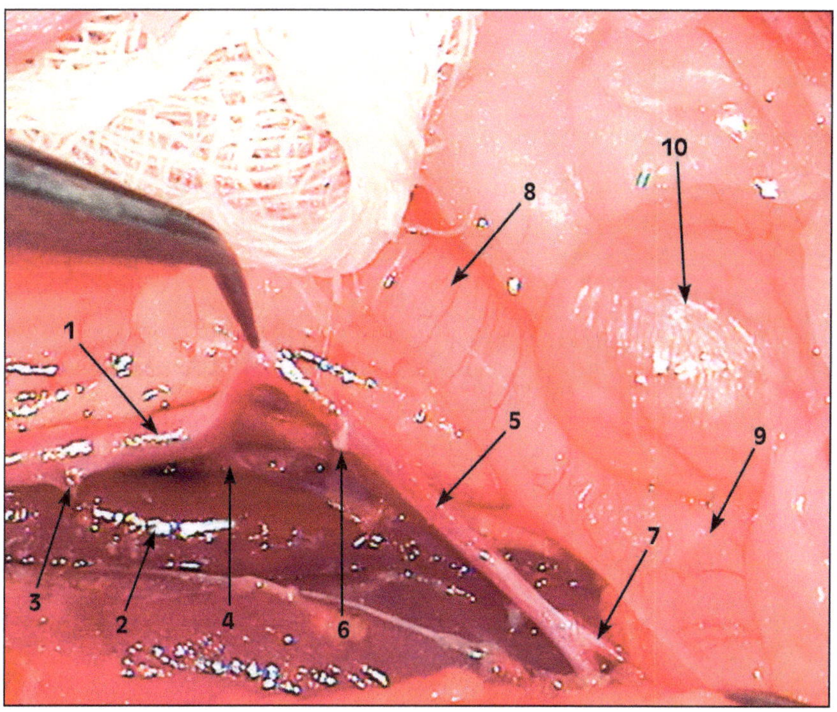

Figure 29-3

Dissection of the aorta at the bifurcation area, continued along the right common iliac artery. The curved microsurgical forceps elevates the right common iliac artery after a lower right lumbar artery and a posterior parietal branch of the right common iliac artery have been cauterized and transected. Another forceps moves the right horn of the uterus laterally (right lower corner of the photo). **1.** aorta, **2.** inferior vena cava, **3.** cauterized lower right lumbar artery, **4.** middle sacral artery, **5.** right common iliac artery, **6.** cauterized posterior parietal branch of the right common iliac artery, **7.** artery of the right horn of the uterus, **8.** left horn of the uterus, **9.** body of the uterus, **10.** urinary bladder. (From author's photo library)

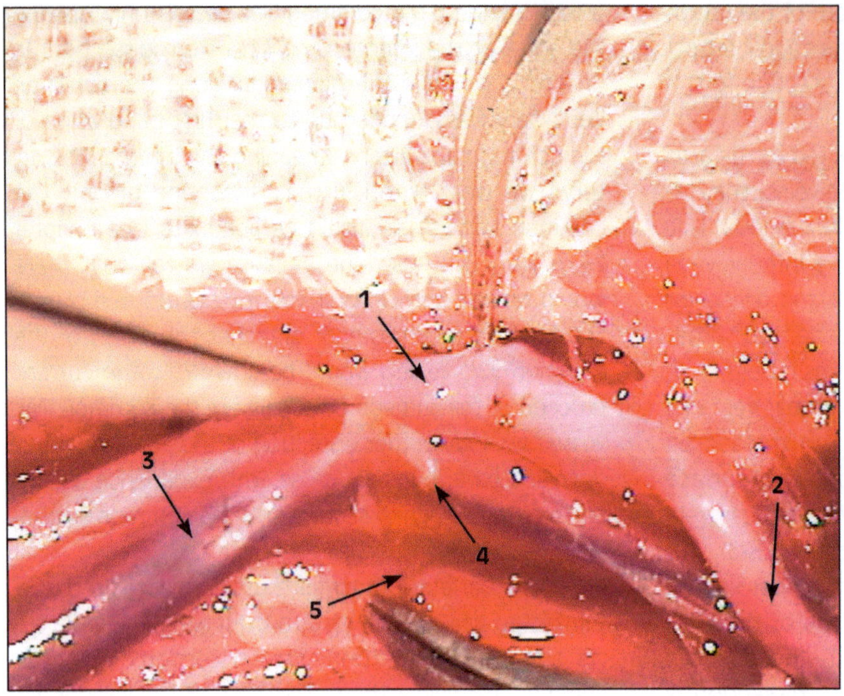

Figure 29-4

Dissection of the inferior vena cava cranial to the confluence of the common iliac veins, approach from the right side. The curved microsurgical forceps elevates the dissected aorta, and the Dumont No. 3 forceps picks up the inferior vena cava after the regional right lumbar vein (4) has been cauterized and transected. The inferior vena cava is pulled to the left with the forceps No 3, and the microsurgical scissors dissect a lower left lumbar vein (5) at its confluence with the inferior vena cava. **1.** aorta, 2. right common iliac artery, **3.** inferior vena cava, **4.** cauterized right lumbar vein, **5.** left lumbar vein. (From author's photo library)

instrumentation in this area; a complication that is not easily managed.

2. Common iliac artery: 'the dissection of the four branches'

- **Posterior parietal branch**
- **Internal iliac artery**
- **Artery of the uterine horn**
- **External iliac artery**

Thus far, we have identified two of the four branches, the *artery of the uterine horn*, given off the anterior surface of the common iliac artery and the *external iliac artery* (**Fig. 29-5**).

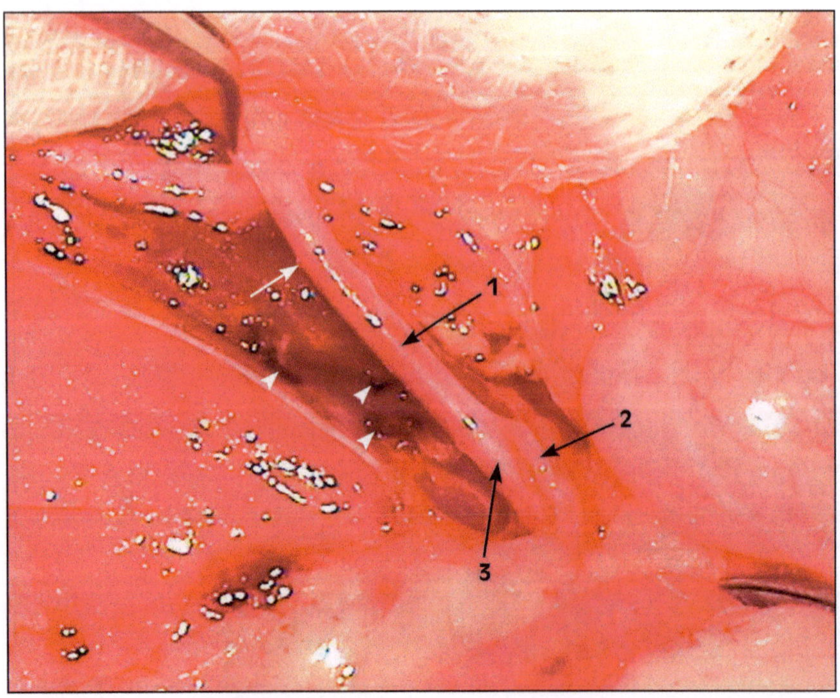

Figure 29-5

Dissected right common iliac artery without dissection of the aorta bifurcation. The curved microsurgical forceps lifts the dissected common iliac artery (the middle sacral artery is not exposed). The artery of ipsilateral uterine horn arises from the anterior surface of the distal part of the common iliac artery. Observe the black markings on the muscles where cauterization of the posterior parietal branches has occurred (white arrowheads); the origin of a cauterized and transected posterior parietal branch can also be seen (white arrow). **1.** common iliac artery, **2.** artery of the uterine horn, **3.** external iliac artery. (From author's photo library)

The remaining two more central branches (located cranially), the posterior parietal branch and the internal iliac artery, are not directly visible because they originate from the posterior surface of the common iliac artery. These branches become evident when the common iliac artery is elevated by the adventitia with a forceps. This maneuver, however, may create a 'false image,' as seen in **Figure 29-6A**. This occurs because the artery of the uterine horn may also be directed posteriorly with traction, thus resulting in three branches that appear to be 'posterior.' The key here is to know the order of the origin of the branches. Running craniocaudally, the *posterior parietal branch* is found first and courses slightly laterally (toward the surgeon). This branch is dissected, double-ligated–proximal and as distal as possible in the field–with 9/0 non-abserbable suture, and divided between the two ligations (**Fig. 29-6B**). The use of diathermy is not advised at all in the current complex configuration of vessels.

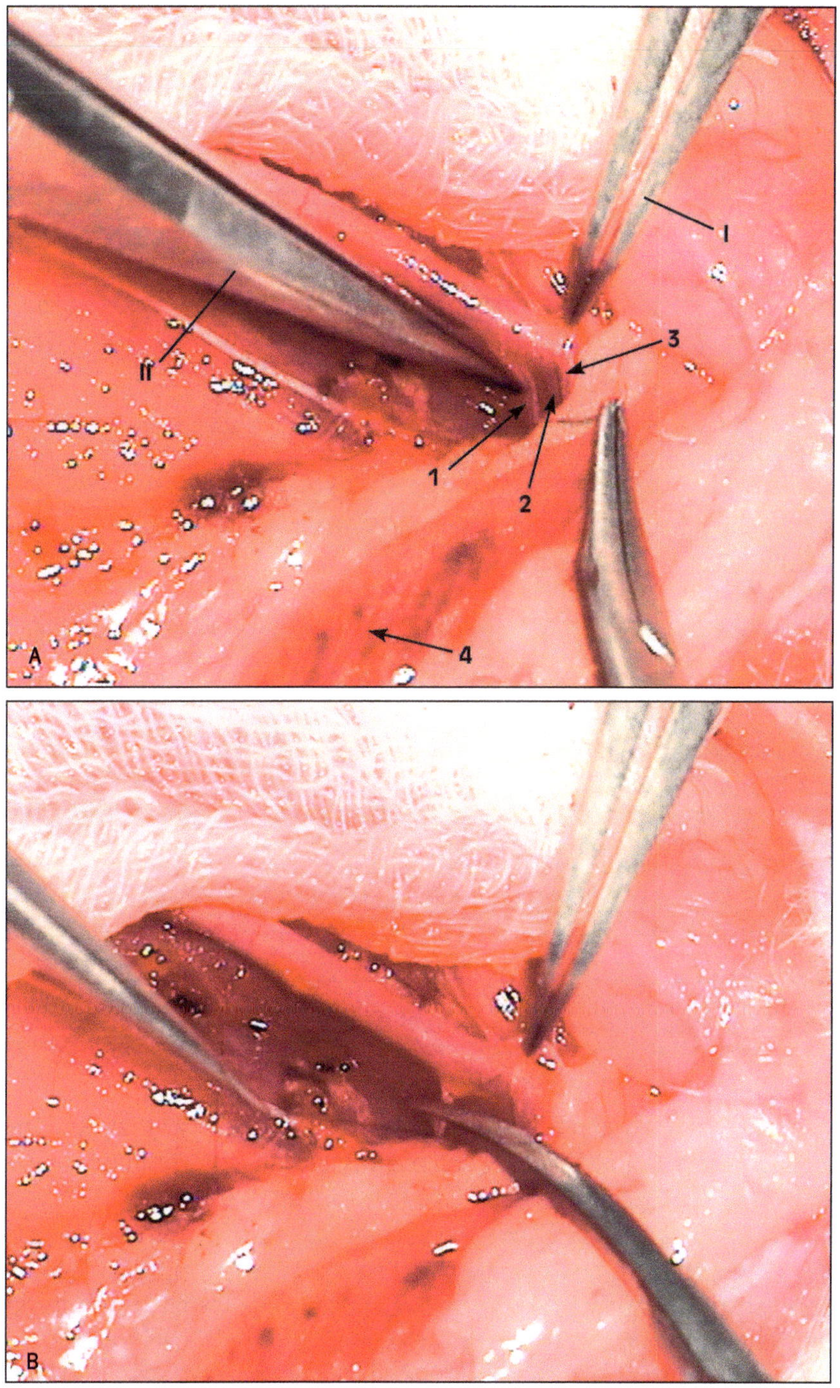

Figure 29-6

Dissection and transection between two ligations of the posterior parietal branch of the common iliac artery. **A.** The Dumont No. 3 forceps (marked I) picks up the common iliac artery just above the origin of the artery of the uterine horn, resulting in a posterior deviation of the latter. The Dumont No. 5 forceps (marked II) grasps the posterior parietal branch from its adventitia. The needle holder is loaded with 9/0 suture, ready to pass the needle around this branch. **B.** The two forceps pull the ends of the suture ligating the posterior parietal branch, which have been left long, and the scissors transect the branch. **1.** posterior parietal branch, **2.** internal iliac artery, **3.** artery of the uterine horn, **4.** small vertical arterial branches and vein tributaries to/from the uterine horn in the mesometrium. (From author's photo library)

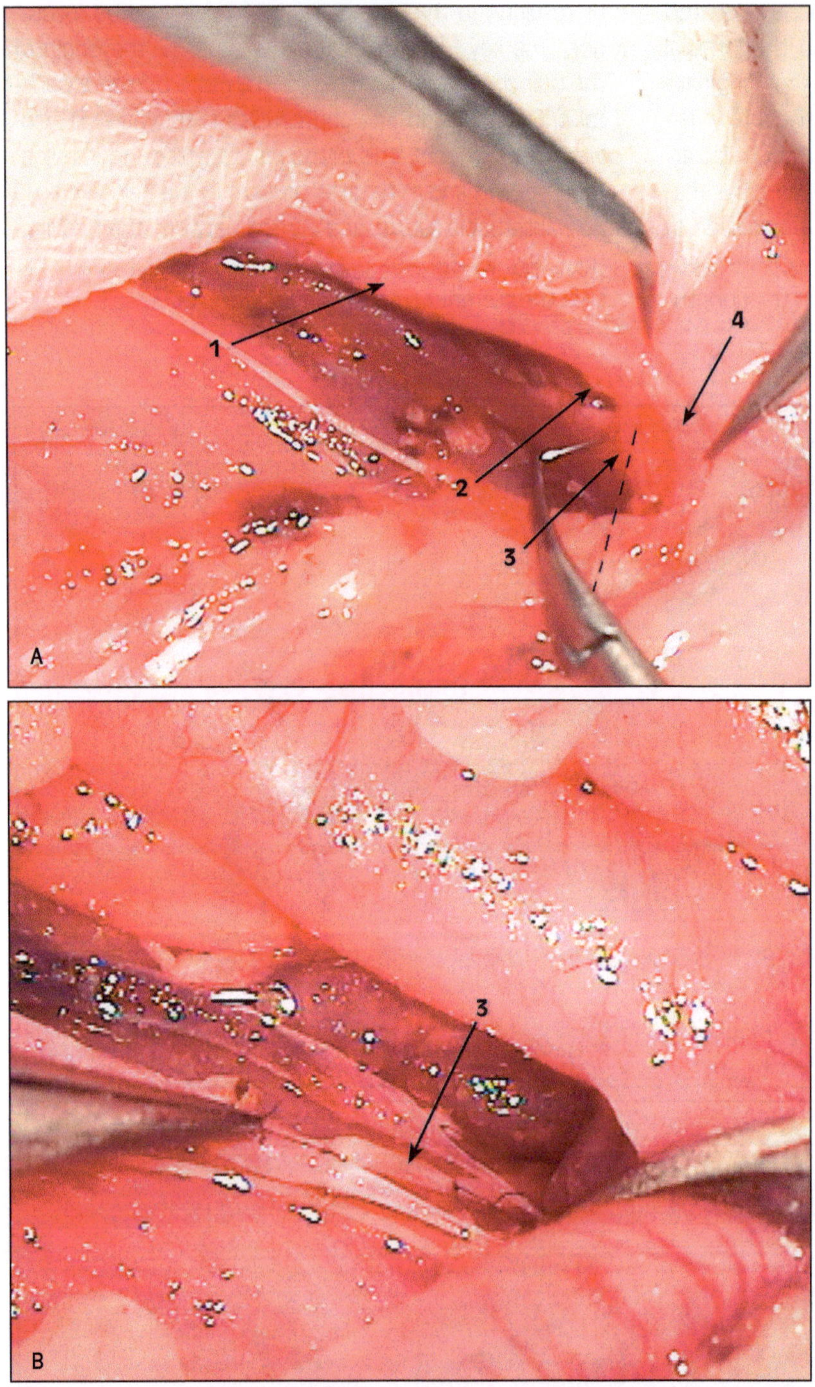

Figure 29-7

Double ligation of the internal iliac artery. **A.** The curved microsurgical forceps elevates the common iliac artery by grasping it just cranial to the origin of the artery of the uterine horn. The Dumont No. 3 forceps holds the mesometrium, where the artery of the uterine horn enters. The needle holder grasps the needle of the 9/0 suture surrounding the internal iliac artery in order to place the proximal ligation (the suture here is highlighted with a dashed line). **B.** The suture of the proximal ligation of the internal iliac artery has been turned toward the pelvis and is pulled towards the abdomen with a Dumont No. 3 forceps. The distal ligation has been placed from the side of the pelvis. **1.** common iliac artery, **2.** stump of the transected posterior parietal branch, **3.** internal iliac artery, **4.** artery of the uterine horn. (From author's photo library)

Running caudally along the posterior surface of the common iliac artery, the *internal iliac artery* is encountered next. As expected, it is much greater in caliber than the posterior parietal branch and courses posteromedially towards the pelvis. By gently lifting the common iliac artery, the internal iliac artery can be dissected bluntly with microsurgical scissors and the proximal ligation (9/0 suture) can be placed close to its origin (**Fig. 29-7A**). The distal ligation can be placed similarly by lifting the common iliac artery, but care should be taken to place the knot deep in the pelvis. Another technique that can be used to achieve this is to turn the proximal ligation toward the pelvis, place traction on it, and follow the course of the internal iliac artery into the pelvis where the distal ligation should be placed (**Fig. 29-7B**). Using this technique prevents having to work in

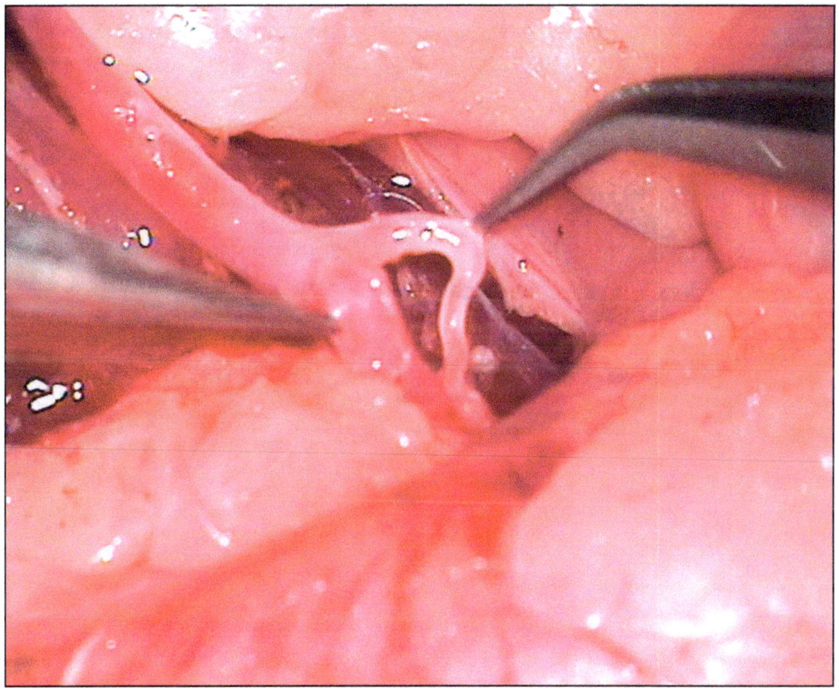

Figure 29-8

Completed dissection of the artery of the uterine horn (held by curved microsurgical forceps) and of the external iliac artery (held by Dumont No. 3 forceps). (From author's photo library)

a deep plane under the common iliac artery and also ensures certainty in correctly identifying the distal internal iliac artery.

Following ligation and division of the internal iliac artery, *the artery of the uterine horn* should be dissected distally until the artery enters the mesometrium of the uterine horn, if possible. The *external iliac artery* should also be dissected distally enough to allow for the ligation and division that will follow (**Fig. 29-8**).

Note that at this stage, the external iliac artery should be dissected only and not ligated. Otherwise, the artery of the uterine horn will be left alone to supply the horn during all the manipulations of the dissections that will follow. Ligation of the external iliac vessels (artery and vein) will be performed subsequently, as described below.

Learning from our mistakes

During the dissection described above, we are confronted with a tripod-like configuration when the common iliac artery is elevated and its three branches (posterior parietal branch, internal iliac artery, and artery of the uterine horn) are exposed (**Fig. 29-6A**). The common iliac artery continues distally as the external iliac artery after the origin of these three branches. Due to the change in relative position of the branches that can occur based on where tension is placed on the common iliac artery or which branch is transected first, mistakes can certainly be made. Here are some examples:

A. In **Figure 29-9**, all of the important branches of the common iliac artery (internal iliac artery, artery of the uterine horn, and external iliac artery) were mistakenly ligated and divided. This mistake ends the operation.
B. In **Figure 29-10** the artery of the uterine horn was mistakenly ligated and divided, again forcing the operation to be prematurely ended.
C. In **Figure 29-11** the external iliac artery has been ligated and transected, and the internal iliac artery is being ligated. If this artery is also double-ligated and transected, the only remaining blood supply to the uterine horn (the artery of the uterine horn) will be at risk during the distal dissection of this artery as well the dissection of the internal iliac vein and its tributaries.

These mistakes happened because the trainee failed to correctly identify all four branches of the common iliac artery before proceeding with double-ligation and division. Such errors show that these branches must be fully dissected and identified before performing any double-ligation and transection of them.

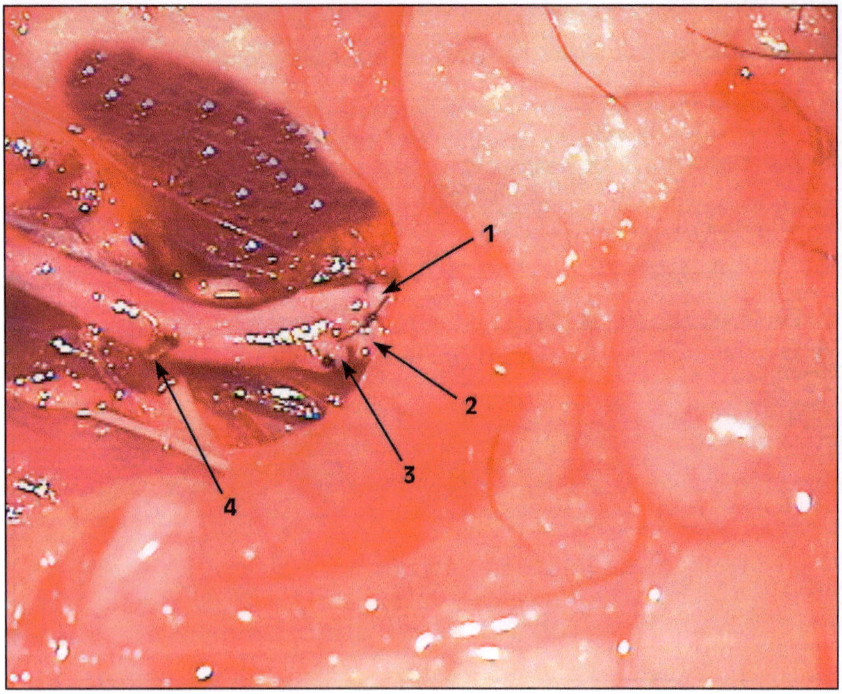

Figure 29-9

Incorrect dissection: all the important branches of the common iliac artery have been ligated and transected. One has to guess in order to name the branches seen in the photo. No. **1** is most likely the stump of the artery of the uterine horn; No. **2** is the stump of the external iliac artery; No. **3** is probably the stump of the internal iliac artery: the size is appropriate, but not the position (found laterally and not medially, as it should). The common iliac artery has most likely rotated medially around its long axis, as indicated by the lateral position of a cauterized posterior parietal branch (**4**), which also explains the position of the internal iliac artery. This parietal branch is located too cranially from the other three branches to be the posterior parietal branch that is a part of the dissection of 'the four branches' (see text). The posterior parietal branch is thus not seen in the picture. (From author's photo library)

3. Common iliac vein

The common iliac vein is expected to have the following tributaries:

- **Internal iliac vein**
- **External iliac vein**
- **Vein of the horn of the uterus**

Note that just three tributary veins are listed for the common iliac vein, as opposed to the four branches that originate from the common iliac artery. This is because it is not certain that a tributary vein corresponding to the posterior parietal branch exists as a standard finding behind the 'trifurcation' of the common iliac arte-

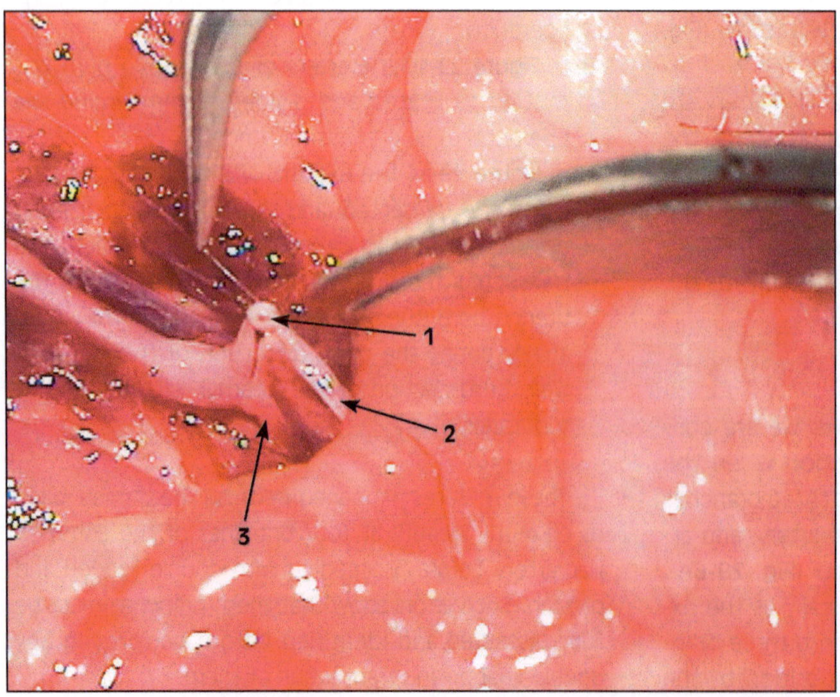

Figure 29-10

Incorrect dissection: ligation and transection of the artery of the uterine horn. The curved microsurgical forceps holds the suture of the proximal ligation, and the scissors have just cut the artery. **1.** stump of the artery of the uterine horn. **2.** external iliac artery, **3.** internal iliac artery. (From author's photo library)

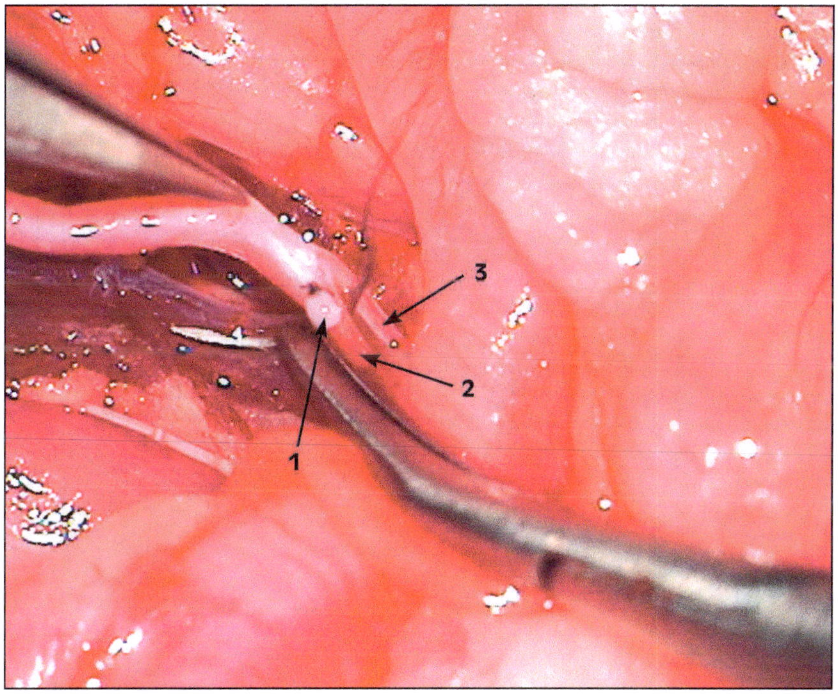

Figure 29-11

Incorrect dissection: ligation of the internal iliac artery after the external iliac artery has been ligated and transected. The forceps lifts the common iliac artery and the needle holder passes the needle under the internal iliac artery for placement of the ligation. With elevation, the common iliac artery has rotated medially around its longitudinal axis; thus, the stump of the internal iliac artery is found lateral and the artery of the right uterine horn has rotated medially. **1.** stump of the external iliac artery, **2.** internal iliac artery, **3.** artery of the right uterine horn. (From author's photo library)

ry. On rare occasions, more that one small posterior parietal tributaries may be found given the unpredictable pattern of veins in the pelvis.

The internal iliac vein is subject to significant amount of variation. In human anatomy, it is established that this vessel does not have a standard pattern of tributary veins. In the rat, the variation of pelvic veins is more pronounced, and even the three tributaries of the common iliac vein may vary. To avoid mistakes, the surgeon should identify every tributary vein during dissection before proceeding to any additional steps.

The common iliac vein and its tributaries are greater in diameter than their respective arteries. Within the surgical field, these veins are found posteromedially to their respective arteries. This relation complicates the dissection as it necessitates working underneath the arteries. In addition, the vein walls are fragile and do not tolerate elevating maneuvers as well as arteries.

To dissect the common iliac vein, the surgeon should handle it in the same way as the inferior vena cava. As an example, the surgeon may, cauterize a parietal tributary vein and use the stump to elevate the common iliac vein in order to develop the plane under its posterior surface. Pay attention to parietal tributary veins, as they may not follow the respective parietal arterial branches.

The common iliac vein should be dissected proximally to distally until the surgeon is near the area of the confluence of the internal iliac vein and the vein of the uterine horn. At this point, the surgeon should move distally along the internal iliac vein and work in a proximal direction along this vessel (as recommended above for the distal ligation of the internal iliac artery). The proximal (cranial) portion of the internal iliac vein allows adequate free space between where it accepts its last tributary and where it enters the common iliac vein. In this space, the surgeon may comfortably dissect, double-ligate and divide in between the internal iliac vein (**Fig. 29-12**). A piece of practical advice at this point is to withdraw the microsurgical scissors that were used to perform the dissection of the posterior surface of the vein, place in the same plane the needle holder carrying the tail of the suture (not the needle), grasp the suture tail with a forceps, and make the peripheral knot at the bottom of the plane developed by the scissors first. Do not advance the suture distally past this point—the tributaries of the internal iliac vein are unpredictable and at risk of trauma if encountered unexpectedly. The proximal ligation of the internal iliac vein should be placed as close as possible to the confluence with the common iliac vein.

Grasping the stump of the internal iliac vein, the surgeon can slightly lift the common iliac vein and ro-

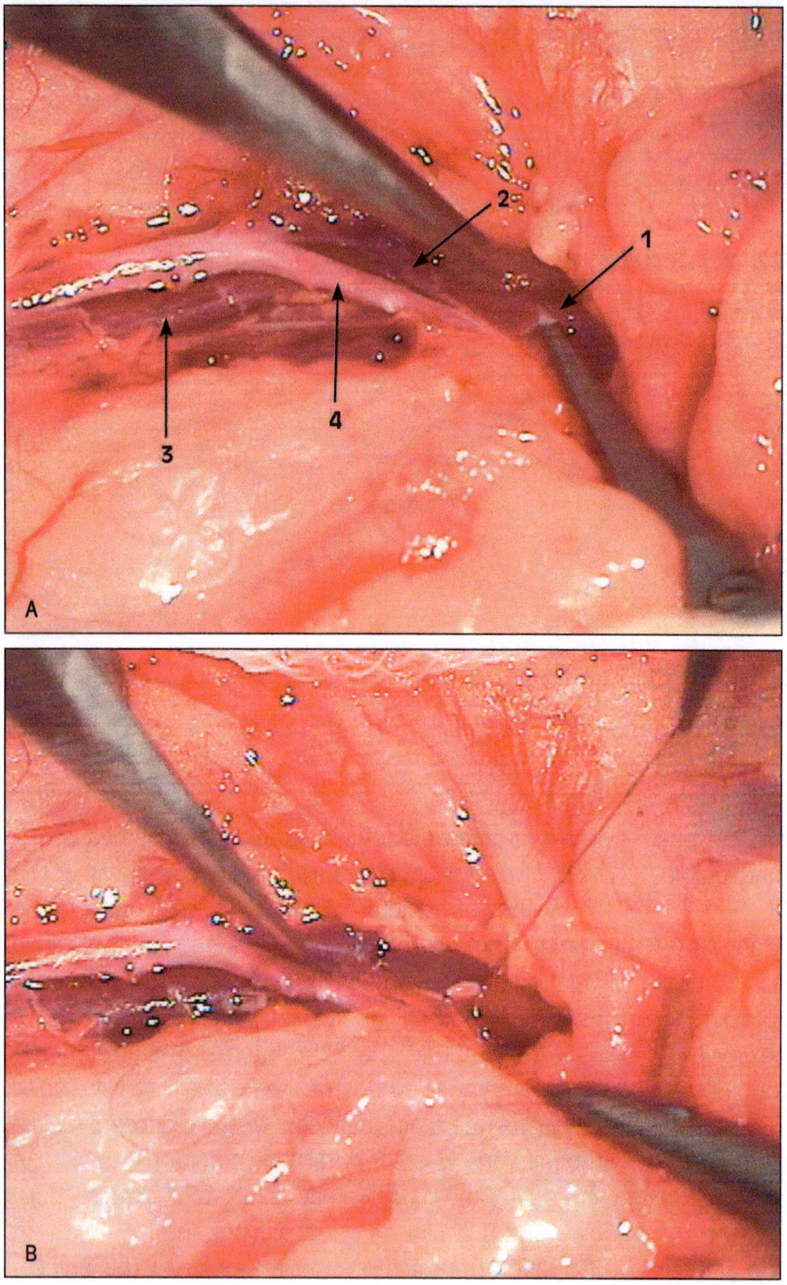

Figure 29-12

Dissection and ligation of the internal iliac vein. **A.** Blunt dissection: the closed microsurgical scissors pass under the internal iliac vein before its confluence with the common iliac vein. **B.** Two ligations have been placed on the vein (the distal first) – the sutures have been left long and are held by the two forceps. The vein is going to be transected between the ligations with the scissors brought in the field. **1.** internal iliac vein, **2.** common iliac vein, **3.** inferior vena cava, **4.** common iliac artery (From author's photo library)

tate it laterally. The common iliac vein can also be rotated medially by lifting the stump of a cauterized parietal tributary vein found posterolaterally. Thus, the surgeon may inspect the posterior surface of the common iliac vein for any tributaries from the confluence with the contralateral common iliac vein to the entrance of the vein of the uterine horn. If any tributaries are found, they should be cauterized or ligated and divided, depending on their size and location.

Working in this way and advancing caudally, the surgeon will reach the exit of the vein of the uterine horn, which should be found on the anterior surface of the common iliac vein. Here, the pattern of the common iliac vein is the same with the homonymous artery; the artery and vein of the uterine horn course in parallel, from their origin/confluence to the point of entrance in the mesometrium of the horn (**Fig. 29-13**).

As the dissection of the vessels of the uterine horn and the external iliac vessels is continued, the surgeon will see that the vein of the horn (which initially looked

Figure 29-13

Dissected right common iliac vessels and vessels of the uterine horn. Here, the s-traight microsurgical forceps moves the body and right horn of the uterus, and the curved forceps (mosquito) points at the vein of the horn. Observe the parallel course of the vessels of the horn from their origin/conflunce at/with the anterior surface of the common iliac vessels until their entrance in the mesometrium of the horn. Their length seems short here, but will increase with further dissection. (From author's photo library)

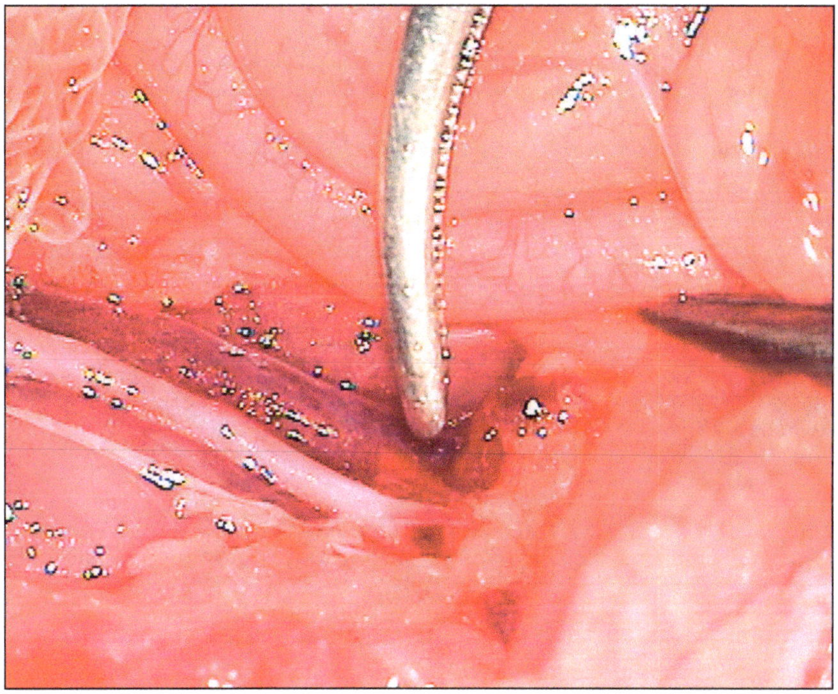

about the same length as the artery) is shorter than the artery. The vein of the horn enters the common iliac vein a few millimeters inferiorly of where the artery takes off from the common iliac artery (**Fig. 29-14**, compare with **Figure 29-13**). Be cognizant of the dissection boundary set by the vein of the uterine horn, i.e. do not try to dissect a length that is equal to the artery of the uterine horn.

Learning from our mistakes

In **Figure 29-15**, the gross mistake of ligating the common iliac vein cranial to the confluence of the tributary

Figure 29-14

View of the surgical field after dissection of the right common and external iliac vessels. The vessels of the right horn of the uterus are partially dissected. Observe that the confluence of the vein of the horn with the common iliac vein is found caudally to the origin of the artery of the horn from the common iliac artery. **1.** right common iliac artery, **2.** right common iliac vein, **3.** right external iliac artery, **4.** artery of the right horn of the uterus, **5.** vein of the right horn of the uterus, **6.** left horn of the uterus, **7.** right horn of the uterus, **8.** urinary bladder, **9.** rectum moved to the left. (From author's photo library)

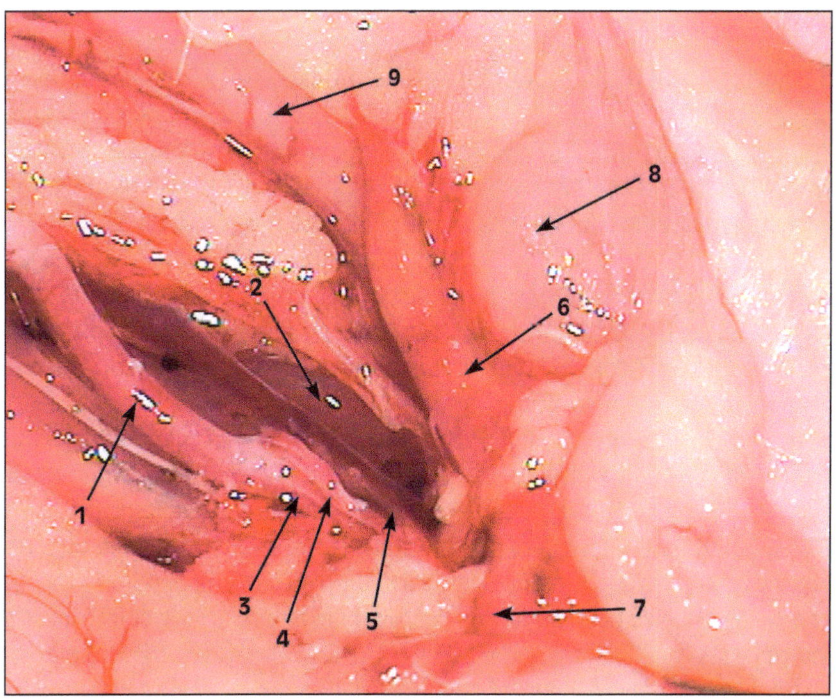

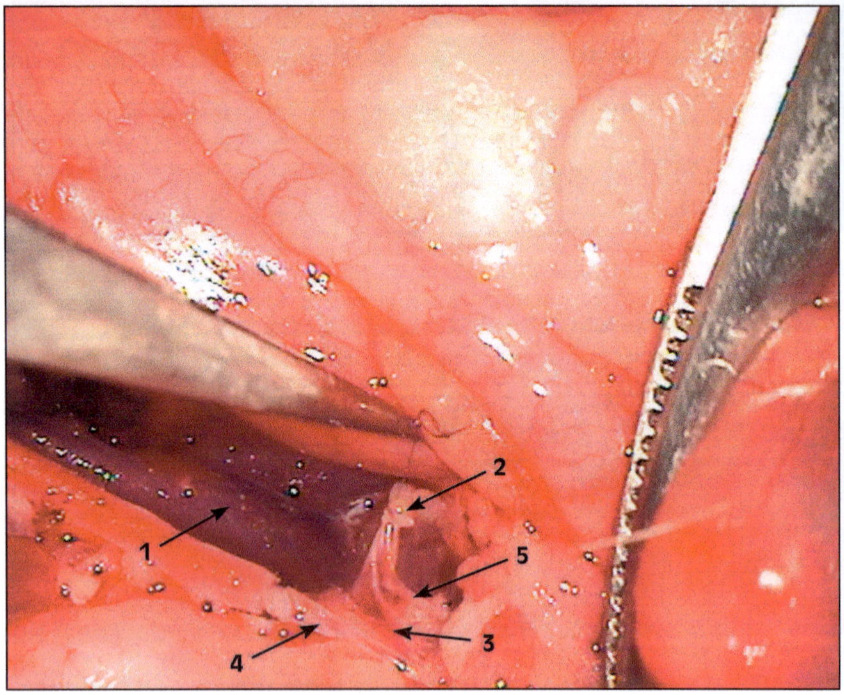

Figure 29-15

Incorrect dissection: obstruction and posterior anchoring of the common iliac vein and premature ligation and transection of the external iliac vein. It is evident that a ligation has been incorrectly placed, obstructing the common iliac vein just cranial to the confluence of the tributaries and also catching the posterior pelvic wall, causing the vein to 'anchor'. Filling of the common iliac vein is mostly retrograde, as indicated by the fullness of the caudal part of the vein (just above the confluence of the tributaries) when compared to the less-filled portion cranially. The tributary veins appear empty due to the tension created between the posterior anchoring of the common iliac vein and the suture of the stump of the external iliac vein elevated by the forceps. **1.** common iliac vein, **2.** external iliac vein, **3.** vein of the uterine horn, **4.** artery of the uterine horn, **5.** internal ilaic vein. (From author's photo library)

veins is shown. The suture of the ligation also seems to anchor the common iliac vein on the posterior pelvic wall. Additionally, the external iliac vein has been prematurely ligated and divided (instead of the internal iliac vein). The operation was terminated at the stage of dissection.

4. Ligation and division of the external iliac vessels

Following the dissection of the common iliac vessels, the vessels of the uterine horn and the external iliac vessels should remain intact. It is at this point that the external iliac vessels will be ligated and divided distally from the origin/confluence of the vessels of the uterine horn. First, the external iliac artery should be divided between two ligations (9/0), as it is lateral and superficial to the external iliac vein, thus being readily accessible (**Fig. 29-16**). Division of the external iliac artery permits a better view of the external iliac vein, which can then be double-ligated and divided (**Fig. 29-17**). As is the case with all veins, the distal ligation should be placed before the proximal ligation, which should go as close as possible to the exit of the external iliac vein.

After ligation and division of the external iliac vessels, rigorously inspect the pelvis for any bleeding. As stated before, the pattern of the tributaries of the common and internal iliac veins is not completely predictable, and the possibility exists that one of the tributary veins may have been inadvertently damaged. Any bleeding from very small vessels can be controlled by careful cauterization under direct visualization (**Fig. 29-18**). Be cautious not to inadvertently damage any surrounding contents of the pelvis or any vessel, especially veins. Also check the entrance of the vessels of the uterine horn into the mesometrium. The first branches/tributaries of the vessels of the uterine horn are found in this area (No. 4, **Fig. 29-6A**). These do have a risk of rupturing and can be cauterized to a limited extent with attention, taking care not to harm the vascularization of the horn (**Fig. 29-18**).

Consequences of transection of the branches of the iliac vessel

It is normal to wonder what the effects of transecting the iliac vessels are. Let us examine the arteries first:

- Transection of a parietal branch of the common iliac artery is of no significance due to the collateral circulation provided by overlapping branches addres-

Figure 29-16

Proximal ligation of the right external iliac artery. The knot is placed immediately caudal to the origin of the artery of the right horn of the uterus. Observe the position of the common iliac vein as the artery is elevated. **1.** common iliac artery, **2.** artery of the right uterine horn, **3.** external iliac artery, **4.** common iliac vein. (From author's photo library)

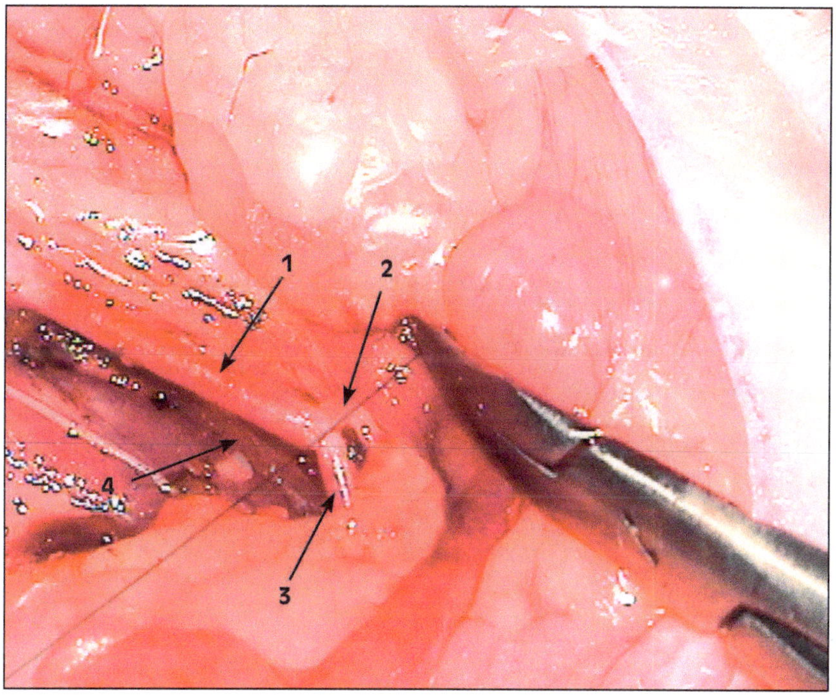

sed to the muscles of the posterior abdomino-pelvic wall.

- Transection of the internal iliac artery has no dramatic consequences either because of the overlap with branches from the contralateral side, which will take over supply for the pelvis and perineum.

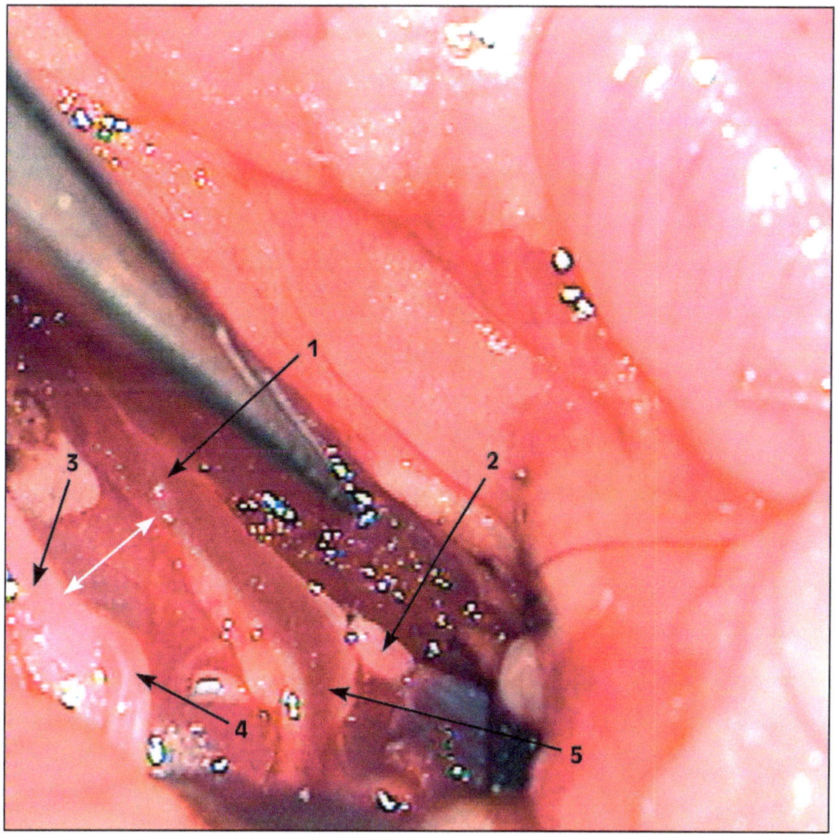

Figure 29-17

Ligations of the external iliac vein prior to transection. Note the adipose tissue left purposefully on the common iliac vein for easy handling. Also, observe the movement of the common iliac artery after transection of the external iliac artery (white bidirectional arrow). **1.** common iliac vein, **2.** double-ligated external iliac vein, **3.** common iliac artery, **4.** artery of the right uterine horn. **5.** vein of the right uterine horn. (From author's photo library)

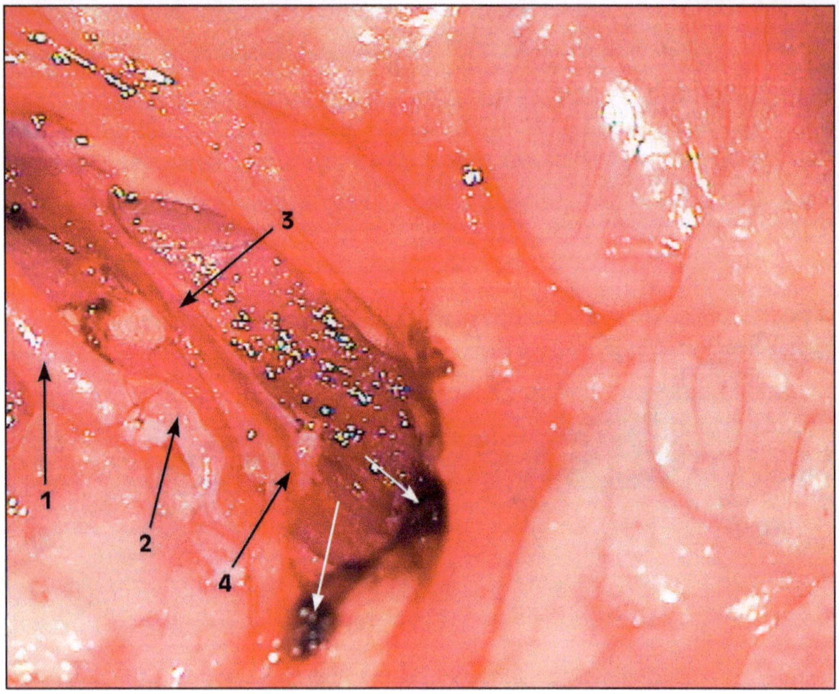

Figure 29-18

View of the surgical field after ligation and transection of the external iliac vessels. Following this, the relative sizes of the vessels have been reversed, with the artery being now of greater caliber than the vein. Observe the sites of cauterization for microhemorrhages in the pelvis (short white arrow) and in the uterine horn, near the entrance of the vessels in the mesometrium of the horn, which most likely involve the first vertical branches of the vessels of the horn (long white arrow). **1.** common iliac artery, **2.** artery of the uterine horn, **3.** common iliac vein, **4.** vein of the uterine horn. (From author's photo library)

- Amazingly, transection of the external iliac artery, as explained in Chapter 15, is compensated by collateral circulation and does not threaten the posterior limb.

The veins have a greater capacity for collateral circulation, especially in the pelvis, where many vein plexuses exist around the viscera.

D. Transection of the common iliac vessels

A yellow plastic background is placed under the common iliac vessels. The double clamp is brought in the field and placed with its basis on the left border of the opened abdominal wall, so that the legs of the clamps point to the right horn of the uterus. The common iliac vessels, have been dissected at this point of the operation and are attached proximally at the bifurcation of the aorta/inferior vena and distally at the entrance to the mesometrium of the uterine horn, and have thus obtained a great degree of freedom. Attention should be paid when placed in the jaws of the clamps to ensure the artery is placed on the lateral side and vein on the medial side (**Fig. 29-19A**). We emphasize this because we have commonly seen the vessels being wrongly positioned with the vein on the lateral side and the artery on the medial side (**Fig. 29-19B**). This should be avoided because the tension on the right common iliac vein, due to the weight of the double clamp and the torsion of the vein, can be transferred to the contralateral iliac vein and its fragile posterior tributaries. Additionally, in this reverse position, there will be greater tension on the subsequent vein anastomosis than in the normal position.

The common iliac vessels are transected midway between the two clamps, and their lumens are irrigated with warm normal saline through a 27G angiocatheter (**Fig. 29-20**).

Following this, the adventitia should be folded at the edges of the stumps of the artery (**Fig. 29-21**) and removed circumferentially from the edges of the vein stumps. The two clamps approach each other and the vessel stumps are ready for anastomoses.

E. End-to-end anastomoses

The technique of the end-to-end anastomoses is presented in detail in Chapter 5.

In autotransplantation of the uterine horn-fallopian tube-ovary, the anastomoses will be performed in the common iliac vessels.

Note that in the normal flow of the operation, the gonadal vessels and vessels of the uterine horn are transected before the anastomosis of the common iliac

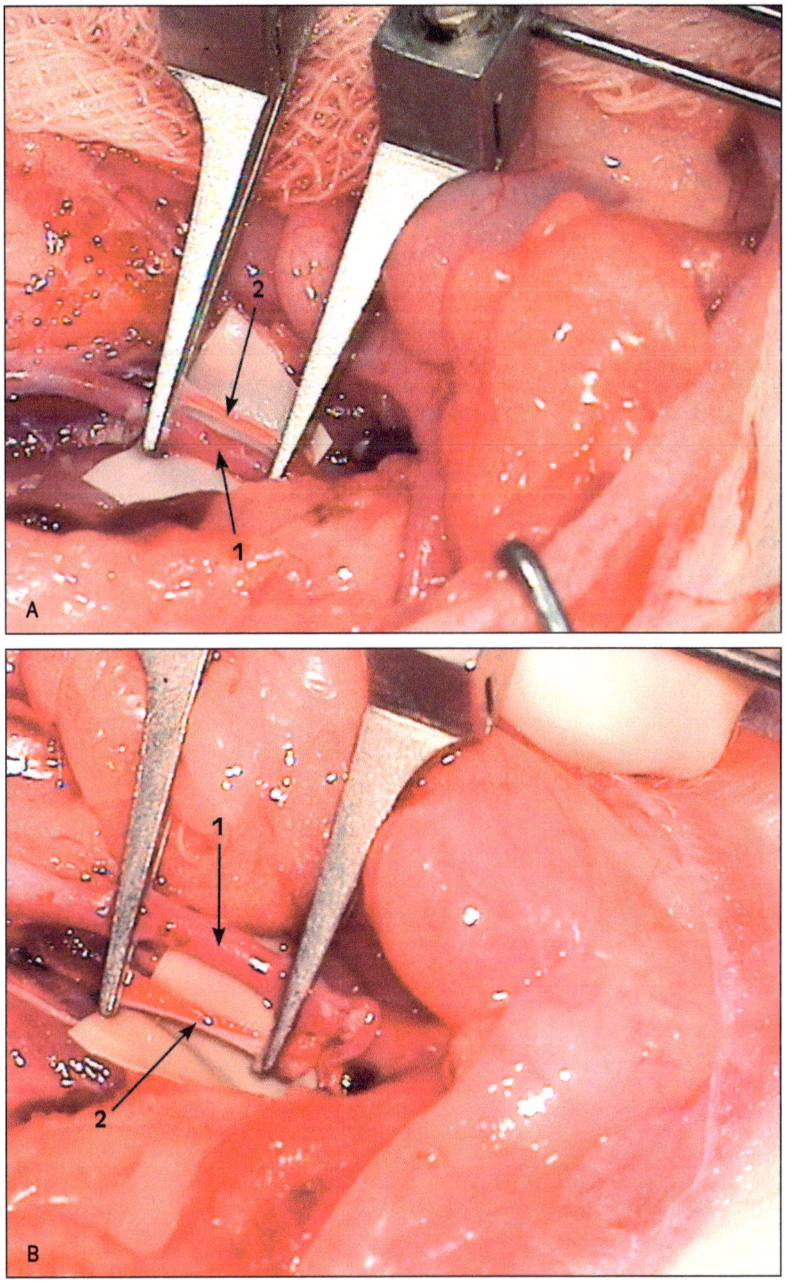

Figure 29-19

Placement of the common iliac vessels in the double clamp. **A.** Correct positioning: artery lateral, vein medial. **B.** Incorrect reverse positioning, which is harmful for the vein because of the tension exerted by the double clamp. **1.** right common iliac artery, **2.** right common iliac vein. (From author's photo library)

vessels. Here the division of these vessels follow the anastomoses of the common iliac vessels (see sections F and G below). In addition, the graft is not removed and repositioned (as should be done in a full-scale operation), but rather the anastomoses are presented in situ while the common iliac vessels are placed in the double clamp.

The following number of sutures are placed:

- **Artery: 8 sutures 10/0**
- **Vein: 8 or 10 sutures 10/0**

The two end-to-end anastomoses of the common iliac artery and vein are performed simultaneously. The anterior surfaces of both vessels are sutured first. The clamp is then rotated, and the posterior surfaces are sutured.

Suturing starts by completing the anterior surface of one vessel and then of the other. It is advised to begin by placing the corner sutures on both vessels first

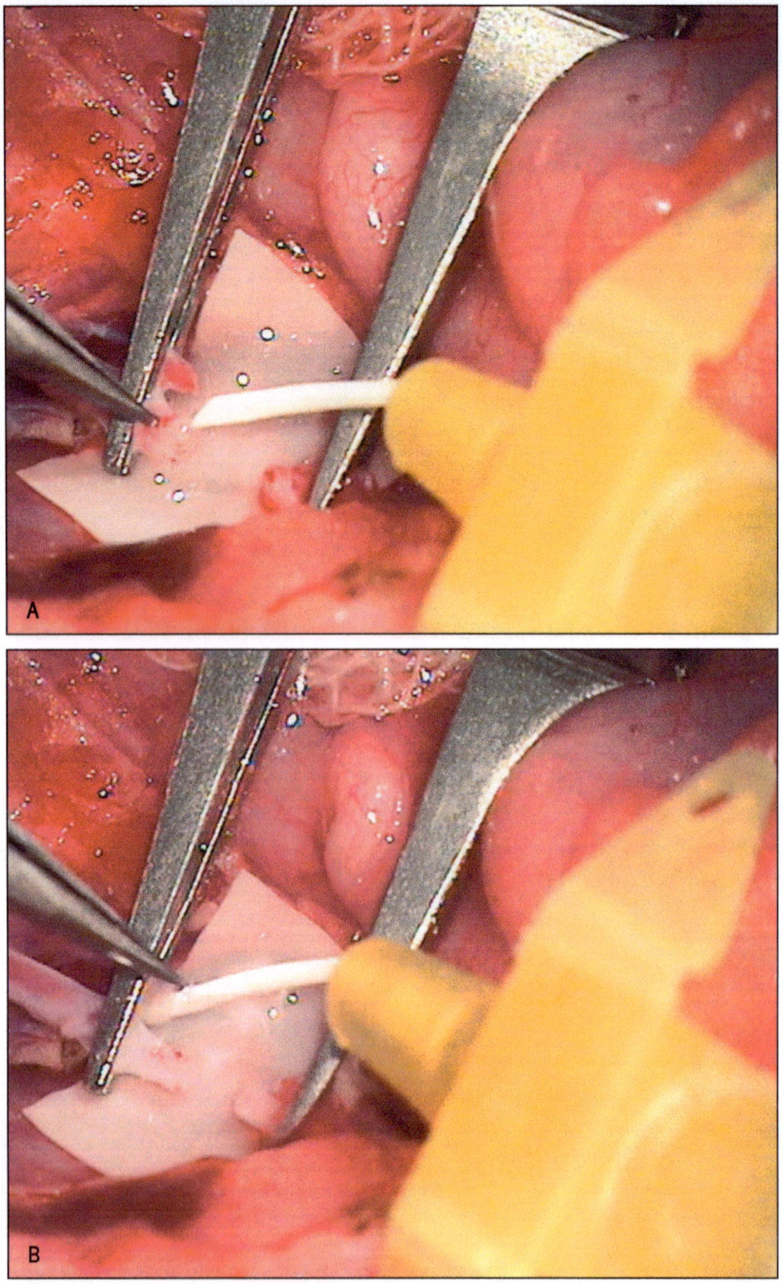

Figure 29-20

Irrigation of the lumens of the common iliac vessels after transection. **A.** The Dumont No. 3 forceps holds the arterial wall while a 27G angiocatheter irrigates the lumen with warm normal saline. **B.** The same forceps holds the vein wall and the catheter enters the lumen and irrigates the vein with attention given not to traumatize the endothelium. (From author's photo library)

to correctly orient them. Here, it might be more comfortable to start with the vein because it is found medial to the artery in the double clamp (**Fig. 29-22**). This is a deviation from prior operations where we have usually started various steps with the artery.

The steps of the end-to-end anastomoses of the common iliac vessels are the following:

1. In the vein, if 10 sutures are needed (this is the usual number of required sutures), the first 2 should be placed as corner sutures. Next, 4 sutures are placed at an equal distance apart on the anterior surface, and the remaining 4 sutures are placed on the posterior surface; on both surfaces, suture placement advances from the corner sutures towards the middle of the semicircle. If 8 sutures are needed (vein or artery), then 3 are placed in the anterior surface and 3 in the posterior, respectively, in addition to the 2 corner sutures; on both surfaces, these 3 are placed 1 in the middle of the semicircle and 1 in the middle of each quadrant.
2. Rotation of the double clamp, and check of the sutures along the anterior surfaces of the anastomoses.

Figure 29-21

The Dumont No. 3 forceps holds the wall of the artery, and the curved forceps inverts the adventitia. Note the incorrect positioning of the vessels in the clamp (artery—medial, vein—lateral). (From author's photo library)

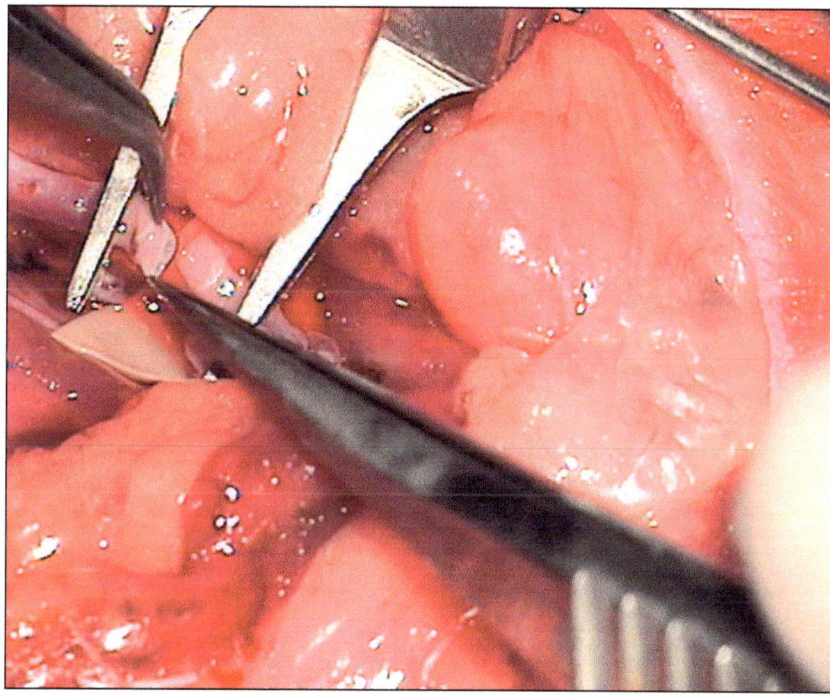

3. Completion of the posterior surfaces of the anastomoses of the vein and artery in the same way as the anterior surface (**Fig. 29-23**).
4. Release of the vessels from the double clamp. We have stated before that the immediate filing of the vessel past the anastomosis (according to blood flow) is indicative of patency. Notably, this observation should not replace the test for patency. In **Figure 29-24**, according to this criterion, the anastomosis of the common iliac artery appears successful.
5. Placement of a wet gauze on the anastomoses for 3 minutes.
6. Patency test is performed, separate for each vessel. The usual patency test is described in detail in Chapter 5 (**Fig. 5-4**). Testing occurs following the flow

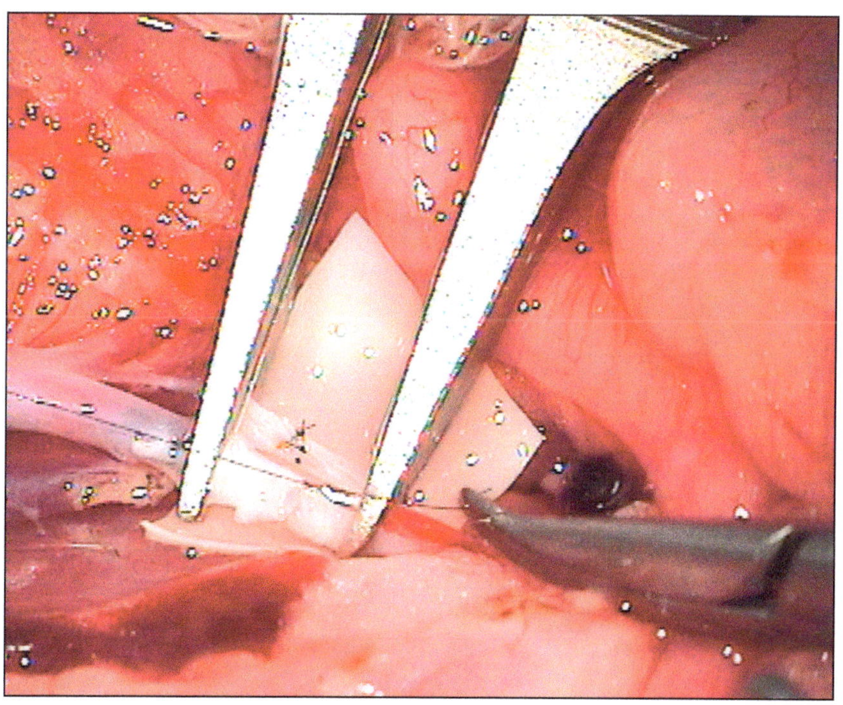

Figure 29-22

Suturing of the anterior surfaces of the common iliac vessels in autotransplantation of the right uterine horn-fallopian tube-ovary. Here, suturing of the anterior surface of the vein has been completed, and a '12 o'clock' corner suture is now being placed on the artery. (From author's photo library)

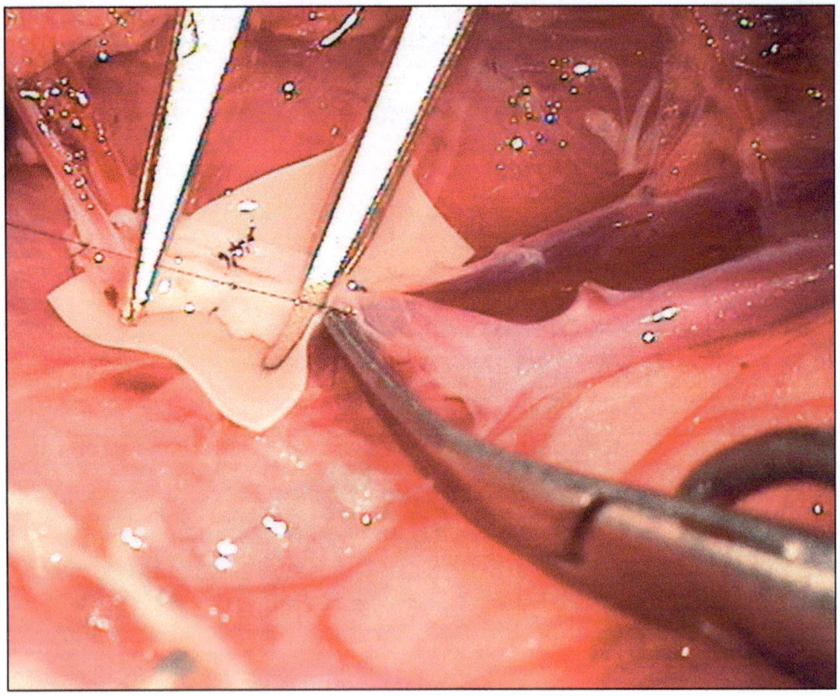

Figure 29-23

Suturing of the posterior surfaces of the common iliac vessels in autotransplantation of the right uterine horn-fallopian tube-ovary. The photo has been taken from the left side of the rat. The double clamp has been rotated to right side of the rat. As can be seen, if the vessels of the uterine horn have been fully dissected up to their entrance in the mesometrium, there is enough space for rotation of the clamp. Here, suturing of the vein has been completed, and the middle suture is being placed in the posterior surface of the artery. (From author's photo library)

of blood: The arterial anastomosis is tested distal to the anastomosis and the venous anastomosis is tested proximal to the anastomosis. In brief, past the anastomosis (according to blood flow), one upstream forceps is used to occlude the blood flow, while a second forceps is placed initially next to the first forceps and then moves downstream while half-closed, thereby 'milking' the vessel, and finally remains closed. The upstream forceps is removed, and if there is patency, the vessel is immediately filled up to the downstream forceps.

We have previously presented a variant of the technique of the patency test that involves placing the upstream forceps before the anastomosis and moving the second forceps downstream over the anastomosis. The same steps are followed—the first

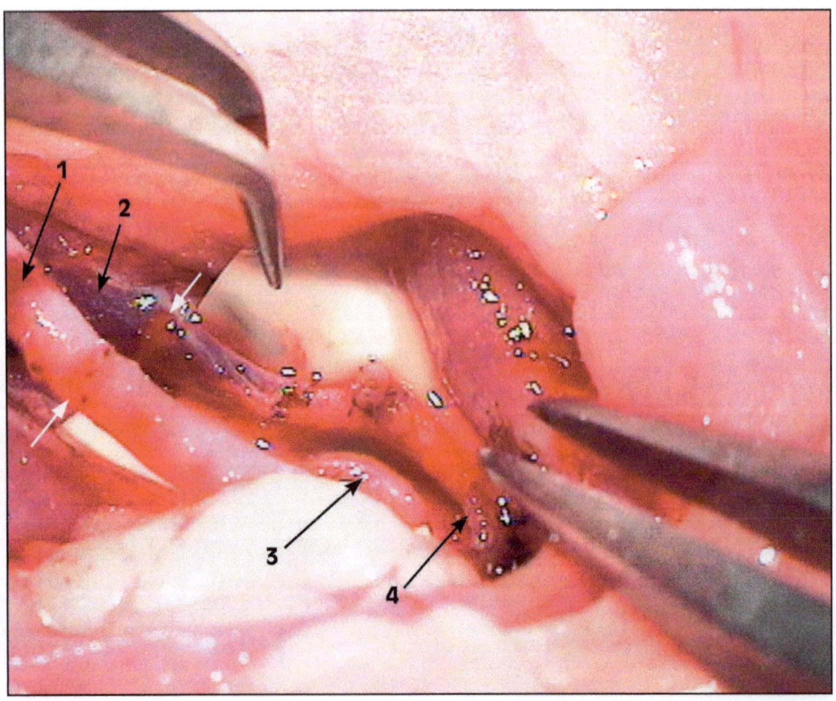

Figure 29-24

View of the anastomosed vessels after removal of the double clamp. The filling of the common iliac artery and artery of the uterine horn indicates that the arterial anastomosis is most likely patent. The anastomosis of the venous return from the uterine horn has not yet been completed (the forceps were freed immediately prior to the moment the photo was taken). Only the vein of the uterine horn can be seen full here. A large part of the common iliac vein is still empty, with the part that is full proximal to the anastomosis likely due to retrograde filling. The anastomoses are noted by white arrows. **1.** common iliac artery, **2.** common iliac vein, **3, 4.** artery and vein of the uterine horn. (From author's photo library) forceps is opened, and flow through the lumen up to the second forceps is observed if the anastomosis is patent. This variant has a disadvantage, however, in that the forceps is drawn over the anastomosis, a maneuver that generally requires experience to avoid damaging the anastomosis.

Here, we present another alternative that does not have this disadvantage. The two forceps are placed on the vessels on either side of the anastomosis. Along the artery (**Fig. 29-25**), one upstream forceps occludes the flow proximal to the anastomosis. A second forceps is applied distal to the anastomosis and is moved half-closed downstream for a short distance before being closed completely. This will place tension on the anastomosis, so it must be performed with caution. The first forceps should then be removed. If the anastomosis is patent, the lumen will immediately fill up to the second forceps. For the vein, the same test should be performed but with opposite positioning (proximal and distal) of the forceps. This variant does not empty the lumen completely as the previous techniques do. If the anastomosis is patent, however, filling of the lumen will be immediately evident. If there is any doubt, the classic test described in Chapter 5 should be attempted.

7. Withdrawal of the yellow plastic backround.

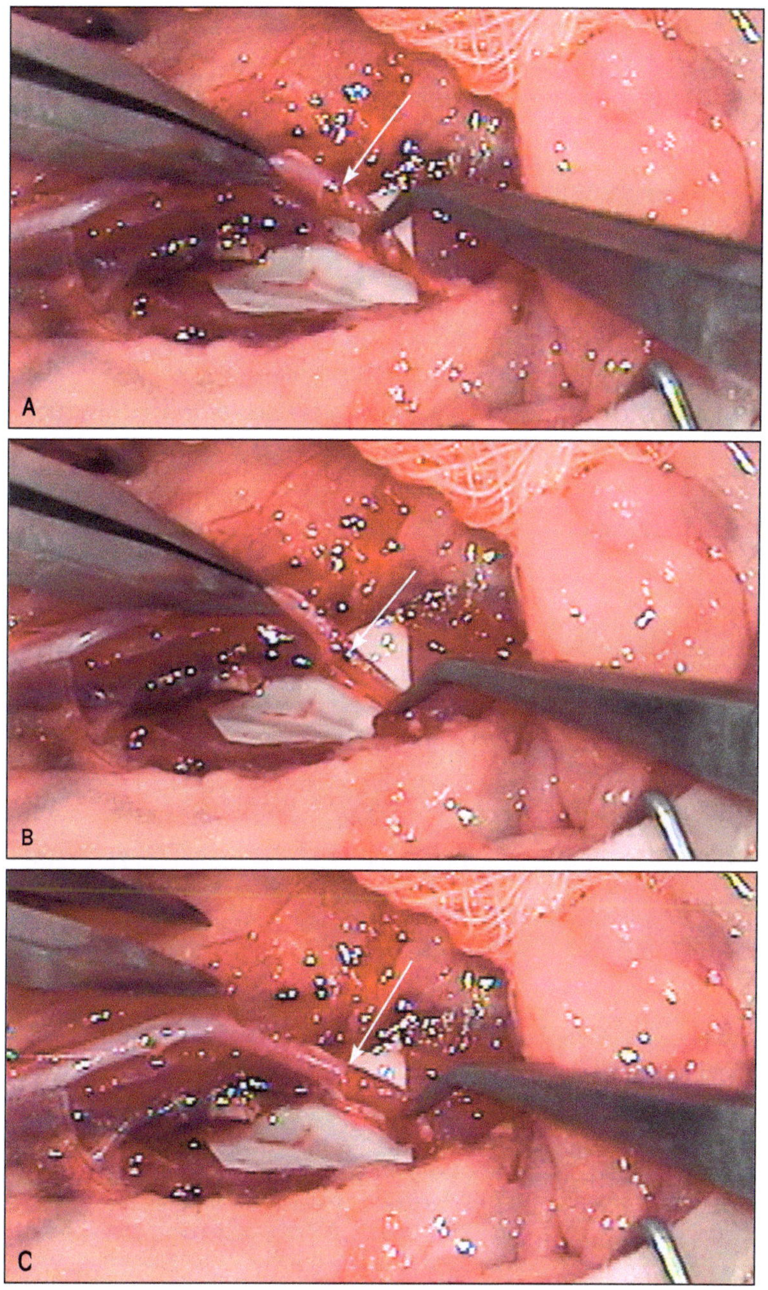

Figure 29-25

Alternative technique of patency testing of the anastomosis of the right common iliac. **A.** The Dumont No. 3 forceps occludes the flow upstream, proximal to the anastomosis, while the curved forceps is applied distal to the anastomosis. **B.** The curved forceps is moved downstream half-closed, partially emptying the lumen before the forceps is stopped and closed. **C.** The Dumont No. 3 forceps is removed. It is evident that the lumen is filled between the anastomosis and the curved forceps (observe the small leak from the anastomosis), indicating a patent anastomosis. The site of the anastomosis is marked with a white arrow. (From author's photo library)

F. Transection of the gonadal vessels

Normally, in the process of the autotransplantation of the uterine horn-fallopian tube-ovary, the transection of the gonadal vessels should follow the transection of the external iliac vessels (**Fig. 29-2**). Here, the transection of the gonadal vessels, and the transection and anastomosis of the uterine horn (see the next section), are left for the end of the operation.

The gonadal vessels will be found extraperitoneally, cranial to the ovary. The reader may not specifically recognize the suspensory ligament of the ovary in the rat (in which the gonadal vessels course), but this is of no significance. The important step is to recognize the gonadal vessels. The artery can be ligated and cut; for the vein, the reader must decide whether to place ligations or cauterize.

G. Transection and anastomosis of the uterine horn

In this Chapter, the transection of the uterine horn should be left until the end of the operation to avoid any hemorrhage. This is due to the fact that the blood supply to the horn comes not only from the vessels of the horn but also from anastomoses in the horn with the vessels of the body of the uterus. This is something that the surgeon becomes aware of while harvesting the uterine horn-fallopian tube-ovary en bloc for implantation.

The transection of the uterine horn is performed with the baby Metzenbaum scissors at the base of the horn. Attention must be paid to make the transection medial to the entrance of vessels into the mesometrium of the horn. Anastomosis of the uterine horn is done with 8 or 10 sutures 9/0 (**Fig. 29-26**).

H. Closure of the surgical trauma

The viscera are positioned back into the abdomen, and the abdominal wall is closed in two layers: the muscles with continuous suturing, and the subcutaneous tissue and skin with interrupted 2/0 non-absorbable sutures.

MOBILIZATION OF THE 'UTERINE HORN-FALLOPIAN TUBE-OVARY' COMPLEX

In the current operation, the 'uterine horn-fallopian

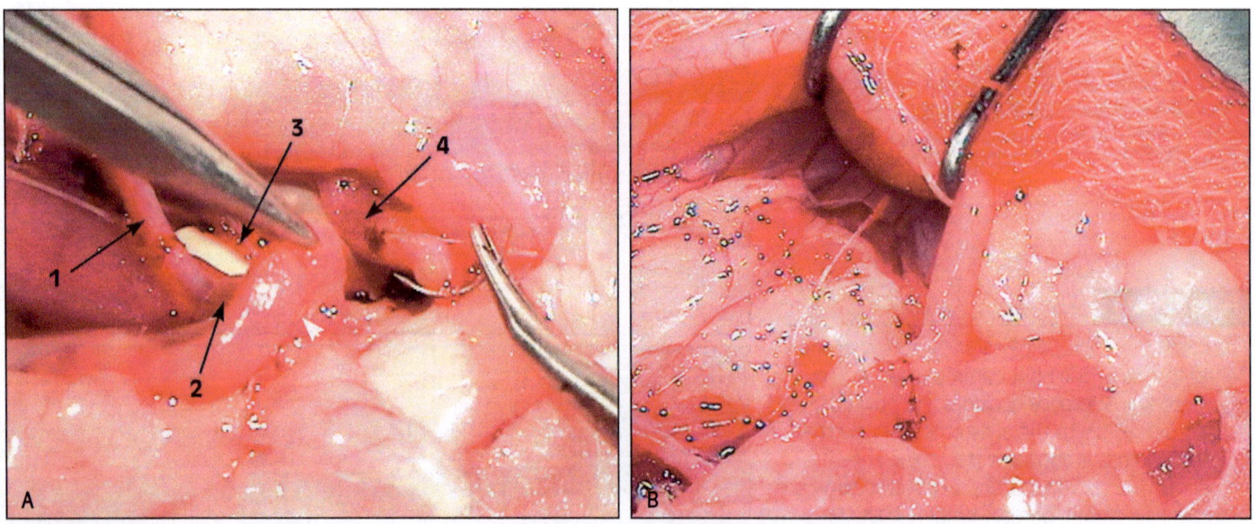

Figure 29-26

Anastomosis of the right uterine horn. **A.** The Dumont No. 3 forceps elevates the distal stump of the right uterine horn, while the needle—loaded in the needle holder—holds the proximal stump. Observe that the transection of the uterine horn has been performed medial to the entrance of the vessels in the mesometrium of the horn. The point of entrance is marked with a white arrowhead on the caudal surface of the mesometrium (note, however, that it is more evident in the cranial surface—see the course of the artery of the horn). **1.** common iliac artery, **2.** artery of the horn of the uterus, **3.** common iliac vein, **4.** body of the uterus. **B.** Completed anastomosis of the uterine horn. (From author's photo library) tube-ovary' complex was not mobilized and transferred; anastomosis of the common iliac vessels and uterine horn was performed in situ. To achieve a full mobilization in order to harvest the complex, the surgeon should transect the mesometrium caudal to the vessels of the uterine horn (**Fig. 29-27**). Understandably, the uterine horn has to be cut at its base and the mesometrium expanded by elevating the horn. The transection of the mesometrium will start from the level of transection of the uterine horn and should be extended cranially along the whole length of the horn; small hemorrhages should be cauterized. Thus, the vessels of the horn (together with the small vertical vessels) will be mobilized and moved en bloc with the uterine horn. A crucial error can happen here: if the transection of the mesometrium takes place between the vessels of the horn and the horn (which will transect the small vertical vessels), there will be no blood supply to the horn, with catastrophic consequences. This takes into account the fact that the gonadal vessels, which could contribute to supply the horn, have been transected.

The transection of the mesometrium will also free the fallopian tube that coils around the cranial part of the uterine horn. As for the ovary, one should remember that the ovary per se is not covered by peritoneum, but rather is connected to the posterior parietal peritoneum by the mesovarium, a double layer of peritoneum. The transection of the mesometrium is extended cranially to the mesovarium, while the ovary, which is quite fragile, is carefully elevated to extend the mesovarium. The incision is extended more cranially in the posterior peritoneum until it meets the point of the preceding transection of the suspensory ligament of the ovary (see F above). After all these maneuvers, the 'uterine horn-fallopian tube-ovary' complex is fully mobilized and connected only by the vessels of the uterine horn.

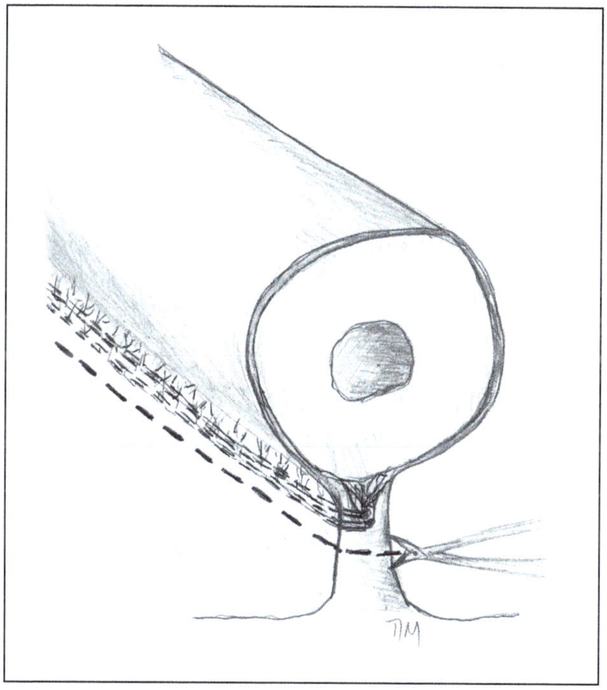

Figure 29-27

Transection of the mesometrium in order to mobilize the uterine horn. The mesometrium is defined as the double-layered peritoneum that contains the uterine horn and its vessels and is continuous with the parietal peritoneum of the posterior abdominal wall. The transection of the mesometrium must be done caudal to the vessels of the horn and is noted here with a bold dashed line. (Drawing by the author)

... of autotransplantation of the uterine horn-fallopian tube-ovary

Synopsis...

A. Positioning of the rat. Dorsal decubitus (supine) with the head on the left of the surgeon. The limbs are immobilized on the working surface with adhesive tape.

B. Preparation of the surgical field. Median incision from the xiphoid process to the pubic symphysis. Mobilization of the small intestine and placement of the intestines, wrapped in a wet gauze, to the left of the rat. Opening of the retroperitoneum, from the renal arteries to the pelvis, using two wet gauzes.

C. Microsurgical dissection

1. Dissection of common iliac vessels (starting from the aorta-inferior vena cava at the area of the bifurcation of the aorta).
2. Dissection of the four branches of the common iliac artery in the area of its bifurcation, in the following order: posterior parietal branch, internal iliac artery, artery of the uterine horn, external iliac artery.
3. Dissection of the respective tributary veins of the common iliac vein (posterior parietal tributary is not expected).
   The dissection of the vessels of the horn is performed up to their entrance at the horn of the uterus.
   Except for the vessels of the uterine horn, all other arterial branches and vein tributaries of the common iliac vessels are transected between two ligations (double-ligated, 9/0 suture) – leaving the vessels of the uterine horn the only branches of the common iliac vessels.
4. The external iliac vessels are ligated and transected immediately peripheral to the origin/confluence of the vessels of the uterine horn.

D. Transection of the common iliac vessels

A yellow plastic background is placed under the vessels. The vessels are placed in the double clamp (the artery laterally, the vein medially), which rests with its base on the left and the jaws pointing to the uterine horn. The vessels are transected, the lumen is irrigated, and the adventitia removed.

E. End-to-end anastomoses

The anastomoses will be done in situ between the stumps of the common iliac vessels.
The following number of sutures are placed:

– Artery: 8 sutures 10/0

– Vein: 8 or 10 sutures 10/0

1. Suturing of the anterior surfaces of the two vessels.
2. Rotation of the double clamp and check of placement of the sutures of the anterior surfaces.
3. Suturing of the posterior surfaces of the vessels.
4. Release of the double clamp
5. Placement of a wet gauze on the anastomoses for 3 minutes.
6. Patency test.
7. Withdrawal of the yellow plastic background.

F. Transection of the gonadal vessels

G. Transection and anastomosis of the uterine horn: 8 or 10 sutures 9/0

H. Closure of the surgical trauma. The viscera are returned to their native position in the abdomen, and the wall is closed in two layers with 2/0 non-absorbable suture (the muscles with a running suture and the subcutaneous tissue and skin with interrupted sutures).

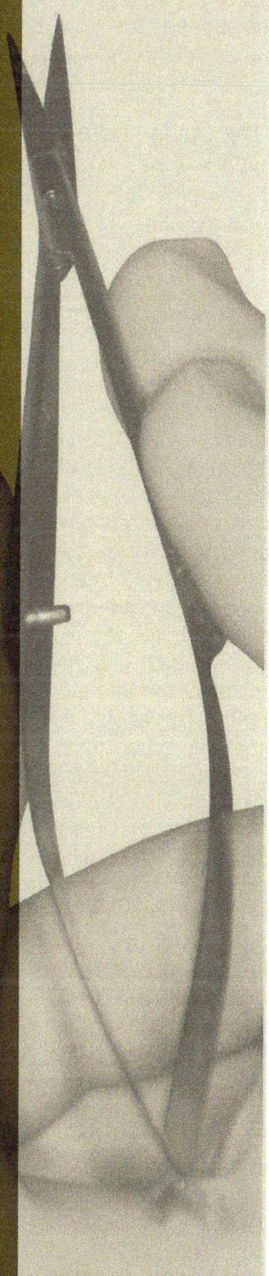

30 Transplantation of the ovary-fallopian tube

The procedure is described in this Chapter as performed on the right side. It can be identically performed on the left side, with the only change being the placement of the intestines to the right side during preparation of the surgical field.

Although this operation refers to transplantation of the ovary and fallopian tube, the cranial part of the uterine horn is included in the complex to be transplanted, because in the rat the fallopian tube coils around the cranial part of the horn and has common blood supply with it. Therefore, we refer hereafter to this complex as 'ovary-fallopian tube-cranial part of the uterine horn'.

I. Preparation of the Donor

The reader is refered to Chapter 29 for sections A and B

A. Positioning of the rat

B. Preparation of the surgical field

C. Microsurgical dissection

The reader is referred to Chapter 29 to study:

1. the vasculature of the pertinent organs (Chapter 29.C.I)
2. the design of the autotransplantation of the complex 'uterine horn-fallopian tube-ovary' (Chapter 29.C.II)

The design of the current operation (**Fig. 30-1**) resembles autotransplantation in that the complex's vascular axis will be the common iliac vessels with sole branch/tributary the vessels of the uterine horn. It differs in that the complex will include only the cranial part of the uterine horn and not the entire horn. Also, all blood needs to be completely flushed from the complex. For this reason, the transection of the common iliac vessels, through which the complex will be irrigated, will be modified (see below).

Following the steps of the design of the autotransplantation, the similarities and the differences in the current operation are as follows:

- Similar to autotransplantation, all branches/tributaries of the common iliac vessels should be ligated and transected except for the vessels of the uterine horn, i.e., the posterior parietal branch (No. 1A, **Fig. 30-1A**), the internal iliac vessels (No. 1B, **Fig. 30-1A**), and the external iliac vessels (No. 1C, **Fig. 30-1A**).
- Also similar to autotransplantation, the supply of the ovary and salpinx from the gonadal vessels should be severed (No. 2, **Fig. 30-1A**).
- The transection of the common iliac vessels should be altered into the following two step procedure:

  a) Initially, the common iliac vein should be ligated cranially and left open cau-daily (No. 3A1, **Fig. 30-1A**), to be used as an exit when the complex is flushed. In addition, the aorta should be ligated (or occluded with a single clamp) caudal to the renal arteries to avoid escape of the fluid cranially (No. 4A, **Fig. 30-1A**); the left common iliac artery must also be ligated to avoid escape toward this vessel (No. 4B, Fig. **30-1A**). After these two ligations, the fluid injected in the aorta is directed solely to the right uterine horn (and the complex) through the right common iliac artery and then through the artery of the horn.

b) After the complex has been flushed, the right common iliac artery will be ligated close to its origin and transected just peripheral to the ligation. The caudal stump of the common iliac artery will be left open and placed together with the peripheral stump of the homonymous vein in the single clamp (No. 3A2, **Fig. 30-1B**).

- The transection of the uterine horn is modified. In the current operation, only about 1 cm of the cranial part of the uterine horn is included in the complex (and not the whole length as in Chapter 29). This is done to ensure that the integrity and blood supply of the transplanted uterine tube will be maintained (the tube is coiled around the tip of the horn until it finally enters the lumen) (No. 5, **Fig. 30-1A**).

To mobilize the upper part of the uterine horn and

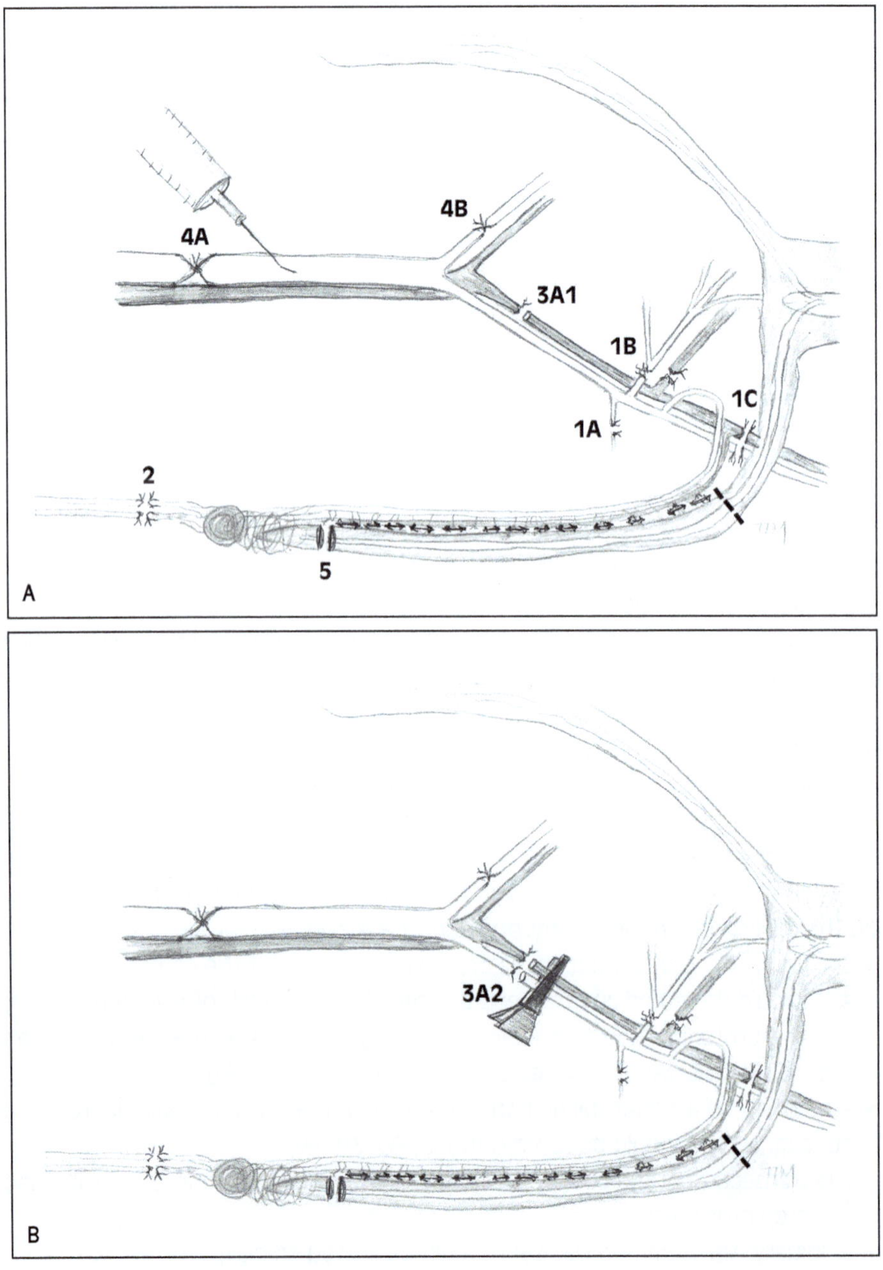

Figure 30-1

Design of the complex harvest. The complex consists of the ovary, fallopian tube, and the cranial part of the uterine horn. **A.** To make the axis 'common iliac vessels-vessels of the uterine horn' the sole source of blood supply the complex, the following are transected: posterior parietal branch (**1A**), internal iliac vessels (**1B**), external iliac vessels (**1C**), gonadal vessels (**2**), and the vertical branches of the vessels of the horn (bidirectional arrows) up to the point of transection at the cranial part. To facilitate the expansion of the mesometrium and the transection of the vertical vessels, it is advised to cut first the horn near its base (heavy dash-line). For flushing the complex, the right common iliac vein is ligated and transected caudally (**3A1**), the aorta is ligated (or clamped) caudal to the renal arteries (**4A**), and the left common iliac artery is ligated (**4B**). Normal saline is injected in the aorta, enters the right common iliac artery and the artery of the horn, washing out the complex, and returns through the vein of the horn to exit from the free caudal stump of the right common iliac vein. The horn is finally cut at the cranial part (**5**). **B.** At last, the right common iliac artery is transected (3A2), and the common iliac vessels are placed in the single clamp. (Drawing by the author) maintain its vasculature, the vessels of the horn must be preserved, but all vertical branches/tributaries to and from the horn should be severed up to the point of transection of the horn (bidirectional arrows, **Fig. 30-1**). Technically, to expand the mesometrium and expose the vertical small vessels, it is advisable to cut the horn near its base first, just prior to the entrance of the vessels in the horn (bold dashed line, **Fig. 30-1**). Once the vertical vessels are cut, the final transection of the horn at the upper part is performed (No. 5, **Fig. 30-1A**).

Note that the above presentation of the steps of harvesting the complex serves to aid in the understanding of the design of the operation. However, the steps of microsurgical dissection will follow a different order than numbering in Figure 30-1.

3. Microsurgical dissection

The reader is referred to Chapter 29.C.III. The following description focuses on the differences in the current operation.

During preparation of the donor, dissection includes all implicated vessels mentioned in Chapter 29, except for the vertical branches of the vessels of the uterine horn, whose dissection and transection is done during harvesting of the complex (see below, section III.F.2)

The microsurgical dissection follows and serves the steps of the design of the operation exposed above (**Fig. 30-1**), but, as mentioned above, the order of steps is different:

1. Dissection of the aorta and the left common iliac artery

- In the current operation, it is imperative that dissection should include the aorta so that the aorta can be ligated for flushing the complex. The dissection of the aorta should start from a point below to the renal arteries, extend caudally and include the aorta bifurcation.

  It could be suggested that the aorta may be dissected only for a short portion caudal to the renal arteries and that a 'window' may be opened between the aorta and the inferior vena cava to pass the suture for ligation. We do not support this technique as during the subsequent dissection of both common iliac arteries two more 'windows' will be opened below them. The creation of these three 'windows' will put the middle sacral artery, the lumbar arteries, and the posterior parietal branches (especially at the edges of the 'windows') at risk. In addition, there will be saline injected in the aorta that will escape toward these vessels. For these reasons, the full dissection of the aorta (division between two ligations or after cauterization of the lumbar, middle sacral and parietal arteries) extended to include the bifurcation and the common iliac arteries is suggested.
- Dissection of the left common iliac artery is necessary to obtain adequate space for ligation. Per the proposed technique, the dissection of the artery will be the continuation of the dissection of the aorta beyond the bifurcation. The dissection is restricted to the proximal part of the common iliac artery for a length that will allow placement of the ligation.

2. Dissection of the right common iliac artery and its 'four branches' near the bifurcation of the internal and external iliac artery

- **posterior parietal branch**
- **internal iliac artery**
- **artery of the uterine horn**
- **external iliac artery**

There are no differences from Chapter 29 in the current operation. In brief, the posterior parietal branch and the internal iliac artery are transected between two ligations (9/0). The artery of the horn remains intact. The external iliac artery is ligated and transected later (see No 4 below).

3. Dissection of the right common iliac vein and tributaries

- **Internal iliac vein**
- **External iliac vein**
- **Vein of the horn of the uterus**

There are no differences from Chapter 29 in the current operation. The internal iliac vein is transected between two ligations. The vein of the uterine horn is kept intact. The external iliac vein is double ligated and transected in the next step.

4. Ligation and transection of the right external iliac vessels

There are no differences from Chapter 29 in the current operation. The external iliac artery is double ligated and transected first.

5. Dissection and transection of the right ovarian (gonadal) vessels

The gonadal vessels will be found retroperitoneally, cranial to the ovary. The artery can be cauterized; as for the vein, you must estimate the size before choosing double ligation or cauterization.

6. Preparation of the aorta and left common iliac artery ligations

To economize time while harvesting the complex, it is wise to pass a 5/0 suture under the dissected aorta, caudal to the renal arteries. A 5/0 suture will also be placed under the dissected left common iliac artery. The needles are removed and the sutures are left long, ready to be tied quickly as the complex is being harvested.

II. Preparation of the Recipient

A. Positioning of the rat

As in the donor.

B. Preparation of the surgical field

As in the donor.

C. Microsurgical dissection

1. Design of complex implantation in the recipient

- The stumps of the common iliac vessels of the complex (Nos. 4 and 5, **Fig. 30-2**) will be anastomosed end-to-side with the recipient's aorta and inferior vena cava (Nos. 1 and 2, **Fig. 30-2**).
- The stump of the donor's uterine horn will be anastomosed end-to-end with the remaining horn of the recipient (Nos. 7 and 8, **Fig. 30-2**), after the complex 'ovary-salpinx-upper part of the horn' of the recipient has been removed; the latter requires transection of the vessels of the horn (No. 9, **Fig. 30-2**) at the upper part of the horn and of the gonadal vessels (No. 10, **Fig. 30-2**).

2. Microsurgical dissection

1. Microsurgical dissection of the aorta and the inferior vena cava

The reader is referred to Chapter 8.C for a detailed description of dissection of the aorta and to Chapter 28,I.D.b for the dissection of the inferior vena cava.

The aorta is meticulously dissected caudal to the left re-

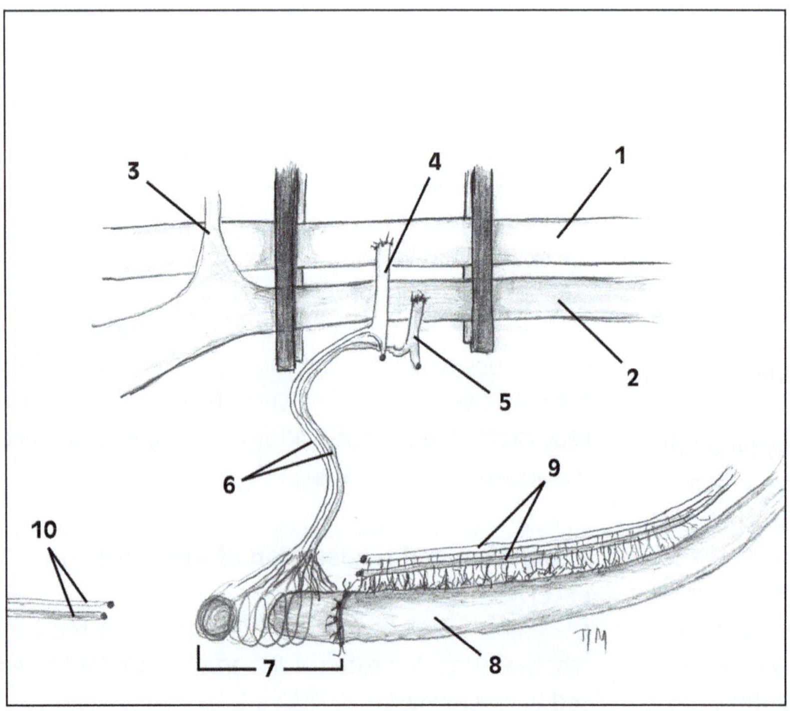

Figure 30-2

Design of the implantation of the complex in the recipient. The ovary, fallopian tube, and the cranial part of the uterine horn are removed in the recipient. This requires transection of the gonadal vessels and vessels of the uterine horn at their upper part (denoted with • on the stumps of the vessels). The stumps of the donor's common iliac vessels are anastomosed end-to-side with the recipient's aorta and the inferior vena cava. The stump of the uterine horn of the donor is anastomosed with the remaining uterine horn of the recipient. **1.** aorta, **2.** inferior vena cava, **3.** left renal vein, **4.** common iliac artery of the donor (stump), **5.** common iliac vein of the donor (stump), **6.** vessels of the uterine horn of the donor, **7.** transplanted complex: ovary-salpinx-upper part of the uterine horn, **8.** remnant of the uterine horn of the recipient, **9.** vessels of the uterine horn of the recipient, transected at the upper part, **10.** gonadal vessels of the recipient, transected caudally. (Drawing by the author) nal vein, and the lumbar arteries and posterior parietal branches are transected between two ligations or after cauterization. By carefully elevating the inferior vena cava, the lumbar veins and the posterior parietal tributaries are dissected, and transected between two ligations.

2. Placement of the aorta and inferior vena cava in the double clamp

A yellow plastic background is placed under the vessels. The aorta and the inferior vena cava are placed in the double clamp. For a right-sided ovary-fallopian tube transplantation, as described here, the double clamp is positioned with its base on the left uterine horn, rectum, and left border of the opened abdominal wall, while the legs of the clamps point at the right uterine horn of the recipient (**Fig. 30-3**).

3. Arteriotomy – Venotomy – Irrigation – Removal of adventitia

As described in Chapter 6, a small transverse incision is made in the aorta and in the inferior vena cava. The two incisions are not made at the same height—a small distance is left between them to facilitate the subsequent anastomoses with the complex's pedicle. The lumen of the vessels is immediately irrigated with warm normal saline (**Fig. 30-4**). The adventitia of the vessels is removed at the periphery of the incisions.

- The complete preparation of the recipient requires the **removal of the complex 'cranial part of the horn-fallopian tube-ovary'** of the right side that will be replaced by the donor complex (**Fig. 30-2**). This step **is deferred until the end of the operation** to avoid the hemorrhage from the stump of the recipient's transected horn, which cannot be cauterized because the surface of the stump must be intact for anastomosis with the donor's stump. It is also unsafe for the anastomosis of the horn to let the hemorrhage organize into clot on the surface of the recipient's stump during the time required for complex harvesting and vascular anastomoses.

III. Graft Harvesting (Donor)

While not technically a graft, we use the terms 'graft' and 'complex' interchangeably to refer to the 'horn-fallopian tube-ovary' complex.

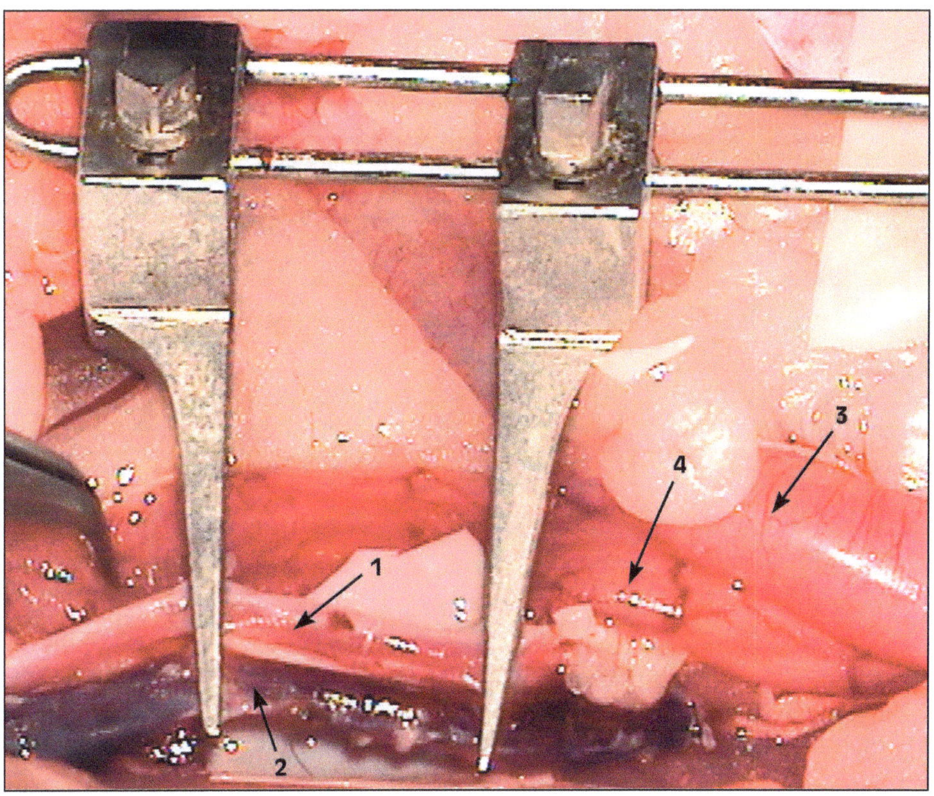

Figure 30-3

Placement of the aorta and inferior vena cava of the recipient in the double clamp (aorta to the left, inferior vena cava to the right). A yellow plastic background has been previously placed under the vessels. The curved microsurgical forceps packs the rectum. **1.** aorta, **2.** inferior vena cava, **3.** left horn of the uterus, **4.** rectum. (From author's photo library)

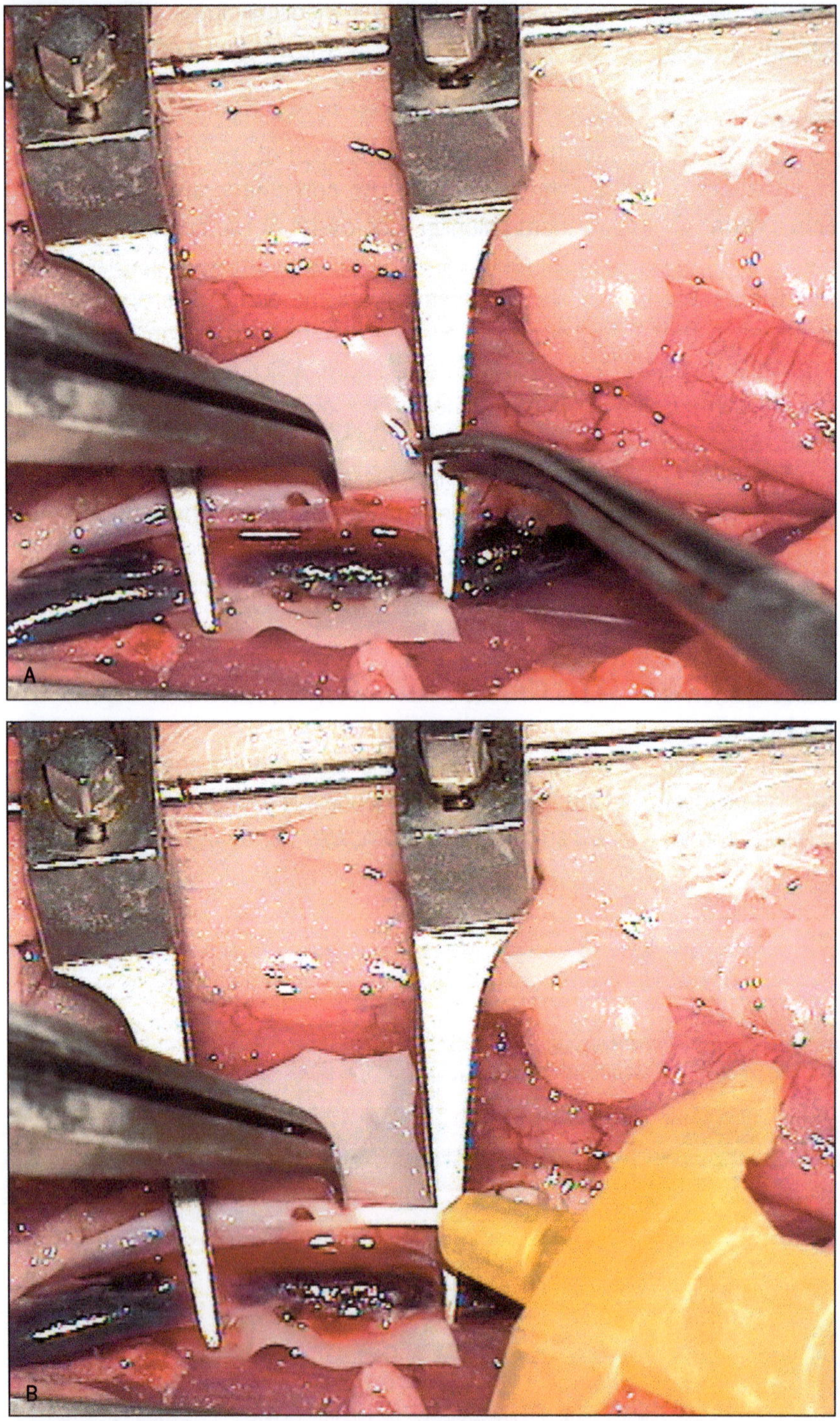

Figure 30-4

Transverse incision and irrigation of the aorta. **A.** The curved microsurgical forceps holds the aorta from the adventitia. The scissors are taken away after the transverse incision on the aorta has been made. **B.** The curved microsurgical forceps lifts the adventitia and the tip of a 27G angiocatheter is inserted in the aorta, injecting warm normal saline in the lumen. (From author's photo library)

A. Ligation of the aorta and left common iliac artery

The 5/0 sutures previously placed under the aorta and the left common iliac artery are tied (Nos. 4A and 4B, **Fig. 30-1A**). Thus, the saline injected in the aorta to flush the complex 'cranial part of the horn-fallopian tube-ovary' will be directed to the right common iliac artery and the artery of the right uterine horn.

B. Ligation and transection of right common iliac vein

The right common iliac vein is ligated cranially, close to

its confluence, with a 5/0 suture and transected just caudal to the ligation (No. 3A1, **Fig. 30-1A**). The caudal stump is left open to allow the saline to flush out. The ligation should be placed at such a distance from the confluence of the common iliac veins that adequate length of vein will be left for the anastomosis of the complex in the recipient.

C. Flushing of the complex

A 5 ml syringe with a 27G needle is used to flush the complex. The needle is bent in its distal part to obtain a course parallel the long axis of the aorta, and is inserted in the lumen. Cold normal saline is slowly injected in the aorta, directed towards the right common iliac artery and the artery of the right uterine horn. The flush returns through the vein of the uterine horn and then the right common iliac vein, exiting from its free stump. Note that since the uterine horn is not yet divided in its cranial part, a small amount of the flush will escape toward the veins communicating with the veins of the uterine plexus, which is drained into the left internal iliac vein (the right was divided previously). The flushing will continue until the entire right uterine horn obtains a whitish color.

It is advised to remove the cold liquid from the peritoneal cavity by absorbing it with pieces of paper towel, and then irrigate the cavity and the splanchna with warm normal saline to prevent the rat from becoming hypothermic.

D. Placement in the single clamp (together with the homonymous vein), ligation and transection of the right common iliac artery

Before being ligated and transected, the right common iliac artery is placed in a single clamp together with the stump of the right common iliac vein (**Fig. 30-5**). The clamp is placed on the common iliac vessels immediately cephalad to the origin/confluence of the vessels of the uterine horn. It is imperative to place the clamp before transecting the right common iliac artery to maintain the relative positioning of the common iliac vessels. If the clamp is placed after transecting the artery, it will shrink and the two vessels must be rearranged in the clamp—waisting time and risking torsion of the free stump of the artery during its placement in the clamp that contains the vein stump.

The positioning of the vessels in the clamp is dicta-

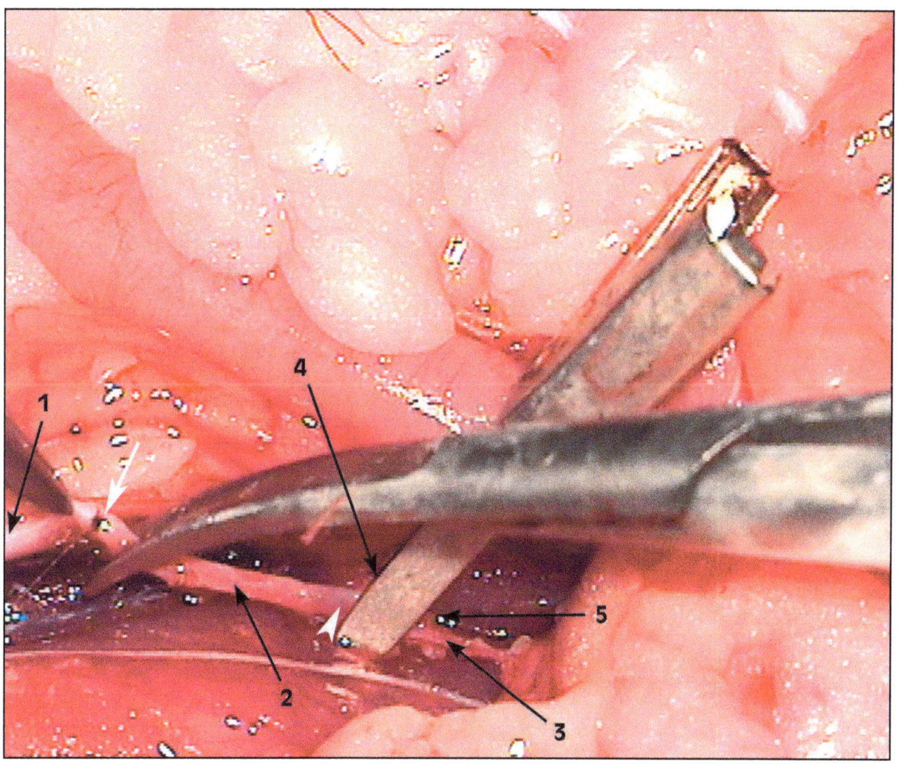

Figure 30-5

Ligation and transection of the right common iliac artery. The ligation (white arrow) is placed close to the aortic bifurcation. The Dumont No. 3 forceps lifts the common iliac artery by grasping it near the aortic bifurcation, before the ligation. The scissors, brought perpendicular to its long axis, cut the artery near the ligation. The single clamp has been placed on the common iliac vessels just before the origin/confluence of the vessels of the uterine horn. The white arrowhead shows the lateral positioning of the artery in the clamp. **1.** aorta, **2.** common iliac artery, **3.** artery of the uterine horn, **4.** stump of the common iliac vein (placed medially in the clamp). **5.** vein of the uterine horn. (From author's photo library) ted by the anatomical location of the vessels: the artery is placed laterally, the vein medially. The stump of the vein must be oriented correctly in the clamp, parallel with the artery.

The ligation of the right common iliac artery (5/0 suture) is placed close to the aortic bifurcation. During transection of the artery that follows, care is taken so that the resulting stump of the artery will be a bit longer than the vein stump. This will ease the end-to-side anastomoses of the complex, since the aorta of the recipient has been placed on the left in the double clamp, and the arteriotomy has been performed at a small distance from the venotomy (**Fig. 30-2**).

E. Irrigation of the lumen of the complex vessels, removal of the adventitia

Even though the right common iliac artery was cleaned during the irrigation of the complex through the aorta, it is necessary to irrigate the lumen of the right common iliac artery immediately after transection (**Fig. 30-6**). Similarly, for the right common iliac vein, another irrigation is reassuring.

Folding the adventitia of the artery (**Fig. 30-7**) and removing the adventitia of the vein is better performed at this point as opposed to just before the anastomoses during the implantation of the complex. The rationale for this is that if the complex is in position and the other end of the vessels are held steady due to the clamp and continuation of the vessels towards the unattached horn. If this step is postponed until the complex is inset, the vessels will be free and handing them will be much more difficult.

F. Transection of the vertical branches/tributaries of the vessels of the proximal uterine horn – Transection of the cranial part of the horn and respective mesometrium

To assure the vascular supply to the complex, we suggest that the transection of the vertical branches of the vessels of the horn should be performed during the harvesting of the complex and not during donor preparation. During the latter, the gonadal vessels are severed and survival of the complex relies on the vessels of the horn. These may be easily jeopardized with transection of the vertical branches of the horn.

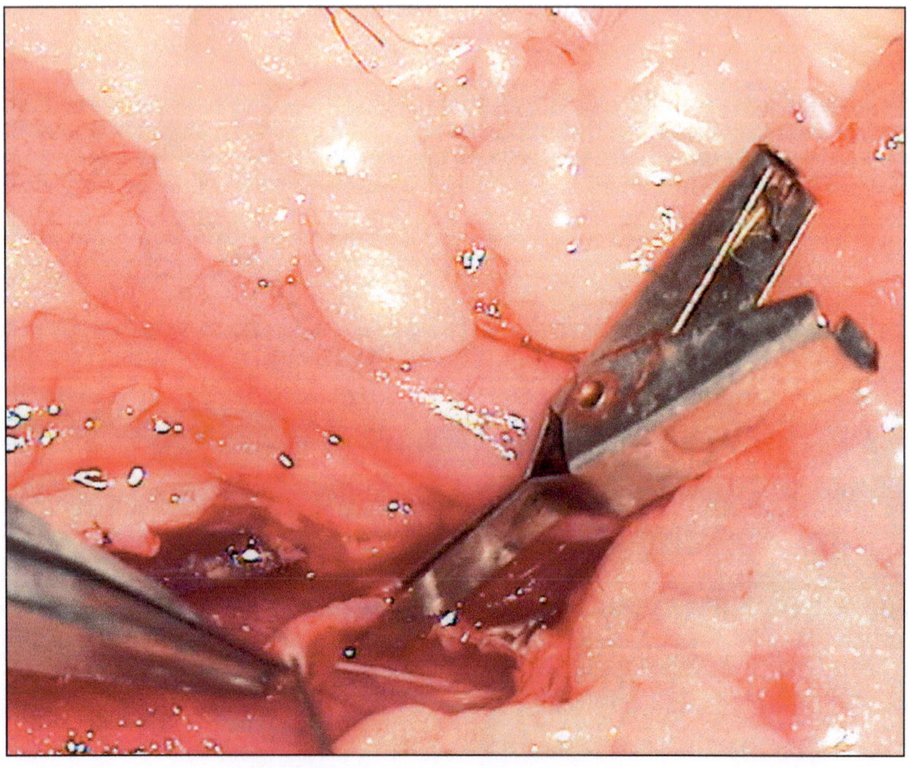

Figure 30-6

Irrigation of the right common iliac artery stump. The Dumont No. 3 forceps holds the artery from the outside surface of the wall, while normal saline is injected through an insulin needle that does not enter the lumen. However, an atraumatic 27G angiocatheter is preferable to use. (From author's photo library)

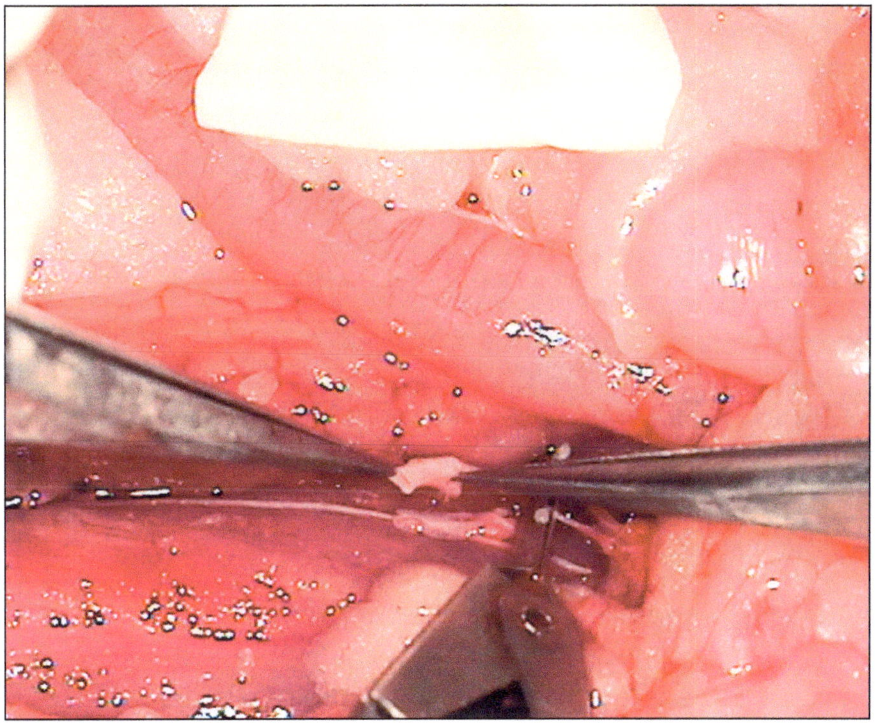

Figure 30-7

Folding the adventitia of the stump of the right common iliac artery. The Dumont No. 3 forceps holds the artery, while No. 5 folds the adventitia. (From author's photo library)

Transecting the vertical tributaries of the vessels of the horn is the most difficult step in the dissection of the vessels of the horn. As a continuation of the common iliac vessels, they will constitute the vascular axis of the complex. This dissection is performed en bloc with the transection of the upper part of the horn that will liberate the complex. In detail, this step of the operation includes 3 actions:

1. Initial transection of the uterine horn near its base

The uterine horn is transected near the base to allow for expansion of the mesometrium and to expose the vessels of the horn and their vertical braches to the horn. The transection of the horn is performed medial to the point of entrance of the vessels in the mesometrium of the horn (**Fig. 30-1** and **Fig. 30-8A**). This point is found at the end of the course of the vessels of the horn as they have been dissected thus far. To ensure the location of the point of entrance of the vessels is correctly identified, follow the course of the vessels of the horn starting from their origin, at the right common iliac vessels.

Transecting the horn near its base means the part of the horn from the base to the cranial part of the horn where the final transection will be performed must be removed. This is because the blood supply has been completely severed: the gonadal vessels have been transected, and the vessels of the horn will stop supplying it after transection of their vertical branches.

To perform the low transection of the horn, the diathermy can be directly applied or cauterization may be used after transection with scissors. No stump of the horn will be anastomosed, so there is no reason to maintain intact surfaces of transection; the cephalad stump of the horn will be removed, while the caudal (toward the base) will remain in the donor.

The transection of the horn must be limited to the horn. It is a tragic mistake here to cut the vessels of the horn or to jeopardize them with the diathermy, because the complex without an intact vascular supply is useless.

2. Transection of the vertical branches/ tributaries of the vessels of the uterine horn

We resume in the drawing of **Figure 30-1**, where the transection of vertical branches of the vessels of the right uterine horn is represented with a series of bidirectional arrows between the vessels of the horn, shown medially, and the horn, shown laterally. Take care not to be misguided by this figure: in the surgical field, when

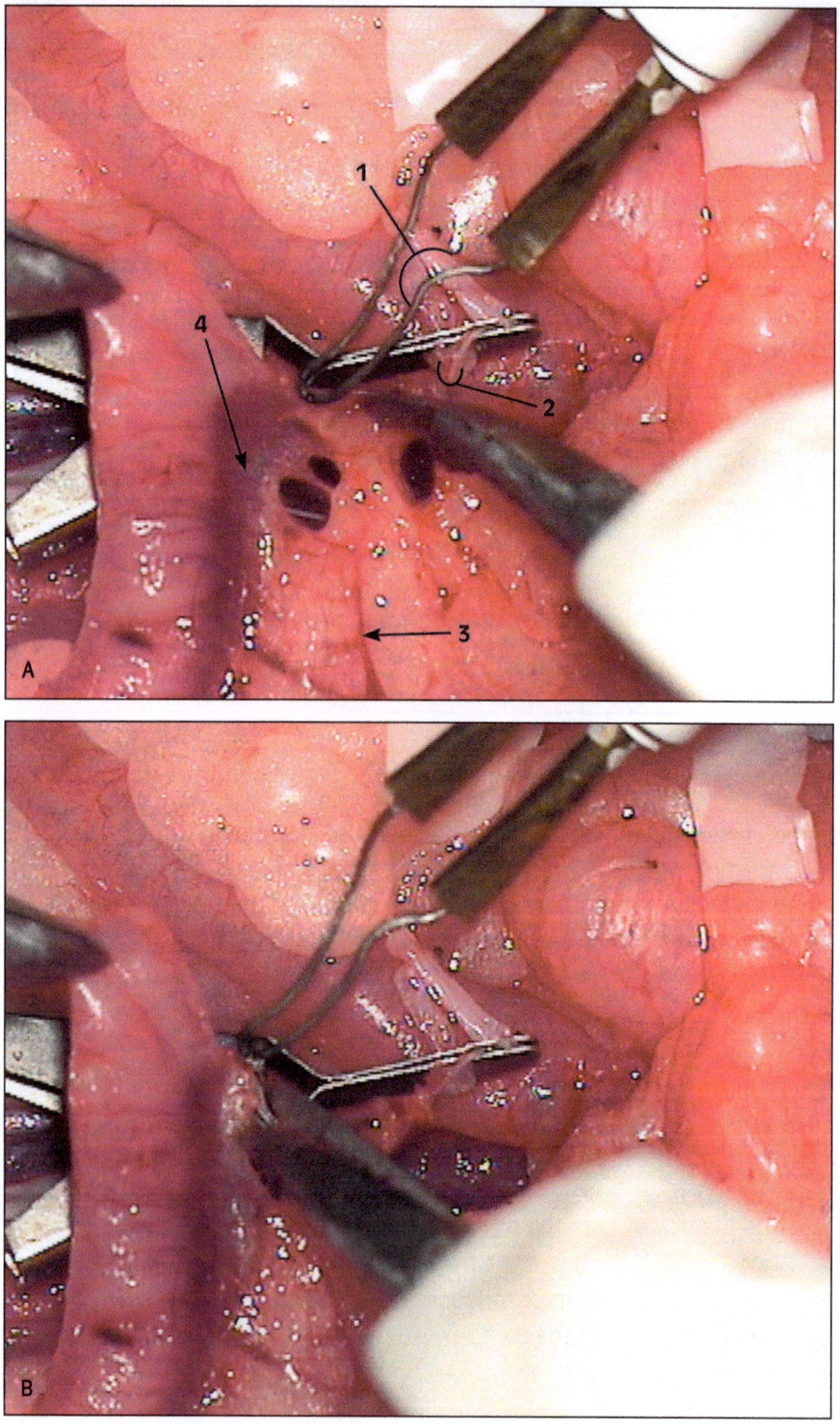

Figure 30-8

Dissection and transection of the vertical branches/tributaries of the vessels of the right horn of the uterus. **A.** To expand the mesometrium and adequately expose the vessels contained in it, the horn has been transected near the base. The stumps of the right common iliac vessels have been placed in the single clamp. The Dumont No. 3 forceps lifts the cranial stump of the horn (on the left of the photo, over the single clamp). The scissors move the vessels of the horn medially, after having opened 'windows' between the vertical branches in the mesometrium. The diathermy is ready to cauterize these branches. **B.** Transection with scissors follows cauterization of the vertical branches. **1.** stumps of the right common iliac vessels, **2.** vessels of the uterine horn, **3.** vein of the horn, **4.** marginal vein (plexus) in the mesenteric border of the horn. (From author's photo library)

elevating the horn at its transected base, this relation is reversed and the vessels of the horn are found lateral and under the horn (**Fig. 30-8A**).

It is also important to perceive the course of the vessels of the horn in the mesometrium, which is not immediately evident. When the stump of the transected horn is lifted, the marginal vein (venous plexus) becomes apparent in the 'mesenteric' border of the horn, i.e. where the mesometrium attaches to the horn (No. 4, **Fig. 30-8A**). The marginal vein plexus is much more obvious compared to the vessels of the horn in the mesometrium, where only the vein of the horn can be seen without further dissection (No. 3, **Fig. 30-8A**). The vertical veins are much smaller and less evident in the fat of the mesometrium, and run vertically between the vein of the horn and the marginal plexus. Nevertheless, the distances between the vertical veins are sufficient to permit microsurgical dissection of these veins in the fatty mesometrium. The vertical veins are closely accompanied by even smaller vertical arterial branches. For this reason, dissection of the vertical vessels is based on the vertical veins.

The dissection between the vessels of the horn, and the horn in the mesometrium, starts bluntly. Open small 'windows' between the vertical veins where the mesometrium seems less fatty with the microsurgical scissors (**Fig. 30-8A**). You will obtain a sense for the location of the vessels of the horn in the mesometrium with this movement of the scissors. The visible vein of the horn already sets the boundary of the length of the 'window' that will be opened between the vertical vessels. You can also find the artery of the horn with very meticulous dissection, but this is not necessary. In the space between the marginal vein and the vein of the horn you may cauterize and transect the vertical vessels coursing between the 'windows' in the mesometriun (**Fig. 30-8B**). This detaches the vessels of the horn from the horn itself and should be followed for the length of the right horn that will be removed. The transection of the vertical vessels stops at the cranial part of the horn that will later be transplanted together with the fallopian tube and the ovary.

3. Final transection of the cranial part of the horn and mesometrium

The uterine horn is finally transected at its cranial part—making the segment that will be transplanted together with the fallopian tube and the ovary approximately 1 centimeter in length. The devascularized part of the horn, from the initial transection at its base to the final transection at the cranial part, is removed. Transection of the horn at the cranial part must be done with scissors, because the surface of the stump of the horn that belongs to the complex should stay intact to be anastomosed with the stump of the horn in the recipient. Any small hemorrhage on the cut surface is welcomed, because it shows the adequate vascular supply to the complex. Do not cauterize it, just absorb the blood with paper and wash with warm normal saline.

To mobilize the stump of the cranial part of the horn along with the salpinx and the ovary, the plane of dissection changes: *transection of the mesometrium is performed caudal to the vessels of the horn* (and not between the vessels of the horn and the marginal vein of the horn up until this point). This retains the blood supply of the upper part of the horn along with the salpinx and the ovary (**Fig. 30-9**). The vessels of the horn together with the vertical vessels of the upper part of the horn are an indispensable part of the complex as they are the only axis of blood supply from the common iliac vessels.

To change the plane of transection of the mesometrium, pull up on the vessels of the horn by lifting the single clamp applied to the stumps of the common iliac vessels (**Fig. 30-9**). This maneuver will bring the vessels closer to stump of the horn, and the tension will provide you with a sense of the location of the vessels in the mesometrium. The transection of the mesometrium should be performed caudally to the vessels of the horn with enough distance to ensure that they are not cut or traumatized. This would of course lead to complete devascularization of the complex, and bring an abrupt end to the procedure.

The transection of the mesometrium will include the length of the upper part of the horn and will be extended cranially behind the salpinx and the ovary to join the opening of the posterior peritoneum for transection of the gonadal vessels (see above, I.C.3.5). This will completely free the complex 'cranial part of the horn-fallopian tube-ovary.'

G. Transfer of the complex

The freed complex is taken together with the single clamp, and is placed in a gauze moistened in cold normal saline on the working surface. Care should be taken to maintain the complex in its correct anatomical position during the transfer to prevent vessel torsion that can occur with accidental rotation of the clamp.

IV. Graft Implantation (Recipient)

The transplanted complex 'cranial part of the horn-fallopian tube-ovary' is transferred to the surgical field of the recipient, and is placed ipsilateral, parallel and at the same height with the right, non-prepared, cranial part of the horn of the uterus, the fallopian tube and the ovary of the recipient. The vessels of the transplanted complex are brought perpendicular to the aorta and inferior vena cava. The edges of the stumps are placed close to the sites of their respecti-

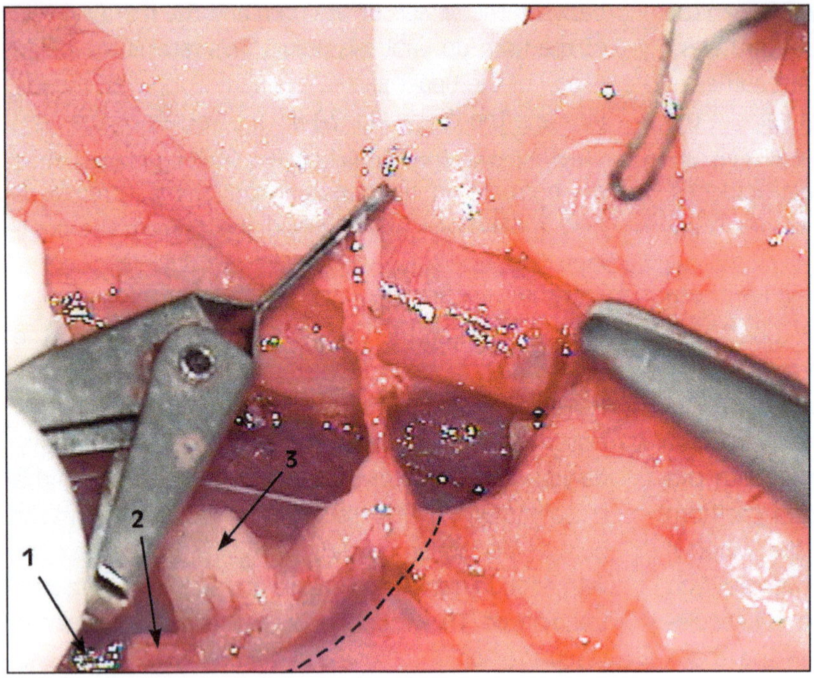

Figure 30-9

Transection of the mesometrium caudal to the vessels of the cranial part of the horn (dashed line), which is extended cranially, behind the fallopian tube and the ovary, to free the complex 'cranial part of the horn-fallopian tube-ovary'. The horn has been transected, the cranial portion remains attached, while the remainder of the horn up to its base has been removed. The single clamp placed on the common iliac vessels pulls up and exerts light tension on the vessels of the horn that will help in detecting them in the mesometrium and defining the proper location of the transection (along the dashed line). Observe how low the 'cranial part of the horn-fallopian tube-ovary' complex is compared with the contralateral side. This is due to the preceding dissection and transection of the gonadal vessels. **1.** ovary, **2.** fallopian tube, coiled around the upper part of the horn, **3.** fat of the mesometrium of the horn, detached to show 2. (From author's photo library)

ve transverse incisions (i.e. the common iliac artery to the aorta and the common iliac vein to the inferior vena cava). Continue to pay careful attention to avoid torsion of the single clamp holding the stumps of the vessels of the complex.

If the stumps of the vessels of the transplanted complex differ much in length, or if the aorta has moved to the left in the double clamp in the recipient, do not hesitate to remove the single clamp of the complex to perform the anastomoses. This will give you freedom while handling the vessels of the complex.

A. End-to-side vascular anastomoses

The reader will find details on end-to-side anastomoses where the clamp can be rotated in Chapter 6.1.

The following number of sutures is placed on the vessels

- **Artery: 10 sutures 10/0**
- **Vein: 10 sutures 10/0**

The anterior surfaces of both anastomoses are sutured first. The single clamp is then reversed together with the complex, and the posterior surfaces are completed.

The arterial and venous anastomoses are commonly recommended to be performed simultaneously, i.e. to place the 9 and 3 o'clock sutures in both vessels. Given the small caliber of the vessels and the difficulty in handling the elaborate complex in the current operation, we often start with the more difficult anastomosis of the vein and then proceed to the artery. Therefore:

1. Suturing of the anterior surface of the vein is performed first. Verify that the adventitia has been removed along the perimeter of the transverse incision in the vena cava. First the corner sutures are placed at 3 and 9 o'clock (**Fig. 30-10A**). Then 4 sutures are placed in the anterior surface, first the more lateral (toward the corner sutures) and next the more central, all equally spaced between themselves and from the corner sutures (**Fig. 30-10B**). The anastomosis of the anterior surface of the artery is performed in the same way. The adventitia should also be removed from around the aorta if this was not done during the recipient preparation (**Fig. 30-11**).
2. Rotation of the complex and single clamp, and check of the sutures along the anterior surface of the anastomosis.
3. Placement of the remaining 4 sutures on the posterior surfaces of the artery and vein.

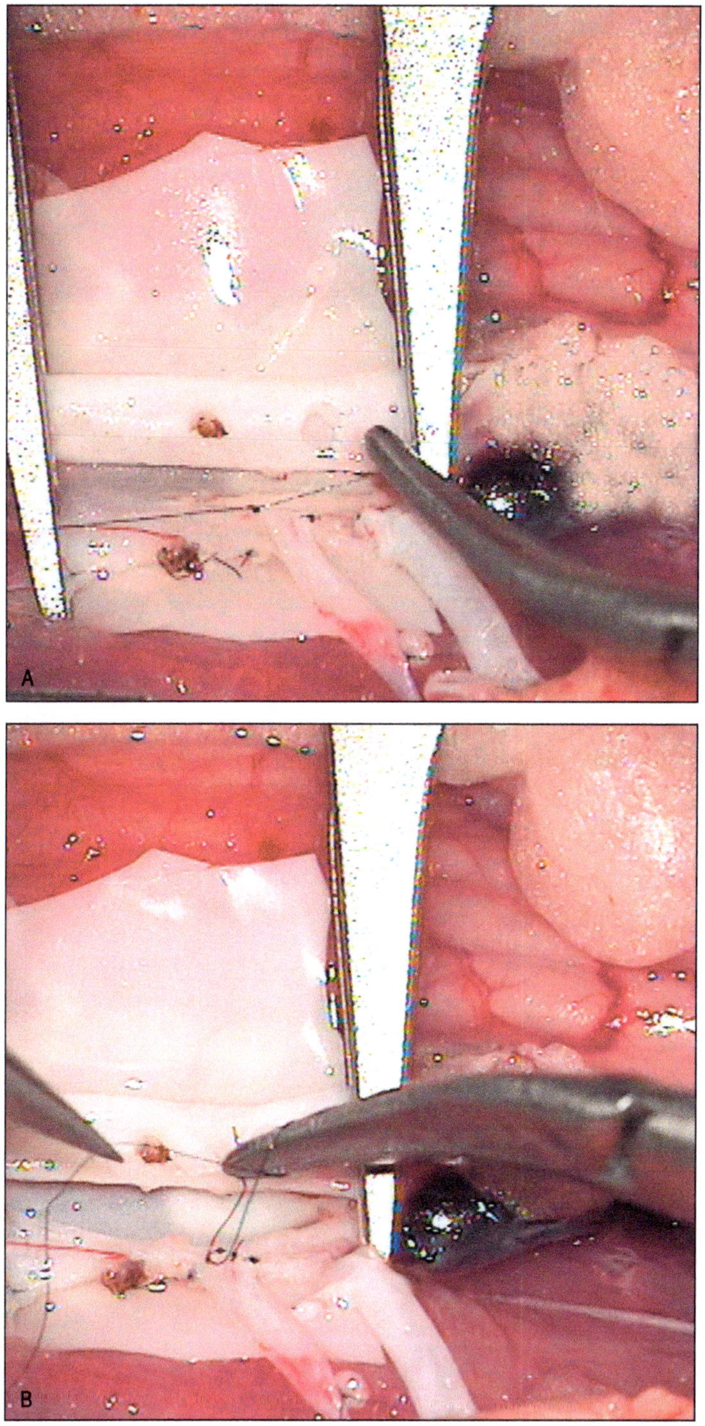

Figure 30-10

Suturing the anterior surface of the vein. **A.** Placement of the 2nd corner suture at 9 o'clock. The suture seen at the '7 o'clock position' does not belong to the venous anastomosis but is a ligated right tributary vein of the inferior vena cava. **B.** Placement of the 3rd out of the 4 sutures of the anterior surface. (From author's photo library)

4. Release of the vessels from the clamps, starting with the single clamp, then the double clamp.
5. Placement of a wet gauze on the anastomoses for 3 minutes.
6. Patency test, separately for each anastomosis, as described for the end-to-side anastomosis; see Chapter 6.9.1 (**Fig. 6-9**) for the artery, and 6.9.2 (**Fig. 6-10**) for the vein.
7. Withdrawal of the yellow plastic background.

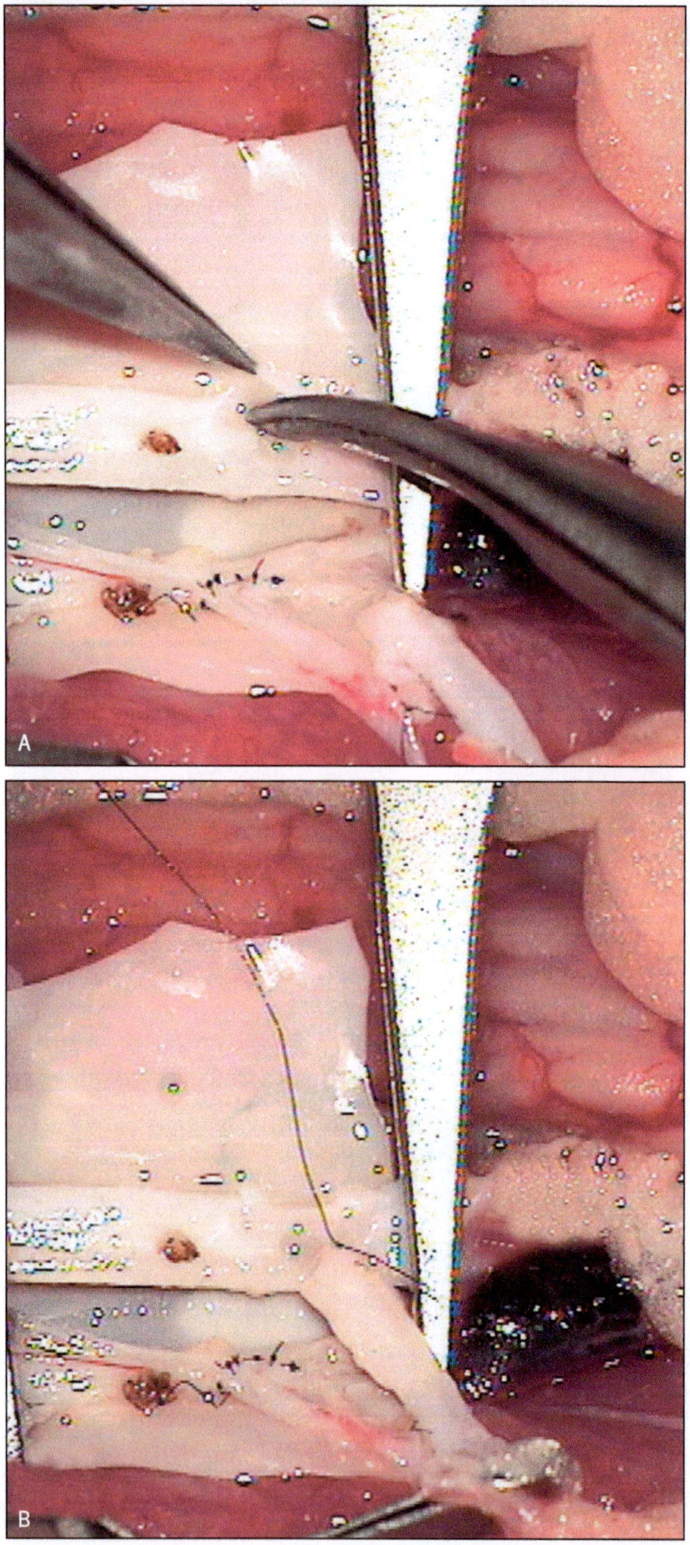

Figure 30-11

Suturing the anterior surface of the artery. **A.** Removal of the adventitia along the perimeter of the transverse incision of the aorta. The Dumont No. 3 forceps lifts the adventitia, while the scissors enter closed underneath it. By spreading outwards with the scissors, the adventitia is detached from the rest of the wall. **B.** Placement of the 3 o'clock corner suture. (From author's photo library)

B. Removal of the complex 'cranial part of the uterine horn-fallopian tube-ovary' of the recipient (right side)

To begin, blood supply to this complex (vessels of the horn and gonadal vessels) must be severed (**Fig. 30-2**).

1. Transection of the gonadal vessels

As in the donor.

2. Transection of the vessels of the uterine horn

The vessels are cauterized and transected at a level corresponding to the site of the subsequent transection of the horn.

3. Transection and removal of the complex 'cranial part of the horn-fallopian tube-ovary'

The transection of the horn will be done sharply with scissors, and not with the diathermy. This is done to prevent harm to the blood supply of the transverse surface of the remaining horn, which will be anastomosed with the horn of the complex.

C. Anastomosis of the stump of the horn of the complex with the remaining horn of the recipient

An end-to-end anastomosis of the horn will be performed using **8-10 sutures 9/0** (**Fig. 29-26**).

V. Closure of the Surgical Traumas

In the recipient and donor, the splanchna are returned into the abdomen, and the incision is closed in two layers with non-absorbable 2/0 sutures. Use a running suture in the muscles, and interrupted sutures in the subcutaneous tissue and skin.

ALTERNATIVE TECHNIQUES

- The procedure can be performed by using the vessels of the uterine horn of the donor (and not the common iliac vessels) for the anastomoses. Due to their miniscule size, however, the difficulty of the operation increases dramatically.
- The vessels of the complex may be anastomosed to the common iliac vessels of the recipient end-to-side. This will also increase the difficulty and duration of the operation.

Synopsis... of transplantation of the ovary-fallopian tube

The transplanted complex (graft) includes the cranial part of the uterine horn as the salpinx coils around it and finally exits in it. The operation is described for the right side.

I. PREPARATION OF THE DONOR

A. Positioning of the rat. Laid on its back, head on the left of the surgeon. The limbs are immobilized on the working surface with adhesive tape.

B. Preparation of the surgical field. Median incision, from the xiphoid process to the pubic symphysis. Mobilization of the small intestine, and placement of the intestines, enveloped in a wet gauze, on the left of the rat. Opening of the retroperitoneum with two wet gauzes.

C. Microsurgical dissection

1. Dissection of the aorta and left common iliac artery.
2. Dissection of the right common iliac artery and its 4 branches found near the bifurcation into internal and external iliac arteries, in the following order: posterior parietal branch, internal iliac artery, artery of the uterine horn, external iliac artery. Transection between two ligations (9/0) of all these branches, except of the artery of the horn and the external iliac artery.
3. Dissection of the right common iliac vein and its respective tributaries (as described above for the artery; a posterior parietal tributary vein is not expected). Transection between two ligations (9/0) of all tributaries except of the vein of the horn and the external iliac vein. Dissection of the vessels of the uterine horn will continue up until their entrance into the mesometrium.
4. Transection between two ligations of the right external iliac vessels.
5. Transection of the right gonadal vessels between two ligations or after cauterization.
6. Preparation of the ligations of the aorta and left common iliac artery: a 5/0 suture, without the needle, is left untied under each vessel.

II. PREPARATION OF THE RECIPIENT

A. Positioning of the rat. As in the donor.

B. Preparation of the surgical field. As in the donor.

C. Microsurgical dissection

1. Microsurgical dissection of the aorta and the inferior vena cava.
2. Placement of the aorta and inferior vena cava in the double clamp.
3. Arteriotomy – Venotomy – Irrigation – Removal of adventitia.

III. GRAFT HARVERSTIG (DONOR)

A. Ligation of the aorta and the left common iliac artery.

B. Ligation and transection of the right common iliac vein (at its confluence).

C. Flushing of the complex: Through a curved insulin needle attached to a syringe, cold normal saline is injected in the aorta, caudal to the ligation. It will exit though the right common iliac vein.

D. Placement in the single clamp (together with the homonymous vein), ligation and transection of the right common iliac artery. The stump of the artery is left a bit longer than the vein.

E. Irrigation of the lumen of the complex vessels, folding/removal of the adventitia.

... of transplantation of the ovary-fallopian tube

Synopsis...

F. Transection of the vertical vessels in the proximal (remaining) part of the horn: The horn is initially transected near its base, medially to the point of entrance of its vessels in the mesometrium. It is pulled to expand the mesometrium and expose the vertical vessels between the marginal vein and the vessels of the horn. The vertical vessels are dissected by bluntly opening 'windows' between them in the mesometrium, then cauterized and transected until the cranial portion of the horn is reached. – **Transection of the cranial part of the horn and its mesometrium:** The mesometrium is transected caudal to the vessels of the horn (and not between vessels and horn as before).

G. Transfer of the complex on the working surface on a gauze moistened with cold normal saline.

IV. IMPLANTATION IN THE RECIPIENT

The transplanted complex is placed parallel and at the same height with the right cranial part of the horn, fallopian tube and ovary of the recipient. The complex vessels are brought perpendicular to the aorta and the inferior vena cava.

A. End-to-side anastomoses between the common iliac vessels of the complex and the aorta/inferior vena cava

The following number of sutures are placed:

Arteries: 10 sutures 10/0

Veins: 10 sutures 10/0

1. Suturing of the anterior surface of the vein is performed first. The corner sutures of 3 and 9 o'clock are placed, followed by 4 more, at equal distances. Same for the anterior surface of the artery.
2. Rotation of the complex and single clamp are rotated, and check of the sutures of the anterior surface.
3. Suturing of the posterior surfaces of the vein and artery is completed.
4. Release of the vessels from the clamps. First the single clamp is withdrawn, then the double clamp.
5. Placement of a wet gauze on the anastomoses for 3 minutes.
6. Patency test, separately for each anastomosis.
7. Withdrawal of the yellow plastic background.

B. Removal of the 'cranial part of the uterine horn-fallopian tube-ovary' complex of the recipient:

1. Transection of the gonadal vessels.
2. Transection of the vessels of the uterine horn.
3. Transection and removal of the 'cranial part of the horn-fallopian tube-ovary.'

C. Anastomosis of the stump of the horn of the donor with the remaining horn of the recipient:

8-10 sutures 9/0.

V. CLOSURE OF THE SURGICAL TRAUMAS

In recipient and donor, repositioning the splanchna in the abdomen and suturing of the abdominal wall in 2 layers with 2/0 sutures, continuous in the muscles, interrupted in the skin.

31 Heterotopic heart transplantation

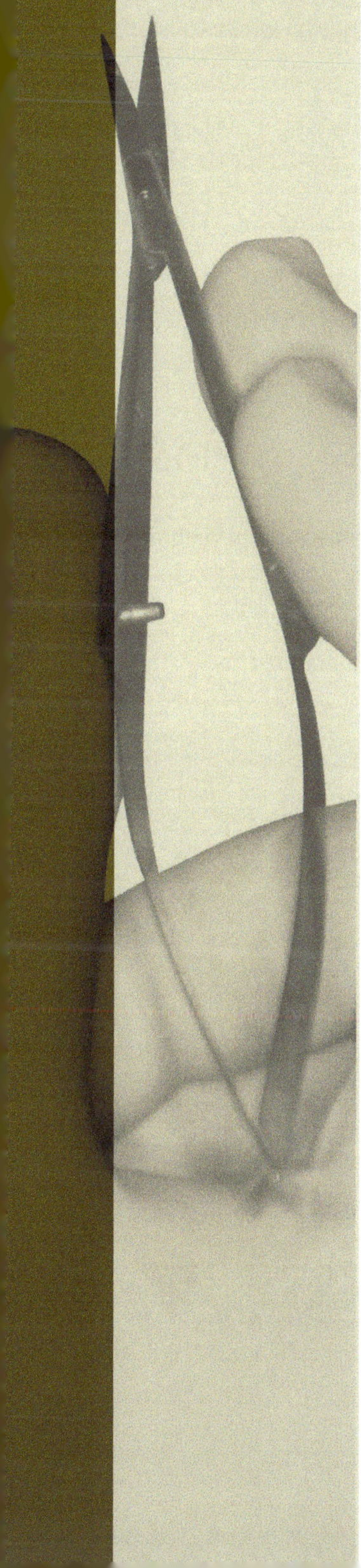

Implantation of the graft in the donor will be performed with end-to-side anastomoses of the graft vessels with the aorta and inferior vena cava, caudal to the origin of the renal arteries.

The design of the operation includes 3 steps:

1) Recipient: dissection of the aorta and inferior vena cava.
2) Donor: thoracotomy, en block removal of the heart and all related vessels, lungs, trachea, and esophagus. Once removed from the donor, the heart is dissected free of splanchna, and all vessels are ligated except the aorta and the left pulmonary artery.
3) Recipient: arteriotomy (aorta) and venotomy (inferior vena cava), heterotopic implantation of the heart in the abdomen, end-to-side anastomoses of the aorta and left pulmonary artery of the graft toward the aorta and the inferior vena cava of the recipient respectively.

I. Recipient Preparation

A. Position of the rat

The rat is placed in dorsal decubitus position with the head on the left of the surgeon. The limbs of the rat are immobilized on the working surface with adhesive tape.

B. Preparation of the surgical field

The reader will find details of the preparation of the field in Chapter 8.B and 8.C.1.

In brief, a median incision is performed from the xiphoid process to the pubic symphysis, and retractors are placed on the edges of the incision. The lobes of the liver are packed with a retractor enveloped in a wet gauze. The intestine is mobilized and moved out of the surgical field enveloped in a wet gauze by placing it on the right side of the rat. The retroperitoneum is opened with two gauzes moistened in warm normal saline.

C. Microsurgical dissection of the aorta and inferior vena cava

The reader is referred to Chapter 8.C.2 for details about the aorta dissection.
The microsurgical dissection of the inferior vena cava is described in detail in Chapter 28.I. D.b.

The aorta and the inferior vena cava are dissected from the origin/confluence of the renal vessels to the area of the aorta bifurcation. The two major vessels are separated, and all branches/tributaries are transected between two ligations. When the two major vessels are fully mobilized and dissected, a gauze is placed on the vessels, and the surgical field is irrigated with normal saline to keep it moist. To avoid occlusion of the aorta and inferior vena cava for a prolonged period of time, the arteriotomy and venotomy will be performed in the 3rd step, after harvesting of the graft and during implantation of the graft in the donor (see below).

The rat is kept warm. The surgical field in the abdomen and the gauze-covered splanchna outside the abdomen are irrigated periodically with normal saline.

II. Donor - Removal and Preparation of the Graft

Before starting the operation, the following materials should be prepared:

1. One Petri dish containing iced normal saline.
2. One Petri dish, with a gauze-covered bottom (or covered by a yellow plastic background), on which dissection of the graft will be performed.
3. Cold normal saline and cold heparin solution.

The Petri dish containing the normal saline is frozen overnight and will serve as a dissection platform. The second dish with the gauze-covered bottom will be placed on top of the iced platform, and the dissection of the graft will be performed on this gauze (the gauze is preferred as it is more stable than the yellow plastic background). It is wise to prepare two or three spare iced normal saline dishes in order to change the dish when the ice begins to melt. This maintains a steady low temperature on which to keep the graft during dissection.

A. Position of the rat

The rat is placed in dorsal decubitus position with the head on the left of the surgeon. The limbs of the rat are immobilized on the working surface with adhesive tape.

B. Preparation of the surgical field

A wide, bilateral U-type thoracotomy is performed, initially with scalpel and then with scissors. The incision is extended laterally on the ribs in order to obtain a wide surgical field (**Fig. 31-1**).

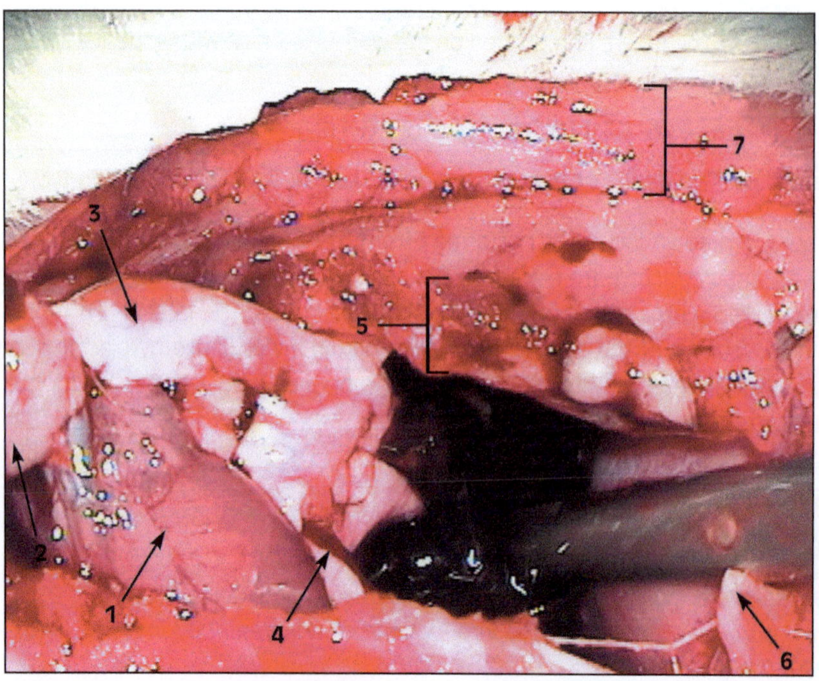

Figure 31-1

Wide U-thoracotomy and en-masse removal of the heart, lungs, and rest of thoracic splanchna. Here the heart is pulled cranially and the hyperdiaphragmatic splanchna (inferior vena cava, aorta, esophagus) are transected with scissors just cranial to the diaphragm. **1.** heart, **2.** right lung, **3.** left lung, **4.** inferior vena cava, **5.** transected thoracic wall, **6.** remnant of the xyphoid process, **7.** skin and superficial fascia. (From author's photo library)

C. Graft harvesting

Removal of the heart is performed en masse together with the lungs, trachea and esophagus (**Fig. 31-1**).

The splanchna seen in the surgical field, including the vessels are presented in **Figure 31-2**.

The following are transected during harvesting of the graft (**Fig. 31-2**):

- the superior vena, leaving a long stump near the heart. This vessel is found in front of the aortic arch.
- the aortic arch, which, together with its three branches, is revealed after moving the stump of the superior vena cava and the left brachiocephalic vein.
- the tree branches of the aortic arch, leaving the maximum possible length at the stump near the heart
  - brachiocephalic trunk
  - left carotid artery
  - left subclavian artery
- the trachea
- the esophagus

and then, just above the diaphragm:

- the inferior vena cava, which passes through the diaphragm in the middle of the dome, anterior to and right of the esophagus
- the esophagus
- the aorta, which passes though the diaphragm posteriorly, behind the esophagus, and near the spine.

The graft harvest must be performed as quickly as possible, with care not to traumatize the graft. Care must be taken to avoid touching the heart during the above maneuvers, and never lift the heart with forceps when cutting the vessels. If the heart needs to be moved, push with a wet cotton-tipped swab. The goal of the en masse removal of thoracic splanchna is to protect the heart as much as possible.

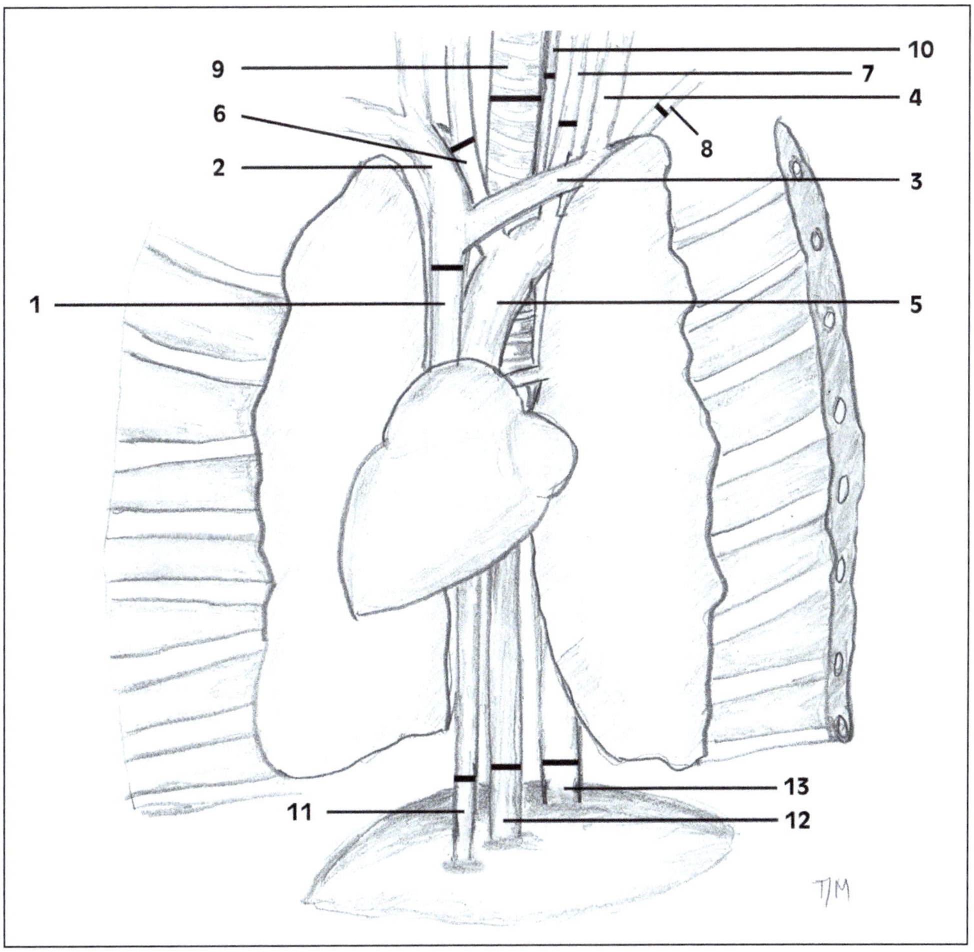

Figure 31-2

Sketch of the view of the surgical field after opening the thoracic wall (rough anatomic relations). The bold lines indicate the sites of transection in order to remove the heart and the rest of splanchna en masse. It is important to acquire long stumps of the big vessels. **1.** superior vena cava, **2.** right brachiocephalic vein, **3.** left brachiocephalic vein, **4.** left internal jugular vein, **5.** aortic arch, **6.** brachiocephalic trunk, **7.** left common carotid artery, **8.** left subclavian artery, **9.** trachea, **10.** cervical esophagus in the neck, **11.** inferior vena cava, **12.** esophagus above the diaphragm, **13.** thoracic aorta. (Drawing by the author)

Comment

In other textbooks and schools of microsurgery, additional techniques are applied prior to harvesting the graft (exsanguination, heparinization, and cardioplegia). However, we believe as others do (Microsurgery 1994; 15:279-81) that these techniques do not offer significant advantages. Nevertherless, they are described below for the reader's awareness, such that after gaining experience, the reader may decide on his/her own preference.

Exsanguination of the rat

A midline incision is made in the abdominal wall. The intestine is enveloped in gauze moistened in warm normal saline and is mobilized to the right of the rat. The retroperitoneum is opened by using two pieces of gauzes to push laterally away from the midline. The aorta and inferior vena cava are exposed with this maneuver. Then, they are transected to allow the animal to exsanguinate. To access the heart, the laparotomy is followed by opening of the diaphragm and lateral thoracotomies as described above.

Heparinization

After opening the abdomen and prior to transection of the aorta and inferior vena cava, 200 units of heparin dissolved in 0.4 ml normal saline are injected into the aorta. The solution is allowed to diffuse for 1 min before the vessels are transected. Details can be found in Microsurgery 2006;26:470-2 and 2005;25: 227-34.

Cardioplegia

In addition to the transabdominally injected heparin solution, a preservation solution for cardioplegia is injected through a 22G angiocatheter into the thoracic aorta, which has been transected. The solution is the Celsior® (Imtix Sangstat Italia, Milan, Italy) and is administered at 10 ml/min. The solution exits from the untransected inferior vena cava, where an opening has been created for this purpose in its supradiaphragmatic part. Ten to 15 mls are injected until the heart turns white and stops beating. Details can be found in Microsurgery 2005;25:227-34.

Other techniques of graft harvest

Some microsurgeons suggest carefully mobilizing the heart with a cotton-tip swab and placing a 4/0 suture (with a double knot ready) to ligate en masse the pulmonary veins and whatever is behind the heart, followed by blind transection (Microsurgery 2005;25:227-34). Others suggest tying the pulmonary veins, the superior and inferior vena cava en block (Microsurgery 1994;15:279-81).

We believe that these techniques are too risky for the trainee to perform safely and accurately. It is preferrable to dissect, identify, and ligate each vessel separately after harvesting the graft, as described below.

D. Microsurgical preparation of the graft

As soon as the graft is removed, it is placed in the gauze-covered dish, which is then placed on the dish with the iced saline serum. The graft is irrigated with abundant cold normal saline. It can be stabilized by pinning the lungs on the gauze. However, we suggest that the graft stays freely moving to allow for more maneuverability with handling. It is strongly suggested that the graft dissection be performed through the surgical microscope, as described here.

- ➢ Before starting the dissection of the graft, it is essential that the graft be flushed with cold normal saline in order to remove the contained blood. The injection is performed via the inferior vena cava (**Fig. 31-3**).

1. Removal of the lungs, esophagus, trachea

The splanchna (esophagus, trachea, lungs) taken from the chest together with the heart are dissected and removed. We start with removal of the lungs.

Removal of the lungs, on either side, is performed by transecting the root of the lungs close to the hilum. The transection is guided by the pulmonary veins, which are evident. In humans, the four pulmonary veins enter the left atrium, in the posterior surface of the heart. In the rat, however, on either side, the two pulmonary veins confluence in a single vein after exiting from the hilum of the lung; thus, in the root of the lung, only one pulmonary vein is encountered (the root of the lung is defined at some distance towards the heart, while the hilum of the lung is defined exactly on the viscerum—the root consists of the structures entering and emerging at the hilum). The most reliable me-

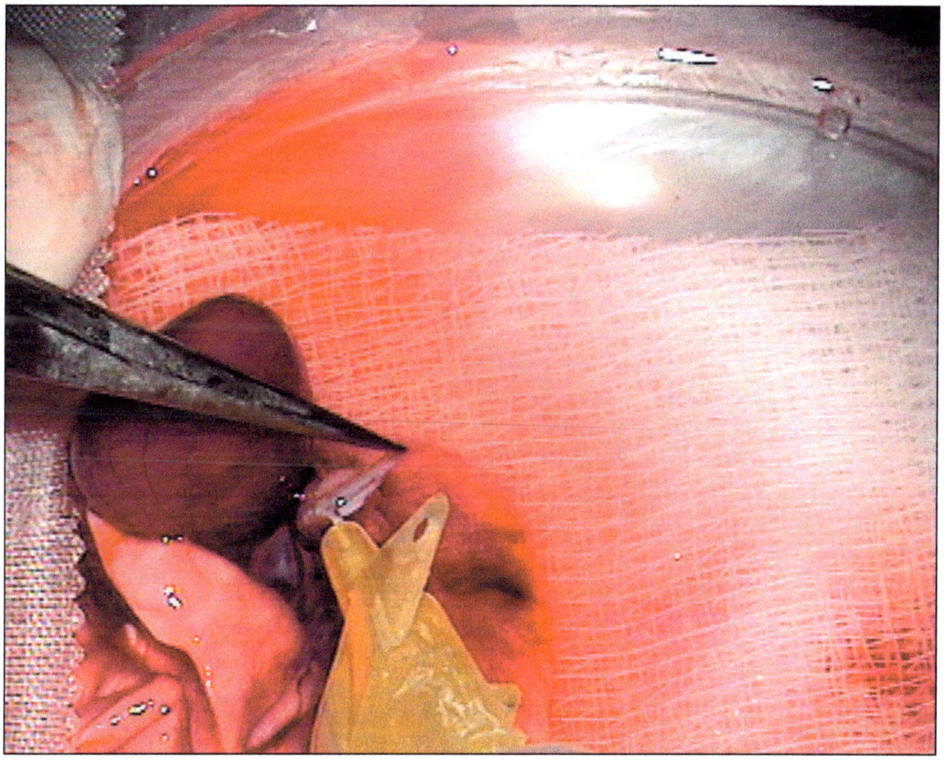

Figure 31-3

Injection of cold normal saline in the inferior vena cava for flushing the graft. The heart is placed on the Petri dish with gauze on the bottom, which is placed on another dish with ice. The two dishes are immobilized with adhesive tape on the working surface (here the left band can be seen). A Dumont No. 3 forceps lifts the stump of the inferior vena cava. The injection is performed through a 27G venocatheter, inserted into the lumen. (From author's photo library)

thod is to follow the pulmonary vein peripherally starting from the heart and to perform the transection close to the hilum of the lung. It is expected to have two veins close to the hilum where the transection is performed (**Fig. 31-4A**). This is not an issue because ligation of the pulmonary vein will be done at the root of the lung where the vein is singular (see immediately below, I.D.2 and **Fig. 31-13A**).

Transection of the root of the lung will be performed en block as close as possible to the hilum, including the pulmonary veins, the main bronchi (and possibly the lobar bronchi if the 2nd class division takes place before the hilum of the lung), and the pulmonary arteries. The bronchi will be evident by their cartilaginous structure and the open lumens (**Fig. 31-4B**).

Our suggestion is to perform the transection of the root of the right lung with the heart reversed and the apex up, while the rest of splanchna are left in place (**Fig. 31-4**). For the pulmonary root of the other lung, you can work with the heart resting on its base because there is already good exposure (**Fig. 31-5**).

The pulmonary arteries will be transected without dissection at the root of the lungs. The wall of the vessel does not help to immediately recognize the pulmonary arteries. Although named 'arteries', the wall is vein-like. It is of extreme importance that the stump of the left pulmonary artery toward the graft be left long (see below), because this will be the 'vein' of the graft. In order to preserve the pulmonary arteries of the graft, transect the contents of the root as close as possible to the hilum for each lung.

Dissection continues with the *removal of the esophagus*. The only attachment of the esophagus is the symphysis between the anterior wall of the esophagus and the posterior wall of the trachea. This attachment is dissected and transected (**Fig. 31-6**), which frees the esophagus to be moved away from the surgical field.

Removal of the trachea follows. Dissection starts from the left side. Connective tissue of the mediastinum connects the trachea to the posterior surface of the aortic arch. With blunt dissection while holding the trachea away from the transected left bronchus, the connection with the aortic arch is detached (**Fig. 31-7**).

In the right side, the trachea is related to the supe-

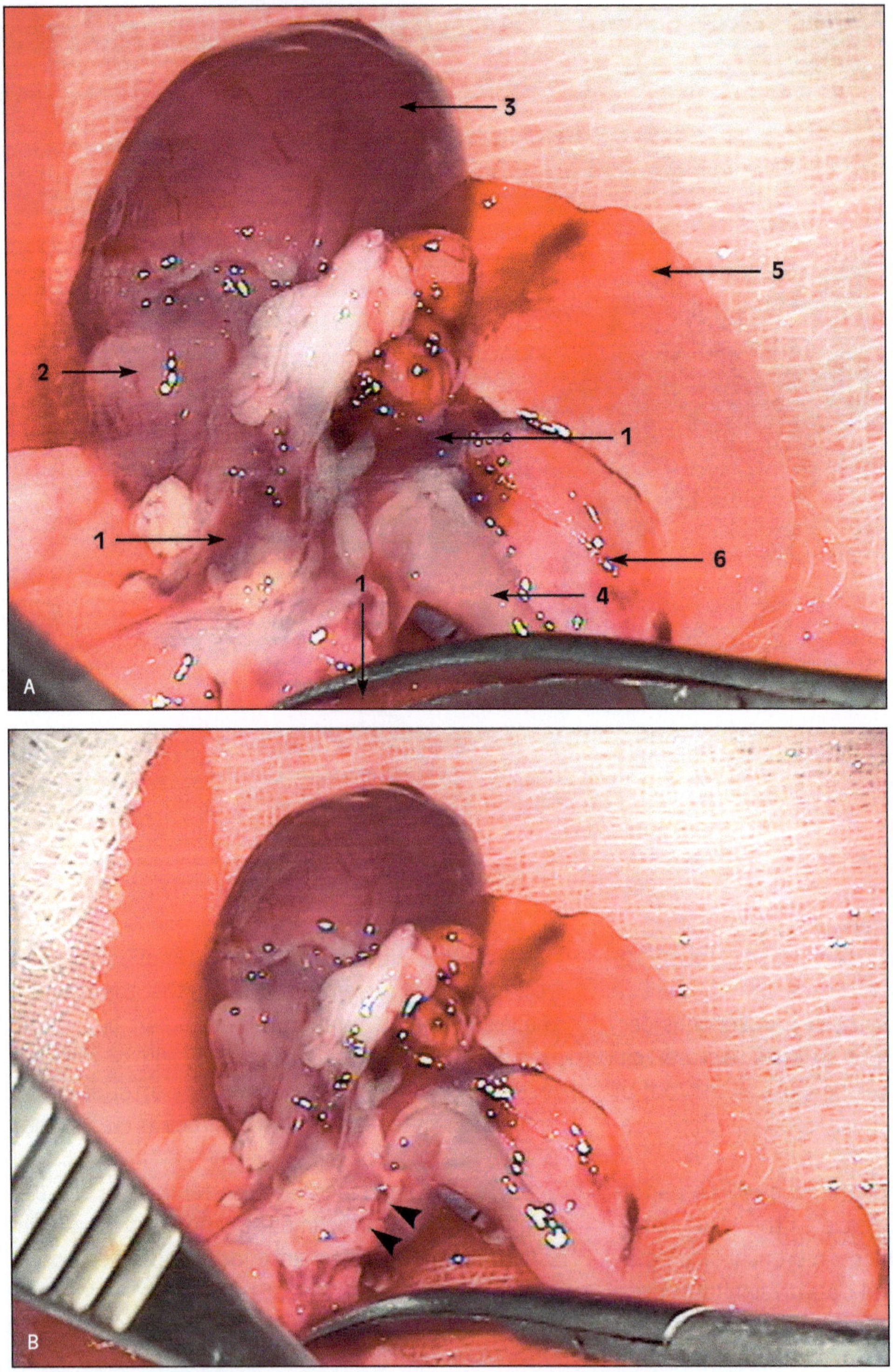

Figure 31-4

Transection of the root of the right lung near the hilum, guided by the pulmonary vein. Near the hilum of the lung, there are two pulmonary veins, which converge into one at the root of the lung close to the heart. The heart has been reversed with the apex up, while the rest of splanchna is left in normal position. **A.** The transection is performed as peripherally as possible, at the hilum of the lung. Here the lower (lobar) pulmonary vein is in the legs of the scissors. **B.** Completed transection of the root segment addressed to the lower lobe of the right lung. Observe the transected bronchi with the lumens wide open (arrowheads). The rest of the root is held by the forceps and the tip of the scissors. **1.** pulmonary vein, **2.** right atrium, **3.** left ventricle, **4.** esophagus, **5.** upper lobe of left lung, **6.** lower lobe of left lung. (From author's photo library)

rior vena cava, which is located in front of it and has to be preserved. The cranial part of the attachment between the superior vena cava and the trachea can be transected with no risk (**Fig. 31-8**). Attention is needed in the lower part of the trachea and especially in the azygos vein, which arches over the right main bronchus to exit in the superior vena cava. After the trachea has been mobilized cranially, dissection will continue toward the root of the lung by pulling the trachea and transecting the attachments close to the

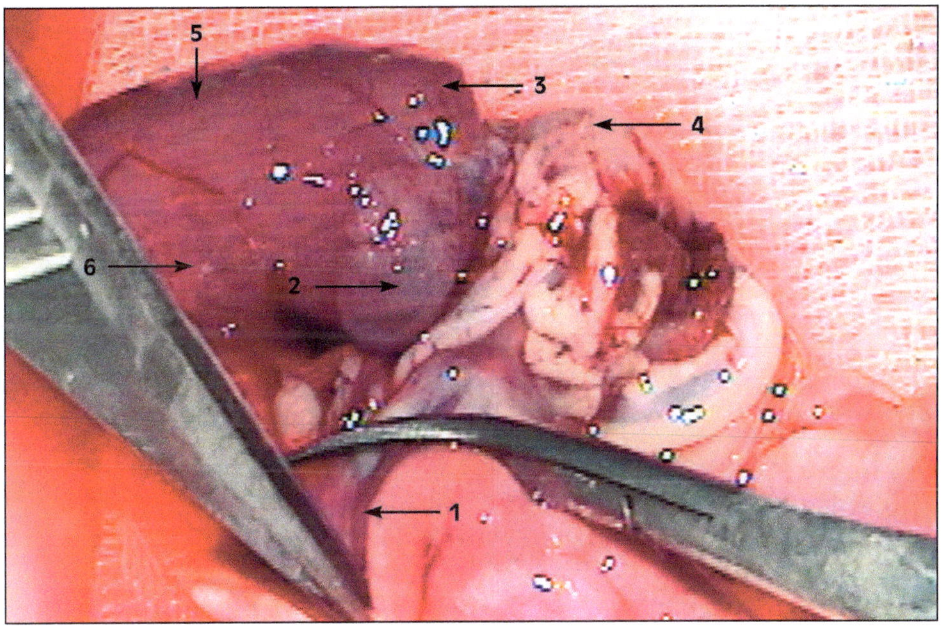

Figure 31-5

Transection of the root of the left lung near the hilum. The heart is normally resting on its base (view from left side). The forceps moves the lung and scissors are used to transect en block the contents of the root as close as possible to the hilum of the lung. **1.** pulmonary vein, **2.** left atrium, 3. right atrium, **4.** superior vena cava, **5.** right ventricle, **6.** left ventricle. (From author's photo library)

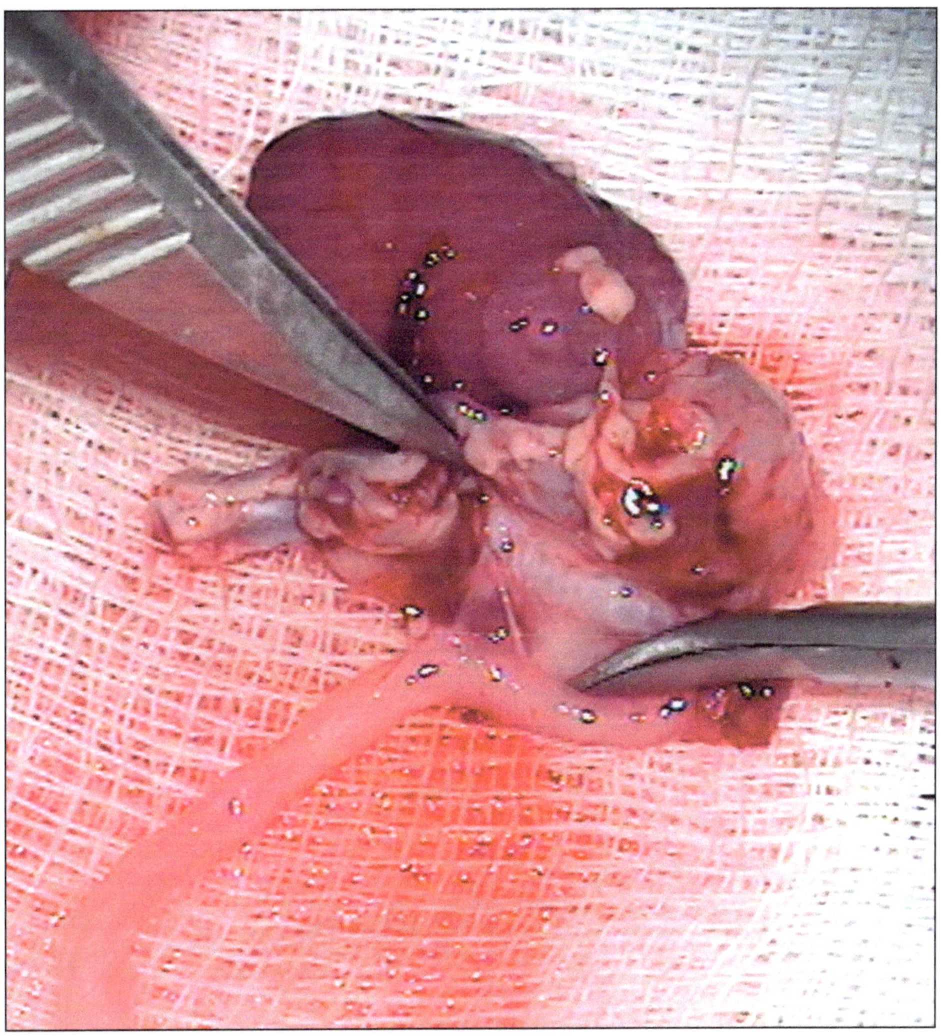

Figure 31-6

Removal of the esophagus. The forceps holds the trachea, while the closed scissors are used to dissect the attachment between the posterior wall of the trachea and the anterior wall of the esophagus. (From author's photo library)

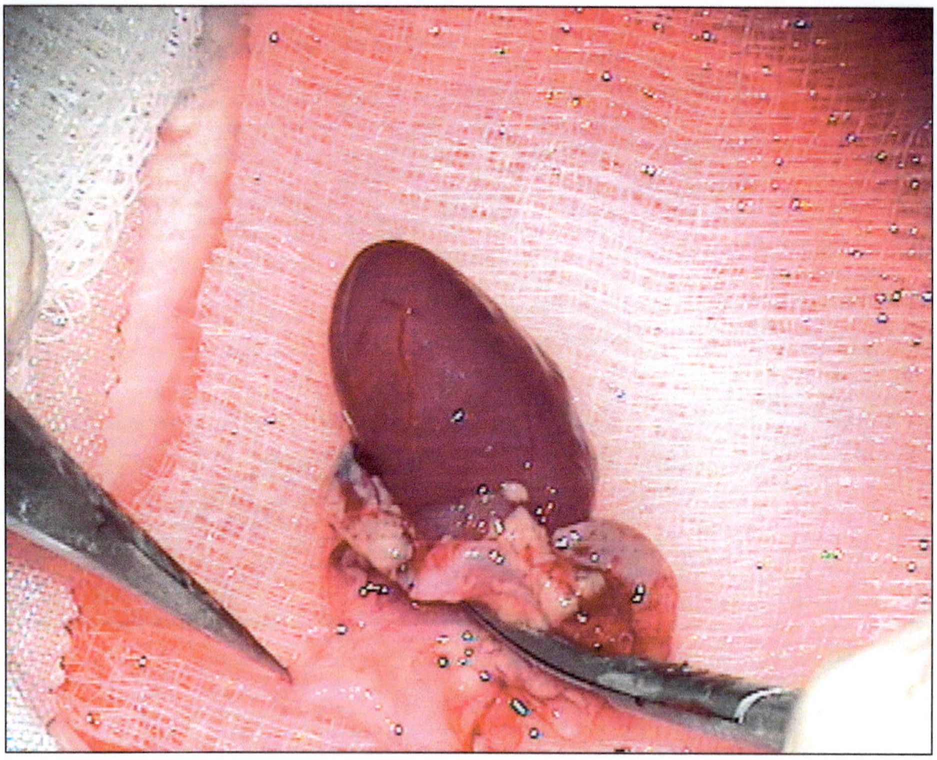

Figure 31-7

Dissection of the trachea stump, left side of the graft. The forceps holds the transected main bronchus while the scissors bluntly dissect the remaining structures of the root of the lung (pulmonary artery and veins) and move them towards the heart. (From author's photo library)

tracheal wall (**Fig. 31-9A**). Finally, the transected right main bronchus can be pulled under the azygos arch and freed from the vessels of the root of the lung (**Fig. 31-9B**). The azygos vein must be preserved, because in the suite, the superior vena cava is going to be ligated just central to the exit of the azygos vein.

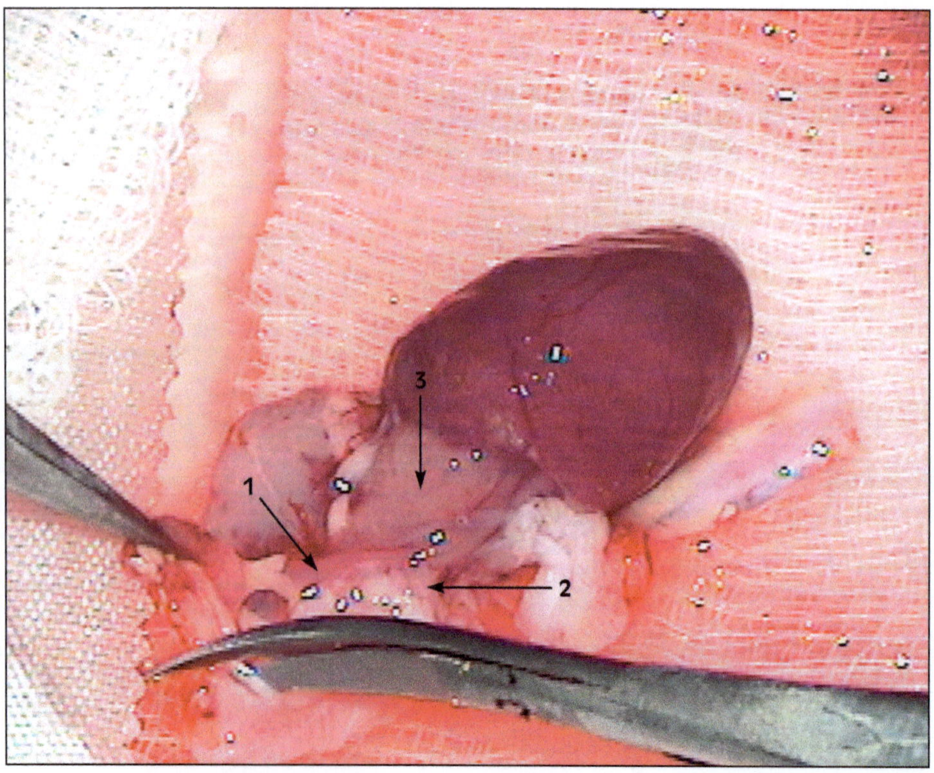

Figure 31-8

Dissection of the cranial part of the trachea on the right side. The trachea is separated by transecting the attachments to the superior vena cava, which is located anterior to it. **1.** superior vena cava, **2.** azygos vein (non-dissected), **3.** right atrium. (From author's photo library)

Figure 31-9

Detachment of the trachea and right main bronchus from the rest of the constituents of the root of the right lung, **A.** Sharp dissection of the trachea with s-cissors, performed close to its wall. **B.** Final step of the dissection. The last attachments of the right main bronchus are transected. (From author's photo library)

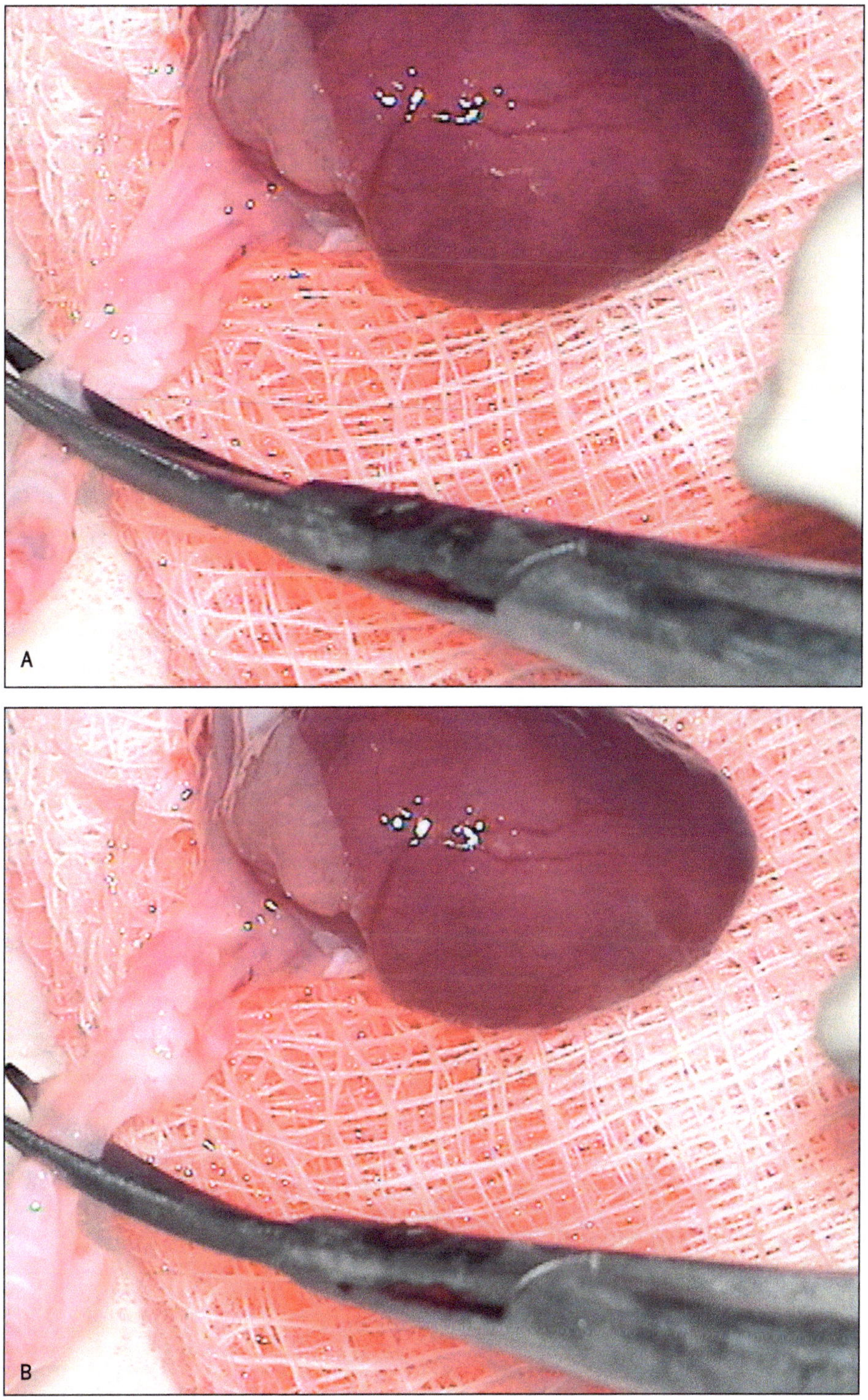

2. Ligation of the vessels of the heart

The following vessels of the heart are ligated (Nylon 5/0) and transected (peripheral to the ligation) in sequence (**Fig. 31-10**):

- superior vena cava
- right pulmonary vein (one in the rat)
- right pulmonary artery
- left pulmonary vein (one in the rat)
- branches of the aortic arch
- inferior vena cava

The vessels that remain and will be used for the anastomoses are:

- the aorta
- the left pulmonary artery

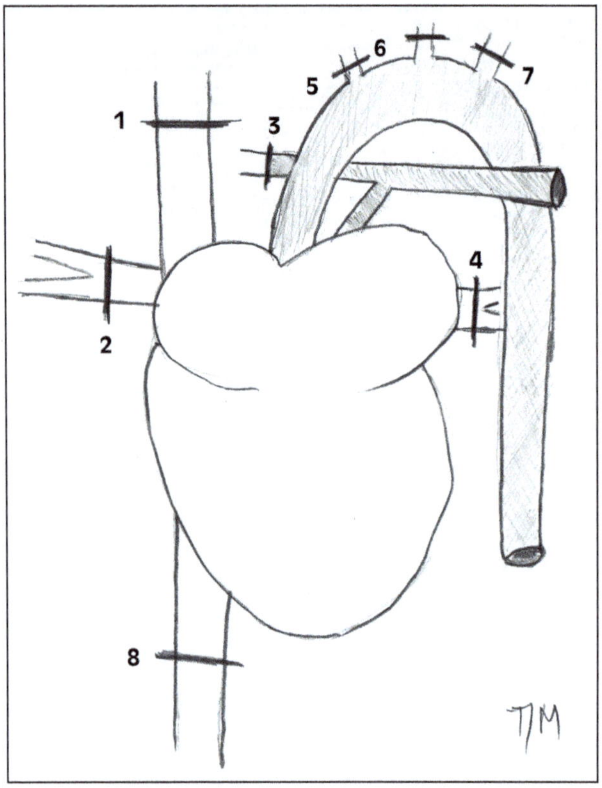

Figure 31-10

Diagrammatic representation of the sites of ligation and transection of the vessels in the heart graft, each noted by a heavy line. Numbers annotate the order of the ligations. **1.** superior vena cava, **2.** right pulmonary vein, **3.** right pulmonary artery, **4.** left pulmonary vein, **5.** brachiocephalic trunk, **6.** left common carotid artery, **7.** left subclavian artery, **8.** inferior vena cava. (Drawing by the author)

In continuation of the dissection described above, *superior vena cava* is ligated first. The ligation is placed between the confluence of the azygos vein and the exit of the superior vena cava into the right atrium (**Fig. 31-11**). If difficulty is encountered in dissecting and identifying the azygos vein, ligate the superior vena cava as close as possible to the right atrium to ensure that the azygos vein is not left open.

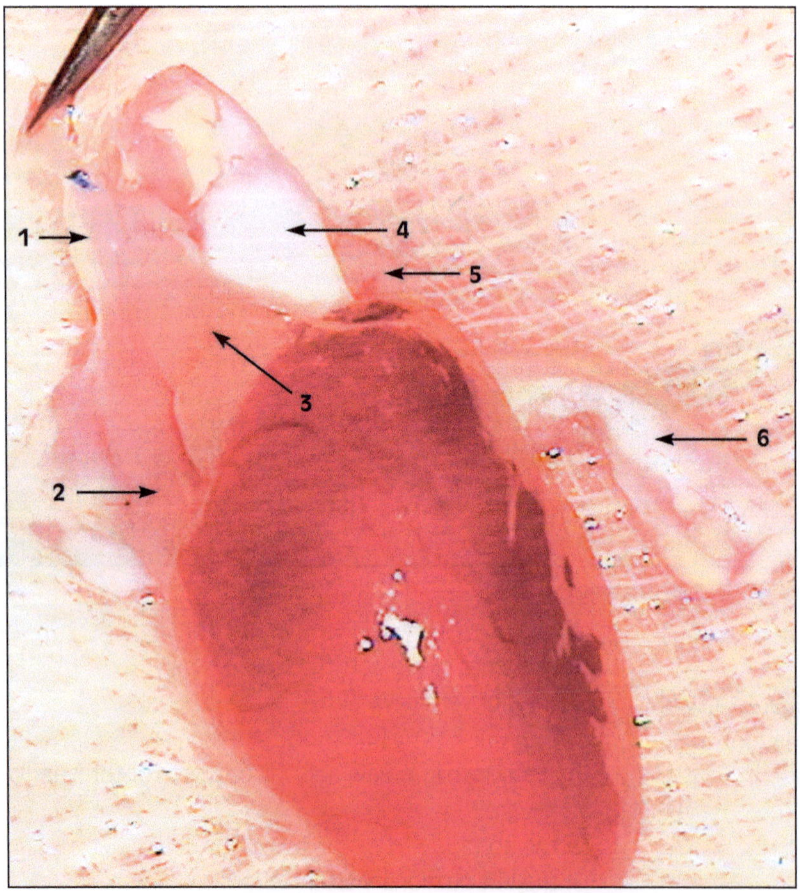

Figure 31-11

Ligation of the superior vena cava. The microsurgical forceps holds the stump of the superior vena cava at the confluence with the azygos vein. The ligation of the superior vena cava has been placed more centrally. The traction also moves the inferior vena cava and partially the right atrium upwards. **1.** superior vena cava, **2.** inferior vena cava, **3.** right atrium, **4.** aortic arch, **5.** pulmonary artery trunk, **6.** thoracic aorta. (From author's photo library)

Dissection continues in the right side of the heart, in the remaining structures of the root of the right lung after removal of the right bronchus, to find the *right pulmonary artery and vein*. With blunt dissection in this 'mass', using microsurgical scissors and forceps (**Fig. 31-12**), the vessels found are dissected and identified. While it sounds simple, these vessels may be difficult to distinguish between pulmonary artery and vein because they are macroscopically similar, and the two cannot be discriminated by 'feeling' the vessel with forceps. This is due to the specific histological structure of pulmonary vessels: the veins have a well-developed media of smooth muscle cells, while the arteries have reduced muscle and elastic elements compared with the rest arteries of the body. Therefore, in order to identify the pulmonary vessels, it is normal to reference memories of human anatomy (what is in front? the arteries or the veins?). However, with the vessels cut and after all the preceding manipulations, this approach may not be possible. Thus, it is necessary to follow the vessels and name them after identifying their course towards the heart when completely dissected.

We reiterate that the pulmonary veins in the rat converge and form one pulmonary vein, where as humans have two with separate exits. On the right side, this vein is relatively wide, short and exits in the left atrium as expected. When the latter is visualized, it confirms correct identification of the *right pulmonary vein*, which is subsequently ligated after the confluence of the two tributary veins, towards the heart (**Fig. 31-13**).

In the root of the right lung, the *right pulmonary artery* is longer and narrower compared with the ipsilateral pulmonary vein. With the heart in normal position, the pulmonary artery is located cranial to the pulmonary vein. When the pulmonary artery is pulled, it becomes evident that it is in close relation with the superior vena cava found immediately anterior to it. The pulmonary artery is ligated as close as possible to the heart to avoid leaving a long stump (**Fig. 31-14**).

For an experienced microsurgeon, the location of

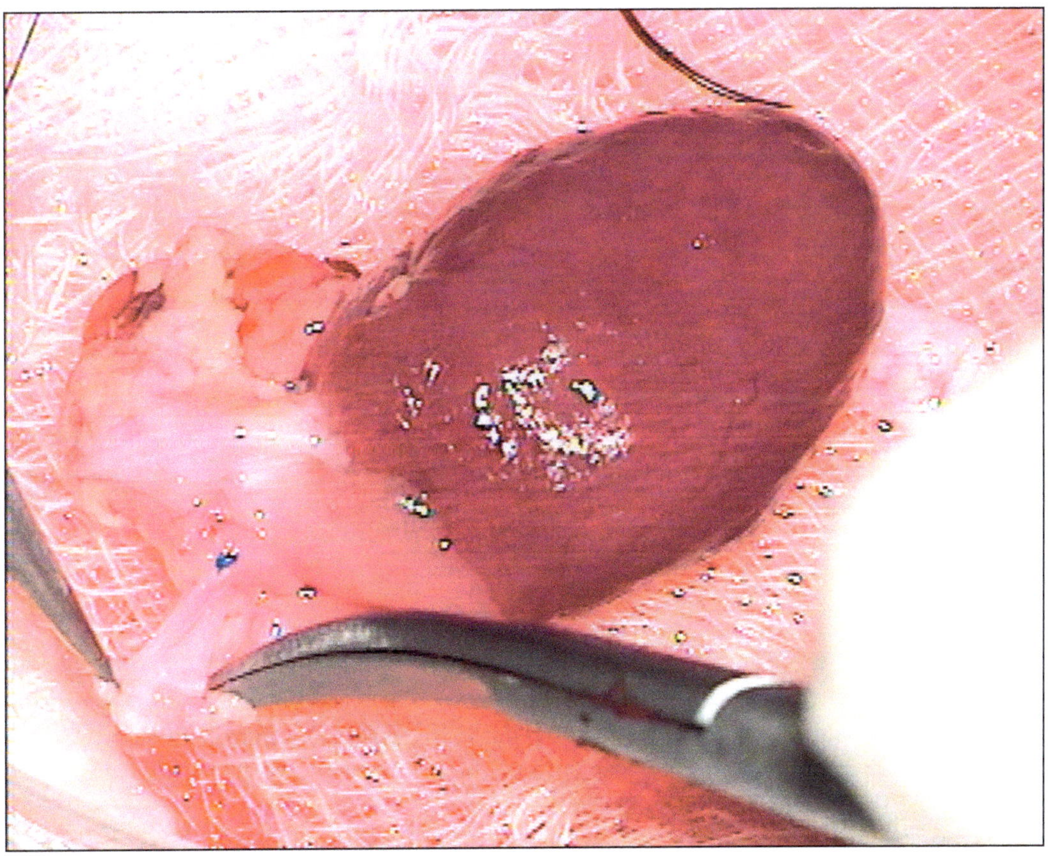

Figure 31-12

Blunt dissection of the remaining structures in the root of the right lung (after removal of the main bronchus and trachea), aimed to find the pulmonary artery and vein(s). The knot seen (blue dot) is the preceding ligation of the superior vena cava. (From author's photo library)

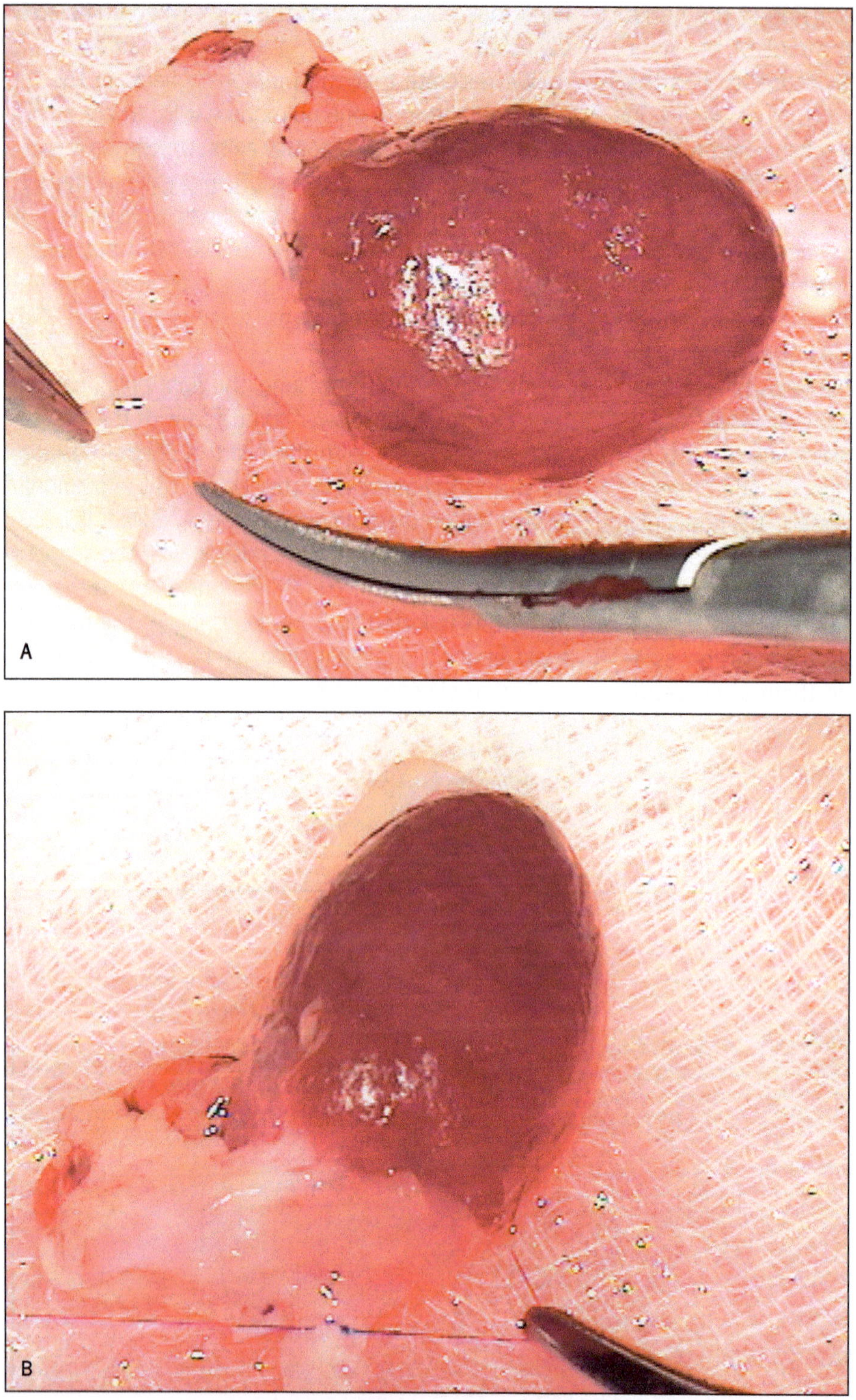

Figure 31-13

Dissection and ligation of the right pulmonary vein. **A.** The two pulmonary veins converge into a single pulmonary vein, which is wide and short. **B.** Ligation on the (single) right pulmonary vein, between the confluence of the two tributary pulmonary veins and its exit into the right atrium (From author's photo library)

the right pulmonary artery immediately posterior to the ligated superior vena cava can direct the dissection into the 'mass' of the root of the right lung (**Fig. 31-15**). If this tactics is followed, the right pulmonary artery is ligated first, and the right pulmonary vein follows after meticulous dissection.

In the left side, the *left pulmonary artery* is preserved while the *left pulmonary vein* is ligated. Since the pulmonary trunk is found under the aortic arch, it may be helpful to move the thoracic aortic stump cranially. This will open the arch and provide a wide view of the pulmonary vessels (**Fig. 31-16**). Dissection and ligation

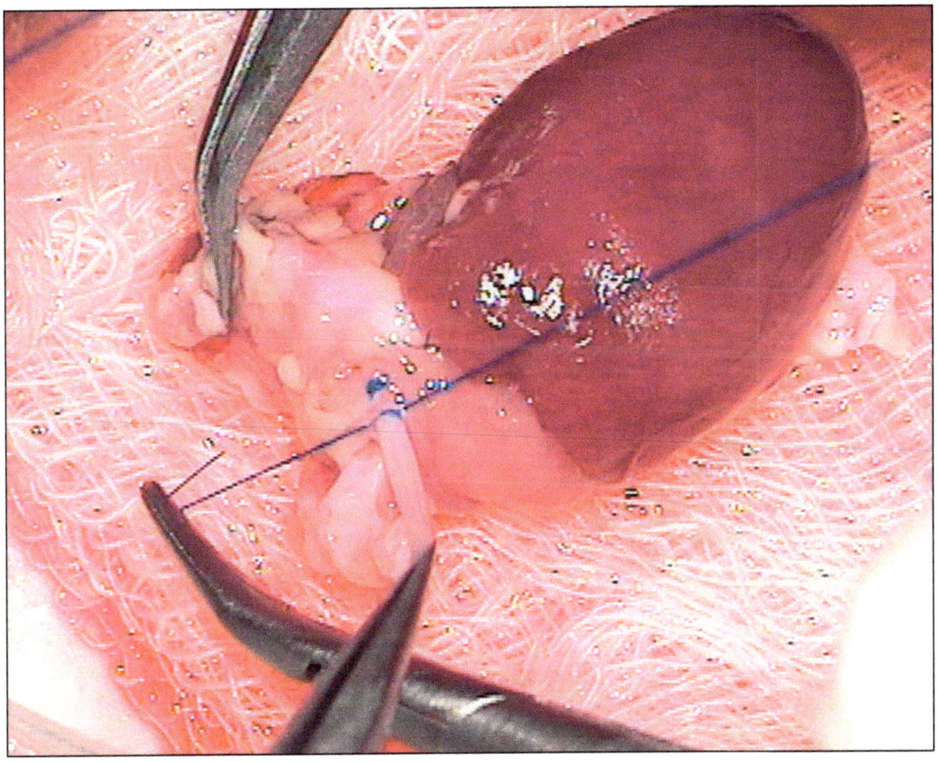

Figure 31-14

Ligation of the dissected right pulmonary artery. The artery is held from the edge and the knot descends as low as possible to the left. Note that the right pulmonary artery is found posterior to the superior vena cava, whose knot can be seen in front of the current ligation. (From author's photo library)

of the left pulmonary vein in the root of the left lung (**Fig. 31-16A**) may prove difficult. Evidently, attention must be paid not to ligate the left pulmonary artery instead of the left pulmonary vein (the artery should stay intact with the graft to serve as the 'vein' of the graft, see below). Meticulous dissection in the root of the lung, with removal of the mediastinal fat, will help to discriminate the two vessels (**Fig. 31-16B**). The left pul-

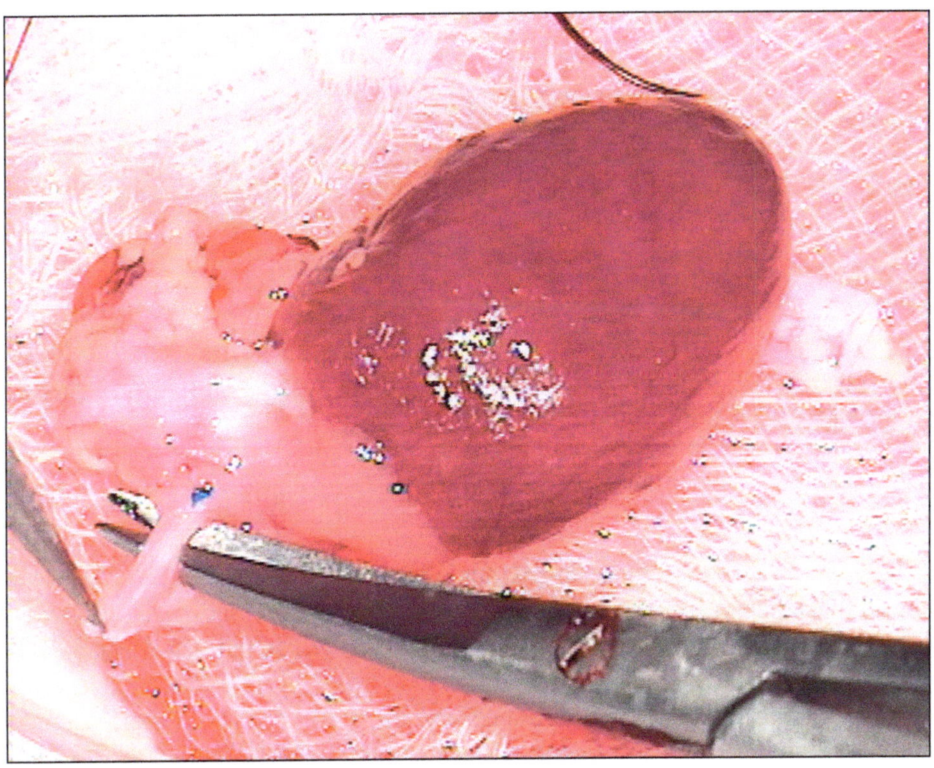

Figure 31-15

Direct dissection of the right pulmonary artery, guided by the ligated superior vena cava (the blue knot) and the fact that the right pulmonary artery courses behind the superior vena cava. The root of the lung is pulled with the forceps and the right pulmonary artery is exposed by blunt dissection with scissors. Here the artery rests on the legs of the scissors. (From author's photo library)

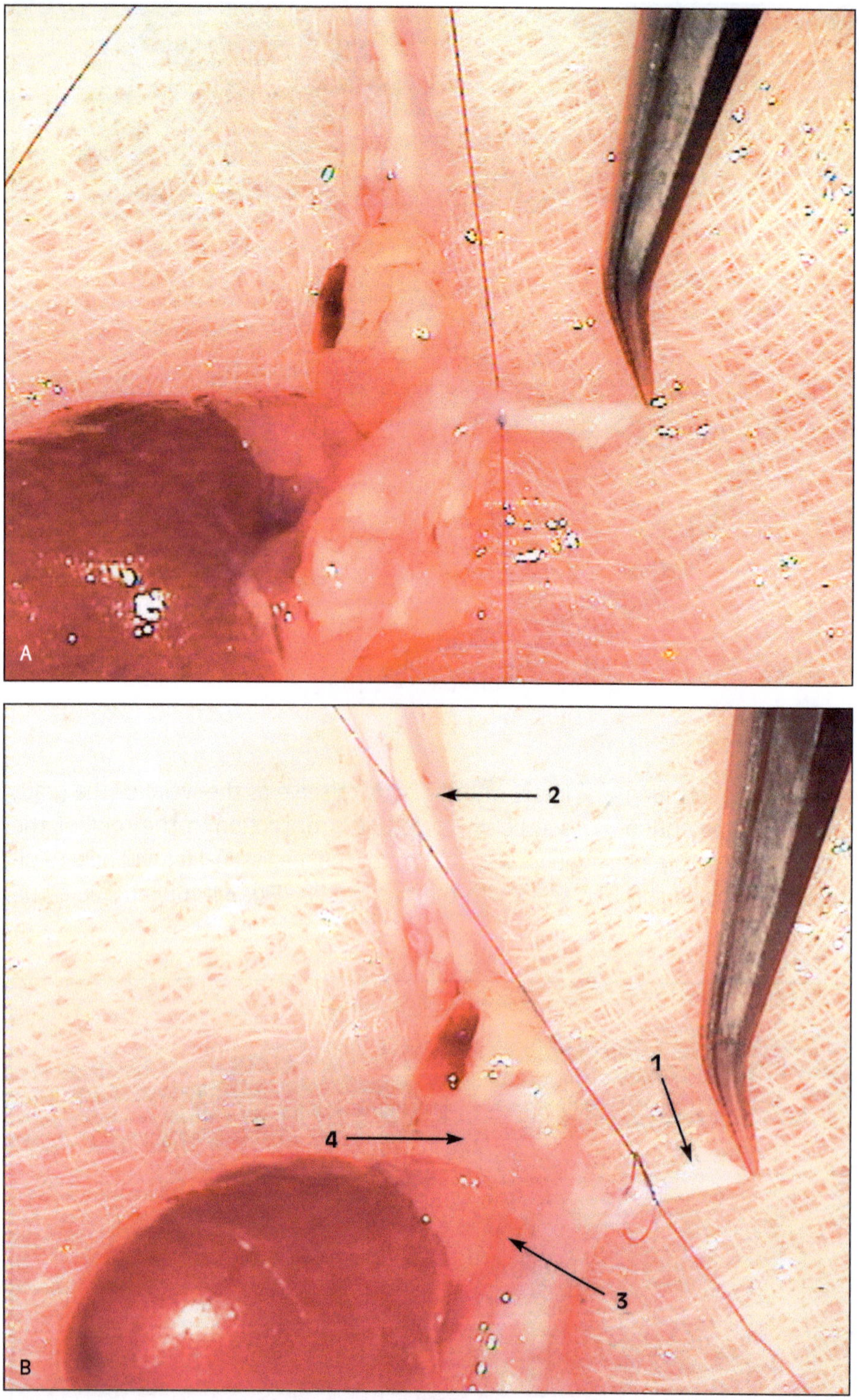

Figure 31-16

Exposure and ligation of the left pulmonary vein (left side view). The thoracic aorta has been rotated cranially, and the aortic arch has been aligned. The curved forceps holds the right pulmonary vein, while the knot is descending. **A.** View after rough dissection of the stump of the root of the left lung. **B.** More detailed dissection after removal of mediastinal fat at the origin/exit of the pulmonary vessels. The left pulmonary artery has been rotated to the right for better exposure of the left pulmonary vein. If the forceps pulls the vein, the tension is transferred to its attachment at the left atrium (verification that the vessel is indeed the pulmonary vein). **1.** left pulmonary vein, **2.** thoracic aorta (reflected cranially), **3.** exit of the left pulmonary vein to the left atrium. **4.** left pulmonary artery (reflected to the right of the graft). (From author's photo library)

monary artery is found cranial to the homonymous vein. In the stump of the root of the lung, the artery is longer than the vein; therefore the stump of the artery overlaps the stump of the vein. Rightward rotation (to the right of the graft) of the left pulmonary artery stump allows visualization and ligation of the stump of the left pulmonary vein (**Fig. 31-16 B**). In any case, it is verified that the vessel to ligate arises off the left atrium (No. 3, **Fig. 31-16B**).

The three branches of the aortic arch, *the brachiocephalic trunk, the left common carotid artery,* and *the left subclaviam artery* are dissected and ligated in order

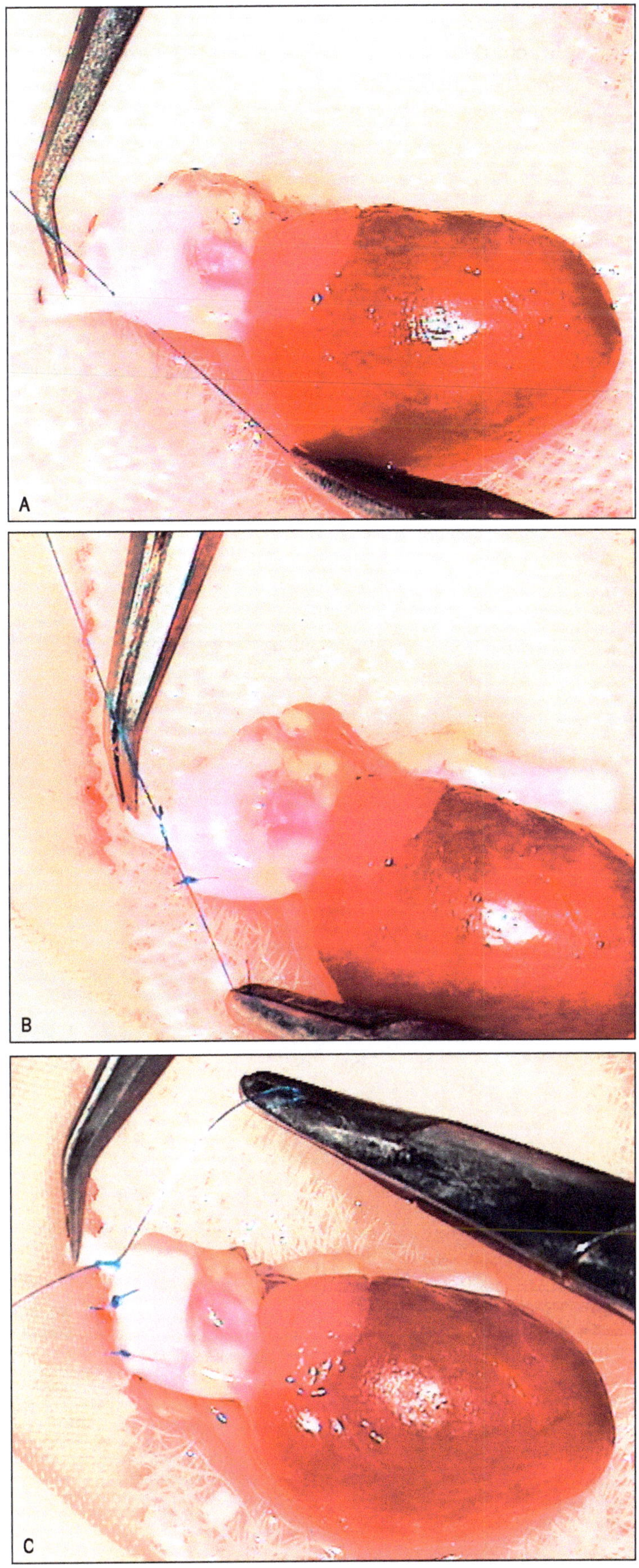

Figure 31-17

Ligation of the three branches of the aortic arch: **A.** brachiocephalic trunk, **B.** left common carotid artery, **C.** left subclaviam artery. (From author's photo library)

(**Fig. 31-17**). The stumps of the vessels can initially be left long to be used for traction while placing the next ligations and then are cut short.

The *inferior vena cava* will be ligated next. Before ligation, the graft is flushed for the last time via the stump of the inferior vena cava (**Fig. 31-18**). Cold heparin solution will be used again. The liquid will pass through the right atrium and right ventricle, and will exit from the open left pulmonary artery; therefore, the left heart is not flushed. Then the inferior vena cava is ligated so that the knot will descend very low at the exit of the vessel in the right atrium, without leaving a residual stump (**Fig. 31-19**). The remaining initial stump of the inferior vena cava is transected peripherally to the ligation and removed from the field.

Then the *thoracic aorta* stump is dissected in its full length. The fat and residues attached to the vessel wall are removed. The dissection is performed in a retrograde order; it starts peripherally with the descending aorta and advances centrally to the aortic arch and the ascending aorta (**Fig. 31-20A**). The dissection is expanded in the adjacent pulmonary trunk in order to free and lengthen the left pulmonary artery (**Fig. 31-20B**).

The dissected stump of the aorta is evidently much longer than that of the left pulmonary artery. These two vessels will be kept in the graft to serve as entrance (aorta) and exit (left pulmonary artery) of the blood stream and will be respectively anastomosed with the aorta and the inferior vena cava of the recipient. The aorta must be cut so that the stump remaining on the graft should a bit longer the stump of the pulmonary

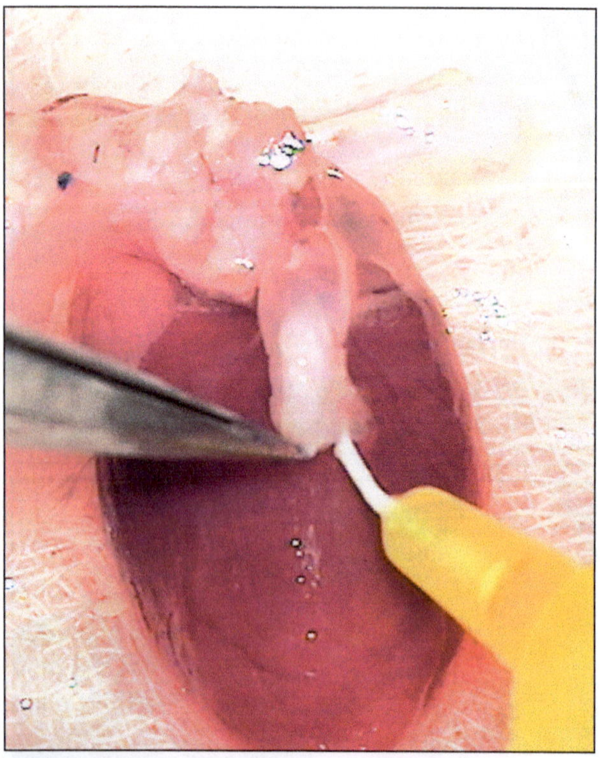

Figure 31-18

Flushing with cold heparin solution through the stump of the inferior vena cava. The posterior surface of the heart is shown. The inferior vena cava enters caudally into the right atrium, which is found on the left here because the heart has been reversed. The forceps holds the adventitia of the vein stump, while the venocatheter 27G injects with pressure the saline without entering the lumen. The fluid washes the right heart and exits from the left pulmonary artery. (From author's photo library)

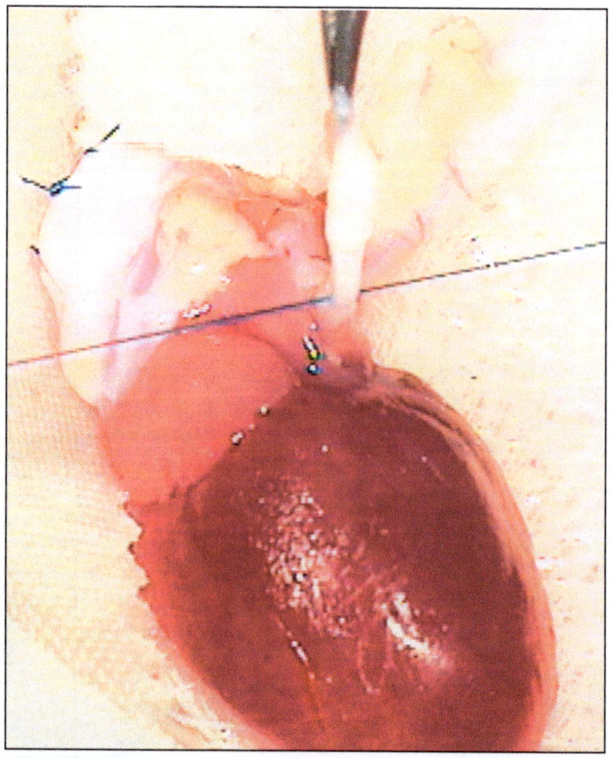

Figure 31-19

Ligation of the stump of the inferior vena cava. The heart has been reversed and the posterior surface is exposed; the descending aorta has been inverted and left on the upper part of the field, thus dislocating the aortic arch (the blue knots of the ligations on the stumps of the three divided branches can be seen). Here, the knot of the ligation descends as proximally as possible to the right atrium. (From author's photo library)

Figure 31-20

Dissection of the aorta stump. **A.** Removal of the fatty tissue from the stump of descending aorta starts peripherally with sharp dissection (forceps-scissors). The curved forceps holds the end of the stump under moderate tension. **B.** During the same dissection the pulmonary trunk is also cleaned. **1.** aortic arch, **2.** pulmonary trunk, **3.** left pulmonary artery, **4.** ligated left pulmonary vein. (From author's photo library)

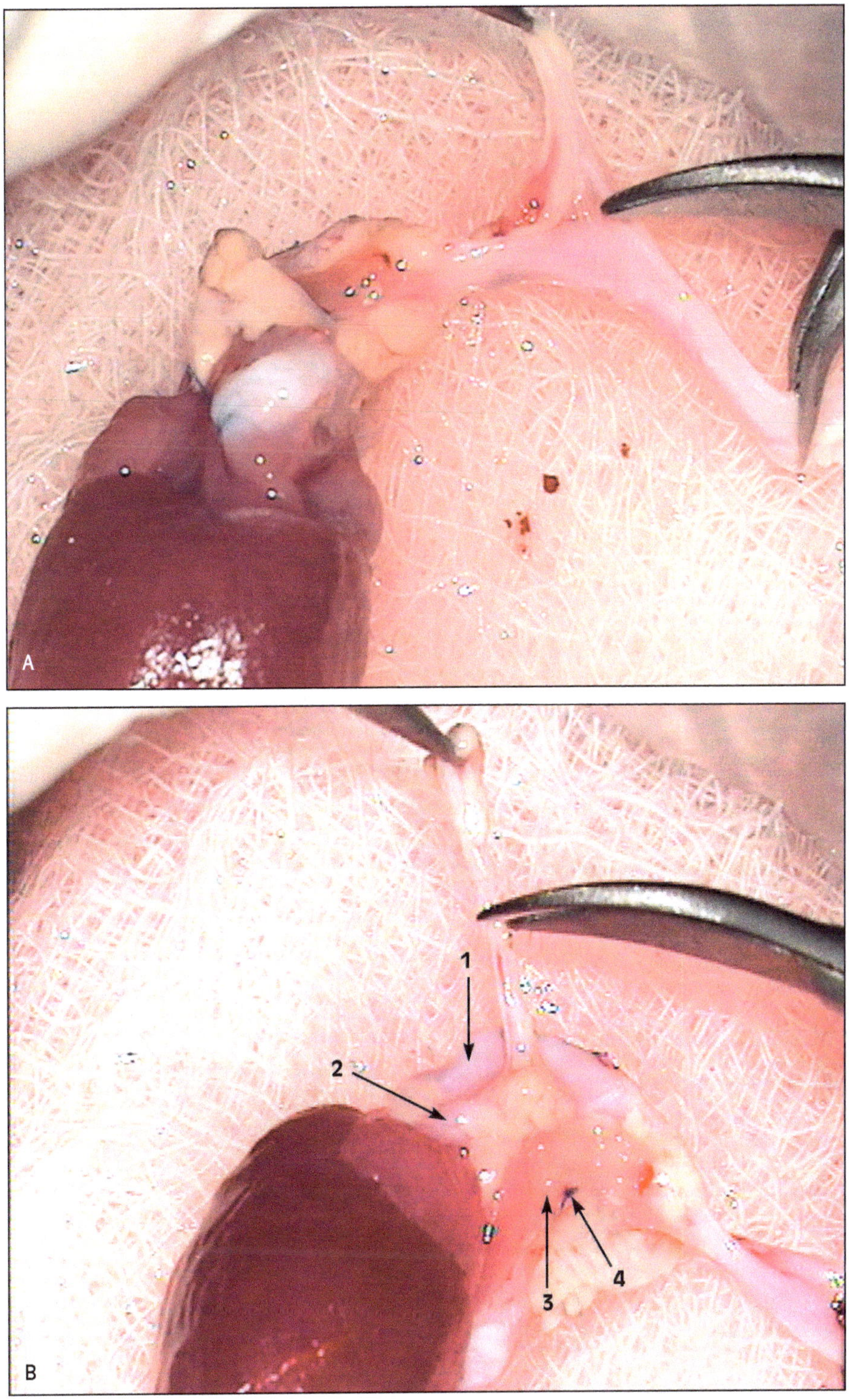

artery (**Fig. 31-21**). This is needed because during implantation of the graft, the recipient's aorta is placed to the right of the inferior vena cava in the double vascular clamp and thus is found more distant to the graft, which is placed in the left side of the recipient (see below). Pay attention to the length of the aortic stump: if the aortic stump is cut too short, this will disturb the positioning of the graft and make the anastomoses difficult due to lack of space. On the contrary, if the stump is left too long, it may undergo kinking or twi-

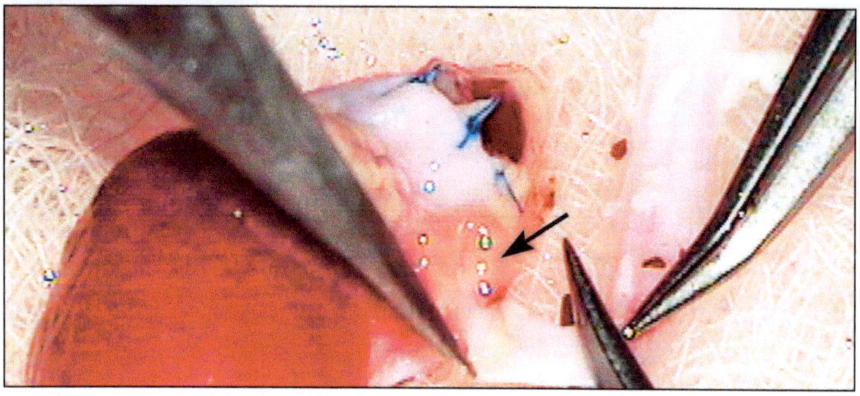

Figure 31-21

Transection of the stump of the descending aorta. The remaining length should be longer than that of the left pulmonary artery, here seen shrunken (arrow). The two forceps hold the aorta from the adventitia, while the scissors are brought perpendicular to the axis of the vessel. The transection should be done with a single cut of the scissors. (From author's photo library)

sting, but this can be repaired before the anastomosis; thus, if there is any doubt, it is better to leave the stump longer than shorter.

After transection, the aortic stump should be irrigated with normal saline using a fine venocatheter (**Fig. 31-22**). Of course, if the aortic valve is normal, the serum will not reach the left ventricle, and the liquid will flow back and exit from the aortic opening. Therefore, the irrigation must be performed slowly and repetitively. The vessel can also be washed at earlier stages (e.g. after transection of the thoracic aorta). After irrigation, the aortic stump will be prepared for the anastomosis by reflecting the adventitia (**Fig. 31-23**).

The *stump of the left pulmonary artery* must also be prepared. Because of the non-arterial structure of the pulmonary artery, it needs to be handled as a vein (e.g. irrigation with serum to keep the lumen open, etc). A final irrigation of the lumen is performed using a 27G venocatheter (**Fig. 31-24**). The adventitia may need to be transected at the perimeter of the edge and be removed. Given that the implantation of the graft in the recipient will be complicated, the lumen of the left pulmonary artery should be dilated at this

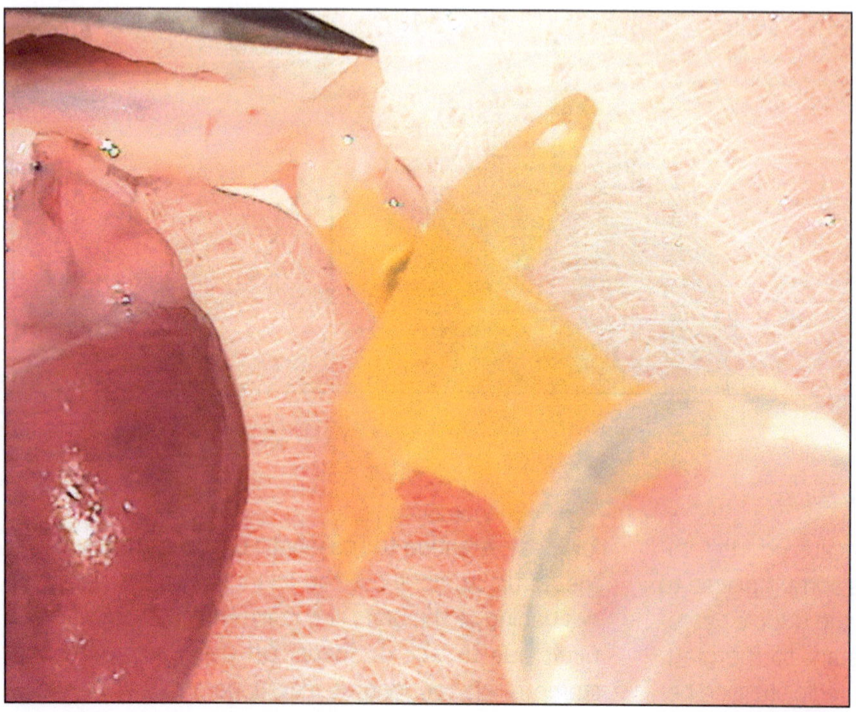

Figure 31-22

Irrigation of the aortic stump before dissection and folding of the adventitia. Normal saline is injected through a 27G catheter inserted carefully into the lumen. Injection is performed slowly and intermittently, because the fluid refluxes back from the entrance as the aortic valve obstructs the flow towards the left ventricle. Here, in order to facilitate the exit of the fluid, the catheter has temporarily been drawn out of the vessel (white item under the aorta). (From author's photo library)

Figure 31-23

Folding of the adventitia of the aortic stump. One forceps holds the external surface of the wall and the other reflects the adventitia. (From author's photo library)

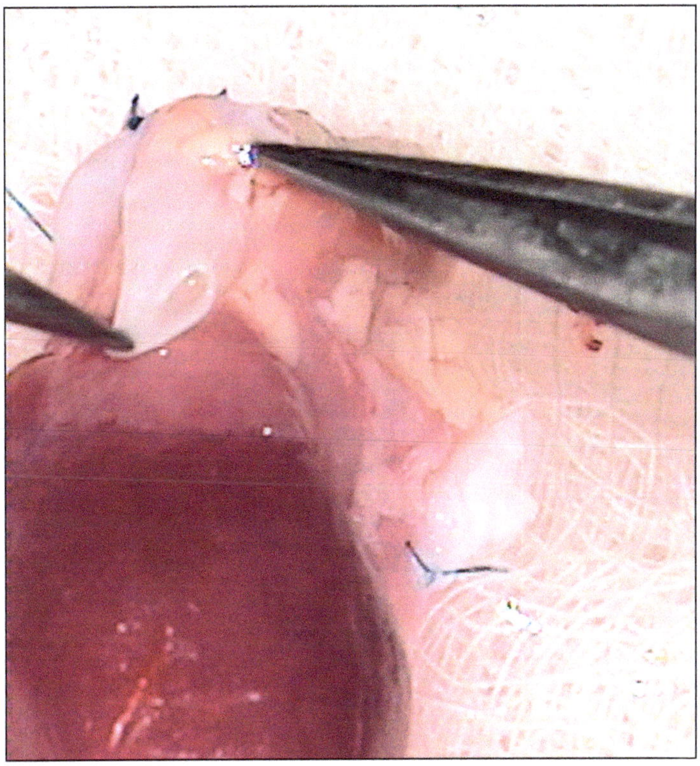

point. To achieve this, a relatively blunt microsurgical forceps enters the lumen and is left to open the lumen gradually (**Fig 31-25**). This maneuver can be repeated a few times.

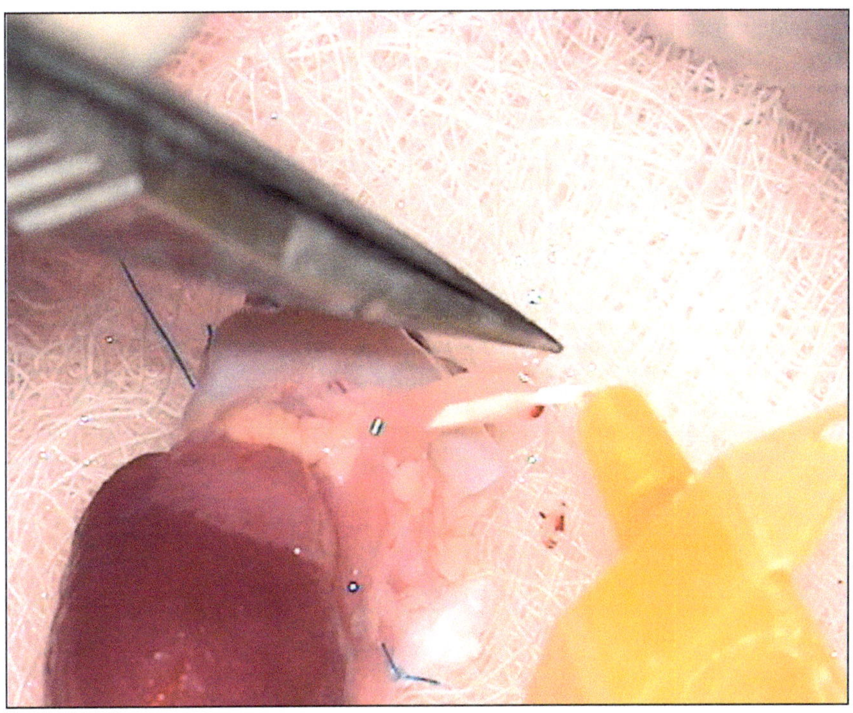

Figure 31-24

Irrigation of the stump of the left pulmonary artery. A Dumont No. 3 forceps lifts the wall of the vessel, while a venocatheter 27G, with its tip bent, enters the lumen and performs the wash of the vessel. Observe the 'venous' structure of the vessel wall: the adventitia held by the forceps is not distinct from the rest of the wall, which is transparent and the catheter can be fully seen. (From author's photo library)

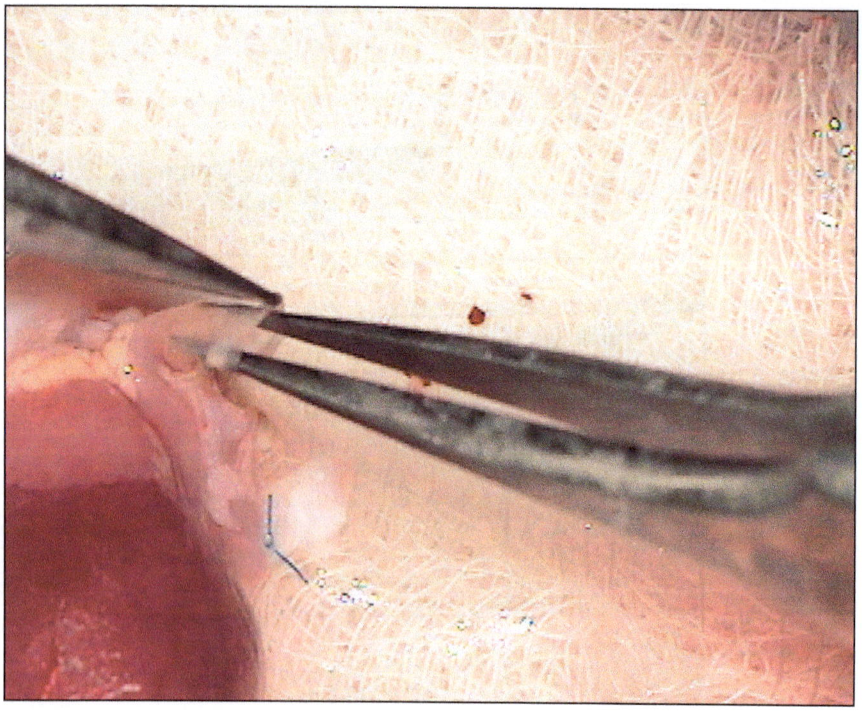

Figure 31-25

Dilation of the lumen of the left pulmonary artery. The Dumont No. 5 forceps holds the pulmonary artery from the external surface of the wall, while the more blunt No. 3 forceps has entered the lumen and is used to open the vessel gradually. (From author's photo library)

III. Recipient - Implantation of the Graft

A. Preparation of the recipient vessels

- **Occlusion of aorta and inferior vena cava with the double clamp**

A yellow plastic background is placed under the aorta and inferior vena cava. The vessels are double clamped simultaneously. The infrarenal aorta which is found anteriorly and to the left of the inferior vena cava, is placed to left, while the inferior vena cava stays in place. In the surgical field, with the rat in dorsal decubitus and head on the left hand of the surgeon, the aorta should be above and the inferior vena cava below (**Fig. 23-26**).

- **Arteriotomy-Venotomy-Irrigation-Removal of adventitia**

A small transverse incision is performed in the aorta and inferior vena cava by lifting each vessel with Dumont No. 3 forceps and using the microsurgical scissors (the technique is described in Chapter 6.3.A) (**Fig. 31-27**). The venotomy is performed more cranially so as to be aligned with the position of the left pulmonary artery of the graft when it is placed in the recipient (**Fig. 31-28**). The lumen of both vessels is irrigated with warm normal saline (**Fig. 31-28**). The adventitia is removed around the edge of each incision.

B. Implantation of the graft

The graft is transferred from the Petri-dish in the peritoneal cavity of the recipient. The heart is placed in the left side of the abdomen, lying on its base, with the apex pointing cranially. It remains on the double clamp. The aortic stump of the graft should freely reach the incision of the aorta of the recipient. Similarly, the pulmonary artery stump should reach the incision of the inferior vena cava of the recipient without tension.

C. End-to-side anastomoses

Please refer to Chapter 6 for the technique of the end-to-side anastomoses, with the possibility of rotation of the clamp (Chapt. 6.6.1) and without the possibility of rotation of the clamp (Chapt. 6.6.2.I).

- **10 or 12 sutures 10/0** are placed **on the anastomosis between the aortic stump of the graft and the abdominal aorta of the recipient.**
- A **mean of 10 sutures 10/0** is placed **on the anasto-**

Figure 31-26

Placement of the aorta and inferior vena cava in the double clamp. The aorta is placed to the left of the inferior vena cava. (From author's photo library)

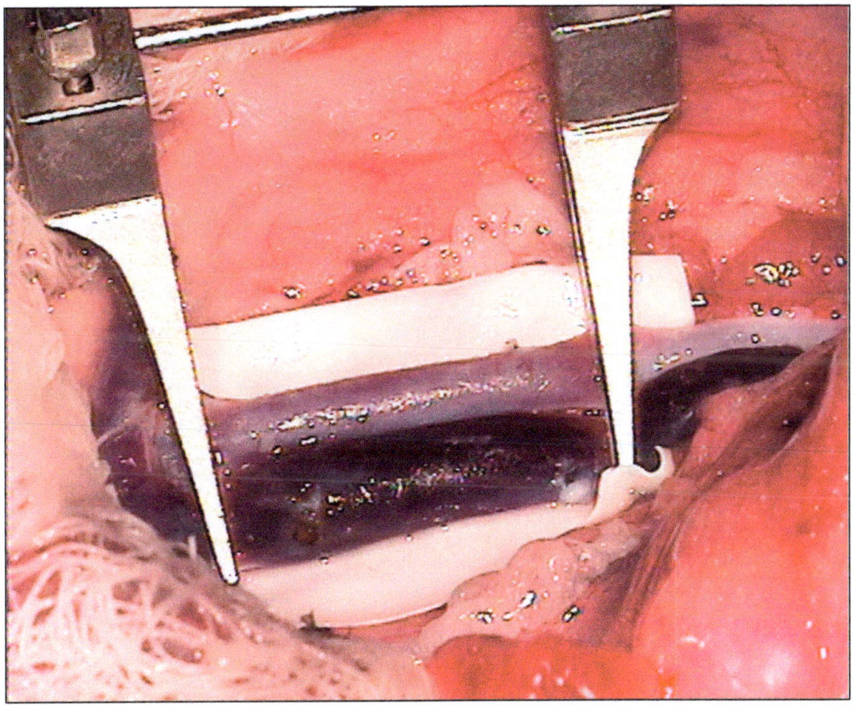

mosis between the left pulmonary artery of the graft and the inferior vena cava of the recipient. Sometimes (as the case presented below) 8 sutures are sufficient. In rare cases, 12 sutures were placed; therefore, it is up to the surgeon's discretion and judgment to put more or less sutures if needed, while keeping the mean of ten.

Although it is technically more difficult, we handle

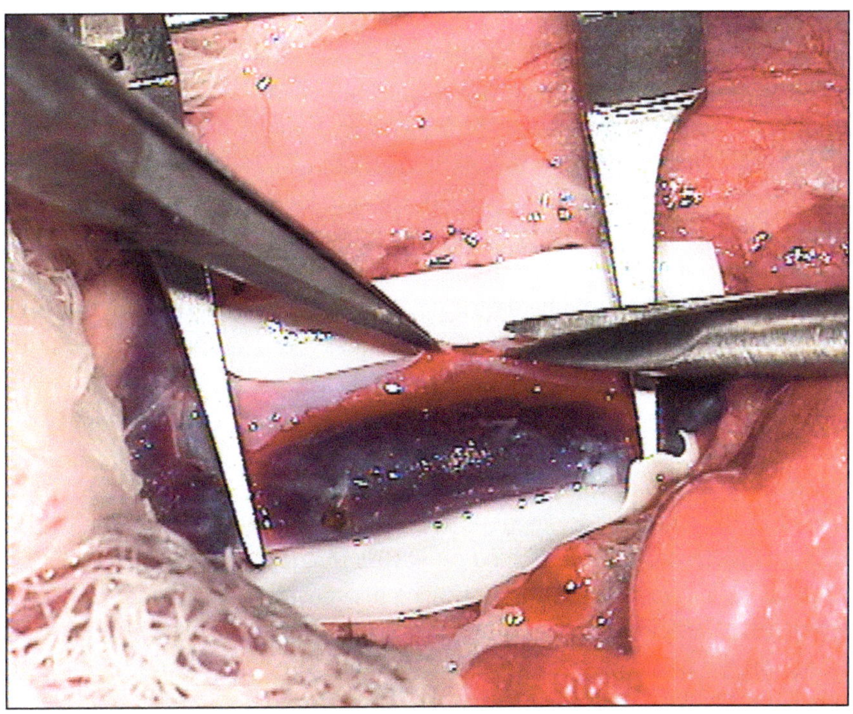

Figure 31-27

Transverse incision of the aorta in the recipient. The Dumont No. 3 forceps lifts the aorta from the adventitia and the microsurgical scissors are ready to make a perpendicular cut in the vessel. (From author's photo library)

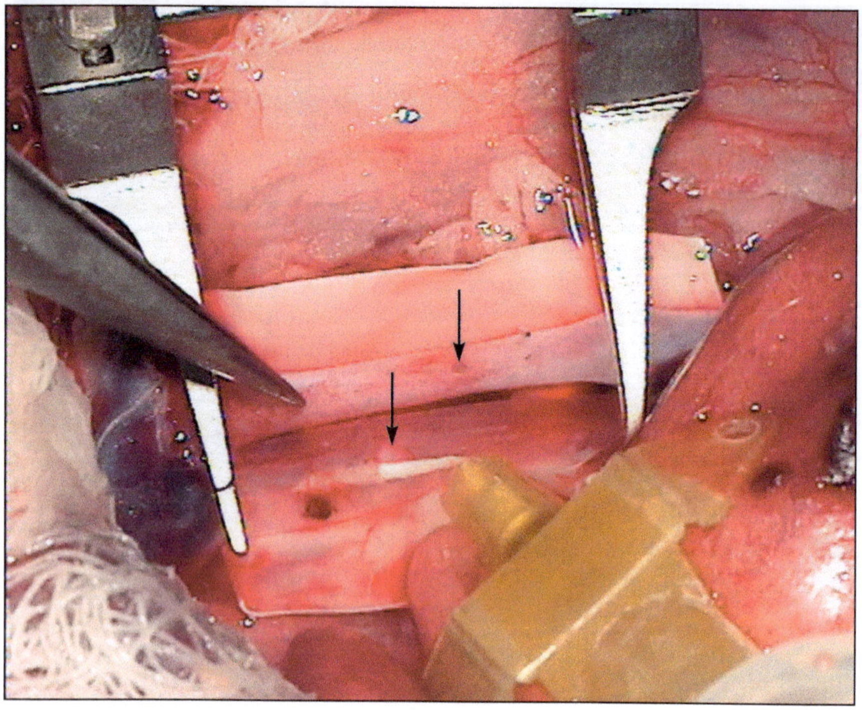

Figure 31-28

Irrigation of the lumen of the inferior vena cava in the recipient. Here, the venocatheter is inserted in the lumen (which is generally avoided), and careful attention is paid to avoid traumatizing the endothelium of the inferior vena cava. Note the distance in the longitudinal axis between the incision in the inferior vena cava from the respective incision in the aorta (arrows). This distance will make the end-to-side anastomoses with the graft vessels more comfortable. (From author's photo library)

these anastomoses as if rotation of the clamp is not possible. We suggest this because reversal of the heart toward the right side will cause the heart to lie on the aortic arch, which results in the pulmonary artery anastomosis being performed under tension due to the relatively shorter stump of the pulmonary artery. Other times, because the abdomen bed is not flat, leaving the heart to sit on the right side of the receiver's abdomen can result in free rotation and twisting of the vessels whose anterior surfaces had been sutured. If the heart is not reversed, it lies on the legs of the double clamp in relatively stable position. However, in many schools and textbooks of microsurgery, it is advisable to perform the anastomoses of the anterior surfaces first, rotate the graft and then complete the suturing of the posterior surfaces (as in the heterotopic transplantation of the kidney). The reader can try both techniques, with rotation of the graft and without.

Following the suggested technique here, the anastomosis starts from the middle of the posterior surface of the aortic stump of the graft (**Fig. 31-29A**). The placement of the sutures is as described in Chapter 6.6.2.I. Since this anastomosis is performed on vessels that retain an open lumen, aorta to aorta, suturing may not be performed by placing sutures on either side of the 1st suture, but by placing the 2nd suture in the middle of the anterior surface (**Fig. 31-29B**) and suturing the two semicircles. The 1st and 2nd suture are left long as stay sutures. First the caudal semicircle (**Fig. 31-29C**) and then the cranial (**Fig. 31-29D**) is sutured as follows: if 12 sutures are placed in total, use 5 sutures per semicircle, the first of which bisects the semicircle, and then 2 per quadrant are placed, at equal distances. If 10 sutures are placed, use 4 sutures per semicircle, symmetrically placed on either side at equal distances, from laterally towards the middle of the semicircle.

The anastomosis of the pulmonary artery with the inferior vena cava (with no rotation of the clamp) will strictly follow the principles described in Chapter 6.6.2.I. The collapsing 'vein-like' wall of the pulmonary artery does not permit any variation of the technique. Therefore, the 1st suture will be placed in the middle of the posterior wall, and the rest in symmetrical pairs on either side, at equal distances from the 1st suture and each other, advancing toward the anterior surface (**Fig. 31-30A, B**). Depending on the total number of sutures in the anterior surface, we complete suturing as follows: if 8 sutures are placed, there are 3 remaining per surface, from which the first is put in the middle of the semicircle (**Fig. 31-30C**), and each of the rest 2 in the middle of each quadrant. Alternatively, as described in Chapter 6.2.I, first place the two lateral sutures and then the central (see **Figure 6-7B**) in order to have a view of the posterior wall. If 10 sutures are placed totally, there are

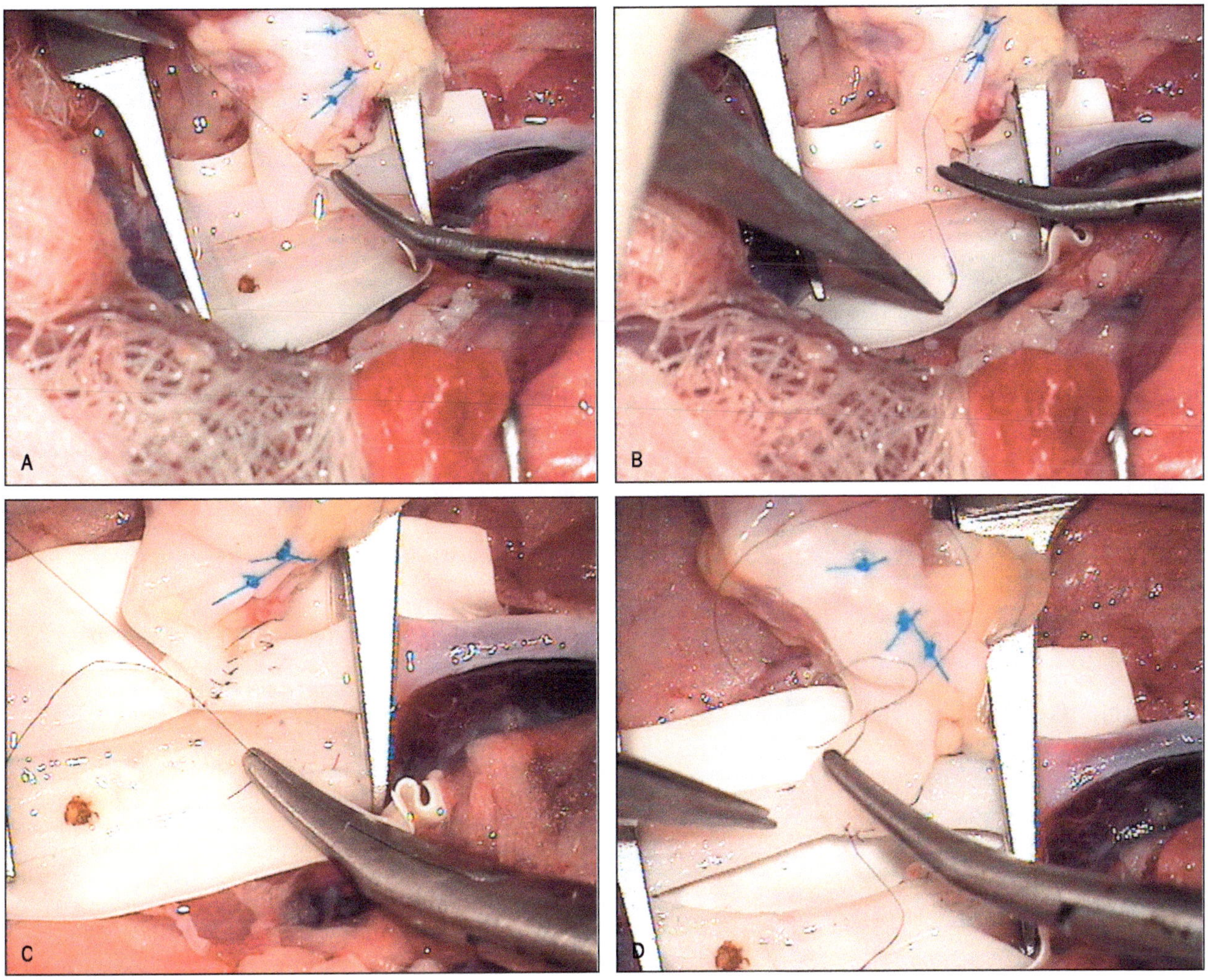

Figure 31-29

Anastomosis between aortic stump of the graft and aorta of the recipient. **A.** Placement of the 1st suture in the middle of the posterior surface. **B.** Placement of the 2nd suture in the middle of the anterior surface. The 1st and 2nd sutures are left long. **C.** Finishing the sutures of the caudal semicircle. **D.** Suturing the cranial semicircle. Observe how easily the suture passes 'blindly' (in one step), without risk of catching the posterior wall, due to the 'self-opening' of the aortic lumens. (From author's photo library)

5 remaining per surface, and we continue with the tactics of the posterior surface (de proche en proche), i.e. first the two laterally, then two more medial and last the central (see **Figure 6-7C**). This is the most secure technique, because the posterior wall is visualized. Another option is to put the central suture first, and then the two on either semicircle.

The aorta and the inferior vena cava are released from the double clamp. A wet gauze is placed on the anastomoses for 3 minutes.

The instant filling of blood into the aorta and pulmonary vein of the graft is very encouraging for the patency of the anastomoses (**Fig. 31-31**). The heart should pulse immediately after removal of the double clamp from the aorta and inferior vena cava in the recipient. The color of the heart will also change to pink.

Patency test follows for each vessel, as described in Chapter 6.9. The blood flow is from the receiver aorta to the donor aorta (see specific paragraph below); therefore, the test is performed as in Chapter 6.9.1 (see **Figure 6-9**): two forceps are applied on the aorta of the graft. One closes centrally, close to the anastomosis, and the other one milks the lumen peripherally toward the graft. The peripheral forceps closes and the central one is removed. If the anastomosis is patent, the lumen

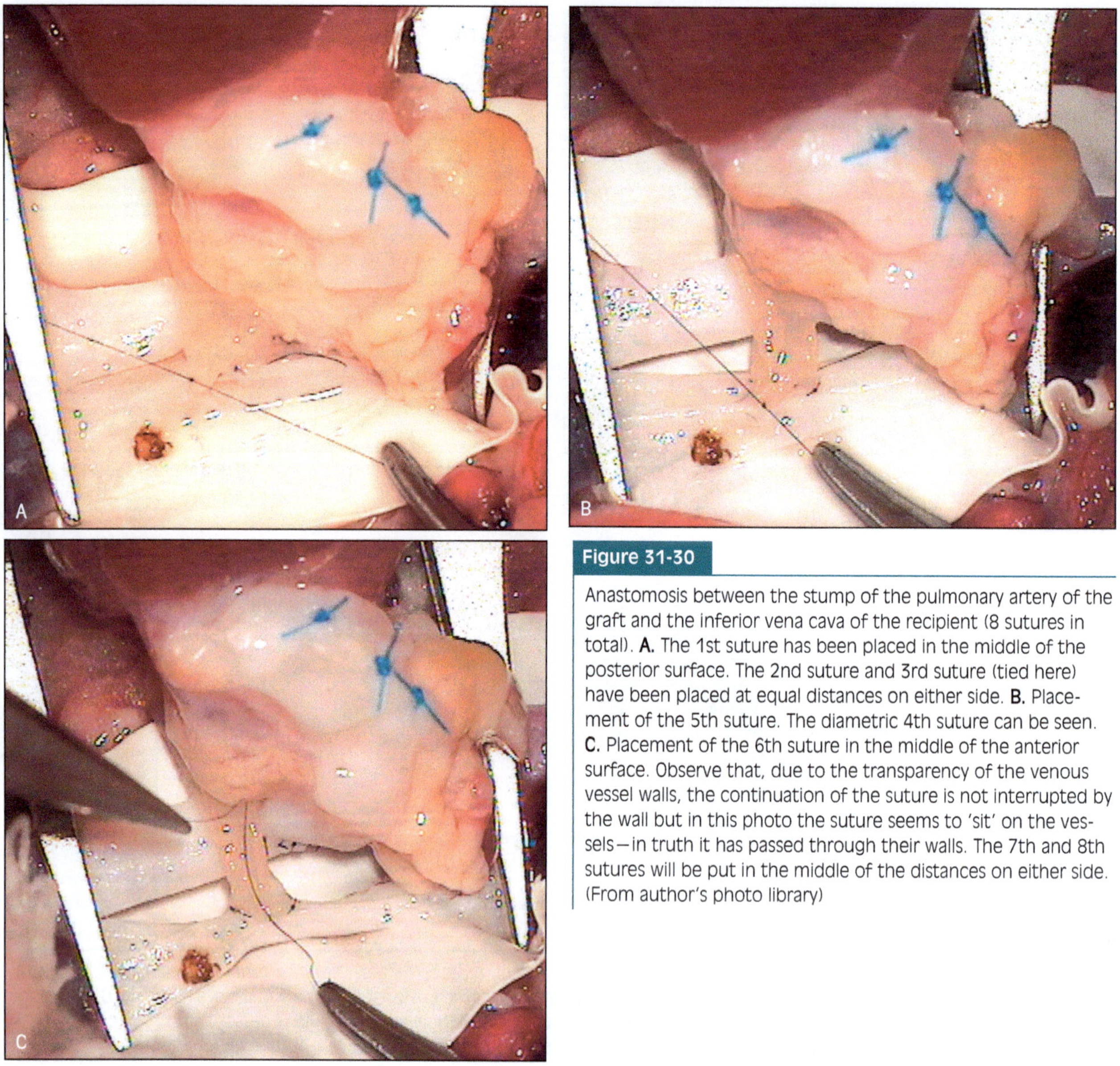

Figure 31-30

Anastomosis between the stump of the pulmonary artery of the graft and the inferior vena cava of the recipient (8 sutures in total). **A.** The 1st suture has been placed in the middle of the posterior surface. The 2nd suture and 3rd suture (tied here) have been placed at equal distances on either side. **B.** Placement of the 5th suture. The diametric 4th suture can be seen. **C.** Placement of the 6th suture in the middle of the anterior surface. Observe that, due to the transparency of the venous vessel walls, the continuation of the suture is not interrupted by the wall but in this photo the suture seems to 'sit' on the vessels—in truth it has passed through their walls. The 7th and 8th sutures will be put in the middle of the distances on either side. (From author's photo library)

of the aorta before the remaining forceps will fill immediately.

The blood flow in the pulmonary artery is toward the inferior vena cava of the recipient. Therefore the test is performed as in Chapter 6.9.2 (see **Figure 6-10**): two forceps are applied in the inferior vena cava and empty the lumen by moving away from each other half-closed. When they re-approximate, the lumen fills in immediately if the anastomosis is patent.

The yellow background is withdrawn.

D. Closure of the surgical trauma

The splanchna of the recipient are brought back in the abdomen, paying attention to avoid twisting of the graft and torsion of the vessels. In addition, the graft should be placed superficially for palpation after closure of the surgical trauma.

The incision is closed in two layers with non-absorbable suture 2/0, one layer on the muscles, and one in the skin and subcutaneous tissue.

E. Follow-up

The everyday follow-up of the recipient is performed with palpation of the pulsating heart in the abdomen.

Blood circulation in the graft

The blood enters the grafted heart from the aorta of

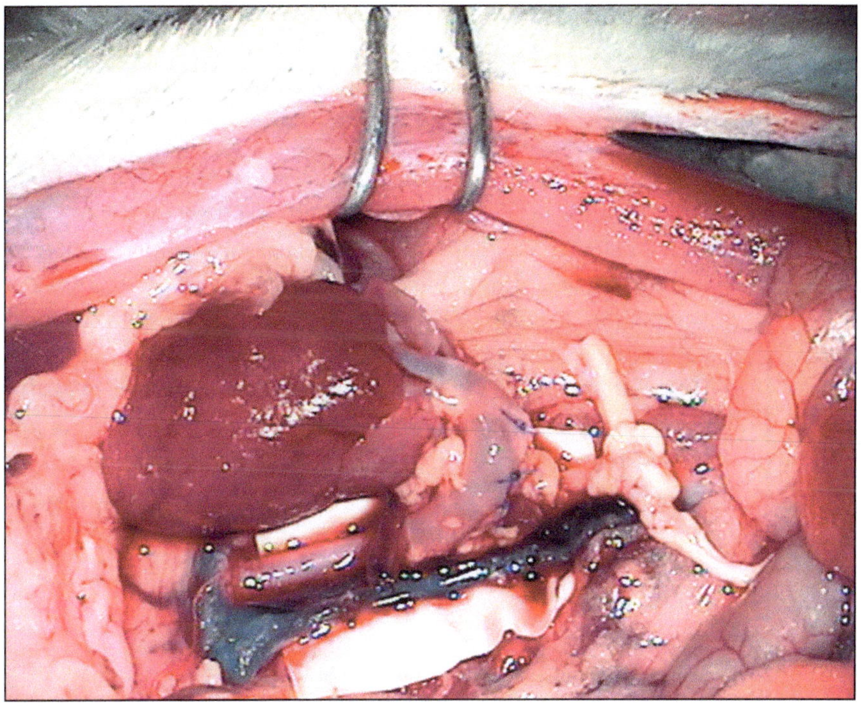

Figure 31-31

Removal of the aorta and the inferior vena cava from the double clamp. The immediate filling of the aorta and pulmonary artery of the graft is indicative of the patency of the anastomoses. The blood flows from the aorta of the recipient to the aorta of the graft, and from the pulmonary artery of the graft to the inferior vena cava of the recipient. (From author's photo library)

the recipient through the anastomosed aortic stump, which is evidently opposite of the normal flow in the aorta. Under the condition that the aortic valve is intact, the blood cannot enter the left ventricle and will deviate toward the coronary arteries. Through these arteries, the myocardium is perfused, and the blood returns via the coronary sinus (exit of the coronary veins) in the right atrium. From there it passes in the right ventricle that expels towards the pulmonary artery trunk. Through the anastomosed left pulmonary artery, the blood returns in the inferior vena cava of the recipient.

It is evident from above that the left heart of the graft is not used at all. If we manage long term survival of the graft, the left heart will become atrophic. The grafted heart has no work load. The blood entering the graft from the aorta returns through the pulmonary artery and is used for supplying the heart itself, which is beating but not pumping.

This model is useful for graft rejection studies and influence of drugs, etc. Of course, there are other models in which the heart is used as a pump (for example, anastomoses: aorta-aorta, inferior vena cava-inferior vena cava, pulmonary artery-iliac artery). Others transplant the heart together with the lungs. Considering the experience of the current model, and with all that you have learned through this book, I could say that I am confident that you will manage to perform any other model, and perhaps make your own model.

Synopsis... of heterotopic heart transplantation

I. RECIPIENT-PREPARATION

A. **Position of the rat:** Dorsal decubitus with the head on the left of the surgeon.The limbs of the rat are immobilized on the working surface with adhesive tape.

B. **Preparation of the surgical field:** Median incision from the xiphoid process to the pubic symphysis. The intestines are mobilized and placed to the right of the rat in a wet gauze. The retroperitoneum is opened with two wet gauzes.

C. **Microsurgical dissection of the aorta and inferior vena cava:** Development of a separation plane between the aorta and the inferior vena cava, from the bifurcation of the aorta to the level of the left renal vein. Dissection and transection of all branches/tributaries between two ligations (9/0) or after cauterization. Complete mobilization of the aorta and inferior vena cava.

II. DONOR – REMOVAL AND PREPARATION OF THE GRAFT

Before the operation, prepare the following: 2-3 Petri-dishes containing normal saline frozen overnight, 1 dish with gauze-covered bottom, cold normal saline and cold heparin solution.

A. **Position of the rat:** Same as in donor.

B. **Preparation of the surgical field:** Bilateral, U-type thoracotomy and opening of the pericardium.

C. **Graft harvesting:** Removal of the heart is performed en block with the lungs, trachea, esophagus. In the upper mediastinum, the following are transected: the superior vena cava with a long stump, the tree branches of the aortic arch, the trachea, and the esophagus. The following are transected just above the diaphragm: the inferior vena cava, the esophagus, and the aorta.

D. **Microsurgical preparation of the graft:** The graft is placed in a Petri-dish covered with gauze. The dish is placed on another dish with iced normal saline. The graft is irrigated with abundant cold normal saline. Immediately flush the graft with cold normal saline via the inferior vena cava.

1. The lungs are removed by transecting the root close to the hilum, the esophagus is removed and then the trachea. Pay attention to the right side in order to smoothly remove the main bronchus from under the arch of the azygos vein without jeopardizing the azygos vein or the inferior vena cava.
2. The following vessels of the heart are ligated (Nylon 5/0), and the stumps are transected (peripheral to the ligation) in sequence:
   - ➢ superior vena cava (central to the exit of the azygos vein)
   - ➢ right pulmonary vein (one in the rat)
   - ➢ right pulmonary artery
   - ➢ left pulmonary vein (one in the rat)
   - ➢ branches of the aortic arch
   - ➢ inferior vena cava: prior to ligation the graft is flushed again with cold heparinized normal saline through the inferior vena cava.

   The aorta and the left pulmonary artery are preserved for the anastomoses. The aorta stump is shortened, but kept longer than the stump of the left pulmonary artery.

... of heterotopic heart transplantation

Synopsis....

III. RECIPIENT – IMPLANTATION OF THE GRAFT

A. **Preparation of the recipient vessels:** After placement of a yellow plastic background under the vessels, the aorta and the inferior vena cava are occluded with a double clamp. A transverse arteriotomy follows, and more centrally a venotomy. The lumens are irrigated, and the adventitia is removed in the perimeter of each incision.

B. **Implantation of the graft:** The graft is transferred into the left side of the abdomen with the apex pointed cranially and lies on the clamps of the double clamp.

C. **Termino-lateral anastomoses between the following**

- aortic stump to aorta, **10 or 12 sutures 10/0** are placed
- left pulmonary artery to inferior vena cava, **10 sutures 10/0** are placed

1. Suturing can be performed in two ways:
   ⇒ First the corner sutures, then the anterior surfaces, followed by rotation of the graft and completion of the posterior surfaces.
   ⇒ Without rotation of the graft, starting from the middle of the posterior surface and then at equal distances on either side advancing toward the anterior surface (recommended technique, especially for the pulmonary artery).
2. Removal of the double clamp. The heart should start beating and revive its color.
3. Placement of a wet gauze on the anastomoses for 3 minutes.
4. Patency tests
5. Removal of the yellow plastic background.

D. **Closure of the abdominal wall in two layers.**

E. **Examine** the heart again by palpating it through the abdominal wall.

Blood circulation in the graft: Circulation starts from the aorta of the recipient, then to the donor aorta, coronary arteries, myocardium, coronary veins, right atrium, right ventricle, pulmonary artery, and ends in the inferior vena cava of the recipient. The left heart is not used. The heart beats but does not work as a pump.